WB
400
Pay

Advancing Dietetics and Clinical Nutrition

Commissioning Editor: Mairi McCubbin
Development Editor: Catherine Jackson
Project Manager: Annie Victor
Designer/Design Direction: Stewart Larking
Illustration Manager: Bruce Hogarth
Illustrator: Gillian Richards

Advancing Dietetics and Clinical Nutrition

Edited by

Anne Payne BSc PhD RD

Professional Lead in Nutrition and Dietetics, School of Health Professions, Faculty of Health, University of Plymouth, Peninsula Allied Health Centre, Plymouth, UK

Helen Barker BSc MPH PGCE RD

Associate Head, Physiotherapy and Dietetics, Faculty of Health and Life Sciences, Coventry University, Coventry, UK

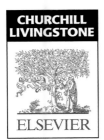

CHURCHILL LIVINGSTONE

ELSEVIER

Edinburgh London New York Oxford Philadelphia St Louis Sydney Toronto 2010

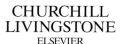

CHURCHILL
LIVINGSTONE
ELSEVIER

First published 2010, © Elsevier Limited. All rights reserved.

ISBN 978 0 443 06786 0
  Reprinted 2010

British Library Cataloguing in Publication Data
A catalogue record for this book is available from the British Library

Library of Congress Cataloging in Publication Data
A catalog record for this book is available from the Library of Congress

Notice

Knowledge and best practice in this field are constantly changing. As new research and experience broaden our knowledge, changes in practice, treatment and drug therapy may become necessary or appropriate. Readers are advised to check the most current information provided (i) on procedures featured or (ii) by the manufacturer of each product to be administered, to verify the recommended dose or formula, the method and duration of administration, and contraindications. It is the responsibility of the practitioner, relying on their own experience and knowledge of the patient, to make diagnoses, to determine dosages and the best treatment for each individual patient, and to take all appropriate safety precautions. To the fullest extent of the law, neither the Publisher nor the Editors assumes any liability for any injury and/or damage to persons or property arising out of or related to any use of the material contained in this book.

The Publisher

Printed in China

Contents

PART 1   Advancing practice

PART 2   Evidence based care

Contents

Preface

The nature of dietetic practice and the roles and responsibilities of the dietitian have undergone major change in the past decade. Within the UK the development of the advanced practitioner and consultant roles and our requirement to demonstrate continued professional development to maintain registration with the Health Professions Council has meant that many more practitioners are engaged in study at Master's level. As dietetics is now soundly established as an evidence-based profession, this book has been developed to provide dietitians with evidence-based information that can be drawn on at the post-registration, postgraduate level.

All the chapters have been written by clinical experts, drawing on existing evidence, their clinical expertise and the emerging evidence where relevant, to explore the use of diet and nutrition therapeutically and the scientific rationale underpinning treatment. Whilst the majority of the chapters have been written by UK authors we have tried to ensure that wherever possible an international perspective has been included.

We hope that the publication of this book will support the academic development of the post-graduate dietitian and that it will be a valuable resource to ensure that patients receive evidence-based care.

Plymouth and Coventry, 2010
Anne Payne
Helen Barker

Contributors

Jaime Aranda-Michel MD
Associate Professor of Medicine, Division of Gastrointerology, Heptology and Liver Transplantations, Mayo Clinic, Jacksonville, Florida, USA

Lynn Clouder BSc(Hons) MA PhD MCSP
Research Fellow and Director of the Centre for Interprofessional e-Learning, Coventry University, Coventry, UK

Avril Collinson BSc PhD RD
Lecturer in Dietetics, Faculty of Health and Social Work, University of Plymouth, Plymouth, UK

Kristine Farrar BSc(Hons) RD
Consultant Dietitian, Salford Community Health, NHS Salford, UK

Karen Green BSc MSc RD
Senior Specialist Dietitian (Neurosciences), Department of Nutrition and Dietetics, National Hospital for Neurology and Neurosurgery, London, UK

Paula Hallam BSc(Hons) RD
Senior Paediatric Dietitian, Nutrition and Dietetics Department, Kingston Hospital, London, UK

Lindsay Harper BSc(Hons) MRPharms DipClin
Principal Clinical Pharmacist, Slaford Royal NHS Foundation Trust, Salford, UK

Mary Hickson BSc DipADP PhD RD
Therapy Research Facilitator, Imperial College Healthcare NHS Trust; Honorary Senior Lecturer, Imperial College; Department of Nutrition and Dietetics, Charing Cross Hospital, London, UK

Linda Hindle BSc(Hons) RD
Consultant Dietitian in Obesity, Birmingham East and North PCT, Birmingham, UK

Lynne D. Hubbard BSc(Hons) MPhil RD
Specialist Dietitian in Burns and Intensive Care, St Thomas' Hospital, London, UK

Simon Igo BSc(Hons) MSc PGCert MCSP
Senior Lecturer, Coventry University, Faculty of Health and Life Sciences, Charles Ward Building, Coventry, UK

Marion Ireland BSc(Hons) RD
Specialist Dietitian, Neurorehabilitation Unit, Astley Ainslie Hospital, Edinburgh, UK

David Kendrik MPhil dflp
Consultant in Bariatric Psycology, UK

Nick Lewis-Barned FRCP FRACP Cert Clin Ed
Consultant Physician (Diabetes and Endocrinology), Northumbria Diabetes Service, Diabetes Resource Centre, North Tyneside General Hospital, North Tyneside, UK

Paula Murphy BSc PhD AdvDipDietetics RD
Team Leader Nutrition Support, Dietetic Department, Derriford Hospital, Plymouth, UK

Lindsay Oliver BSc(Hons) RD
Consultant Dietitian, National Training Lead for Year of Care Programme, Diabetes Resource Centre, North Tyneside General Hospital, North Shields, UK

Hari Krishnan Parthasarathy MBBS MRCP
Specialty Training Registrar in Cardiology, Department of Cardiology, Papworth Hospital, Cambridge

Katherine E. Paterson BSc(Hons) RD
Clinical Lead Specialist Cardiology Dietitian, Department of Nutrition and Dietetics, Norfolk and Norwich University Hospitals NHS Foundation Trust, Norwich, UK

Anne Payne BSc PhD RD
Professional Lead in Nutrition and Dietetics, School of Health Professions, Faculty of Health, University of Plymouth, Peninsula Allied Health Centre, Plymouth, UK

Cathy Payne BSc MSc PhD RD
Joint Lecturer in Palliative Care for Allied Health Professionals, Northern Ireland Hospice Care and Ulster University, Belfast, UK

Dympna Pearson RD
Freelance Dietitian & Behaviour Change Trainer

Ursula Philpot BSc MSc PGDip RD PGCHE
Senior Associate Lecturer, Faculty of Health, Leeds
Metropolitan University; Advanced Practitioner in Eating
Disorders, Yorkshire Centre for Eating Disorders, Seacroft
Hospital, Leeds, UK

Isma Rafiq MBBS MRCP
Specialist Training Registrar in Cardiology, Basildon,
Essex, UK

Michelle M. Romano RD LDN CNSD
Assistant Professor of Nutrition, College of Medicine, Mayo
Clinic, Jacksonville, Florida, USA

Isabel Skypala BSc PGDip RD
Director of Rehabilitation and Therapies, Royal Brompton
and Harefield NHS Trust, London, UK

Clare Stradling BSc(Hons) RD
Specialist HIV Dietitian, Department of Infection and
Tropical Medicine, Birmingham Heartlands Hospital,
Birmingham, UK

Max Watson BD MBChB MRCGP MSc DCH DRCOG DMH
Consultant Palliative Medicine/ Lecturer in Palliative
Care, Northern Ireland Hospice and University of Ulster,
Belfast, UK

Rebecca White BSc MSc MRPharms(IPresc) BCNSP
Pharmacy Team Manager, Nutrition and Surgery,
Oxford Radcliffe Hospitals NHS Trust, Oxford, UK

Kenneth C-W Wong BChir MA MB MRCP
Department of Cardiology, Norfolk & Norwich University
Hospitals NHS Foundation Trust, Norwich, UK;
Department of Clinical Oncology, Prince of Wales Hospital,
Shatin, New Territories, Hong Kong

Introduction

Quality Improvement and Research in Advancing
Dietetics and Clinical Nutrition

Mary Hickson

Improving quality in clinical care is the current remit of healthcare providers worldwide. While methods of achieving this may vary, common elements of quality improvement focus on the promotion of better partnership working among patients, frontline medical staff and clinical experts.[1,2] The process of identifying and auditing relevant outcome measures, or quality metrics, is also at the heart of quality improvement to provide evidence to inform, develop and sustain 'best practice'.

To advance dietetics and clinical nutrition it is recognised that practitioners require the ability to blend evidence of what works with current practice, to promote best practice and so improve quality of care. An ability to critique literature is an essential skill for a practitioner who promotes 'evidence-based practice'. The application of new knowledge to influence change in practice is a skill that develops with experience and is enhanced through engagement in research.

Today's focus on quality improvement (QI) is embedded in the concept of clinical governance that was established in the late 1990s to provide a framework where real accountability could be given for the safe delivery of health services.[3,4] At this time there was a need to address both the public's and professionals' perception of systemic failings in the provision of healthcare. QI and clinical governance are about patient safety and the quality of clinical services provided and as such patients are central to every aspect of the process.

A wide range of activities contribute towards improving quality in care. These include:

- Patient, public and carer involvement— Analysis of patient–professional involvement and interaction, including strategy, planning and delivery of care;
- Strategic capacity and capability—Planning, communication and governance arrangements from a strategic perspective, including aspects of cultural behaviour;
- Risk management—Incident reporting, infection control, prevention and control of risk;
- Staff management and performance— Recruitment, workforce planning, appraisals;
- Education, training and continuous professional development—Professional re-validation, management development, statutory training, personal development;
- Clinical effectiveness—Clinical audit management, planning and monitoring, learning through research and audit;
- Information management—Patient records, confidentiality and data protection;
- Communication—Patient and public, external partners, internal, board and organisation-wide;
- Leadership—Throughout the organisation, including Board, Chair and non-executive directors, chief executive and executive directors, managers and clinicians;
- Team working—Within the service, senior managers, clinical and multidisciplinary teams, and across organisations; and
- Research—The basis of evidence-based practice and as such ensures the best available treatments to patients can be provided.

This list illustrates the wide range of activities that promote QI and clearly shows how it must be an ongoing collaborative effort. Different organisations will manage QI in different ways and some aspects are more relevant than others to dietitians and clinical nutritionists at various stages of their career.

Although much of QI addresses the process that makes healthcare happen and the importance of communication and working together, underpinning these activities are the facts on which treatment decisions are based. In order to provide the best care new treatments need to be tested and evaluated, new areas of application must be explored and new knowledge of disease and metabolic processes must be discovered. In order to progress the profession and find better ways of treating people research is essential and is a fundamental part of dietetic practice and clinical nutrition.

The UK National Health Service research strategy 'Best Research for Best Health' includes a goal to 'attract, develop and retain the best research professionals to conduct people-based research'.[5] This strategic approach may help promote new opportunities for dietitians and clinical nutritionists to be involved in research in the future. To be in a position to capitalise on such opportunities it is paramount that practitioners advance their research skills, so that they can develop the evidence upon which to base their practice.

Research can be incorporated into clinical practice at all stages of a dietetic career and the British Dietetic Association has produced a framework outlining the knowledge and skills required at different stages of a career pathway.[6] This document splits involvement with research into four stages:

Stage 1: Understand, interpret and apply research

At qualification, all dietitians and clinical nutritionists should have achieved the knowledge and skills required to understand, interpret and apply research and should maintain or improve upon these throughout their career.

Stage 2: Active involvement in research

Having met the above criteria, the dietitian may wish to achieve the knowledge and skills required to become more actively involved in research, including identifying appropriate research questions and planning, under supervision, research projects.

Stage 3: Leading research

The dietitian may then wish to achieve the knowledge and skills required to lead research. This would entail the planning and preparation, obtaining appropriate approvals, running the study and managing data collection, through to analysis and publication of findings.

Stage 4: Supervision and leadership in research

The final stage includes the knowledge and skills required to provide supervision and leadership in research. This would include developing and pursuing a programme of funded research, educating others about research and supervising and mentoring colleagues to facilitate their progress to the next stage.

All dietitians and clinical nutritionists should be competent at the first stage, which is about using research. The key skills they should be able to demonstrate are:

- Understand the difference between research and audit and the role of these within the clinical effectiveness cycle and its impact on practice.
- Identify research needs within a general area. This requires an awareness of research within their specialist field and the level of evidence it provides, and to question their practice in the context of changing healthcare systems and requirements.
- Undertake a comprehensive literature search. Literature searching ideally needs to be done in a systematic and comprehensive way. Undertaking a quick and dirty search for a particular piece of information is not difficult to do with today's advances in technology and access to online bibliographic databases, but it is more demanding to produce a search that includes all known literature relevant to a particular clinical question. If dietitians are to work to the best available evidence then they must have the skills to undertake this type of search.
- Understand research methodology and research methods. This should include an understanding of quantitative (e.g. randomised controlled trials, case-control studies) and qualitative (focus groups, semi-structured interviews) approaches and their advantages and disadvantages. The level of knowledge required is to enable dietitians to decide whether appropriate methods and research designs have been used in original research, and thus is part of critical appraisal skills.
- Understand and interpret basic data analysis. This should include descriptive (e.g. means, medians, percentages, 95% confidence intervals), distribution (e.g. standard deviations, normal distribution) and comparative (e.g. P values, t-tests, chi-squared test) statistics. As above, dietitians need enough knowledge to judge whether analysis

has been done appropriately and to accurately interpret the findings of quantitative research.

- Interpret research through critical appraisal of the scientific literature. Critical appraisal is a key skill which all dietitians need to develop in order to keep up to date with new evidence and research. An understanding of statistics and methodology as outlined above is essential but critical appraisal is also about applying research findings and deciding whether findings are relevant and applicable to the patients under their care.
- Apply research evidence into their practice. This aspect is discussed in more detail in Chapter 1, entitled Evidence-Based Practice.
- Understand the ethical framework in which research should be conducted and be aware of research governance issues. A basic appreciation of ethics within research is required at this first stage and an understanding that research in the NHS is governed by a framework to ensure quality and safe practice.

It is important that all dietitians, particularly those working at an advanced level, maintain and use their skills as described in this first stage. Those who wish to pursue a more active involvement in research will need to find support within their organisation and education at Masters or ideally Doctorate levels, to gain the skills and experience required to reach the fourth stage in this framework.

This book does not set out to provide the knowledge required to move from the first stage onwards; this is the aim of other books, such as the *Research Handbook for Healthcare Professionals*,[7] and of postgraduate education at Masters or Doctorate levels.

Other aspects of clinical governance of particular relevance to dietitians and clinical nutritionists are discussed in Part I of this book. These include evidence-based practice (EBP); the use of 'reflection' in advancing practice; motivational interviewing; and transition to adult care.

All the clinical areas covered in the second part of this book addresses key specialist fields in dietetic practice and clinical nutrition, many written jointly with a clinical dietitian and a medical practitioner to provide a holistic review of patient care. It should be recognised that each clinical field has gaps in knowledge where better evidence is required or areas where improvement in treatment is needed.

All recent advances and changes seen in the practice of dietetics have been driven by research evidence. This is clearly illustrated in the care of people with diabetes. Dietary advice has changed from a semi-starvation diet of the pre-insulin era, to restricted carbohydrates and carbohydrate exchanges, to today's far more flexible regimens, the incorporation of glycaemic index and an emphasis on patient education to enable them to match their diet to their chosen lifestyle.

To advance our professional practice we need to undertake research to answer the gaps in our knowledge and questions. It is important that advanced practitioners have the skills to use research but also choose to focus their expertise on establishing the high-quality evidence required to improve patient care.

References

1. Department of Health. *High Quality Care for All—NHS Next Stage Review Final Report*. London: DOH; 2008.
2. Parker LE, Kirchner JE, Bonner LM, et al. Creating a Quality-Improvement Dialogue: utilising knowledge from frontline staff, managers and experts to foster health care quality improvement. *Qual Health Res*. 2009;19:229–242.
3. Department of Health. *A First Class Service*. London: DOH; 1997.
4. Scally G, Donaldson LJ. The NHS's 50 anniversary. Clinical governance and the drive for quality improvement in the new NHS in England. *Br Med J*. 1998;317(7150):61–65.
5. Department of Health. *Best Research for Best Health: A New National Health Research Strategy*. London: DOH; 2006.
6. British Dietetic Association. *Dietitians and Research: A Knowledge and Skills Framework*. Birmingham: BDA; 2007.
7. Hickson M. *Research Handbook for Healthcare Professionals*. Chichester, UK: Blackwell; 2008.

PART 1

Advancing practice

Evidence-based practice

Defining the nature of best evidence
for policy and practice

Simon Igo

Introduction

Evidence-based practice (EBP) is a ubiquitous term
in dietetic practice and has become a major policy
theme in the modernisation of the British National
Health Service. One of the biggest challenges for
the modern-day healthcare professional, manager
and policy maker is to apply the principles of
evidence-based practice in a changing and complex
clinical, political and economic healthcare arena.

An evidence-based approach in dietetic practice is
founded on 'a model of clinical reasoning that uses
a systematic process to integrate best evidence
(research) with clinical expertise and patient values
to optimise patient care'.[1-3] Engaging with clinical
research and other forms of 'best evidence' widens
the professional knowledge base, contributes towards
improved patient care, leads to economic savings in
healthcare practice and improves knowledge and skill
development in dietetic practice.[4]

Despite the perception of being ubiquitous, some
authors argue that EBP has not achieved the acceptance that it set out to accomplish; common reported
barriers that preclude the application into clinical
practice include an inflexible organisational culture,
inadequate resources (time, staffing or finance),
insufficient skills and limited knowledge.[5-8] In addition to these political, economic and organisational
barriers there are fundamental philosophical concerns that relate to the theoretical framework that
underpins EBP. Essentially, the process of EBP is
grounded on the premise that best evidence in the
form of high-quality research will enable sound clinical decision-making. However, critical debate as to

what constitutes best evidence and how to apply
evidence remains, at best, confusing. Thus healthcare
practitioners and policy makers remain uncertain
about the nature and application of an EBP approach
to healthcare decision-making.[9,10]

This chapter will revisit the notion of best evidence and will offer a pragmatic and practical classification that will help dietitians to understand the
nature of best evidence and to understand how to
apply best evidence in healthcare practice.

From evidence-based medicine to evidence-based practice

In its simplest form evidence-based medicine (EBM)
is an approach to clinical problem solving: it is
defined as 'the conscientious, explicit and judicious
use of current best evidence in making decisions
about the care of individual patients';[1] a process of
systematically finding, appraising and using research
findings to inform healthcare practice, and follows
four basic steps:

1. Formulate a clear clinical question from a
   patient's problem;
2. Search the literature for relevant clinical
   articles;
3. Evaluate (critically appraise) the evidence for
   its validity and usefulness; and
4. Implement useful findings in clinical
   practice.[11]

Liberati and Vineis trace the origins of EBM back
to mid-nineteenth-century Paris where proponents

of a new movement called 'medicine d'observation' were attempting to reject the notion of medical care-based speculation[12]; however, it is widely accepted that modern contemporary practice originated at McMaster's University in 1981. The faculty of the Department of Clinical Epidemiology and Biostatistics published a series of articles for the *Canadian Medical Association Journal* that taught clinicians how to critically appraise medical literature, and developed an awareness of the relationship between research and clinical practice.[13]

This philosophical approach was formalised in 1992 in a paper written by the Evidence Based Medicine Working Group (EBMWG) the authors present the reader with two alternatives for clinical decision-making.[14] The first, 'the way of the past', novice physicians seek expert and experienced opinion from authorities higher in the medical hierarchy: expert opinion and past precedent informs practice. However, a second and more robust option is presented, one that represents a shift away from opinion towards the critical use of medical literature to enable physicians to make sound clinical judgements; this method was seen as 'the way of the future' and the term 'evidence-based medicine' was coined.

Understanding the origins and history of the evidence-based medicine movement identifies that EBM evolved within a biomedical philosophy and has been shaped by key thinkers in the medical, biological, epidemiological and statistical sciences. Early adopters developed EBM within a positivist research framework, the premise being that the use of empirically based quantitative research methodologies would answer patient dilemmas and solve the issue of using non-substantiated evidence in the form of personal opinion.

The term evidence-based 'medicine' was rejected by healthcare professions such as dietitians and other professions allied to health on the grounds that the medical model of clinical decision-making did not reflect the different scientific philosophies, professional values and approaches to healthcare.[15,16] Professions allied to health have different professional identities and values that are paradigmatically different to that of medicine. Subsequently, an alternative term was adopted, one that accepted other forms of evidence and enabled clinical decision-making in a wider professional context. The term 'evidence-based practice' was created, a process that evolved from the school and teachings of EBM but recognised a broader selection of evidence within the context of healthcare.[13]

Defining best evidence

So what do we mean by best evidence in dietetic practice and how should we apply best evidence in the clinical setting? Traditionally evidence has been categorised into hierarchies constructed within an empirically based positivist research paradigm. Hierarchies classify evidence in terms of how valid the results are for determining the effectiveness of an intervention. Systematic reviews, randomised controlled trials (RCTs) and other quantitative-based approaches are used to help determine the effectiveness of clinical practice; the more robust the research method, the more valid the result. Moore proposed one such hierarchy of evidence combining primary and secondary research methods and, to date, it still underpins the use of quantitative-based research in EBP (Table 1.1).[17]

A brief critical review of such hierarchies quickly reveals the noticeable absence of other sources of evidence including qualitative naturalistic research. This raises some fundamental questions for practising dieticians: How appropriate are such hierarchies and are we missing other sources of important evidence? What about the nature of interpretive research paradigm using qualitative research methodologies and where does clinical knowledge fit into the EBP framework? To answer these questions it is necessary to revisit what we mean by best evidence and consider other forms of clinical research, our clinical knowledge and practice experience, and the notion of reflective practice when we attempt to apply and use best evidence.

Table 1.1 Moore's original evidence hierarchy

I	Strong evidence from at least one systematic review of multiple well-designed randomised controlled trials.
II	Strong evidence from at least one properly designed randomised controlled trial of appropriate size.
III	Evidence from well-designed trials without randomisation, single-group pre-post cohort, time series or matched case controlled studies.
IV	Evidence from non-experimental studies from more than one centre or research group.
V	Opinions of respected authorities, based on clinical evidence, descriptive studies or reports from expert committees

The nature of best evidence

The previous section has identified that the use of ordered quantitative-based evidence is useful but perhaps limited for the complex clinical arena that constitutes dietetic practice. The philosophy that clinical research should be used to inform practice is at the heart of the EBP movement, but it needs to be defined so that it can be applied within the context of clinical practice.

Fundamentally research, or research-based knowledge,[18] can be categorised into two broad camps, the 'empirico analytical paradigm' and the 'interpretive paradigm'.[19] Evidence associated with the former includes methods associated with quantitative research methodology but also incorporates biological and pathological theory.[10] Evidence that sits in this framework of knowledge is invaluable for informing practice and policy relating to treatment, therapy and diagnosis.

Evidence associated with the 'interpretative paradigm' includes research approaches framed within qualitative methodology including studies allied to humanities and social science. The importance of such evidence is no less important than its quantitative cousin but it seeks to answer different clinical questions. Using evidence, framed within the interpretive paradigm, allows policy makers and clinicians to understand the nature of the healthcare experience and will allow for a deeper understanding of healthcare behaviour.

So when faced with a particular clinical dilemma or situation classifying the nature of evidence into an 'empirico analytical' or 'interpretive' framework begins to narrow down the type of evidence that could be used to help understand the key issues in clinical practice; identifying the type of evidence for clinical decision-making is elaborated in the next section.

Methods for translating evidence into practice: choosing the right question

The previous section briefly summarises two separate research paradigms; understanding where evidence falls within these frameworks is the key to applying best evidence. But how should evidence be applied?

Mulhall recognises the need for using appropriate sources of evidence and offers an intuitive approach, an approach commensurate with clinical reasoning.[20]

Mulhall suggests that the clinical question dictates the choice of evidence. Like research questions the clinical question can be categorised in terms of their purpose and the purpose of the clinical question can be aligned to one of the research paradigms indicating a choice of evidence to help inform clinical practice.[21] Examples of three types of clinical questions, explanatory, exploratory and descriptive, are given below.

Explanatory clinical questions

Explanatory clinical questions are created and constructed within the empirico-analytical paradigm; these questions are specific, and they seek to answer clinical issues that relate to testing an idea or hypothesis relating to clinical effectiveness. Consequently, research designs grounded in quantitative research methodology are used to answer these types of clinical questions.[21] An example explanatory clinical question is given below.

'Does taking vitamin supplements improve cognitive function in the elderly population?'[22]

Research methods that could be used to answer such explanatory questions include the following:

Primary research

- Experimental studies (to enable the detection of direct causal relationships):
  - Randomised controlled trials;
  - Comparative studies;
  - Uncontrolled trials; and
  - $n = 1$ trials.
- Observational studies (to investigate causal associations):
  - Cohort studies;
  - Prospective cohort;
  - Case-control studies;
  - Retrospective cohort.

Secondary research

- The systematic review (a systematic appraisal and summary of primary research).

Exploratory clinical questions

Exploratory clinical questions have a function different to that of explanatory questions and consequently are grounded in a separate research paradigm, in this case the interpretive paradigm. Here the clinical question seeks to find answers that aim to explain human activity and behaviour within a healthcare context.[21] Exploratory-type questions are answered through critical engagement with research approaches grounded in qualitative methodology. An example exploratory clinical question is given below.

'What are the problems with mothers breastfeeding their children?'[23]

Developing an understanding of the lived experiences of mothers feeding their children would give valuable insight into the joys and real world problems and benefits of breastfeeding. Understanding the context in which this health behaviour operates would inform the direction of clinical practice and dietary advice. To answer such questions qualitative methodologies need to be considered and include:

- Phenomenology;
- Ethnography;
- Grounded theory; and
- Action research.

Descriptive clinical questions

The descriptive clinical question blends both the empirical analytical paradigm and the interpretive paradigm to underpin the construction of this type of question. Descriptive questions provide a descriptive account of a phenomenon within an established framework of knowledge, rather than establishing a cause-and-effect relationship or providing an exploration into healthcare behaviour.

Methods associated with answering descriptive clinical questions relate to 'survey' approaches to research and include the notion of clinical audit.[21] An example descriptive question is detailed below:

'What are the current dietetic practices for the management of overweight and obese clients?'[24]

Evidence that should be considered to answer such questions would include:

- Non-analytical observational studies (descriptive studies);
- Cross-sectional studies (surveys);
- Longitudinal studies (surveys); and
- Clinical audit.

The above account identifies that evidence sits within a body of espoused knowledge and that two research paradigms support the notion of what constitutes best evidence. It has been argued that evidence grounded in positivism is only a small portion of the professional knowledge base and that other forms of research evidence are available, including methods in qualitative research and methods associated with survey research and clinical audit. Constructing a clinically focused question and framing it within a theoretical context allows the evidence-based practitioner and policy maker to judiciously select appropriate best evidence from within a body of professional knowledge.

Widening the knowledge base: the role of reflection in EBP

Finding, selecting and critically appraising evidence in preparation for practice is only part of the EBP process; the next step is to apply and translate the evidence to a particular clinical situation. Rolfe and Gardner identify that advice from the original EBMWG paper suggests that the practitioner should use evidence in a stepwise process and only look at lower forms of evidence in the hierarchy if more robust methods have not been conducted.[25] This stepwise application of evidence into clinical practice is perhaps too simplistic and counterintuitive to the clinical reasoning process. Rolfe and Gardner suggest that there is confusion as to how evidence should be applied and Rycroft-Malone discuss that standards for determining whether research or evidence is appropriate and how it should be applied for a particular patient context have not yet been developed.[26] The stepwise application of evidence may be suitable as a foundation for applying evidence but is perhaps too dogmatic and is based on the notion that evidence determines practice. Mantzoukas as well as Mantzoukas and Watkinson argue that despite the objectivity of the EBP method (identification of a problem, searching the literature, critically appraising best evidence and implementing findings into practice), paradoxically, requires the subjective interpretation of the evidence to a particular situation, the very process, one of intuition and opinion, that the original proponents of EBP aimed to distance themselves from.[27,28] Thus, the final step in the EBP process, the subjective application of evidence into practice, throws the philosophy of EBP into disarray!

Schön acknowledges this type of issue and argues that in reality [clinical] practice is complex, conflicting and uncertain.[29] The simplistic method of EBP (or as Schön describes it 'the technical rational approach to decision making') does not reflect the complex milieu in which healthcare professions work. This is true when attempting to apply evidence in healthcare practice; the clinician must contend with the ethical framework that governs practice and the political, economic technical and social factors that affect the decision-making process. The clinician also must apply the complex principles of EBP as well as acknowledging the needs and requirements for the patient/client group. Therefore, the final step of the EBP process, applying evidence, does not provide answers for practitioners nor does it guarantee best practice; it becomes subjective and does not adhere to the conscientious and judicious approach espoused by the proponents of EBP.

So how should healthcare practitioners and policy makers contend with this final philosophical issue? Higgs and Titchen argue that the subjective application of evidence is *not* bereft of a theoretical foundation; in fact it represents the artistry, wisdom and intuition of clinical practice.[19] This artistry and wisdom encompasses practical expertise and skills based on experiential knowledge, knowledge gained from practice: a body of knowledge termed practical craft knowledge or aesthetic knowledge.

The idea that intuition and artistry in the form of practical craft knowledge should be used to apply evidence in the complex reality of clinical practice is contrary to the notion of a conscientious and judicious approach to EBP.[15,27] To counter this and to ensure that practitioners operationalise the final stage of applying evidence within the philosophy of EBP, it is important to recognise that intuition, artistry and wisdom play a significant part in the evidence application process. The mechanism by which this can be incorporated into the philosophy of EBP lies with the concept of reflective practice.[27,28] Through the process of reflection, practitioners are empowered to explain and justify their decision-making process and rationalise their choice of evidence for supporting clinical practice; this reflective approach will enable the practitioner to think consciously and judiciously and will enable the selection and application of best evidence. The process of reflection will also ensure that the complex legal, ethical, social and technological issues that underpin the complex milieu of dietetic practice are considered when applying evidence; this reflective approach will ensure that the application of best evidence remains within the philosophy of EBP.

In summary this chapter has proposed that the type of clinical question should determine the nature of evidence used in clinical practice and that the process of reflection should be used to apply best evidence, in conjunction with clinical experience, in a conscientious and judicious way. Evidence should be considered in its broadest sense and it should be recognised that the evidence from a paper, per se, does not determine the treatment approach but the critical and systematic appraisal of its usefulness, blended with clinical interpretation, does.

References

1. Sackett DL, Rosenberg WM. On the need for evidence-based medicine. *Health Econ.* 1995;4(4):249–254.
2. Sackett DL, Rosenberg WMC, Gray JAM, Haynes RB, Richardson WS. Evidence based medicine: what it is and what it isn't. *Br Med J.* 1996;312(7023):71–72.
3. Sackett DL, Rosenberg WMC, Gray JAM, Haynes RB, Richardson WS. Evidence based medicine: what it is and what it isn't. 1996. *Clin Orthop Relat Res.* 2007;455:3–5.
4. Whelan K. Knowledge and skills to encourage comprehensive research involvement among dietitians. *J Hum Nutr Diet.* 2007;20(4):291–293.
5. French B. Contextual factors influencing research use in nursing. *Worldviews Evid Based Nur.* 2005;2(4):172–183.
6. Cameron KA, Ballantyne S, Kulbitsky A, Margolis-Gal M, Daugherty T, Ludwig F. Utilization of evidence-based practice by registered occupational therapists. *Occup Ther Int.* 2005;12(3):123–136.
7. Salbach NM, Jaglal SB, Korner-Bitensky N, Rappolt S, Davis D. Practitioner and organizational barriers to evidence-based practice of physical therapists for people with stroke. *Phys Ther.* 2007;87(10):1284.
8. Byham-Gray LD, Gilbride JA, Dixon LB, Stage FK. Predictors for research involvement among registered dietitians. *J Am Diet Assoc.* 2006;106(12):2008–2015.
9. Miles A, Loughlin M, Polychronis A. Medicine and evidence: knowledge and action in clinical practice. *J Eval Clin Pract.* 2007;13(4):481–503.
10. Tonelli MR. Integrating evidence into clinical practice: an alternative to evidence-based approaches. *J Eval Clin Pract.* 2006;12(3):248–256.
11. Rosenberg W, Donald A. Evidence based medicine: an approach to clinical problem-solving. *BMJ.* 1995;310(6987):1122–1126.
12. Liberati A, Vineis P. Introduction to the symposium: what evidence based medicine is and what it is not. *J Med Ethics.* 2004;30(2):120–121.

13. Gray GE, Gray LK. Evidence-based medicine: applications in dietetic practice. *J Am Diet Assoc.* 2002; 102(9):1263.

14. EBMWG. Evidence-based medicine. A new approach to teaching the practice of medicine. *J Am Med Assoc.* 1992;268(17):2420–2425.

15. Page S, Meerabeau L. Hierarchies of evidence and hierarchies of education: reflections on a multiprofessional education initiative. *Learning in Health and Social Care.* 2004;3(3):118–128.

16. Swinkels A, Albarran JW, Means RI, Mitchell T, Stewart MC. Evidence-based practice in health and social care: where are we now? *J Interprof Care.* 2002;16(4): 335–347.

17. Moore A, McQuay H, Gray JAM. Evidence based everything. *Bandolier.* 1995;1(12):1.

18. Scott-Findlay S, Pollock C. Evidence, research, knowledge: a call for conceptual clarity. *Worldviews Evid Based Nurs.* 2004;1(2):92–97.

19. Higgs J, Titchen A. The nature, generation and verification of knowledge. *Physiotherapy.* 1995; 81(9):521–530.

20. Mulhall A. Nursing research and the evidence. *Evid Based Nurs.* 1998; 1(1):4–6.

21. Sim J, Wright C. *Research in Health Care: Concepts, Designs and Methods.* Cheltenham: Stanley Thornes; 2000.

22. Jia X, McNeill G, Avenell A. Does taking vitamin, mineral and fatty acid supplements prevent cognitive decline? A systematic review of randomized controlled trials. *J Hum Nutr Diet.* 2008;21(4):317–336.

23. Stewart-Knox B, Gardiner K, Wright M. What is the problem with breast-feeding? A qualitative analysis of infant feeding perceptions. *J Hum Nutr Diet.* 2003;14(4):265–273.

24. Cowburn G, Summerbell C. A survey of dietetic practice in obesity management. *J Hum Nutr Diet.* 1998;11:191–195.

25. Rolfe G, Gardner L. Towards a geology of evidence-based practice—a discussion paper. *Int J Nurs Stud.* 2006;43(7):903–913.

26. Rycroft-Malone J, Seers K, Titchen A, Harvey G, Kitson A, McCormack B. What counts as evidence in evidence-based practice? *J Adv Nurs.* 2004; 47(1):81–90.

27. Mantzoukas S. A review of evidence-based practice, nursing research and reflection: levelling the hierarchy. *J Clin Nurs.* 2008;17(2):214–223.

28. Mantzoukas S, Watkinson S. Redescribing reflective practice and evidence-based practice discourses. *Int J Nurs Pract.* 2008;14(2): 129–134.

29. Schön D. *The Reflective Practitioner: How Professionals Think in Action.* New York: Basic Books; 1983.

The use of reflection in advancing practice

2

Lynn Clouder

Introduction

> Reflective practice is like a pool of blue, inviting water. The pool has a shallow end where the bottom is visible and a deep end where the blue is deep and the bottom unknown.[1]

I open this chapter by referring to the words of Christopher Johns, a well-known devotee of reflection from the nursing world because it is my perception that the pool provides an apt metaphor for discussing the status of reflection in the contemporary practice of dietitians. Having recently interviewed several highly experienced practising dietitians in the UK, my impression is that they are floating tentatively at the shallow end with an unfounded lack of confidence in venturing into deeper water to claim to be reflective practitioners, notwithstanding overwhelming evidence to the contrary.

Discussions with practitioners have highlighted that the perceived inadequacy of reflective skills can be attributed to lack of formal teaching about reflection and little or no experience of it, which is in agreement with other research findings.[2] This inadequacy is exacerbated by the sense that undergraduate students, for whom practitioners are frequently responsible on placement, are perceived to be better equipped to engage in reflection which is promoted in undergraduate curricula. The current UK Health Profession Council's (HPC) Standards of Proficiency for Dietitians explicitly highlight the requirement to understand the value of reflection for clinical practice and the need to record the outcome of such reflection.[3] While this stipulation aligns with continuing professional development (CPD) requirements, it necessitates the acquisition of additional skills in written reflection, which practitioners can find challenging. These factors appear to conspire to create uncertainty and ambivalence about reflection and its potential benefits for practitioners.

Perhaps the most powerful driver encouraging the uptake of some form of reflective dialogue within teams and departments is the necessity to demonstrate competence through CPD.[4] This requirement is not confined to dietitians, but includes other health professions and extends worldwide. The Dietitians Association of Australia Accredited Practising Dietitian programme is a self-regulatory strategy, which actively promotes reflective practice as a means of ensuring high-quality practice and service delivery.[5] Dietetic colleagues in the USA and Canada are already familiar with and have embraced the necessity to submit a professional development portfolio based on a reflective learning cycle for recertification every five years. From 2010 dietitians renewing their registration in the UK will be chosen at random and asked to produce a profile of evidence, taken from a professional CPD portfolio and stemming from work-based learning, underpinned at least partially by reflective practice.

Dietitians keen to learn more about reflection are confronted with a dearth of literature in dietetics, previously highlighted.[2] Fade provides a useful account of models and structures used to support the development of reflection within the dietetics curriculum. However, she emphasises the challenge faced by the profession to develop its own research-based literature. A limited literature around the experiences of completing the professional development portfolio in the USA and Canada informs this

2010, Elsevier Ltd.

account. However, given that the research base currently remains inadequate I draw on research and conceptual thinking across a wide range of professions to suggest ways in which practising dietitians might engage in reflection. My aim is to clarify what is meant by reflection, to explore the potential value of reflection for dietitians and the profession and its juxtaposition with evidence-based practice (EBP), as well as discussing a variety of approaches to facilitating reflection in practice. I hope to persuade colleagues that establishing a departmental or unit framework for reflection is achievable, useful and sustainable in the context of contemporary healthcare.

Some definitions

> Reflection is a specialized form of thinking that requires technical mastery of a subject plus active analysis of the purposes and consequences of decision-making.[6]

It seems to be worth briefly exploring what we mean by the terms *reflection* and *reflective practice*, which tend to be used interchangeably. Conceptions vary and both terms have been defined from a range of perspectives. For instance, Johns' definition of reflective practice as 'the practitioner's ability to access, make sense of and learn through work experience, to achieve more desirable, effective and satisfying work', emphasises the focus on self, as well as its developmental potential.[7] Boud et al.'s definition focuses pragmatically on the process by which 'people recapture their experience, think about it, mull it over and evaluate it' in a relatively straightforward and unproblematic way.[8] However, Mezirow's notion of reflection as 'seeing through habitual ways of interpreting everyday experience' suggests greater complexity and a necessity to venture beyond the shallows to transcend this basic appraisal.[9] The purpose of reflection is ultimately to come to new understanding and appreciation, opening the way for transformational learning that 'changes the way people see themselves and their world'.[10] However, this capacity for reflection to act as a catalyst for change might operate at a range of levels, whether it leads to a new way of doing something, the clarification of an issue, the development of a skill or the resolution of a problem.[11]

One might ask whether reflection is different to *analysis*. My response is to suggest that they are synonymous but belong to different paradigms or ways of viewing the world. Analysis refers to a cognitive or behavioural process where the person undertaking the analysis adopts a position of objectivity an separateness in an attempt to establish 'truth' claims. Alternatively, reflection involves affective as well as cognitive and behavioural domains, and therefore acknowledges subjectivity. The person is actively involved in developing understanding of self and others in a particular context, which is consistent with a professional artistry view of the world. As individuals and professionals, we all differ in how we view the world. However, health professionals tend to be driven down a scientific route, which influences their approach to their work not least because they have been persuaded by the discourse of *evidence-based practice*.

EBP has been defined as the means by which the scientific credentials of health are re-established,[12] and the movement has grown within the health professions internationally,[13] despite criticism that the only evidence for EBP is reliance on the very same introspection and intuition for which reflection is condemned.[14] In fact, reflective practice complements the EBP discourse by providing a means of addressing the 'messiness' of the real world of health and social care practice. It has become widely accepted as the means by which the self of the practitioner, the context of the lived experience and humanistic aspects of practice are made explicit. EBP supports development of propositional knowledge whereas reflective practice acknowledges the importance of personal knowledge. The two discourses, although presented as oppositional, are highly congruent. Johns argues that to value personal knowledge 'challenges the view of the practitioner as a largely uncritical receiver and user of knowledge produced by others', challenging the dominance of EBP in favour of a more balanced view that values both approaches.[7]

Plath acknowledges critical analysis as integral to the effective use of research evidence in social work practice, emphasising the need for practitioners to become less rigid in their interpretation of what counts as evidence.[13] This echoes messages conveyed by colleagues in dietetics,[15,16] advocating reflection on the biases created by personal values and assumptions in order to evolve from practising in 'black and white' to being comfortable practising 'in grey'.[16] Personal knowledge and that produced by others complement rather than oppose one another and need to be valued in their own right.[12] Developing Plath's suggestion I argue that they can be assimilated through the notion of *criticality* or *critical reflection*.

Criticality is the 'willingness to challenge, recreate and re-imagine in a manner that is searching, persistent and resolute'.[17] The consideration of evidence as one resource to be judged alongside other ways of knowing in practice, provides a healthy compromise and an essential means of confronting, understanding and resolving what Johns refers to as 'the contradictions between what is desirable and actual practice'.[18] Brookfield highlights that in order to become critically reflective it is necessary to be able to identify and challenge assumptions, to challenge the importance of context and to imagine and explore alternatives, which he believes leads to 'reflective scepticism'.[19]

The value of reflection in advancing practice

Brookfield suggests that non-reflexive learning, lacking a critical element, often takes place in action contexts that are easily equated with healthcare practice.[20] Conjure up an image of the practice setting and the practitioner, coping with increasing service demands and the consequences of poor staffing levels, trying to deal with heavy patient workloads, as expeditiously as possible. The suggestion that the ability to engage in critical reflection is a matter of social determination certainly seems to ring true here. Submission 'without resistance to rules of debate, argument assessment, and decision-making processes that the dominant culture favors [sic]' feels all too familiar in the type of context described.[20] Whether the all too common organisational context is the cause of a lack of reflection in dietitians' day-to-day practice,[2] or it is attributed to professional cultural beliefs about what counts as valuable knowledge, it seems that dietitians need to be alert to the potential for critical reflection to advance practice.

Such advancement of practice can occur on several fronts. First, critical reflection provides a means of improving practice through the development of personal knowledge, professional expertise and competence. In other words, there is potential for professional and individual growth. Recognising this potential allows practitioners to identify their own learning needs and to take increased responsibility for their own learning.[21] Furthermore, critical reflection encourages us to scrutinise our own implicit, unexamined assumptions, which might limit or undermine intended or espoused practice.[22] By reflecting

and deconstructing our own interpretations of a situation we may be able to challenge internal barriers in our thinking that preclude other possible conceptualisations or options.[23] For example, a dietitian asked to see a new cancer patient might decide that nutrition support is the best treatment for the patient. Finding that s/he is more concerned with quality rather than length of life and being cared for at home might mean a compromise, which could prove challenging in terms of what is clinically appropriate. Space for reflection allows greater depth of thinking about the psychosocial perspectives of care and tensions with evidence-based clinical decision-making. In broader terms the case potentially raises issues of human rights and healthcare ethics and at an individual level it might provoke thoughts about personal and professional values and beliefs. This example illustrates the interaction between different areas of work interest served by reflection.[4] Namely it is the overlap between instrumental/evaluative interests (getting the job done), personal growth and development (searching for greater understanding) and ethical interest (confronting moral or ethical dilemmas and being empowered to take action).

Secondly, advancement of practice will occur if assumptions on which practice is based are questioned. This is of particular importance in organisational contexts not necessarily conducive to critical practice, namely, the contexts in which most dietitians work. Morley suggests that critical reflection 'forces us to reflect on how we subjectively position ourselves within certain contexts and discourses'.[23] For example, within the health- and social care context, the medical model with attendant hierarchical structures and working relationships based on traditional power differentials forms the dominant discourse with which there seems to be an imperative to identify. Practitioners quickly learn to find their level in the hierarchy and sink into habitual practice, failing to question whether things could be bettered when it might be argued that it is their professional responsibility to challenge structural barriers of this nature. Part of advancing practice might be to make the invisible, such as alternative approaches, visible and valued.[7] Current changes in the healthcare practice offers more opportunities than ever before for dietitians and other health professionals to re-imagine systems and practices to exploit new ways of working. Guided reflection offers a means of negotiating new roles and new identities.

Approaches to facilitating reflection

Johns is adamant that reflective practice always needs to be guided in some way.[7] His rationale is that lone reflection can be difficult because practitioners tend to focus narrowly on disturbing experiences, and find it difficult to know what to reflect upon and what factors need to be attended to. He maintains that without some guidance much of 'normal' practice is not rendered problematic and hence does not become the focus for reflection, limiting potential for increased understanding and learning. I have argued elsewhere that lone reflection serves to maintain the status quo rather than promoting change, so is less effective and desirable than reflection that includes some form of dialogue.[24]

There are a number of approaches for facilitating reflection in practice that are discussed at present. However, reflection is essentially individualistic; therefore finding the optimal means of structuring it probably comes down to individual preferences regarding models and strategies. Griffin highlights the need to take into account a number of assumptions when selecting facilitation methods.[25] For instance, she stresses that reflection is developmental in nature, that writing is a critical lever for learning and that dialogue can help externalise thinking by 'enrich[ing] internal conversations'.[26]

Given insufficient space to discuss the wide range of models and frameworks that might help to structure reflection, a reading list is provided at the end of the chapter. Popular models tend to incorporate similar stages of awareness, description, evaluation, new awareness, learning and action.[21] Research suggests that simple practical guidance works best.[27] However, Jones warns against the repeated use of guides, which can become ritualistic, leading to superficial learning.[28] Such habitual practice might be avoided by using a variety of different facilitation techniques over time within the reflective framework adopted by a department or unit. What seems important in the departmental context is that reflection is undertaken systematically.[29]

Clinical supervision

Of the various means of engaging in reflective practice one approach debated in the dietetics literature is that of clinical supervision.[30,31] Burton favours the NHS Management Executive definition of clinical supervision, which seems both to stress its potentially regulatory function and to promote CPD:

> a formal process of professional support and learning which enables individual practitioners to develop knowledge and competence, assume responsibility for their own practice and enhance consumer protection and the safety of care in complex situations. It is central to the process of learning and to the expansion of the scope of practice and should be seen as a means of encouraging self assessment and analytic and reflective skills.[32]

This definition is consistent with Proctor's 'three function interactive model', which identifies the related functions that clinical supervision might serve (Table 2.1).[33]

Proctor confines reflection to the formative function; yet it is clearly inherent to the other functions especially given that they are interrelated and are likely to overlap depending on individual needs, which of course will develop and change. In principle, clinical supervision provides an ideal milieu for the guidance of reflective practice, which in turn helps to structure the clinical supervision process.[7] Kirk et al. express some ambivalence about the feasibility of clinical supervision and its appropriateness in all areas of dietetic practice.[31] Its potential supportive function in the mental health field is acknowledged. However, more generic educative benefits, which Kirk et al. equate with management regulation, are weighed against staff shortages and heavy workload commitments. Clinical supervision seems to be presented as a necessary evil, when in fact there is evidence to suggest that practitioners are enthusiastic about it and benefit greatly from it.[34]

Table 2.1 The three-function interactive model of clinical supervision

Normative	Formative	Restorative
Managerial focus	Developmental focus	Supportive focus
Upholding standards	Education	Peer support
Concerned with competence	Personal development	Active listening
	Reflection	Guidance and counselling

Adapted from Proctor.[33]

One-to-one supervision is the most frequently cited structural model within nursing,[35] although group or multidisciplinary supervision is well used across other health professions.[36] Shepherd and Rosebert report on the setting up of a *reflective practice group* for a multidisciplinary community mental health team.[37] The group, which was led by a clinical psychologist, seems to adopt a clinical supervision approach. Aside from pragmatic considerations such as the importance of management support, negotiating timing and establishing understandings about the learning opportunities that are afforded, the motivation to want and to see the benefits of the group are highlighted as essential if clinical supervision is to be successful. The key message seems to be that staff must want and see the value in clinical supervision and managers must give it their full support. Sellars' research suggests that notwithstanding informal mechanisms that might exist, a formal system is necessary in the current healthcare climate to ensure that dedicated time is used productively.[34] Perhaps most significantly, she stresses again the need for unequivocal management support if a system of clinical supervision is to be implemented successfully.

Within a supervisory-type framework a number of techniques might be used to facilitate and structure reflection. *Critical incident* or *significant event analysis* is used extensively in the teaching profession but is equally applicable in the healthcare professions. Tripp identifies four steps to conducting a critical incident analysis (Box 2.1).[38]

Selecting a suitable incident for analysis is a frequent block. Tripp suggests choosing something that 'amused or annoyed', while Posner favours choosing an event that provoked an 'aha or ouch' response.[39] By focusing on the meaning rather than the experience the incident is rendered critical. I would argue that in itself its capacity to promote depth of critical reflection is limited and only through subsequent analysis through conversation with a supervisor,

mentor or group might this be deepened. Research on the use of critical incident analysis with pre-service teachers suggests that it increases capacity for critical and reflective thinking.[25] *Critical case review*, which again draws on clinical supervision, reflective practice and action learning, provides an alternative means of structuring reflection. Describing how critical case reviews were implemented in a leadership programme for experienced critical care practitioners from a range of health professions, Crofts attributes their success to the problem approach and a strong patient focus.[40]

Preceptorship

Preceptorship might be considered to provide a hybrid form of clinical supervision. Morley's evaluation of a preceptorship programme for new occupational therapists recommends it as an alternative means of structuring reflection, which preceptors rated more highly than supervisory practice.[41] The success of the preceptorship programme is attributed partially to its close alignment with the NHS Knowledge and Skills Framework (KSF),[42] against which reflective accounts and other sources of evidence can be mapped during the first year of practice. Written evidence towards the KSF also contributes to the practitioner's ongoing CPD portfolio. Although the findings of the preliminary evaluation are limited, initial impressions are that preceptorship provides a robust structure within which reflection can be facilitated and learning recorded as part of ongoing CPD for new graduates.

Portfolio building

The approach to facilitating professional development through reflection, which has been embraced by the American Dietetics Association, and that fits most closely with the CPD initiative developed by the HPC in the UK, is that of portfolio keeping. Although health professionals are probably quite good at collecting evidence of their CPD, in the form of certificates of attendance on courses and other factual material, the CPD framework suggests that this is not enough. Moreover, research amongst nurses suggests that portfolios are rarely kept up to date and there is limited understanding of the nature of reflection.[40] Nevertheless, building portfolios is a popular method of fostering reflective practice commended

Box 2.1

Four steps to critical incident analysis

1. Describe and explain an incident
2. Find a general meaning and classification for the incident
3. Take a position with regard to the meaning
4. Describe actions to be taken

Adapted from Tripp.[38]

to students, practitioners and teachers as a means of making better sense of what they are doing and planning for continuous improvement stimulated by continuous self-assessment of what has been done.[43]

The Commission on Dietetic Registration (CDR) implemented the professional Development Portfolio in the USA in 2001, publishing a portfolio guide to help practitioners understand and embark on the portfolio process. A national pilot study conducted shortly after the launch of the scheme, exploring how well the process was working, found that practitioners had a positive perception of reflection as the first step in the portfolio process.[44] A smaller subsequent study, which sought to explore 'how' dietitians reflect,[45] found that reflection was characterised by informal non-structured processes. Although participants recognised that it was part of a 'job requirement' there was no formal system for reflection and no time commitment to it. Weddle et al. recommended that practitioners needed to give sufficient time to the reflection process and also needed to find appropriate tools for facilitating and structuring reflection.

Notwithstanding the use of the reflective portfolio for renewal of registration, it can serve other purposes such as preparation for personal development appraisal, and regrading or job applications, therefore, might include a wide range of evidence. Cross et al. suggest including a log of CPD activities mapped to evidence, standards and outcomes, reflective statements and evidence to support claims relating to fulfilment of outcomes and action plans for ongoing development.[4] To this list can be added SWOT analyses repeated at regular intervals, reflections on critical incidents, supporting statements and feedback from line managers, peers, students or clients.

Paschal et al. advocate the move to using technology and electronic portfolios, which would enable the collection of an even broader range of artefacts such as audio, video, and graphics as well as text.[43] The e-portfolio has the benefit of being easily editable and modified for different audiences, making it attractive to busy practitioners.

Looking to the future

The arguments in favour of dietitians having a system of CPD in place underpinned by reflective skills are persuasive. However, there is an imperative to ensure that if reflection is to inform practice it needs to be guided in some way. I have provided a brief overview of popular approaches to facilitating reflection with which colleagues might experiment. However, whichever tools or approaches are adopted it is important that the activity is deliberate and that it leads to changes in practice. In terms of meeting the challenges of contemporary practice and advancing practice, it is my belief that the value of reflective practice for dietitians should not be underestimated.

References

1. Johns C. Foreword. In: *The Higher Education Academy Health Science and Practice Subject Centre, the Development of Critical Reflection in the Health Professions*. London: LTSN; 2004:3.

2. Fade S. Reflection in the dietetic curriculum. In: *The Higher Education Academy Health Science and Practice Subject Centre, the Development of Critical Reflection in the Health Professions*. London: LTSN; 2004:76–81.

3. Health Professions Council. *Standards of Proficiency for Dietitians*. London: Health Professions Council; 2003.

4. Cross V, Liles C, Conduit J, Price J. Linking reflective practice to evidence of competence: a workshop for allied health professionals. *Reflective Practice*. 2004;5(1):3–31.

5. Daniels LA, Magarey A. The educational and vocational role of peer assessment in the training and professional practice of dietitians. *Aust J Nutr Diet*. 2000;57(1):18–22.

6. Dewey J. *How We Think*. Boston: Heath; 1933.

7. Johns C. The value of reflective practice for nursing. *J Clin Nurs*. 1995;4:23–30.

8. Boud D, Keogh R, Walker D. *Reflection: Turning Experience into Learning*. London: Kogan Page; 1985.

9. Mezirow J. *Transformative Dimensions of Adult Learning*. San Francisco: Jossey Bass; 1991.

10. Baumgartner LM. An update on transformational learning. *New Directions for Adult and Continuing Education*. 2001;89:15–22.

11. Boud D, Keogh R, Walker D, eds. *Reflection: Turning Experience into Learning*. London: Kogan Page; 1994.

12. Taylor C. Narrating practice: reflective accounts and the textual construction of reality. *J Adv Nurs*. 2003;42(3):244–251.

13. Plath D. Evidence-based practice: current issues and future directions. *Aust J Soc Work*. 2006;59(1):56–72.

14. Rolfe G. The deconstructing angel: nursing, reflection and evidence-based practice. *Nurs Inq*. 2005;12(2):78–86.

15. Lean MEJ, Anderson AS. The nature of evidence. *J Hum Nutr Diet*. 2004;17:291–292.

16. Morrison T, Foisy S. Being comfortable practising 'in grey': an exercise in reflexive practice. *Can J Diet Pract Res*. 2007;68(2):8.

17. Curzon-Hobson A. Higher learning and the critical stance. *Studies in Higher Education*. 2003;28(2): 201–212.

18. Johns C. *Becoming a Reflective Practitioner: A Reflective and Holistic Approach to Clinical Nursing, Practice Development and Clinical Supervision*. Oxford: Blackwell Science; 2000.

19. Brookfield SD. *Developing Critical Thinkers*. Milton Keynes: Open University; 1987.

20. Brookfield SD. *The Power of Critical Theory for Adult Learning and Teaching*. Maidenhead: Open University; 2005.

21. Cooney A. Reflection demystified: answering some common questions. *Br J Nurs*. 1999;8:1530–1534.

22. Brookfield SD. Using critical incidents to explore learners' assumptions. In: Mezirow J, ed. *Fostering Critical Reflection In Adulthood*. San Francisco: Jossey Bass; 1990:177–193.

23. Morley C. Engaging practitioners with critical reflection: issues and dilemmas. *Reflective Practice*. 2007;8(1):61–74.

24. Clouder DL. Reflective practice: realizing its potential. *Physiotherapy*. 2000;86:517–522.

25. Griffin ML. Using critical incidents to promote and assess reflective thinking in preservice teachers. *Reflective Practice*. 2003;4(2):207–220.

26. Costa AL, Kallick B. Getting into the habit of reflection. *Educational Leadership*. 2000;57:60–62.

27. Clarke A. Enabling learning through reflective tutorials in the nursing practice setting. In: *The Higher Education Academy Health Science and Practice Subject Centre, the Development of Critical Reflection in the Health Professions*. London: LTSN; 2004:54–62.

28. Jones I. Using reflective practice in the paramedic curriculum. In: *The Higher Education Academy Health Science and Practice Subject Centre, the Development of Critical Reflection in the Health Professions*. London: LTSN; 2004:39–46.

29. Burton J. Reflective practice revisited. *Work Based Learning in Primary Care*. 2006;4:297–300.

30. Burton S. A critical essay on professional development in dietetics through the process of reflection and clinical supervision. *J Hum Nutr Diet*. 2000;13:323–332.

31. Kirk SFL, Eaton J, Auty L. Dieticians and supervision: should we be doing more? *J Hum Nutr Diet*. 2000;13:317–322.

32. NHS Management Executive. *A Vision for the Future: The Nursing, Midwifery and Health Visiting Contribution to Health and Health Care*. London: Department of Health; 1993.

33. Proctor B. Supervision: a cooperative exercise in accountability. In: Marken M, Payne M, eds. *Enabling and Ensuring: Supervision in Practice*. Leicester: National Youth Bureau; 1987.

34. Sellars J. Learning from contemporary practice: an exploration of clinical supervision in physiotherapy. *Learning in Health and Social Care*. 2004;3(2):64–82.

35. Butterworth T, Carson J, White E, Jeacock J, Clements A, Bishop V. *It Is Good to Talk: An Evaluation Study in England and Scotland*. University of Manchester: School of Nursing, Midwifery and Health Visiting; 1997.

36. Hawkins P, Shohet R. *Supervision in the Helping Professions*. Milton Keynes: Open University; 2000.

37. Shepherd E, Rosebert C. Setting up and evaluating a reflective practice group. *Clinical Psychology Forum*. 2007;172:31–34.

38. Tripp D. *Critical Incidents in Teaching: Developing Professional Judgement*. London: Routledge; 1993.

39. Posner GJ. *Field Experience: A Guide to Reflective Thinking*. 5th edn. New York: Longman; 2000.

40. Crofts L. Learning from experience: Constructing critical case reviews for a leadership programme. *Intensive Crit Care Nurs*. 2006;22:294–300.

41. Morley M. Building reflective practice through preceptorship: the cycles of professional growth. *Br J Occup Ther*. 2007;70(1):40–42.

42. Department of Health. *The NHS Knowledge and Skills Framework (NHS KSF) and the development review process, Final Version*. London: Department of Health; 2004.

43. Paschal KA, Jensen GM, Mostrom E. Building portfolios: a means of developing habits of reflective practice in physical therapy education. *J Phys Ther Educ*. 2002;16(3):38–53.

44. Keim KS, Gates GE, Johnson CA. Dietetics professionals have a positive perception of professional development. *J Am Diet Assoc*. 2001;101(7):820–824.

45. Weddle DO, Himburg SP, Collins N, Lewis R. The professional development portfolio process: setting goals for credentialing. *J Am Diet Assoc*. 2002;102(10): 1439–1444.

Further reading on models and frameworks for structuring reflection

Atkins S, Murphy K. Reflection: a review of the literature. *J Adv Nurs*. 1993;18:1188–1192.

Boud D, Keogh R, Walker D. *Reflection: Turning Experience into Learning*. London: Kogan Page; 1985.

Fish D, Twinn S, Purr B. *Promoting Reflection: The Supervision of Practice in Health Visiting and Initial Teacher Training*. London: West London Institute; 1991.

Jarvis P. *Adult Learning in the Social Context*. London: Croom Helm; 1987.

Johns C. Framing learning through reflection within Carper's fundamental ways of knowing. *J Adv Nurs*. 1995;22:226–234.

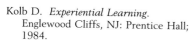

Kolb D. *Experiential Learning.* Englewood Cliffs, NJ: Prentice Hall; 1984.

Mezirow J. *Fostering Critical Reflection in Adulthood: Guide to Transformative and Emancipatory Learning.* San Francisco: Jossey Bass; 1990.

Moon JA. *Reflection in Learning and Professional Development: Theory and Practice.* London: Kogan Page; 1999.

Moon JA. *A Handbook of Reflective and Experiential Learning.* London: Routledge Falmer; 2004.

Schön DA. *The Reflective Practitioner: How Professionals Think in Action.* New York: Basic Books; 1983.

Schön DA. *Educating the Reflective Practitioner.* San Francisco: Jossey Bass; 1987.

Changing behaviour

3

Dympna Pearson

Introduction

This chapter describes the importance of the application of behaviour change principles to improve health and well-being. It focuses on achieving change at the individual level while recognising that this needs to be part of an overall strategy involving interventions at population and community levels.

Context

Human behaviour has been defined as 'the product of individual or collective human actions, seen within and influenced by their structural, social and economic context'.[1]

Behaviour can have a major impact on mortality and morbidity, and behaviour change interventions have the potential to significantly alter disease patterns.[1] It is recommended that changes in behaviour, and the social, economic and environmental contexts in which unhealthy behaviours take place, should be at the heart of all disease prevention strategies.[2]

Whilst acknowledging social inequalities as a key determinant of health, NICE suggests that changes in behaviour may be more achievable than changes to social circumstances, at least in the short term.[1] Nevertheless, behavioural changes are hugely challenging for both the individual and the healthcare professional involved.

Interventions to achieve behaviour change can be directed at the individual, community or population level. Changes at any one level can lead to changes at another level—the so-called ripple effect. For example, individuals who change their eating behaviour may have an impact on the rest of the household or other individuals in the community, whilst population strategies to increase activity may encourage individuals to become more active. Clearly a coherent overall strategy operating at all levels is the most desirable. It needs to have clear aims and be based on sound principles and available evidence, and methods for monitoring the effects should be developed hand in hand.

Models of behaviour change provide a framework for planning and delivering behavioural interventions. Relevant theories originating from the world of behavioural sciences include resilience, coping, self-efficacy, planned behaviour, structure and agency, 'habitus' and social capital.[1] Over the past few decades, although a number of behaviour change models have been described, the evidence does not tend to support any one model over and above another. On the whole, these models do not satisfactorily capture the complexities and contradictions in human behaviour and, because they have been developed to explain aspects of the individual's behaviour, they fail to capture population-level dynamics.[1]

Therefore, even though some psychological constructs can be helpful and interesting when considering an individual's behaviour, behaviour change interventions are best focused upon therapeutic skills rather than on specific theoretical constructs. Programme development needs to draw on current evidence and be subjected to ongoing evaluation. No single approach will suit everyone. So any intervention should be tailored to the individual, community or population.

The focus of the rest of this chapter is interventions with the individual patient or client.

A behavioural approach

'The main principles of this approach include the modification of current behaviour patterns, new adaptive learning, problem solving and a collaborative relationship between client and the therapist.'[3] A behavioural approach seeks to empower clients—to equip them with the knowledge and skills to bring about and sustain desired changes.[4] It supports self-efficacy by building competence and self-belief in one's ability to make changes.[5] It acknowledges that change is complex and is influenced by the environment in which someone lives as well as their attitude, level of knowledge and skills. Changing habits that have often been acquired over a long period of time requires a degree of effort, energy, time and commitment. There is no quick fix Collaborative problem solving is the essence of a behavioural intervention.

A problem-solving approach has five easily identified steps:

1. Identify the problem (often described as the 'assessment');
2. Explore all possible options for dealing with it;
3. Explore pros and cons of each option;
4. Identify which one is a realistic next step; and
5. Try out the option and review progress.

The next section will focus on the *process* of helping based on a problem-solving approach. The approach differs from the traditional advice-giving approach in that the client is very much involved in the whole process and ultimately makes the decision to change (or not) and makes the choices for their preferred options.

The process

Assessment

This should start with building rapport, outlining the purpose of the intervention and checking that the person wishes to be involved. In traditional healthcare the assessment has focused on the clinical picture. Using a behavioural approach, the clinical picture is explored along with the aspects likely to influence health behaviour: the reason for the intervention, the targeted behaviour(s), the story so far (history of condition, previous attempts at change, successes/what did not work), motivation, expectations of the

intervention and outcomes, current lifestyle including social aspects, possible difficulties. This assessment needs to be undertaken in a skilled and sensitive manner involving the client throughout the process, although guided by the practitioner in order to ensure that a complete picture evolves. Once the assessment has been completed, it is then important to clarify the client's agenda (preferred outcome) and to be clear about what the practitioner can offer. Both parties can then move forward with a shared agenda.

Explore the options

This involves checking what the client already knows or has tried and often involves providing information to help the person make an informed decision. Providing information needs to be undertaken in a structured manner, firstly, checking what the person knows and indeed if they would like some information (this is part of the respectful nature that threads through the intervention). Provide the information in a way that makes sense to the person and tailoring it to their needs; avoiding jargon and allowing for questions and comments so that it becomes a two-way process; checking what the person thinks of the information as this is likely to influence their decision-making. People may want guidance on what research shows or what works best for others in similar situations, but ultimately, they are the best judge of what will work best for them.

Choose an option (goal setting)

Most practitioners are familiar with the principles of goal setting; yet in practice, this is poorly executed. SMART (specific, measurable, achievable, realistic and time specific) goals can be achieved in practice through the collaborative development of a *Change Plan*.[6] This involves paying attention to the detail of the Change Plan.

- *What* is the overall target? (desired outcome)
- *How* is this going to be achieved? (specific behavioural goals/sub-goals)
- *What* needs to be in place? (e.g. correct food in cupboards, trainers in the car)
  - ○ Support—where from and how to elicit this
  - ○ Rewards—for ongoing effort and achieving new behaviours
  - ○ Monitoring progress
- *When* is it going to start
- Review.

Implement the plan

Efforts to change do not necessarily succeed at the first attempt. A detailed Change Plan is more likely to help the person succeed but even then, unforeseen difficulties may crop up or simply the effort required to change ingrained habits may be greater than initially realised. Trying it out is the only way to check whether the plan is right for that person. The plan will need to be regularly reviewed and revised throughout the change process. The role of the practitioner is to support clients in developing a realistic Change Plan and to convey optimism and a willingness to re-examine. Efforts to change need to be acknowledged and affirmed. Clients should be encouraged to seek support from significant others and to reward themselves for changes in behaviour. Self-monitoring is a key behavioural tool and it often requires coaching and practice to develop this skill.

Review the plan

Ongoing review is part of the problem-solving process, so it is important to build a regular review into the Change Plan. For the majority of people, it is not enough to discuss it and then expect them to do it. Time needs to be devoted to discussing ongoing review and how this can be tailored to the individual.

Maintenance

When changes have been achieved, maintaining these changes provides a new challenge. The nature of change is that people are likely to lapse back into old habits and therefore they need to be equipped with the skills to deal with lapses. Ongoing support is an important component of maintaining changes and how this is arranged will need to be agreed.

There are many strategies or tools which can be used as to modify behaviour. These include exploring motivation, eliciting information on current behaviours, exchanging information, exploring options, goal setting, self-monitoring, identifying unhelpful behaviours and problem-solving ways to overcome them. Methods for using these tools are described in detail elsewhere.[6] All of the above tools need to be used with skill and underpinned by the spirit of a person-centred approach which relies heavily on the use of reflective listening and good communication skills. Cognitive restructuring where unhelpful patterns of thinking promote the continuation of unhelpful behaviours is an advanced skill requiring further training and supervision.

Motivation

Motivation is a key aspect of changing behaviour—the person has got to want to do it and believe in their ability to achieve the desired change. Motivation needs to be present throughout the change process—not just at the beginning. The person facilitating change needs to check (and not assume) that the client *does* want to change their behaviour in order to achieve the desired outcome. Often a person may *want* the desired outcome but may be less willing to make the necessary changes to their behaviour. Resistance to change is normal.[7] Change is difficult—it requires effort, energy and commitment. Life's competing priorities may get in the way. The practitioner can help reduce resistance to change by ensuring that they truly listen to the client and help explore any difficulties they are experiencing, whilst respecting that the decision-making lies with the client.

Lack of confidence in their ability to change is often at the heart of the difficulty. The practitioner can support individuals by checking that they feel able to undertake the proposed change, what might get in the way and what might help overcome any difficulties. Self-efficacy or a belief in their ability to change can be supported through a problem-solving approach, remembering to build on previous achievements, acknowledge any effort and help clients to develop a realistic step-wise Change Plan. Conveying optimism is a guiding principle of a behavioural approach. This is not meant to be interpreted as an 'of course, you can do it' approach, but conveyed as a genuine belief that everyone has within themselves the ability to change. It is also important to acknowledge efforts, including past efforts to change, along with any achievements, however small.

Scaling questions can be used to 'assess' motivation, but care needs to be taken that these are used skilfully and in a collaborative manner to help explore the client's current situation. It is not the practitioner's role to decide whether this person is 'ready or not'. The nature of motivation is that it fluctuates and it is influenced by many factors, so maintaining motivation throughout the change process is a challenge for clients and practitioners. Clients often experience feelings of ambivalence about change ('I want to, but I can't') and simply exploring these ambivalent feelings can enhance motivation. This is done by helping the client look at all aspects of change/no change from their perspective. Going through this process can often help clarify thinking.

A person-centred approach and the use of reflective listening skills underpin motivational interviewing. Miller and Rollnick found that the health practitioner's way of working or therapeutic style strongly influences the intervention outcome.[7]

Patient-centredness

Background

The traditional medical model is characterised by an expert-led, advice-giving style. Implied in this way of working is the expectation that once people are told what to do, they will follow advice. However, research shows that giving advice alone does not automatically change behaviour.[8–10] Whilst behavioural interventions address the processes of change, it can be just as expert-led as the traditional medical model. Behavioural interventions need to take on board a 'patient-centred' orientation. A patient-centred approach, developed by Stewart and colleagues,[11] has been advocated for modern clinical consultation across disciplines. This approach aims to focus on the person rather than the problem in isolation; it incorporates the psycho-social aspects of care.

Modern approaches to chronic disease management and prevention, e.g. diabetes, coronary heart disease, renal disease, are based on a patient-centred approach. The challenge is for healthcare professionals to appreciate the health-related behavioural issues in context, and work with it to influence change in a positive direction.

Stewart et al. outline key aspects of a patient-centred approach.[11] These are:

- Professionals actively seek to enter into the patient's world to understand his or her unique experiences. They can demonstrate this through effective listening skills.
- How patients feel and what they expect from practitioners is taken into account. Patients are experts about themselves and their situation and are therefore best placed to make their own decisions about change, with support from practitioners.
- How the illness affects patients' lives is taken into account.
- The importance of practitioners and patients finding common ground and working together to define the problem and establish

goals, whilst being clear about each other's roles within the helping relationship, is highlighted.

An integrated, client-centred approach demands intervention skills to address the processes of lifestyle change.[6] Such an approach aims to:

- Collaborate with the person to decide on the next concrete, practical step to change eating behaviour or other behavioural aspects of his or her lifestyle.
- Combine information exchange with motivational, behavioural and cognitive approaches.
- Emphasise the most relevant strategies at any given time, e.g. motivational or behavioural.
- Take into account the world in which the individual lives, what matters to him or her, how eating and activity fit into the person's life, and the factors likely to influence change processes.
- Recognise that the skills and mindset of the practitioner will influence how effective they are as a behaviour change agent. The need for practitioners to engage in increasing self and other awareness is explicitly acknowledged.

The evidence

A review of the evidence based on 21 studies undertaken by Stewart and colleagues showed that a patient-centred approach:[11]

- Improves clinical outcomes;
- Increases patient satisfaction;
- Improves compliance with medication; and
- Reduces patients' concerns.

Interpersonal skills

The importance of good communication skills in facilitating change has been highlighted and there is good evidence to support this. The single most important factor that influences change is the practitioner's possession of strong interpersonal skills.[12] A review of the literature undertaken by Stewart concluded that 'good communication is good evidence-based medicine'.[11] Modern medicine encourages evidence-based practice and this is applied to most clinical procedures. However, good communication skills are often taken for granted. These skills are essential within an integrated approach to health behaviour change and may be variably described as counselling, consultation skills, interviewing, active listening, reflective listening and communication or interpersonal skills. Many practitioners are naturally good listeners; others develop their listening skills through years of practice. However obtained, these skills need to be continually developed and refined.

Core practitioner qualities

The qualities that a practitioner working in a patient-centred way needs to take to a consultation are often described as the core qualities of a client-centred approach. As described by Rogers and reiterated by Gable,[13,14] these are:

- Empathy—every effort is made to understand the situation from the client's point of view and this understanding is conveyed to the client through the use of effective listening skills.
- Genuineness—honesty is key to an effective helping relationship and this is built on trust. Clients are unlikely to enter into a helping relationship if trust is not present.
- Acceptance—being non-judgemental can at times be challenging for practitioners who can themselves be influenced by the prejudices that exist in the society in which they live.

The importance of reflecting on one's own attitudes and beliefs when working with individuals in a helping relationship cannot be understated. Working in a behavioural way often requires change on behalf of the practitioner as well as the client. Continuous reflective practice with accompanying clinical supervision is essential. Often when things do not go well in a helping relationship, i.e. the patient does/does not want to change, it is easy to place the blame with the patient. A behavioural approach encourages practitioners to look at their own approach.

Important principles for helping relationships

- Client responsibility—whilst it is widely accepted that people are responsible for their own health (and parents are responsible for their children's health), this does not mean that once people have been given information

'it is up to them' and healthcare professionals can abdicate any further responsibility for influencing change. It is important to try to gain an understanding of the difficulties that each individual is experiencing with change and to tailor the intervention to suit their needs, whilst respecting the person's right to make decisions about their own health. It is about paying full attention to the client's agenda.

- Social responsibility—healthcare professionals have an agenda to influence health and this can be very powerful even in a short space of time. What is important is that when time is limited it is used to maximum effect. The temptation is to provide as much information as possible, accompanied by advice-giving. However, this tends to make clients into passive recipients of information. It is important to ensure that the person feels truly heard and understood which in turn is more likely to make them receptive to change.
- Collaboration—the principle of collaboration helps to accommodate both the client's agenda and the healthcare professional's agenda. It recognises that two people with expertise have met—one with expertise about themselves (the client) and one with expertise in the topic area, along with specific 'helping skills' (the healthcare professional). A collaborative helping relationship is built on trust and mutual respect; it considers both parties as equals in exploring the possibilities for change.

Practitioner development

This chapter has described the complexity of applying behavioural interventions within a client-centred framework. Such a way of working requires skills development on the part of the client and the practitioner. It is critical that practitioners should continue to reflect on their level of skills and knowledge and their needs for further training and supervision. Their increased awareness of their own attitudes and beliefs and the way in which these could impact on their professional interactions will also stand to benefit patients. The self-reflection will need to be an ongoing process and is in line with the recommendation for health professionals to be lifelong learners.[15] NICE recommends an education and training strategy to support the development needs of those involved in helping to change people's behaviour (both in NHS and non-NHS settings) in order to improve effectiveness.[1] National training standards to reflect skills and competencies would support their implementation.

Evaluation

Interventions aimed at changing individual behaviours need to take into account the needs of the individual as well as being part of an overall coordinated and strategic approach. NICE recommends the evaluation of all behaviour change interventions and programmes, both locally and as part of a larger project and where possible, evaluation should include an economic component. This will enable future planning of interventions to be based on the best available evidence and cost-effectiveness.

Summary

Changing health-related behaviour is a challenging and complex task for patients and health professionals. A high level of behaviour change skills drawn on sound principles is important. However, these skills need to be applied within a client-centred framework for clinical practice, which requires long-term development supported by our professional and organisational contexts.

References

1. National Institute for Clinical Excellence. *Behaviour Change at Population, Community and Individual Levels*. 2007.

2. Wanless D. *Securing Good Health for the Whole Population: Final Report*. London: HM Treasury; 2004.

3. Health Development Agency. *The Management of Obesity and Overweight: An Analysis of Reviews of Diet, Physical Activity and Behavioural Approaches*. London: HDA; 2003.

4. Funnell MM, Anderson RM, Arnold MS, et al. Empowerment: an idea whose time has come in diabetes education. *Diabetes Educ*. 1991; 17(1):37–41.

5. Bandura A. *Social Learning Theory*. Englewood Cliffs, NJ: Prentice Hall; 1997.

6. Rapoport L, Pearson D. *Changing Health Behaviour in Manual of Dietetic Practice*. Oxford: Blackwell; 2007:46–48.

7. Miller WR, Rollnick S. *Motivational Interviewing: Preparing People to Change Addictive Behaviour*. New York: Guilford Press; 2002.

8. Thomas J. New approaches to achieving dietary change. *Curr Opin Lipidol*. 1994;5:36–41.

9. Contento J, Balch GI, Bronner YL, et al. The effectiveness of nutrition education and implications for nutrition education policy, programs, and research: a review of research. *J Nutr Educ*. 1995;27(6).

10. Thorogood M, Hillsdon M, Summerbell C. Changing behaviour. *Clin Evid*. 2002;8:37–59.

11. Stewart M. Studies of Health Outcomes and Patient-Centred Communication. In: Stewart M, Brown JB, Weston WW, McWhinney IR, McWilliam CL, Freeman TR, eds. *Patient-Centered Medicine Transforming the Clinical Method*. London: Sage; 1995:185–190.

12. Najavits LM, Weiss RD. Variations in therapist effectiveness in the treatment of patients with substance use disorders: an empirical review. *Addiction*. 1994;89:679–688.

13. Rogers CR. *Client-Centered Therapy*. Boston: Houghton Mifflin; 1951.

14. Gable J. *Counselling Skills for Dietitians*. London: Blackwell Science; 2007.

15. Department of Health. *Core Curriculum for Nutrition in the Education of Health Professionals*. London: Department of Health; 1994.

Transition to adult care

Paula Hallam

Introduction

The simple matter of transferring care from pae-diatricians to adult physicians has been challenged in the past decade by the notion of 'transition', emphasising the need for the change to adult care to be a guided educational and therapeutic process, rather than an administrative event.[1]

Older adolescents are in the midst of many life changes related to physical and emotional develop-ment, education and career choices, family and peer relationships and the presence of a chronic disease only adds an additional burden. At this stage of devel-opment, transfer of care to an adult facility becomes a major challenge for the adolescent, parents and paediatric and adult care providers.[2]

The term 'transfer' is often used to describe the handover from children's services to adult ser-vices. However, this terminology refers to a single event, whereas the handover should be a planned and managed process which is much better described using the word 'transition'.[3]

Transition can be defined as a 'purposeful, planned process that addresses the medical, psycho-social, educational and vocational needs of adoles-cents and young adults with chronic physical and medical conditions as they move from child-centred to adult-orientated health care systems'.[4]

The importance of transition of young people with chronic health conditions from paediatric to adult care is finally being recognised but it still needs to be addressed in a coordinated and integrated way.[5] Adolescence is not an easy time for young people. However, if you have a chronic health condition coupled with the usual turmoil of adolescence, it makes it that much harder to cope with. What is clear, both anecdotally and with some modest support in the literature, is that the journey faced by young people with chronic and disabling condi-tions is a complex one.[5,6] Arranging efficient and caring transfer for adolescents from paediatric to adult care is one of the greatest challenges facing paediatrics—and indeed the healthcare services—in the coming century.[1]

Adolescent health issues, including transitional care, have been identified as a major priority area of health in the UK in a recent document of the Children's National Service Framework:

> Current gaps in adult health services need to be addressed to make the transition to adult services easier for young people at risk from, or who have genetic diseases. Paediatric services for rare conditions are frequently more highly developed than adult services, making transition particularly problematic in areas where little adult expertise exists.[7]

There are two main reasons why these gaps exist:[7]

a) New treatments mean that for the first time, children and young people are surviving into adulthood where there is often an absence of, or limited services.

b) Young people will normally have experienced a more comprehensive approach to their problems through paediatric care, whereas adult services are frequently organ- or system-specific. As many genetic diseases affect several organ systems, the coordination of adult medical care can be problematic.

Communicating with adolescents

It is very important to communicate with adolescents at an appropriate level so as not to be too patronising but also to ensure they understand what is being explained. By far the most important issue in the eyes of young people is communication.[3] Working with adolescents needs different consultation skills from those needed for children or older adults in addition to the clinical knowledge and skills required in each speciality.[3]

The following are some practical points for communicating and working with adolescents:[8]

- See young people by themselves as well as with their parents. Ensure that you do not exclude the parents but also make it clear that the adolescent is the centre of the consultation.
- Be empathetic, respectful and non-judgemental especially when discussing behaviours such as substance misuse.
- Assure confidentiality at all times.
- Be yourself—don't try to be too 'cool' or 'hip'!
- Try to explain concepts in a manner appropriate to their development—avoid abstract concepts and examples too far in the future.

Why transition to adult services?

The burden of chronic illness in adolescence is increasing in all developed countries as larger numbers of chronically ill children survive into their second and third decades.[1] The prevalence of cystic fibrosis over 15 years of age in the UK more than doubled between 1977 and 1985 and currently over 85% of children with chronic illnesses survive to adult life.[1]

It is important to note that the change from paediatric to adult healthcare is difficult for any young person as well as those with a chronic illness.[1] Young adults often do not register with a general practitioner and frequently drop out of the healthcare system after they leave home and leave behind childhood surveillance such as immunisations, growth monitoring and development.[1] These young people often only make contact with the medical profession in an emergency situation or crisis which could have been avoided if regular contact with the medical profession had been maintained.[1] Good transitional

Box 4.1

Attendance of young people at four diabetes services averaged 94% before transfer to an adult clinic but fell to 57% two years after transfer. There was large inter-district variation in clinic attendance 2 years post-transfer (29% to 71%) with higher rates seen in districts where young people had the opportunity to meet the adult diabetes consultant prior to transfer.[14]

planning and implementation could hopefully prevent such situations from arising.

The particular dangers of the period of moving from paediatric to adult services are illustrated by reports of 'near misses' occurring when adult cardiologists treated grown-up congenital heart patients.[9] However, there is some anecdotal evidence that transition programmes in cystic fibrosis,[10,11] diabetes,[12,13] and arthritis[2] improve health outcomes and patient quality of life.

To illustrate how different models of transition can affect patient care, an example from a diabetes service is discussed in Box 4.1.

Aims of transition

The goals or aims of an organised, coordinated and uninterrupted transition to adult healthcare for young adults with chronic conditions are:[3,6]

- To optimise health;
- To facilitate each young person's attainment of their potential;
- To involve each young person in the decisions; and
- To reinforce positive attitudes of growing up/adulthood.

Principles of successful transition

Despite the paucity of meaningful data, there are several fundamental principles or elements of transition that have received recognition/endorsement:[6,15,16]

- There should be a written policy between paediatric and adult services.
- The timing of transition should depend on the developmental readiness and health status of the individual adolescent.

- Transition should have an early start—when children enter a paediatric service, they should know that they are expected to leave it at some stage.
- Services need to be appropriate for chronological age *and* developmental attainment of the adolescent.
- Transition should not occur before the young person can manage their illness largely on their own, independent of parents/carers and staff, and can function in an adult clinic. In order to achieve this, preparation for transition needs to begin well before the anticipated transition time. Some suggest an individualised transition plan should be in place by age 14, created with the young person and their family and under regular review.
- Common health problems experienced by adolescents should be addressed, such as growth and development, sexuality, mental health disorders, substance use, and other health promoting and damaging behaviours.
- Transition programmes need to be flexible enough to meet the needs of a wide range of young people but also individualised to meet specific needs of young people and their families.
- The transition should be a coordinated process, including a visit to the adult clinic and one or more joint paediatric–adult clinic visits.
- There should be a designated professional or key worker who, together with the patient and family, takes responsibility for the transition process. This person should be able to act as an advocate for the patient and family and help streamline the transition process.
- Administrative support is key to the process, including provision of a medical summary that is portable and accessible.
- A successful transition to adult services should enhance autonomy, facilitate self-reliance and help the young person develop a sense of personal responsibility for their health.

When?

I do not believe that one particular age for transition can be set for all adolescents with a chronic illness, as the timing must depend on the developmental readiness of the individual adolescent. The timing should also take into account young adults with learning difficulties who may require additional support to be in place before the transition process can begin. The most important point about the timing of transition is the need for flexibility.

Transition should not occur before the young person is able to function in an adult clinic—that is, they should have the necessary skills and education to enable them to largely manage their illness independently of their parents and healthcare staff.[1] In order to achieve this, preparation for the transition process should begin many years before the anticipated time, preferably in early adolescence. A series of educational sessions should include discussions on understanding their illness, the treatment rationale, the source of symptoms, recognising deterioration and taking appropriate action and most importantly, how to seek help from health professionals.[1]

See Box 4.2 for common factors that often precede a decision to transfer to adult services.

Planning for transition

Improving transition needs time, resources and commitment,[3] but these are small compared to what is invested in each young person throughout their childhood.[1] Therefore it makes sense to ensure that this investment is not wasted due to poor transition.

The following issues should be considered when planning for transition services:[1,3]

- Address professional and managerial attitudes;
- Recognise the differing perspectives of paediatricians, physicians and GPs;

Box 4.2

Common precipitants for transfer[1,15]

- Leaving school
- Pregnancy
- Embarrassment at attending a paediatric clinic
- Patient refusal to attend paediatric clinic
- Suicide attempt
- Drop out of healthcare system
- Non-adherence to treatment

Threatening an adolescent with transfer to adult services should not be used as a form of punishment for non-compliance.

- Establish a dialogue between clinicians, management and commissioners and other agencies;
- Appropriate environment;
- Consultation with users;
- Agree a policy on timing of transfer;
- Set up a preparation period and education programme for the young person and parents;
- Identify interested and capable adult services;
- Identify a coordinator;
- Consider information transfer;
- Monitoring and 'fail-safe' mechanisms;
- Ensure primary care involvement; and
- Administrative support.

Barriers to transition

There are many barriers to a successful transition to adult services and these may deter adolescents, their families and doctors from the whole process. It is important to recognise these barriers and then try to work around these issues.

- One barrier to effective transition is the reluctance of some paediatric professionals to 'let go' and trust either the independence of the adolescent or the skills of the adult services; and parents may be reluctant to let go for the very same reasons.[15]
- Another barrier to transition may arise from the adolescents themselves, their parents and from the receiving adult services.[1] There is little incentive for adolescents to leave a paediatric service that has served them well for many years. Moving to adult services may also be seen as a step closer to disease complications and even death, particularly in cystic fibrosis and diabetes.[1,15]
- Adult services themselves frequently present obstacles to successful transition. This is because adult physicians may have little interest in 'paediatric' diseases in adult life.[1,15]
- One of the biggest barriers is the complete lack of an adult specialist in the locality: for example, though paediatric services for cystic fibrosis are well provided, most districts in the UK do not offer a service for adults and some patients must travel long distances to regional centres which could be a major deterrent.[15] Another example is that of inherited metabolic

Box 4.3

Connexions

Connexions is the advice and guidance service for young people aged 13–19 years and is available to young people with learning difficulties and disabilities up to the age of 25 in the UK. It provides support to all young people with additional needs during their transitions to adulthood. Young people with disabilities or long-term conditions may have a statement of special educational needs (SEN) and Connexions can help with the transition plan for young people with SEN which begins in Year 9 of schooling, around the age of 14.[3]

diseases, where a service for adults is not yet available in all regions of the country.

- Structural hospital problems may be equally important deterrents to transition, as few hospitals have well established and reliable communication channels for transfer of medical records and imaging results.[1]
- The adolescent may feel scared of transferring and may fear the unknown of the adult clinic. Their fears can be overcome by encouraging the adolescent to visit the adult hospital before their first appointment, perhaps with a trusted health professional from the paediatric environment, such as a clinical nurse specialist.
- A multiagency approach for a range of young people with special needs/learning difficulties/disabilities should be the core of the transition process for this group of young people. Connexions can offer advice and guidance for this specific group—see Box 4.3.

Models of transition

The most prevalent model for a transition service is not transition at all but rather a transfer of young people to what looks like the most relevant adult clinic. Or worse still, discharge from the children's clinic with instructions for the GP to refer to adult services.[3]

Models for transition such as disease-based programmes and other more generic programmes where transition is coordinated by generalists such as adolescent physicians or general practitioners have been suggested.[1] However, the value of different programmes and their suitability for different patient and disease groups has also not been shown conclusively.[1]

The models include:

1. Follow-up service

A dedicated follow-up service is provided within the adult setting without a combined paediatric–adult clinic and with no direct input or continuity from paediatric services.[3] This is the simplest model but in order for it to work well, there needs to be good communication between the adult and paediatric teams including nurse specialists taking young adults to clinics and meetings between adult and paediatric clinical staff.

2. A 'seamless' clinic

This model begins in childhood or adolescence and continues into adulthood, with both child and adult professionals providing ongoing care as appropriate.[17] This is a joint approach which allows patients to benefit from both experts in paediatric diseases and the appropriate management of fertility, cardiovascular health, psychological disorders and other 'adult' problems. It also allows both paediatric and adult specialists to continue learning from each other and the patient's experiences. The duration of joint care will vary depending on the specialities.[3]

3. Life-long follow-up in paediatric setting

This approach ensures continuity of care and may sometimes be appropriate in conditions with limited life expectancy. However, it may also make it more difficult for the young person to access expertise on contraceptive and fertility problems, for example, or on vocational and benefit issues and to develop more appropriate independent living alongside their peers.[3]

4. Generic 'transition team' within a children's hospital

This approach involves having 1–2 dedicated nurse specialists who have the expertise to ensure that all young people in different specialities go through appropriate transitions.[3] The coordinating team could also have a role to play in ensuring young people have the necessary skills to function in the adult environment.[1] An example of this model was developed at the British Columbia Children's Hospital, Vancouver, Canada.

5. Generic 'transition coordinators'

This model involves large geographical regions and may be appropriate for conditions which are relatively rare or for coordinating links between Children's Hospitals and local General Hospitals. The Department of Health in New South Wales, Australia, has recently developed such a model.[5]

6. Disease-based programmes

The greatest experience with transition comes from specific disease programmes, which have been developed where strong adult services exist, most notably in diabetes and renal disease.[18–20] More recently, the increasing survival of childhood chronic illnesses has led to the growth of adult services in cystic fibrosis and congenital heart disease with the consequent development of new transition programmes.[9,10]

This type of model offers the advantage of being able to individualise the transition to the particular needs of the speciality patients.[1] For example, it may not be appropriate to transfer an adolescent to a general diabetes clinic as there are many elderly, sick patients often with complications such as amputations, renal disease and cardiovascular disease. In this situation a 'young adult diabetic clinic' may be a more appropriate environment as a preliminary to the full adult clinic.[21] However, in contrast, adult cystic fibrosis clinics consist mainly of younger adults and intermediary clinics may not be useful in this speciality.[1]

Unmet training and education needs

A lot of research about transitional care has been conducted in the speciality of juvenile idiopathic arthritis (JIA). The British Paediatric Rheumatology Group conducted a postal survey to identify the transitional needs of adolescents with JIA from the perspectives of professionals involved in their care.[22] They found that the specific areas of training need were:

- Mental health issues;
- Sexual health issues;
- Vocational issues;
- Multidisciplinary and interagency working; and
- Communication skills.

In summary, a variety of unmet education and training needs of healthcare professionals was identified in this study of transitional care. There is now a need to provide an educational programme aimed at imparting the core knowledge and skills required by all health professionals to provide developmentally appropriate transitional services for adolescents.[22] An example of an innovative programme is the European Teaching in Effective Adolescent Care and Health initiative (http://www.euteach.com).

Summary

- Transitional care requires careful, coordinated and planned consideration;
- Communication is key when working with adolescents—make sure your consultation skills are appropriate to the age and developmental stage of the individual adolescent;
- Transition to adult services has been shown to improve patient quality of life but beware of possible resistance from the adolescent, their family and paediatric health professionals;
- There is no 'one size fits all' approach as to when is the correct time to transfer to adult services—be flexible in your approach and work with the individual adolescent and their family;
- Start planning for the transition long before you plan to 'hand over' your patient—most of the literature suggests the age of 14 to begin discussing the process;
- Be aware of the many barriers to transition;
- Consider the different models of transition and adapt the one most appropriate for your speciality and setting; and
- Consider the training needs of the adult healthcare staff and try to work with them to ensure a successful transition for the adolescent and their family.

References

1. Viner R. Transition from paediatric to adult care: bridging the gaps or passing the buck? *Arch Dis Child.* 1999;81: 271–275.
2. Rettig P, Athreya BH. Adolescents with chronic disease. Transition to adult health care. *Arthritis Care Res.* 1991;4(4):174–180.
3. National Service Framework for Children, Young People and Maternity Services. *Transition: Getting it Right for Young People. Improving the transition of young people with long term conditions from children's to adult health services.* UK: Department of Health; 2006.
4. Blum RWM, Garrell D, Hodgman CH, Slap GB. Transition from child-centred to adult health-care systems for adolescents with chronic conditions: a position paper of the Society for Adolescent Medicine. *J Adolesc Health.* 1993;14:570–576.
5. Bennett DL, Towns SJ, Steinbeck KS. Smoothing the transition to adult care. *Med J Aust.* 2005;182(8):373–374.
6. Blum RWM, Britto M, Sawyer SM, Siegel DM. Transition to adult health care for adolescents and young adults with chronic conditions: position paper of the Society for Adolescent Medicine. *J Adolesc Health.* 2003;33: 309–311.
7. National Service Framework for Children, Young People and Maternity Services. UK: Department of Health; 2004.
8. Christie D, Viner RM. ABC of adolescence. Adolescent development. *Br Med J.* 2005;330:301–304.
9. Somerville J. Near misses and disasters in the treatment of grown-up congenital heart patients. *J R Soc Med.* 1997;90:124–127.
10. Nasr S, Campbell C, Howatt W. Transition program from pediatric to adult care for cystic fibrosis patients. *J Adolesc Health.* 1992;13:682–685.
11. Cappelli M, McGrath P, Heick C, MacDonald N, Feldman W, Rowe P. Chronic disease and its impact. *J Adolesc Health Care.* 1989;10: 283–288.
12. Salmi J, Huupponen T, Oksa H, Oksala H, Koivula T, Raita P. Metabolic control in adolescent insulin-dependent diabetics referred from pediatric to adult clinic. *Ann Clin Res.* 1986;18:84–87.
13. Sawyer SM. Transition to adult health care. In: Werther G, Court J, eds. *Diabetes and the Adolescent.* Melbourne: Miranova; 1998:255–268.
14. Kipps S, Bahu T, Ong K, et al. Current methods of transfer of young people with Type 1 diabetes to adult services. *Diabet Med.* 2002;19:649–654.
15. McDonagh JE, Viner RM. Lost in transition? Between paediatric and adult services. *Br Med J.* 2006;332: 435–436.
16. David TJ. Transition from the paediatric clinic to the adult service. *J R Soc Med.* 2001;94(8):373–374.
17. Tucker LB, Cabral DA. Transition of the adolescent patient with rheumatic disease: issues to consider. *Paediatr Clin N Am.* 2005;52: 641–652.
18. Court J. Issues of transition to adult care. *J Paediatr Child Health.* 1993;29(suppl 1):53–55.
19. Cameron J. The continued care of pediatric patients with renal disease into adult life. *Am J Kidney Dis.* 1985;6:91–95.
20. Watson AR, Shooter M. Transitioning adolescents from pediatric to adult dialysis units. *Adv Perit Dial.* 1996;12:176–178.
21. *Bridging the Gaps: Health Care for Adolescents.* London: RCPCH; 2003.
22. McDonagh JE, Southwood TR, Shaw KL, on behalf of the British Paediatric Rheumatology Group. Unmet education and training needs of rheumatology health professionals in adolescent health and transitional care. *Rheumatology.* 2004;43(6): 737–743.

PART 2

Evidence based care

The control of food intake and absorption of nutrients

5

Anne Payne

LEARNING OBJECTIVES

By the end of this chapter, the reader will be able to:

- Explain both the hormonal and neural control of appetite and food intake;
- Define the role of the stomach, small intestine and colon in the absorption of food and fluids;
- Describe the process for the absorption of fat, protein, carbohydrate, key micronutrients and fluid at the mucosal membrane; and
- Identify immunological cells that confer protection in the gut.

Introduction

The gastrointestinal tract is not a single entity but a system of highly specialist organs working in synergy to enable maintenance of energy balance, nutritional status and physical function. It's associated immunological and microbiological activity support maintenance of gut health and homeostasis. This chapter will briefly review the process of food intake and nutrient absorption and is intended to link with subsequent chapters to explain and contextualise, for example, drug-nutrient interactions, the complications of enteral and parenteral nutrition, the causes and consequences of symptoms of irritable bowel disease and colorectal cancer and the consequence of surgical intervention in short bowel syndrome.

Overview of the control of food intake

Intake of food is a bio-behavioural response controlled by hunger, the taste and smell of food and psychological effects. Longer-term appetite regulation may be influenced by hormones such as insulin and leptin and governed by the size of adipose stores. Shorter-term regulation and the duration of meals may be influenced by numerous gastrointestinal peptides such as cholecystokinin (CCK), peptide YY, ghrelin and glucagon-like peptide 1 secreted in repose to nutrient stimulation/inhibition. Integration of these systems at the level of the hypothalamus can then control the release of various neuropeptides influencing appetite regulation. When food is eaten it is ground to a paste in the mouth, mixed with saliva secreted by the salivary glands and then swallowed by reflex action into the oesophagus from where it is passed rapidly by peristaltic motion into the stomach. Saliva contains mucins to lubricate food and salivary amylase to initiate starch digestion. The process of swallowing food is achieved by the musculature of the tongue, pharynx and oesophagus. Difficulty in swallowing, known as dysphagia, is further discussed in Chapter 20, Management of Stroke.

The structure of the GI tract is shown in Figure 5.1.

The stomach

In the stomach food is mixed with gastric juice and further churned into a bolus termed chyme. The stomach is a highly acidic environment, with a typical pH of 3.0 due to the secretion of hydrogen ions (H^+) by the parietal cells of the stomach. The rate of secretion of H^+ and thus acidity of the stomach is related to both the oral stage of food intake and distension of the stomach by food, with pH decreasing after a meal. The oral stage stimulates the vagus

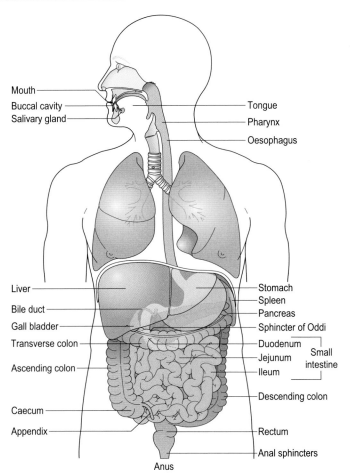

Figure 5.1 • The gastrointestinal tract. From Clancy J and McVicar AJ (eds) *Physiology and Anatomy: A Homeostatic Approach*, 2nd edn. London: Arnold, 2002: 236, Fig 10.2.

Labels in figure: Mouth; Buccal cavity; Salivary gland; Tongue; Pharynx; Oesophagus; Liver; Stomach; Spleen; Pancreas; Bile duct; Gall bladder; Sphincter of Oddi; Transverse colon; Duodenum; Jejunum; Ileum; Small intestine; Ascending colon; Descending colon; Caecum; Appendix; Rectum; Anal sphincters; Anus

nerve to produce acetylcholine and histamine to activate secretion of H^+. Distension of the stomach also activates secretion of H^+ via the release of the hormone gastrin from G cells in pyloric glands.

The resultant hydrochloric acid produced in the stomach has several actions. It converts inactive pepsinogens, secreted by the chief cells of the gastric glands, into active pepsin enzymes to commence the digestion of protein. It also has a front line role in protection from ingested pathogens as it kills the majority of ingested micro-organisms. Protection of the stomach from its acidic content is achieved by secretion of an alkaline mucus gel, known as the gastric mucosal barrier, onto the surface of the mucosa by gastric epithelial cells. A key function of the stomach is the synthesis and secretion of intrinsic factor by the parietal cells in the lower region of the stomach wall, essential for the subsequent absorption of vitamin B_{12} in the ileum of the small intestine. Surgical bypass of the lower stomach due to either stomach carcinoma

or bariatric treatment for obesity may require intramuscular vitamin B_{12} therapy to avoid the development of symptoms of pernicious anaemia.

The rate of release of the stomach contents into the duodenum is influenced by the volume of food and fluid taken at a meal and by hormonal and neural feedback mechanisms, including that of CCK. The presence of fatty acids in the distal parts of the small intestine also influences food intake and gastric emptying. For example, fatty acids in the ileum stimulate the release of CCK and peptides to inhibit gastric motility and thus reduce the rate of gastric emptying. CCK also stimulates intestinal motility and the secretion of bile and pancreatic enzymes.

The GI tract is predominantly under parasympathetic neural control by the vagus nerve of the autonomic nervous system. This runs from the oesophagus to the upper portion of the colon and is largely composed of sensory neurons. Gastric activity, pancreatic secretions and gall bladder contraction are all under vagal control by the action of sensory receptors to monitor the distension of the GI tract and to respond to changes in concentration of secretions in the lumen. Neurotransmitters include serotonin, noradrenaline and acetylcholine. When a meal is eaten neurotransmitter feedback contributes to a feeling of fullness and satiety to control food intake.

The small intestine

The small intestine is a long coiled tube of approximately 6–10 m in length, comprising the duodenum (25 cm), jejunum (> 2.5 m) and ileum (> 3.5 m). The inner surface is often described as having a velvety texture as the highly absorptive villi lining the lumen give its surface a similar physical appearance. Figure 5.2 gives a cross-sectional view of the structure of the small intestine. The large surface area of the mucosa and the abundant capilliary network enmeshed within its mucosa and submucosa aid the rapid adsorption of nutrients. The powerful circular and longitudinal musculature of the intestine propels the food bolus along the length of the GI tract, under the influence of hormones such as CCK, stimulated by the vagus nerve.

Bile from the gall bladder is released into the duodenum via the bile duct. The pancreatic duct also joins the small intestine at the duodenum. The pancreas secretes the following enzymes:

- Trypsin, chymotrypsin and carboxypeptidase, released as zymogens prior to activation in the duodenum for the digestion of protein;
- Lipases to promote the digestion of lipid; these include triacyglycerol hydrolase, phospholipase and cholesterol ester hydrolase; and
- Alpha-amylase, secreted in an active form to promote the digestion of starch.

The absorption of protein

The process of protein degradation, commenced in the stomach, is continued in the duodenum. Pancreatic enzymes are released into the duodenum as inactive zymogens prior to activation by the pro-enzyme trypsin, to proteases. Free amino acids and both di- and tripeptides are then actively absorbed into the enterocytes of the villi of the jejunum and ileum.

The absorption of fat and fat soluble vitamins

Bile salts emulsify dietary fats in the duodenum, increasing the rate of lipid digestion by pancreatic lipase into monoglyceride and free fatty acids. Bile salts then bind with monoglyceride, free fatty acids,

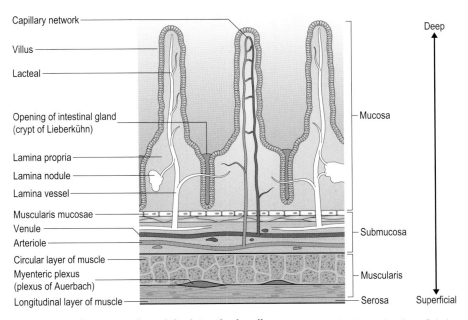

Figure 5.2 • Cross-section of the intestinal wall. The above figure has been taken from: Geissler C and Powers H (eds) *Human Nutrition*, 11th edn. London: Elsevier Churchill Livingstone, 2007: 53.

cholesterol, fat soluble vitamins and phospholipids to form micelles, having a hydrophobic nutrient core. Micelles present this hydrophobic nutrient core to the surface apical membrane of the enterocytes of the jejunum, for absorption.

Within the enterocytes, monoglycerides and free fatty acids are re-esterified into triglyceride and incorporated into lipid droplets coated in lipoprotein, called chylomicrons. These are too large to enter blood capillaries and so chylomicrons diffuse into lacteals, entering the venous circulation in lymph fluid, via the thoracic lymphatic duct.

Bile salts are not directly absorbed at this stage but retained within the lumen of the small intestine and later reabsorbed at the lower portion of the ileum. Normally a small proportion of bile salts are excreted daily in faeces.

Short and medium chain fatty acids (C6–C12), such as MCT oil, are better tolerated by those with bile acid insufficiency or steatorrhoea as they are less hydrophobic than long chain fatty acids and so water soluble. These are readily absorbed into the systemic blood without the aid of bile salts.

The absorption of carbohydrate

Starch is initially hydrolysed by salivary amylase and pancreatic amylases into oligosaccharides and disaccharides. As carbohydrate can only be absorbed as monosaccharides, the brush border of the mucosa secretes the disaccharidase enzymes, lactase, maltase and sucrase, to further hydrolyse carbohydrate to monosaccharides. The absorption of monosaccharide occurs in the upper part of the jejunum, coupled with the uptake of sodium and water, derived partly from intestinal fluids and partly from ingested fluids.

The monosaccharides glucose and galactose compete for active transport across the apical membrane of the enterocyte, aided by the sodium dependant protein transporter SGLT1 and pass across the basal membrane with the aid of a carrier protein GLUT2, for uptake into the capillary network, as outlined in Figure 5.3. A fructose-specific transporter, GLUT5, aids uptake of the monosaccharide fructose. As this is a passive process, when a large dose of fructose is ingested (> 10 g) it may not be completely absorbed, leading to osmotic diarrhoea. Monosaccharides and other water-soluble nutrients pass via the basal membrane of cells into micro-capillaries in the villi and then into the circulatory system via the hepatic portal vein.

The enzyme lactase is produced by mature cells at the tips of villi. Synthesis of lactase and thus absorption of the disaccharide lactose is impaired when the small intestine is inflamed and hence acquired lactose intolerance is an early symptom of mucosal damage. The unabsorbed lactose exerts an osmotic

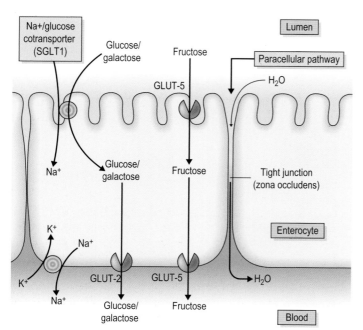

Figure 5.3 • Transport of monosaccharides (glucose, galactose and fructose) across the enterocyte membrane. From: Kumar P and Clark M (eds) *Clinical Medicine*, 6th edn. London: Elsevier Saunders, 2005: 295, Fig 6.21.

effect in the small intestine, inhibiting the absorption of fluid, precipitating diarrhoea. If unabsorbed lactose enters the colon, fermentation by colonic bacteria produces hydrogen gas that can be detected in exhaled breath (hydrogen breath test) and symptoms include abdominal distension, pain and further exacerbation of diarrhoea.

The absorption of minerals

The duodenum is normally the main site of absorption of minerals, such as iron, calcium, zinc and copper. Uptake is by diffusion into enterocytes where they bind with proteins to aid their transfer into the circulation. Chronic inflammation of the upper portion of the small intestine leads to malabsorption of minerals, with symptoms of malnutrition that may have an immediate clinical consequence or be of a subclinical nature with delayed manifestation. For example, microcytic anaemia is an early symptom of malnutrition due to the impaired absorption of iron, whereas osteoporosis develops over many years due to the defective absorption of calcium.

In the surgical treatment of disease, if the duodenum or part of the jejunum is bypassed or removed there are few lasting consequences as the jejunum has an impressive ability to adapt by hypertrophy of the remaining portion to maintain functional homeostasis. However, extensive resection of the ileum causes severe malabsorption that may require artificial nutritional support, as discussed in Chapter 6, Short Bowel Syndrome.

The ileum has a key role to play in the maintenance of gut homeostasis. It is uniquely the site of absorption of vitamin B_{12} and uptake of bile salts for recycling by the liver. If the recycling of bile salts is disrupted by disease or resection of the ileum there are permanent nutritional consequences and their severity depends on the length of the ileum that remains. A failure to reabsorb bile salts in the ileum causes them to be flushed into the colon. This inhibits the absorption of fluid, sodium and potassium from the colon, leading to diarrhoea. A failure to reabsorb bile salts also impacts on the production of bile by the liver, reducing its output of bile and bile salts, leading to a reduction in the absorption of fats and consequently, steatorrhoea (> 6 g fat excreted in the stools daily). Reduced bile acid absorption may be a symptom of Crohn's Disease and other conditions such as coeliac disease, cystic fibrosis and gastroenteritis which cause malabsorption. Medical treatment includes use of the resin cholestyramine to bind bile acids in the colon.

Fluid and nutrient absorption from the colon

From a physiological perspective, the key function of the colon is the absorption of water and the electrolytes sodium and potassium. The colon is also the site of absorption of vitamin K from the remaining food bolus, often referred to as the 'food stream'. Unlike the small intestine, the surface of the colon does not contain villi and so is flat. The distension of the colon by the food stream induces peristaltic propulsion to promote the absorption of water and electrolytes and the evacuation of faeces. The 'normal' rate of passage/transit time of the food stream is 24–48 hours, though highly variable from person to person, with diarrhoea at one extreme and constipation at the other. Both can occur in health and may also be symptomatic of disease. Uptake of water is stimulated by the presence of short chain fatty acids (SCFA) in the colon, derived from the anaerobic degradation of dietary fibre by the microflora of the colon. The main dietary fibre substrate for SCFAs is non-starch polysaccharides and resistant starch fermented by the action of the microflora into a range of SCFAs, including butyrate, acetate and proprionate. The relationship between dietary fibre, transit time and the gut microflora in maintainance of health has been extensively studied over the past 20 years. At present there is considerable interest in the role of prebiotic nutrients, such as fructo-oligosaccharide in the maintenance of GI health and in the efficacy of probiotic microorganisms, such as lactobacilli, in the treatment of disease.

Immune protection in the gut

The warm, moist, nutrient-rich environment of the gut is the perfect host for micro-organisms to thrive. Not surprisingly, the gut has developed an array of innate and adaptive defence mechanisms to protect against pathogens. The small intestine is not normally colonised in the healthy state, unlike the colon where bacteria thrive and perform a vital role as an integral component of gut homeostasis.

Immunocytes within the small intestine include goblet cells, scattered on the surface of villi and immunological cells and tissues embedded within the lamina propria of the mucosa of the GI tract, in the form of lymph nodules, Peyers patches, plasma cells, B cells, T cells and macrophages. These provide a rapid response to antigenic or microbiological invasion, producing antimicrobial peptides and enzymes, such as lysozyme, to protect against bacteria, fungi, viruses and other pathogens. They also assist activation of innate immunity via the secretion of cytokines. For example, immunoglobulin antibodies, secreted by plasma cells into the lumen of the gut, are the first line of defence against antigens. Over 70% of antibodies secreted are immunoglobulin A (IgA) together with IgG and IgM. Their secretion is promoted by the releases of cytokines from T cells and macrophages.

Normally the gut mucosa is able to distinguish between harmless food and foreign protein particles, but when a food protein triggers an immunological response, food hypersensitivity in the form of food allergy may be the outcome, as discussed in the chapter on food allergy and food intolerance. The surface of the mucosa becomes inflamed and malabsorption results. While coeliac disease is known to be the result of an inappropriate immunological reaction to the gliadin component of gluten in wheat, rye and barley, the aetiology of many other conditions of the bowel, such as inflammatory bowel disease (IBD), is yet to be established. It is known that mucosal inflammation is promoted by T lymphocytes in IBD and there are raised levels of lymphocytes and macrophages in the lamina propria.

The nutritional consequence of GI disease

Although most of us rarely experience persistent symptoms of GI upset, beyond those brought about by the occasional bout of gastroenteritis or overindulgence, we are all well familiar with the most common symptoms of GI disease, in the form of nausea, vomiting, diarrhoea and abdominal cramps. Both acute and chronic disease can cause dehydration, weight loss and varying degrees of clinical malnutrition. Whilst the cause of symptoms and hence their nutritional consequences can vary, the universal nature of GI symptoms can render a degree of ambiguity to the underlying pathology of a GI

condition and so incur many weeks or months of tests. For the majority of mild conditions, symptoms resolve within hours or days but in the case of chronic conditions they can wax and wane with a relapsing–remitting pathway and thus prolong diagnosis. Likewise, the onset of malnutrition can be insidious with subclinical nutritional deficiencies developing over a period of months or years and may, as in the case of iron deficiency anaemia, be the presenting symptom of a condition.

The nutritional management of GI disease therefore needs consideration of both the immediate symptoms and long-term consequences with appropriate short- and long-term goals set for patient care. This is further discussed in the chapters on food allergy and food intolerance, inflammatory bowel disease and colorectal cancer, short bowel syndrome, enteral nutrition and parenteral nutrition.

Key points

- Appetite and food intake are controlled by a complex feedback mechanism involving the vagus nerve of the autonomic nervous system and the secretion of hormones such as gastrin, leptin and cholecystokinin by the stomach and small intestine, in response to changes in nutrient concentration in the lumen.

- The stomach prepares food for absorption, creating an acidic chyme that activates pepsin enzymes and inhibits the growth of pathogens. It also releases intrinsic factor to promote the absorption of vitamin B_{12} in the ileum.

- Following degradation of macronutrients by pancreatic enzymes, the large surface area of the small intestine enables the rapid absorption of nutrients, by either passive diffusion or active transport, across the membrane of enterocytes on the surface of the mucosa. While the gut is able to adapt to extensive disease or removal of the duodenum or jejunum, resection of the ileum can cause severe malabsorption.

- The colon is the main site for the absorption of water and electrolytes in the gut. Fluid uptake is stimulated by SCFA such as butyrate, acetate and proprionate, derived from the microbiological degradation of dietary fibre.

- The gut has developed both innate and adaptive defence mechanisms to protect against pathogens. Immunocytes within the small intestine protects against pathogens such as bacteria, viruses and fungi and assist the activation of innate immunity via the secretion of cytokines.

- The common nature of symptoms of GI disease can delay diagnosis. Malnutrition is a frequent consequence of both acute and chronic disease and requires consideration of both short- and long-term goals for effective patient care.

Further reading

Berne RM, Levy MN, Koeppen BM, Stanton BA, eds. *Physiology*. 5th edn. Edinburgh: Elsevier Mosby; 2004.

Calder PC, Field CJ, Gill HS. *Nutrition and Immune Function*. Wallingford: CABI; 2002.

Geissler C, Powers H, eds. *Human Nutrition*. 11th edn. London: Elsevier Churchill Livingstone; 2005.

Kindlen S, ed. *Physiology for Health Care and Nursing*. 2nd edn. Edinburgh: Elsevier Churchill Livingstone; 2003.

Kumar P, Clark M, eds. *Kumar and Clark: Clinical Medicine*. 6th edn. London: Elsevier Saunders; 2005.

Thomas B, Bishop J, eds. *Manual of Dietetic Practice*. 4th edn. Oxford: Blackwell; 2007.

Drug–nutrient interactions

6

Rebecca White

Rebecca White

LEARNING OBJECTIVES

By the end of this chapter the reader will be able to:

- Explain the effect of nutritional status on drug metabolism;
- Demonstrate awareness of the effect of drug therapy on nutritional intake;
- Define drug effects on specific nutrients: vitamins, minerals and macronutrients;
- Discuss nutrient effects on drug therapy;
- Identify drug administration issues in enteral nutrition; and
- Identify patients 'at risk' of drug-nutrient interactions.

Introduction

A drug–nutrient interaction is any interaction between a drug and specific nutritional compound or a drug-induced effect on nutritional intake; these can be both positive and negative in clinical consequence and vary in significance. There are many mechanisms by which these interactions can occur.

Drugs that affect nutrition can be broadly categorised as drugs that affect oral intake, drugs that affect nutrient absorption and drugs that affect nutrient metabolism.

The effect of nutritional status or specific nutrients on drug therapy has been extensively researched and falls into two main categories: the effect of nutritional status on drug metabolism and storage and the effect of nutrient intake on drug metabolism.

Drug metabolism occurs in four steps: absorption, distribution, metabolism and excretion. A drug–nutrient interaction can occur at any stage in this process.

This chapter aims to give clinically relevant examples of drug–nutrient interactions in all these areas.

Effects of nutritional status on drug metabolism

Effects of malnutrition

It has long been known that malnutrition per se reduces the ability to effectively metabolise drugs and increases the incidence of adverse effects.[1]

Malnutrition can significantly affect drug distribution, as a severely malnourished patient will have reduced plasma proteins for drug binding, increasing the free circulating concentrations; an increase in total body water, increasing the volume of distribution of water-soluble drugs; decreased fat stores, decreasing the volume of distribution for fat-soluble drugs; and reduced microsomal enzyme activity and reduced substrates available for metabolism.[2] These factors should be considered, particularly when dosing drugs with narrow therapeutic ranges.

Effects of obesity

Drug metabolism in obesity is a growing research area as the prevalence of obesity increases. Drug disposition in obese individuals is dependent on body composition, where 60–80% of the excess weight may be adipose tissue.[3] However, it is the lean body mass that correlates with total body water, metabolic activity and drug clearance. Therefore loading doses of drugs may be affected by lean body mass, and maintenance doses affected by excess fat mass.

Weight-based dosing is a cause for discussion in obese individuals. However, there are many other aspects of drug dosing that need consideration. There are no data to suggest that intestinal absorption of drugs in this patient group is any different to those with normal body weight. There are also no data relating to transdermal and intralipomatous drug delivery in this patient group.

It should not be assumed that lipophilic drugs will have a larger volume of distribution in obese individuals.[4]

Recommendations on the use of actual body weight and adjusted body weight vary depending on the drug. For example, it is recommended that neuromuscular blocking agents should be dosed on lean body weight; an adjusted body weight plus 40% is recommended for gentamicin dosing,[5] whereas total body weight is recommended for vancomycin dosing.[6] Particular care should be taken when using actual body weight to calculate body surface area for chemotherapy dosing.[7]

Effect of drug therapy on nutritional intake

There are many ways that drug therapy can compromise nutritional intake. Gastrointestinal disturbances are the most commonly reported side effects of drug therapy.[8] These commonly include abdominal discomfort, nausea, vomiting, constipation, diarrhoea, taste disturbances and anorexia, all of which may have an adverse effect on nutritional intake.

There are also circumstances where appropriate use of drug therapy can improve nutritional intake such as the use of steroids as appetite stimulants or prokinetics to aid toleration of enteral nutrition. At the other extreme, drug therapy is also used in the management of obesity.

There are many drugs that have specific dietary guidance relating to dosing. Several antibiotics are recommended to be taken 'on an empty stomach' or 'half an hour before food'; others are recommended 'not to be taken at the same time as milk'. These restrictions are necessary to optimise the oral absorption of these therapies due to a significant drug nutrient interaction. These can reduce oral intake

due to concerns about taking medication on an empty stomach.[8]

The bisphosphonates alendronate and risedronate are required to be taken on waking, half an hour before food, as co-administration with food reduces the absorption to negligible levels.[9] This may affect nutritional intake at breakfast, considered by some to be the most important meal of the day.

Nausea and vomiting

Most drugs are capable of causing nausea or vomiting depending on how and when they are taken. However, there are several classes of drugs with a high incidence of nausea and vomiting, the cytotoxic agents being the most extreme example.

Drugs can cause vomiting through a direct action on the chemoreceptors located in the stomach, jejunum and ileum; these are the same receptors that respond to other toxins. This neuronal pathway leads to the vomit centre, which is where multiple neuronal pathways meet, including those from the chemoreceptor trigger zone (CTZ), higher cortical centres, vagal sensory pathways and the labyrinths (Box 6.1).

Drugs can also act directly on the serotonin and dopamine receptors in the CTZ, the CTZ being outside the blood–brain barrier and therefore can respond to stimuli from both the blood or the cerebrospinal fluid.

The emetic effect of local irritants such as the potassium and iron salts can be minimised when the drugs are taken with food. The emetic effects of other therapies are usually managed with co-prescription of anti-emetic medication.

Box 6.1

Drugs commonly associated with nausea and vomiting

Chemoreceptors in GI tract
- Cytotoxics
- Potassium
- Iron preparations
- Antibiotics

CTZ
- Cytotoxics
- Anaesthetics
- Opiates
- Nicotine
- Levodopa
- SSRI (newer antidepressants e.g. fluoxetine)

Taste disturbances

Altered taste sensation or loss of taste can significantly affect nutritional intake by changing food choice patterns or reducing food intake.

Changes to the sense of taste may be broadly divided into either loss or alteration of taste. Loss of taste may be either incomplete, hypogeusia, or complete, ageusia. Taste alteration, dysgeusia, may occur as aliageusia in which stimuli such as food or drink produce an inappropriate taste or as phantogeusia, sometimes referred to as gustatory hallucination, in which an unpleasant taste is not associated with an external stimulus.

Taste disturbances have many causes including infections, metabolic or nutritional disturbances, radiation, CNS disorders, neoplasms and drug therapy, or may occur as a consequence of normal aging. Management primarily consists of treatment of any underlying disorder. Numerous drugs are associated with taste disturbances, usually described as metallic or bitter; withdrawal of the drug is commonly associated with resolution but occasionally effects persist and may require treatment (Box 6.2).[10]

Effects on gastrointestinal motility

Both a decrease in motility leading to bloating and fullness or an increase in motility causing loose stools or diarrhoea can affect nutritional intake.

Box 6.3a

Drugs associated with reduced intestinal motility

Anticholinergic
- Tricyclic antidepressants e.g. amitriptyline
- Oxybutynin
- Propantheline
- Benzhexol
- Benztropine
- Procyclidine
- Dicyclomine

Opiate
- Morphine
- Codeine
- Ondansetron

Drugs commonly associated with decreased GI motility are the opiates and drugs with anticholinergic activity (Box 6.3a).

Drug therapy can cause diarrhoea by a number of mechanisms. Increasing gut motility, alteration of gut flora or disturbance of the mucosal surface can all result in diarrhoea. A large number of drugs are associated with diarrhoea, which may result in a decrease in oral intake as the patient attempts to minimise this side effect (Box 6.3b).

Box 6.2

Drugs commonly associated with taste disturbance

Fluconazole	Sulphonylureas
Metformin	Terbinafine
Azelastine	Idoxuridine
Zidovudine	Selenium (toxicity)
Zinc (deficiency)	Propafenone
Clindamycin	Levamisole
Zopiclone	Linezolid
Metronidazole	Sodium aurothiomalate
Amiodarone	Amitriptyline
Levodopa and	
combination drugs	Captopril
Losartan	Simvastatin
Sulfasalazine	Griseofulvin
Lithium	Rifampicin
Allopurinol	Penicillamine

Box 6.3b

Drugs associated with diarrhoea
- Prokinetics; erythromycin and metoclopramide
- Antibiotics
- Auranofin (affects 50%)
- Misoprostil (affects 8%)
- Proton pump inhibitors, e.g. lansoprazole (affects 1–3%)
- Antivirals; adefovir, tenofovir, lamivudine
- Magnesium salts
- Iron
- Lithium (sign of toxicity)
- Digoxin (sign of toxicity)
- Acarbose
- Sevelamer
- Metformin
- Colchicine (sign of toxicity)

Box 6.4

Drugs associated with weight gain

Amitriptyline	Chlorpromazine
Clozapine	Olanzapine
Lithium	Valproic acid
Mirtazapine	Beta blockers
Insulin	Oral contraceptives
Oestrogen	Testosterone and derivatives
Anabolic steroids	

 Box 6.5

Drugs associated with anorexia

- Metformin
- Procainamide
- Spironolactone
- Digoxin
- Penicillamine
- Amantadine
- Fluoxetine

Weight gain

Weight gain secondary to drug therapy can be either a desirable or an undesirable outcome.

Psychotropic medication is the most common group associated with clinically significant weight gain; however, there are other commonly used medications which are also associated.

Drugs causing weight gain through stimulation of appetite are used clinically in the management of anorexia and cachexia secondary to cancer and HIV. The corticosteroids remain the most commonly used agents in the UK for appetite stimulation in cancer cachexia.[11] There is increasing evidence for the use of anabolic steroids in HIV-associated cachexia (Box 6.4).[12]

Weight loss

Weight loss secondary to drug therapy is predominantly due to two reasons: loss of appetite, anorexia, leading to reduced nutritional intake, or an increase in the basal metabolic rate.

Anorexia is a commonly reported side effect of many drugs; however, there are a few examples where this is severe enough to be associated with significant weight loss (Box 6.5).

Drug effects on specific nutrients

Drug therapy can affect nutrients at every stage of their metabolism in the same way that nutrients can affect drugs at any point in the metabolic process. Most reports of drug–nutrient interactions relate to absorption. Drugs can cause the malabsorption of nutrients in several different ways. They can bind directly to the nutrient and prevent or reduce its absorption, they can compete for the active transport pathway used by the nutrient or they can reduce absorption through a direct effect on the intestinal mucosa.

Drugs such as the antacids which contain aluminium, magnesium or calcium salts and foods rich in copper, calcium, zinc, magnesium and iron are most often responsible for drug chelation or the formation of insoluble salts, usually preventing the absorption of both drug and nutrient components, e.g. quinolone antibiotics and calcium, cholestyramine and iron.

It is also not surprising that there are distinct interactions between specific nutrients and drug compounds in the metabolic pathway as many drugs owe their pharmacological activity to their interaction with a specific nutrient, such as the dihydrofolate reductase inhibitors, or require vitamin components for their metabolism.

Vitamins

Vitamin A

Vitamin A deficiency leads to visual problems, suppressed immune function, diarrhoea and kidney stones. The mechanism of interaction affecting vitamin A is that of malabsorption (Box 6.6).

 Box 6.6

Drugs associated with vitamin A deficiency

- Ethanol
- Cholestyramine
- Mineral oil
- Neomycin

Thiamine (Vitamin B$_1$)

The co-enzyme thiamine pyrophosphate is essential for decarboxylation and transketolase reactions. Classical signs of thiamine deficiency are lactic acidosis, cardiovascular, cerebral and peripheral neurological impairment. The extent of symptoms that would be seen with subclinical deficiency is uncertain.

There are several studies demonstrating a measurable thiamine deficiency in patients taking furosemide for heart failure.[13,14] Researchers were able to demonstrate an improvement in left ventricular ejection fraction using thiamine supplementation (200 mg daily) in this patient population.[15] However, the direct causal effect of furosemide on thiamine status is not understood and a subsequent study could not confirm earlier findings.[16] At present there is insufficient evidence to recommend routine supplementation of thiamine in this patient population (Box 6.7).[17]

Riboflavin (Vitamin B$_2$)

Riboflavin in its active form is required for the electron transport system, and overt deficiency causes rough scaly skin, angular stomatitis, cheilosis, glossitis and stomatitis. Experimental evidence suggests that drugs such as chlorpromazine, imipramine, amitriptyline and Adriamycin may cause riboflavin depletion.[19] Such drugs could increase the risk of deficiency when the dietary intake is poor (Box 6.8).

Nicotinic acid (Niacin, Vitamin B$_3$)

The precursor of niacin is dietary tryptophan. Niacin is used therapeutically in the management of dyslipidaemias at doses of 1.5–3 g daily. Niacin acts on multiple levels of lipoprotein metabolism, by reducing transport of free fatty acids to the liver and decreasing liver triglyceride synthesis. The adverse effect of excessive niacin is flushing and dyspepsia which is aggravated by coffee or tea; it can also cause hepatotoxicity at high doses.

The important co-factors in oxidation–reduction reactions, NAD and NADP, are formed from nicotinic acid. Pellagra, a syndrome of dermatitis, diarrhoea and dementia, is a result of nicotininc acid deficiency. Pellagra-like symptoms have been associated with isoniazid treatment.[21] This is due to pyridoxine antagonism, inhibiting the conversion of tryptophan to niacin. Nicotininc acid deficiency has also been associated with sodium valproate and glibenclamide therapy (Box 6.9).[22,23]

Pyridoxine (Vitamin B$_6$)

Pyridoxine is part of the co-enzymes pyridoxal phosphate (PLP) and pyridoxamine phosphate (PMP) used in amino acid and lipid metabolism. It is also a co-factor for the conversion of tryptophan to niacin and serotonin and involved in the production of red

Box 6.8

Drugs associated with riboflavine deficiency

- Aminoglycosides
- Doxorubicin[20]
- Cephalosporins
- Fluoroquinolones
- Oral contraceptives
- Phenothiazines
- Sulphonamides
- Tetracyclines

Box 6.7

Drugs associated with thiamine deficiency

- Aminoglycosides
- Cephalosporins
- Digoxin[18]
- Ethanol
- Fluoroquinolones
- Loop diuretics
- Phenytoin
- Sulphonamides
- Tetracyclines

Box 6.9

Drugs associated with nicotinic acid deficiency

- Aminoglycosides
- Cephalosporins
- Fluoroquinolones
- Isoniazid
- Sulphonamides
- Tetracyclines
- Valproic acid
- Pyrazinamide[24]
- Fluorouracil[25]

blood cells. Deficiency leads to anaemia, peripheral neuropathy, dermatitis and a sore tongue.

It is well documented that isoniazid causes clinically significant pyridoxine deficiency leading to peripheral neuropathy; pyridoxine (10 mg daily) is routinely added to antituberculosis therapy on a prophylactic basis.

Pyridoxine metabolism is affected by theophyllines effect on liver enzymes,[26] and pyridoxine deficiency has been reported in patients on theophylline.[27] Attenuation of the side effects of theophylline with pyridoxine therapy has been demonstrated in both animal models and patients (Box 6.10).[28,29]

Vitamin B_{12}

Vitamin B_{12} depletion is associated with a megaloblastic anaemia, cognitive impairment and peripheral neuropathy. B_{12} deficiency is also a causative factor in the development of hyperhomocysteinaemia.

The majority of drugs that affect vitamin B_{12} status do so through their effect on its absorption from the gut. There are data to show that up to 30% of patients taking the antidiabetic metformin malabsorb vitamin B_{12};[30,31] this interaction is also seen with phenformin, and there have been reports of megaloblastic anaemia as a result of this interaction.[32]

The proton pump inhibitor group of drugs, such as omeprazole, and the histamine receptor antagonists, such as ranitidine, reduce the secretion of intrinsic factor and impair the absorption of B_{12} although the extent of this interaction is not yet clear.[33]

Nitrous oxide inactivates B_{12}, causing both neurologic and haematological abnormalities. This interaction is only significant if there is chronic exposure to nitrous oxide. The high doses used in anaesthesia are not considered to have a significant effect if exposure is less than 6 hours (Box 6.11).[34]

Box 6.11

Drugs associated with B_{12} malabsorption
- Aspirin[35]
- Colchicine
- Cholestyramine
- Ethanol
- Trifluoperazine
- Allopurinol
- Methyldopa

Folate

There are a significant number of drugs that interact with folate; indeed many of them owe their therapeutic activity to this drug–nutrient interaction. This group of drugs are the dihydrofolate reductase (DHFR) inhibitors. Drug therapy may also inhibit the reduction of dietary polyglutamate to monoglutamate, thereby preventing its intestinal absorption. Drugs with a significant affect on pyridoxine and B_{12} may also affect folate as both are involved in the demethylation of methylfolate.[36] Drug therapy such as carbamazepine or phenobarbital may accelerate folate metabolism, thereby causing deficiency.[37]

Folate deficiency is easily detected as it has a profound effect on haematological parameters; because of its involvement in DNA synthesis a deficiency is also associated with neural tube defects in the developing foetus.

Treatment of the deficiency state depends on the drug involved. If a therapeutic effect is required from the interaction, as in the case of methotrexate therapy in chemotherapy, then the timing of rescue therapy is critical.

Folate can be administered as folic acid or folinic acid (calcium leucovorin). Folic acid requires conversion and therefore is also subject to the inhibitory effects of the dihydrofolate reductase inhibitors, whereas folinic acid is a derivative of the active metabolite tetrahydrofolic acid and therefore is biologically active even in the presence of these drugs.

Concomitant folinic acid therapy can be used to prevent the deficiency-induced side effects of pyrimethamine and trimethoprim without affecting the therapeutic efficacy of the drug on the bacterial cells as they cannot utilise this form of folate.

In the case of sulphasalazine the induced folate deficiency and resultant macrocytic anaemia respond better to folinic acid than folic acid.[38]

Box 6.10

Drugs associated with pyridoxine deficiency or increased requirements

Aminoglycosides	Cephalosporins
Oestrogen	Ethanol
Fluoroquinolones	Hydralazine
Isoniazid	Loop diuretics
Oral contraceptives	Penicillamine
Phenelzine	Phenytoin
Sulphonamides	Tetracyclines
Theophylline[26,27]	

Box 6.12

Drugs associated with folate deficiency

DHFR inhibitors	Impaired absorption or utilisation
• Methotrexate	• Alcohol
• Trimetrexate	• Carbamazepine
• Pentamidine	• Metformin
• Proguanil	• Nitrofurantoin
• Pyrimethamine	• OCP
• Trimethoprim	• Phenobarbitone
• Triamterene[40]	• Phenytoin[41]
	• Primidone
	• Sulphasalazine[38]

The use of supplements to treat anticonvulsant-induced folate deficiency is controversial. If phenytoin and folate therapy is initiated concurrently it overcomes the problem of folate deficiency and the phenytoin levels reach steady state sooner than without supplements (Box 6.12).[39]

Vitamin C

There are limited data to support drug–nutrient interactions resulting in a significant effect on ascorbic acid. Deficiency of ascorbic acid causes scurvy, usually due to dietary deficit, which is now rare.

Reduced concentrations of ascorbate have been observed in women taking oral contraceptives; however, the mechanism is unclear.[42] Low levels have also been found in alcoholics;[43] reduced intake may be a contributing factor.

Vitamin D

As the majority of vitamin D is produced in the skin it is unsurprising that deficiency has been reported in chronic sunscreen users and institutionalised individuals.[44,45]

The anticonvulsants are the most prominant group of drugs with a significant association with vitamin D deficiency, resulting in osteoporosis.[46] It has been suggested that these effects are secondary to effects on hepatic hydroxylation of vitamin D_3 to the active form 1,25-hydroxycholecalciferol.[47]

Cholestyramine has also been associated with vitamin D deficiency and has been associated with an increased risk of osteoporosis.[48,49]

Vitamin E

Vitamin E plays an important role in maintenance of cell membrane integrity. There have been few reports of drug–nutrient interactions involving vitamin E. Cholestyramine appears to reduce vitamin E levels but the clinical significance of this is unknown. It has also been suggested that anticonvulsants may affect vitamin E status, but these claims have not been substantiated.

Vitamin K

Drug–nutrient interactions affecting vitamin K are evident through their effect on prothrombin time and clinical signs such as excessive bruising and bleeding.

Warfarin, and the other coumarins, owe their clinical activity to their effect on the enzymatic reduction of vitamin K. Alterations in the dietary intake of vitamin K can influence the clinical effectiveness of anticoagulant therapy.[50]

Vitamin K_2 is synthesised by gut flora in the colon; therefore broad spectrum antibiotics affecting these bacteria can indirectly cause deficiency and affect clotting time.[51]

Carnitine

Carnitine is a nonprotein amino acid that is present in tissues with high energy requirements such as the skeletal muscle and myocardium. It is also present in large amounts in such tissues as the liver, kidney and adrenal glands. The major function of carnitine is to transport long-chain fatty acids into the mitochondrial matrix for their oxidation. Carnitine deficiency is a recognised side effect of long-term dialysis;[52] signs and symptoms include muscle cramps, weakness and cardiomyopathy.

Sodium valproate is associated with carnitine deficiency, and although it is unclear whether carnitine supplementation is of value in patients receiving valproate, some neurologists consider it justified in selected cases.[53] There is also evidence suggesting that the hepatic injury caused by sodium valproate may be related to the carnitine deficiency;[54] there is also report of treatment of valproate-induced hyperamonaemia using carnitine.[55]

Some cephalosporin and carbapenem antibiotics inhibit the renal tubular resorption of carnitine, although the clinical significance of this is still uncertain.[56,57]

Minerals

Drug–nutrient interactions affecting trace elements are rarely reported due to lack of awareness of clinical signs of isolated trace element deficiency or toxicity and difficulty in measuring and interpreting biochemical tests. Like the vitamins, they are co-factors in many enzymatic processes and therefore it is unsurprising that they may be influenced by drug therapy.

Aluminium

There are no reports of aluminium deficiency in the literature. All associations between drug therapy and aluminium are of toxicity. The symptoms of aluminium toxicity mimic those of Alzheimer's disease and osteoporosis. Aluminium is a recognised contaminant of large volume parenteral preparations,[58] and high levels are seen in dialysis patients and those on parenteral nutrition. Antacid preparations, and those used as phosphate binders in renal patients, are also associated with aluminium toxicity.[59]

Copper

Penicillamine is used clinically in the management of Wilson's disease due to its ability to reduce copper levels by increasing urinary excretion;[60] this accounts for reports of alopecia and loss of taste in patients with rheumatoid arthritis treated with this drug.

Copper deficiency has also been reported in patients taking zinc supplements.[61,62]

Iron

The majority of drugs associated with iron deficiency are those that cause blood loss anaemia. This is a significant side effect of drugs such as the non-steroidal anti-inflammatory drugs and anticoagulants.

There are few reports of iron deficiency induced by drug therapy.

Several drugs sequester iron and are used therapeutically in the management of iron overload in patients who receive repeated transfusions, such as those with thalassaemia or haemophilia. Desferrioxamine is a parenteral therapy, and deferiprone is given orally; both chelate iron and allow it to be excreted in the urine or faeces.

Selenium

Selenium deficiency is rare; symptoms include cardiomyopathy. Sodium valproate reduces plasma selenium levels in patients chronically treated with this drug.[63] Valproate also decreases levels of glutathione peroxidase, a selenium-dependent enzyme, in children experiencing serious adverse reactions to drug therapy.[63,64] Hepatotoxicity and other adverse effects may be related to diminished antioxidant capacity due to depleted selenium and glutathione levels.

Zinc

Thiazide diuretics, steroids, cisplatin and captopril increase the urinary excretion of zinc and may lead to deficiency.[65–68] The taste disturbance reported in patients taking captopril is similar to that reported in zinc deficiency.[69]

The interactions between the trace elements are complex. Excess iron in the diet can decrease zinc absorption,[70,71] as can preparations containing high quantities of aluminium, such as antacids.[72]

Electrolytes

Drug–nutrient interactions with a clinical effect on electrolytes are easily detectable. Plasma and urinary levels are easily monitored.

Calcium

Calcium homeostasis is predominantly controlled by parathyroid function and vitamin D status; however, thyroid function, corticosteroids and growth hormone can also influence the plasma calcium level. These substances exert their effect via the kidney, bone and intestine; however, the kidney plays the predominant role.

Drug-induced hypercalcaemia through oversupplementation is becoming increasingly common as calcium carbonate supplementation is used routinely for the prevention of osteoporosis and as calcium salts are used as phosphate binder in renal disease.[73] Hypercalcaemia is usually asymptomatic at levels below 3.5 mmol/L; diagnosis from clinical symptoms can be difficult as they are insidious and include nausea, vomiting and lethargy (Box 6.13a).

In severe cases hypocalcaemia can cause tetany and cardiac arrest. In most circumstances mild

Box 6.13a

Drugs associated with hypercalcaemia

Increased absorption from intestine

- Milk-alkali syndrome (excessive oral calcium salt intake especially carbonate)
- Vitamin D

Increased mobilisation from bone

- Vitamin A and derivatives
- Vitamin D
- Calcipotriol, tacalcitriol

Decreased renal excretion

- Calcium-channel blockers
- Lithium
- Thiazides
- Tamoxifen
- Theophylline

hypocalcaemia causes tingling of the peripheries. Treatment involves discontinuation of the causative drug and supplementation using oral or, if severe, intravenous calcium (Box 6.13b).

Magnesium

The kidneys are the major organ that controls magnesium homeostasis. Hypermagnesaemia is very rare as the kidneys are capable of excreting excess magnesium rapidly by reducing tubular reabsorption. Despite this, hypermagnesaemia has been reported, rarely, due to the excessive ingestion of antacids containing high levels of magnesium.

Hypomagnesaemia can be induced by several drugs, most through their effect on the kidney.

Box 6.13b

Drugs associated with hypocalcaemia

- Altered vitamin D metabolism
- Alcohol, anticonvulsants
- Decreased bone mobilisation
- Calcitonin, bisphosphonates, mithramycin
- Increased renal excretion
- Loop diuretics, magnesium sulphate
- Complexing of calcium
- Foscarnet, neomycin, phosphate

Box 6.14

Drugs associated with hypomagnesaemia

- Adrenaline
- Salbutamol, terbutaline
- Theophylline
- Diuretics
- Amphotericin[75]
- Gentamicin, tobramycin, amikacin
- Ciclosporin
- Cisplatin
- Foscarnet

The most common cause of transient hypomagnesaemia is ingestion or infusion of glucose, either with or without insulin, as seen in refeeding syndrome.

Diuretics are associated with mild, usually asymptomatic, hypomagnesaemia.

Cisplatin can cause profound hypomagnesaemia;[74] post chemotherapy hydration regimens usually contain magnesium to minimise this effect (Box 6.14).

Phosphate

Drugs can affect plasma phosphate levels by two mechanisms affecting either intracellular and extracellular distribution or renal excretion. The most common cause of hypophosphataemia in hospitalised patients is due to an acute intracellular shift following exogenous glucose infusion; this is usually during initiation of enteral or parenteral nutrition with inadequate phosphate included, or in the acute management of diabetic ketoacidosis.

The increase in glycogenolysis from catecholamines and beta-adrenergic agents contributes to the hypophosphataemia in critically ill patients.[76]

Mild hypophosphataemia is usually transient and does not require replacement therapy. Prolonged or severe hypophosphataemia can be managed with phosphate supplements (Box 6.15).

Potassium

As much as 98% of the total body potassium is intracellular. Drug therapy can affect plasma potassium concentrations by altering the distribution in the cells or affecting renal excretion. Cellular distribution of potassium is controlled by the sodium–potassium pump in the cell membrane.

Box 6.15

Drugs associated with hypophosphataemia

- Theophylline (especially high levels)
- Glucocorticoids (pharmacological doses)
- Acetazolamide
- Paracetamol (in overdose)
- Foscarnet
- Anticonvulsants

Box 6.16b

Drugs associated with hypokalaemia

- Beta-adrenergic agonists
- Insulin
- Diuretics
- Mineralocorticoids
- Penicillins
- Amphotericin

Acute hyperkalaemia due to drug therapy can be due to altered cellular distribution. Chronic hyperkalaemia due to drug therapy is always associated with impaired renal excretion (Box 6.16a).

Drug-induced hypokalaemia can be due to an intracellular shift or due to increased renal excretion. Insulin increases potassium uptake into the cells by stimulating the sodium–potassium pump.

Beta-agonists such as salbutamol and terbutaline, dopamine, dobutamine and theophylline all promote potassium uptake by the liver and muscle.

Non-potassium sparing diuretics cause an increased loss of potassium from the kidney. Hypokalaemia has been demonstrated in up to 25% of patients taking diuretics.[77]

Amphotericin causes hypokalaemia by causing renal tubular acidosis, thereby increasing renal losses.[78] Amiloride is used to reduce the renal losses of potassium during amphotericin treatment (Box 6.16b).

Sodium

Sodium and water balance are linked. Therefore drugs affecting water homeostasis will also affect sodium.

An increase in plasma sodium can be due to an increase in sodium intake or a loss of water. Rapid infusion of hypertonic saline or sodium bicarbonate can cause a transient hypernatraemia, which is prolonged if the kidneys have a reduced excretion as in acute illness or the postoperative phase. Steroids with a mineralocorticoid effect can cause an increase in plasma sodium.

Dehydration due to excessive lactulose or sorbitol ingestion can cause a hyperosmolar hypernatraemia. Excess water can be lost when the kidneys are unable to appropriately concentrate the urine as in the case of diabetes insipidus; this is the mechanism by which lithium and demeclocycline cause hypernatraemia.[79,80]

Hyponatraemia is the most common electrolyte abnormality in hospitalised patients; it can arise from volume depletion (loss of both sodium and water) or from an inability to excrete, as in SIADH. This topic has been recently reviewed.[81]

There are many drugs associated with low plasma sodium. Hyponatraemia is a common side effect of diuretic therapy, the thiazides having the most pronounced effect,[82] an effect which is dose related (Box 6.17).

Box 6.16a

Drugs associated with hyperkalaemia

- Cardiac glycosides
- Beta-blockers
- Angiotensin-converting-enzyme inhibitors
- NSAIDs
- Heparin
- Ciclosporin
- Tacrolimus
- Amiloride
- Spironolactone
- Triamterene
- Trimethoprim

Box 6.17

Drugs associated with hyponatraemia

- Diuretics
- Cisplatin, carboplatin
- Fluoxetine, fluvoxamine, paroxetine
- Carbamazepine, oxcarbazepine
- Phenothiazines, trifluoperazine, thioridazine
- NSAIDs
- Desmopressin
- ACE inhibitors

Carbamazepine is a common cause of hyponatraemia, with a reported incidence of up to 40%, with elderly patients being at most risk.[83]

Treatment of drug induced hyponatraemia involves discontinuation of the causative agent and appropriate treatment of the cause, either fluid restriction or rarely sodium supplementation.

Macronutrients

Drug effects on lipid metabolism

Cholesterol and triglycerides are transported in plasma by combination with phospholipids and apoproteins. Fatty acids are bound to albumin and transported. There are many drugs that can affect lipid metabolism and cholesterol and triglyceride profile. However, the mechanisms by which these changes occur are very poorly understood.

Thiazides and related diuretics cause a transient rise in cholesterol and triglyceride concentrations.[84]

Beta-blockers have a variable effect on lipid profile. Non-cardioselective beta-blockers such as propranolol have adverse effects, resulting in raised serum triglycerides and reduced HDL-C levels.[85] Cardioselective beta-blockers, such as pindolol or acebutolol, or those with both alpha and beta activity, such as labetalol, appear to have no effects on lipid profile.[86] Newer agents such as celiprolol appear to have beneficial effects on lipid profile with a decrease in both cholesterol and triglycerides.[87]

An extensive review of the effect of antihypertensives on lipid profile found calcium channel blockers to have either a neutral or positive effect, prazosin to have a favourable effect, and ACEI to have a predominantly neutral effect although some may have a positive effect.[88]

Corticosteroid therapy is associated with increased levels of cholesterol and triglycerides.[89] Transient hyperlipidaemia has been reported with ciclosporin.[90]

Didanosine has been reported to cause raised triglyceride levels in one-third of patients.[91]

The changes in lipid profile caused by oestrogens and progestogens appear to be clinically unimportant.[92] Lipid profile changes have also been reported for carbamazepine, phenobarbital, valproic acid, phenytoin, ritonavir, itraconazole and ketoconazole.[93–98]

Drug effects on glucose metabolism

Corticosteroids are the group of drugs most commonly associated with hyperglycaemia; they decrease the peripheral utilisation of glucose, promote

---

Box 6.18

Drugs associated with hyperglycaemia

- Alcohol
- Caffeine
- Growth hormone
- Nicotine
- Thiazide diuretics
- Calcium channel blockers
- Ciclosporine
- Tacrolimus
- Sympathomimetic amines
- Theophylline

---

gluconeogenesis and increase the synthesis of glucose. Beta-blockers are also associated with hyperglycaemia due to inhibition of insulin release (Box 6.18).

Diazoxide is used therapeutically due to its ability to induce hyperglycaemia.[99]

Exogenous insulin sources and sulphonylureas are the most common cause of drug-induced hypoglycaemia. Other drugs associated with hypoglycaemia are anabolic steroids, ACEI, calcium channel blockers, tetracycline and warfarin, with varying clinical importance.

Nutrient effects on drug therapy

Drug absorption, distribution, metabolism, and excretion is a complex sequence of enzymatic processes; it is therefore unsurprising that there are so many ways in which specific nutrient components can affect any of these aspects.

Effects of dietary composition

The hepatic mixed-function oxidase enzyme system is the predominant pathway by which drugs are metabolised. A low-protein diet has been demonstrated to reduce the function of this enzyme system,[100,101] and conversely a high protein, low carbohydrate diet has been shown to induce hepatic enzymes and increase the clearance of drugs such as theophylline.[102]

Electrolytes and metals

Electrolytes, particularly the divalent ions such as calcium and magnesium, can affect drug absorption by chelating with the drug. This is most evident in the interactions between medication and milk,

Box 6.19

Drugs whose absorption is reduced by milk or antacids

- Tetracyclines e.g. doxycycline, tetracycline
- Quinolones e.g. ciprofloxacin, levofloxacin
- Ketoconazole[105]

Box 6.20

Oral drugs with increased bioavailability due to grapefruit juice administration

Drugs used in the management of infections

- Albendazole
- Artemether
- Erythromycin
- Halofantrine
- Praziquantil
- Saquinavir

Steroids and hormones

- Methylprednisolone
- Ethinylestradiol

Cholesterol lowering drugs

- Atorvastatin
- Lovastatin
- Simvastatin

Cardiovascular drugs

- Amiodarone
- Carvedilol
- Felodipine
- Nifedipine
- Nimodipine
- Nicardipine
- Nisoldipine
- Nitrendipine
- Verapamil

Drugs used in erectile dysfunction

- Sildenafil
- Tadalafil
- Vardenafil

CNS drugs

- Buspirone
- Carbamazepine
- Diazepam
- Midazolam
- Scopolamine
- Sertraline
- Triazolam

Immunosupressants

- Ciclosporin
- Tacrolimus

iron or indigestion preparations. These interactions are well documented and instructions are routinely included on the drugs that are affected.

In the case of the tetracyclines and quinolones this interaction can be clinically important with a significant reduction in both the peak plasma levels achieved and the total dose absorbed.[103] Even the small amounts of milk added to tea or coffee can be sufficient to significantly reduce the absorption of these drugs (Box 6.19).[104]

Grapefruit juice

CYP3A are a family of drug-metabolising enzymes found predominantly in the apical enterocytes in the small intestine and in the liver. Grapefruit juice contains furanocoumarins and other substances that can inhibit CYP3A; however, this only affects the intestinal CYP3A and therefore drugs administered intravenously are not affected. It is also thought that grapefruit juice may affect intestinal drug transporters such as p-glycoprotein, which may be the mechanism for the interaction with ciclosporin.

The effect of grapefruit juice on drug absorption was first reported in 1989;[106] subsequent research has identified many drugs affected by this interaction.[107,108] The predominant indicator appears to be a moderate to low oral bioavailability, indicating significant pre-systemic metabolism in either the intestine or the liver. There is now a vast amount of literature on this drug–nutrient interaction.

Any form and quantity of grapefruit should be considered sufficient to produce an interaction. As much as 200 ml of grapefruit juice has been shown to produce a clinically significant increase in drug bioavailability,[109] and a high consumption may also affect hepatic enzyme function.[110]

Cisapride and terfenadine have been withdrawn from the market due to the consequence of their interactions with grapefruit juice.[111]

There are several major drug groups affected by this drug–nutrient interaction (Box 6.20).

Cholesterol lowering drugs

The bioavailability of atorvastatin, lovastatin and simvastatin is increased by grapefruit juice. Restricted intake of grapefruit juice is recommended for simvastatin and lovastatin as the increase in absorption can be up to 15-fold.[112,113] The bioavailability of the other drugs in this class, pravastatin, fluvastatin and rosuvastatin, are unaffected by this interaction.[114]

The possible consequences of an increased level of these drugs are diffuse myalgia and elevated creatine phosphokinase and possibly severe rhabdomyolysis (skeletal muscle breakdown) and associated acute renal failure.

Cardiovascular drugs

The bioavailability of the calcium channel blockers felodipine, isradipine, lacidipine, lercanidipine, nifedipine, nimodipine, nicardipine, nisoldipine, and verapamil is increased by grapefruit juice. amlodipine and diltiazem are not affected. The resultant increase in bioavailability may increase risk of hypotension leading to headache, ankle oedema and facial flushing; severe hypotension may cause symptomatic hypotension or myocardial infarction.

Erectile dysfunction

The phosphodiesterase type-5 inhibitors sildenafil, tadalfil and vardenafil are all affected by grapefruit juice. The resultant increase in bioavailability may result in symptomatic hypotension, myocardial infarction or even sudden death; although no reports of such have been published it is recommended to avoid grapefruit juice.

Immunosuppressants

The group with possibly the most serious consequence of this drug–nutrient interaction are the immunosuppressants ciclosporin and tacrolimus.[115] Grapefruit juice should be avoided by patients on these drugs.

Cranberry

There have been several case reports published suggesting a possible interaction between cranberry and warfarin resulting in an increased INR;[116,117] however, neither a RCT or a pharmacokinetic study has been able to reproduce or elicit a mechanism to explain these case reports.[118,119] Until further information is available a cautious restriction on the intake of cranberry juice is still advocated in patients on warfarin therapy.

Pomegranate juice

The possible mechanism and effect of pomegranate juice on drug metabolism is the subject of current research. It is possible that it affects another of the CYP enzyme family, CYP2C9.[120] This enzyme is also inhibited by the drug fluconazole; it is possible that drugs affected by fluconazole may also be affected by pomegranate juice.

Tyramine

The mono-amine oxidase (MAO) inhibitors are predominantly used in refractory depression. Due to their side effect profile their use has been largely superseded by newer agents. However, there is still significant use in elderly patients and those with severe depression. The MAO inhibitors are phenelzine, tranylcypromine, and isocarboxazid; these inhibit both MAO-A and MAO-B.

The side effects experienced by patients on these medications who ingest tyramine-containing food is a consequence of inhibition of MAO-A. MAO-A is the enzyme responsible for metabolism of noradrenaline and serotonin, located in peripheral adrenergic neurons. When tyramine, a phenylethylamine, is ingested orally it is normally deaminated by the mono-amine oxidases in the intestine and liver. Inhibition of MAO prevents this deamination and allows systemic absorption of the phenylethylamines and subsequent displacement of noradrenaline from storage vesicles in the nervous system. This results in severe headaches, hypertension and an irregular heartbeat.

There are several other drugs that also have some MAO-inhibiting activity. Moclobamide is referred to as a reversible inhibitor; it affects predominantly MAO-B. Linezolid, a new antibiotic being increasingly used for the treatment of MRSA, has a dietary tyramine response similar to that of moclobemide.[121,122] Selegiline is used in the management of Parkinson's disease. It does not cause a response to tyramine at the doses used for Parkinson's; however, doses above 20 mg will elicit a pressor effect from oral tyramine.[123] A new preparation licensed in the USA uses a transdermal delivery system which avoids the effect on intestinal MAO; however, dietary restrictions are still recommended for the higher doses.[124]

Procarbazine, used in the management of Hodgkin's lymphoma,[125] and isoniazid, used for treatment of TB, are both weak MAO inhibitors and dietary restriction is not considered necessary.[126]

In clinical practice only foods with a high tyramine content should be restricted; all other foods are considered safe in moderation.[127]

Drug administration issues in enteral nutrition

There is significant potential for interaction between drug therapy and enteral nutrition, particularly when administration is simultaneous via the same device. There are two types of interaction, the physical interaction that results in the alteration of the consistency of the enteral feed, and the chemical interaction between the drug and the nutritional components of the feed.

Physical interactions

These interactions are due to a physical interaction between the drug and a component of the feed or the feed formulation itself. They result in a physical change in the consistency of the feed and can result in enteral feeding tube blockage or in extreme cases physical obstruction of the GI tract.[128] These concretions, called bezoars, have been reported with sucralfate where the aluminium in the sucralfate binds to the protein in the enteral feed.

Most enteral feeds are stabilised emulsions; therefore anything that destabilises the emulsion will affect the consistency of the feed. Medication formulations with extremely high or low pH or with high electrolyte content can decrease the stability of the emulsion and cause flocculation.

Reduced absorption with enteral feed

There are reported interactions between many drugs and individual components of the diet, for example elements such as calcium and iron, which bind to the drug and change its molecular size or solubility and thereby reduce absorption.

Tetracyclines readily chelate with divalent and trivalent metal cations such as calcium, magnesium and iron—these are present in higher concentrations in enteral feed and milk-based diets than in a normal diet and therefore the potential for interaction is greater. Tetracycline absorption is decreased by 80% by co-administration with feed, whereas for doxycycline the reaction is not considered clinically important.

| Box 6.21 |

Interactions with enteral feed
- Ciprofloxacin
- Tetracycline
- Rifampicin
- Theophylline
- Warfarin
- Phenytoin

Ciprofloxacin absorption is decreased 50% by enteral feed, the reaction with levofloxacin and ofloxacin is less significant, and food does not have any effect on the absorption of moxifloxacin.[129]

The interactions reported with phenytoin and warfarin highlight the potential for a drug to bind to protein in the diet and thereby reduce drug absorption. As yet there are no reports comparing the interaction with whole protein as opposed to amino acid-based feeds (Box 6.21).

Where possible the contact between drug and feed should be minimised. This is achieved through flushing the tube adequately and allowing a break between stopping the feed and giving the drug and then restarting the feed. Close communication between all members of the healthcare team is necessary to ensure that the feed and drug regimen can be optimised.

Identification of 'at risk' patients

The effective use of drug therapy underpins modern medicine. Polypharmacy is widespread particularly in the elderly, and the risk of drug–nutrient interactions is compounded by pre-existing nutritional status and chronic illness.[130] It has been proven that there is a direct linear relationship between the number of drugs a patient is taking and the number of drug–nutrient reactions for which the patient is at risk.[131] Those patients with chronic illness and the elderly should be considered high risk for the effects of drug–nutrient interactions and careful monitoring undertaken to identify and treat any deficiencies that develop.

However, a lack of knowledge of drug–nutrient interactions and a lack of awareness of the symptoms of specific deficiencies leads to underreporting of these potentially clinically important interactions.

An accurate record of drug therapy and records of weight, body mass index (BMI) and appetite changes should be maintained in order to identify potential drug–nutrient interactions and facilitate appropriate prevention or early intervention.

Methods of intervention

A clear understanding of the nature and consequence of the interaction between drug and nutrient is necessary before appropriate steps can be taken. A balance of risk and benefit must be undertaken before drug therapy is stopped or changed. Targeted supplementation of specific nutrients may be appropriate in some cases providing that it does not change the therapeutic effect of the drug.

When interactions result from the direct binding of the drug to a nutrient in the gut, simply modifying dosage times may reduce the effect, for example not drinking milk with drugs such as the quinolones or tetracyclines. Clear communication and documentation is required to ensure that all professionals and carers involved in the care of these patients understand the importance of these interventions.

Summary

There are many ways that drug therapy can affect nutritional status and also many ways in which nutrition and specific nutrients can affect the efficacy of drug therapy. Knowledge of drug–nutrient interactions and the consequences of nutrient deficiencies is necessary to identify patients at risk and make appropriate interventions.

As our understanding of the mechanisms of drug absorption increase so does our ability to identify the mechanisms by which drug–nutrient interactions occur. There is increasing interest in p-glycoprotein as a drug transport enzyme and also organic anion transporting polypeptides (OATPs).

All healthcare professionals have a responsibility to optimise patients nutritional status; a knowledge of drug–nutrient interactions will contribute to nutritional care.

Key points

- Drug metabolism occurs in four steps: absorption, distribution, metabolism and excretion. A drug–nutrient interaction can occur at any stage in this process.

- Malnutrition can significantly affect drug distribution, as a severely malnourished patient will have reduced plasma proteins for drug binding, an increase in total body water, decreased fat stores, reduced microsomal enzyme activity and reduced substrates available for metabolism.

- Gastrointestinal disturbances are the most commonly reported side effects of drug therapy. They include abdominal discomfort, nausea, vomiting, constipation, diarrhoea, taste disturbances and anorexia, all of which may have an adverse effect on nutritional intake.

- There are several classes of drugs with a high incidence of nausea and vomiting, the cytotoxic agents being the most extreme example.

- Numerous drugs are associated with taste disturbances, usually described as metallic or bitter; withdrawal of the drug is commonly associated with resolution but occasionally effects persist and may require treatment.

- A large number of drugs are associated with diarrhoea, which may result in a decrease in oral intake as the patient attempts to minimise this side effect.

- Drugs can cause the malabsorption of nutrients by binding directly to the nutrient and prevent or reduce its absorption; they can compete for the active transport pathway used by the nutrient or they can reduce absorption through a direct effect on the intestinal mucosa.

- Drug absorption, distribution, metabolism and excretion is a complex sequence of enzymatic processes. There are so many ways in which specific nutrient components can affect any of these aspects.

- Patients with chronic illness and the elderly should be considered high risk for the effects of drug–nutrient interactions and careful monitoring undertaken to identify and treat any deficiencies that develop.

- A clear understanding of the nature and consequence of the interaction between drug and nutrient is necessary before appropriate steps can be taken. A balance of risk and benefit must be undertaken before drug therapy is stopped or changed.

References

1. Cambell TC, Hayes JR. Role of nutrition in the drug metabolism enzyme system. *Pharmacol Rev.* 1974;26(3):171–197.

2. Krishnaswamy K. Drug metabolism and pharmacokinetics in malnutrition. *Clin Pharmacokinet.* 1978;3:216–240.

3. Forbes GB, Welle SL. Lean body mass in obesity. *Int J Obes.* 1983;7:99–107.

4. Bickel MH. Factors affecting the storage of drugs and other xenobiotics in adipose tissue. *Adv Drug Res.* 1994;25:55–86.

5. Leader WG, Tsubaki T, Chandler MHH. Creatinine-clearance estimates for predicting gentamicin pharmacokinetic values in obese patients. *Am J Hosp Pharm.* 1994;51:2125–2130.

6. Blouin RA, Bauer LA, Miller DD, Record KE, Griffin WO. Vancomycin pharmacokinetics in normal and morbidly obese subjects. *Antimicrob Agents Chemother.* 1982;21:575–580.

7. De Jonge ME, Mathot RAA, Van Dam SM, Beijnen JH, Rodenhuis S. Extremely high exposures in an obese patient receiving high-dose cyclophosphamide, thiotepa and carboplatin. *Cancer Chemother Pharmacol.* 2002;50:251–255.

8. Bateman DN, Aziz EE. Gastrointestinal disorders. In: Davies DM, ed. *Textbook of Adverse Drug Reactions.* 5th edn. London: Lippincott-Raven; 1998:259–274.

9. Fosamax (MSD). Summary of Product Characteristics, 30 March 2009.

10. Henkin RI. Drug-induced taste and smell disorders. Incidence, mechanisms and management related primarily to treatment of sensory receptor dysfunction. *Drug Saf.* 1994;11(5):318–377.

11. Yavuzsen T, Davis MP, Walsh D, LeGrand S, Lagman R. Systematic review of the treatment of cancer-associated anorexia and weight loss. *J Clin Oncol.* 2005;23(33):8500–8511.

12. Mwamburi DM, Gerrior J, Wilson IB, et al. Comparing megestrol acetate therapy with oxandrolone therapy for HIV-related weight loss: similar results in 2 months. *Clin Infect Dis.* 2004;38:895–902.

13. Seligmann H, Halkin H, Rauchfleisch S, et al. Thiamine deficiency in patients with congestive heart failure receiving long-term frusemide therapy. A pilot study. *Am J Med.* 1991;91:151–155.

14. Zenuk C, Healey J, Donnelly J, Vaillancourt R, Almalki Y, Smith S. Thiamine deficiency in congestive heart failure patients receiving long term furosemide therapy. *Can J Clin Pharmacol.* 2003;10(4):184–188.

15. Shimon I, Almog S, Vered Z, et al. Improved left ventricular function after thiamine supplementation in patients with congestive heart failure receiving long-term frusemide therapy. *Am J Med.* 1995;98:485–490.

16. Yue QY, Beermann B, Lindstrom B, Nyquist O. No difference in blood thiamine diphosphate levels between Swedish Caucasian patients with congestive heart failure treated with frusemide and patients without heart failure. *Intern Med.* 1997;242:491–495.

17. Sica DA. Loop diuretic therapy, thiamine balance, and heart failure. *Congest Heart Fail.* 2007;13(4):244–247.

18. Zangen A, Botzer D, Zangen R, Shainberg A. Furosemide and digoxin inhibit thiamine uptake in cardiac cells. *Eur J Pharmacol.* 1998;361(1):151–155.

19. Pinto J, Huang YP, Rivlin RS. Inhibition of riboflavin metabolism in rat tisues by chlorpromazine, imipramine and amitriptyline. *J Clin Invest.* 1981;67:1500.

20. Ogura R, Ueta H, Hino Y, Hidaka T, Sugiyama MJ. Riboflavin deficiency caused by treatment with adriamycin. *J Nutr Sci Vitaminol (Tokyo).* 1991;37(5):473–477.

21. Meyrick TRH, Payne RCM, Black MM. Isoniazid-induced pellagra. *Br Med J.* 1981;ii:278.

22. Gillman MA, Sandyk R. Nicotinic acid deficiency induced by sodium valproate. *S Afr Med J.* 1984;65(25):986.

23. Berova N, Lazarova A. Pellagra-anliche verandertungen nach Glibenklamid-Behandlung bei einer Patient- in mit diabetes mellitus und vitiligo. *Dermatol Monatsschr.* 1988;174(1):50–51.

24. Jørgensen J. Pellagra probably due to pyrazinamide: development during combined chemotherapy of tuberculosis. *Int J Dermatol.* 1983;22:44–45.

25. Stevens HP, Ostlere LS, Begent RH, Dooley JS, Rustin MH. Pellagra secondary to 5-fluorouracil. *Br J Dermatol.* 1993;128(5):578–580.

26. Delport R, Ubbink JB, Serfontein WJ. Vitamin B6 nutritional status in asthma: the effect of theophylline therapy on plasma pyridoxal-5-phosphate and pyridoxal levels. *Int J Vitamin Nutr Res.* 1998; 58:67–72.

27. Shimizu T, Maeda S, Mochizuki H, Tokuyama K, Morikawa A. Theophylline attenuates circulating vitamin B6 levels in children with asthma. *Pharmacology.* 1994;49:392–397.

28. Glenn GM, Krober MS, Kelly P, McCarty J, Weir M. Pyridoxine as therapy in theophylline-induced seizures. *Vet Hum Toxicol.* 1995;37:342–345.

29. Bartel PR, Ubbink JB, Delport R, Lotz BP, Beckjer PJ. Vitamin B6 supplementation and theophylline-related effects in humans. *Am J Clin Nutr.* 1994;60:93–99.

30. Tomkin GH, Hadden DR, Weaver JA, Montgomery DAD. Vitamin B12 status in patients on long term metformin therapy. *Br Med J.* 1971;2:685–687.

31. Adam JF, Clark JS, Ireland JT, Kesson CM, Watson WS. Malabsorption of vitamin B12 and intrinsic factor secretion during biguanide therapy. *Diabetologia.* 1983;24:16–18.

32. Callaghan TS, Hadden DR, Tomkin GH. Megaloblastic anaemia due to vitamin B12 malabsorption associated with long-term metformin treatment. *Br Med J.* 1980;280:1214.

33. Carmel R. Malabsorption of food cobalamin. *Baillieres Clin Haematol.* 1995;8(3):639–655.

34. Weimann J. Toxicity of nitrous oxide. *Best Pract Res Clin Anaesthesiol.* 2003;17(1):47–61.

35. Van Oijen MG, Laheij RJ, Peters WH, Jansen JB, Verheught FW. BACH study, Association of aspirin use with vitamin B12 deficiency (results of BACH study). *Am J Cardiol.* 2004;94(7):975–977.

36. Lee GR. Nutritional factors in the production and function of erythrocytes. In: Lee CR, Bithell TC, Forster J, et al. *Wintrobe's Clinical Haematology.* Philadelphia: Lea and Febinger; 1993.

37. Kishi T, Fujita N, Eguchi T, Ueda K. Mechanism for reduction of serum folate by antiepileptic drugs during prolonged therapy. *J Neurol Sci.* 1997;145(1):109–112.

38. Pironi L, Cornia GL, Ursitti MA, et al. Evaluation of oral administration of folic acid and folinic acid to prevent folate deficiency in patients with inflammatory bowel disease treated with salicylazosulfapyridine. *Int J Clin Pharmacol Res.* 1988;8(2):143–148.

39. Lewis DP, Van Dyke DC, Willhite LA, Stumbo PJ, Berg MJ. Phenytoin-folic acid interaction. *Ann Pharmacother.* 1995;29:309–315.

40. McInnes GT. Diuretics. In: Dukes MNG, ed. *Myler's Side Effects of Drugs.* Amsterdam: Elsevier; 1996.

41. Carl GF, Smith ML. Phenytoin-folate interactions. Differing effects of the sodium salt and free acid of phenytoin. *Epilepsia.* 1992;33: 372–375.

42. Tyrer LB. Nutrition and the pill. *J Reprod Med.* 1984;29(7 suppl): 547–550.

43. Wood B, Nicholls KM, Breen KJ. Nutritional status in alcoholism. *J Hum Nutr Diet.* 1992;5:275.

44. Matsouka LY, Wortsman J, Hanifan N, Holick MF. Chronic sunscreen use decreases circulating concentrations of 25-hydroxy-vitamin D. A preliminary study. *Arch Dermatol.* 1998;124:1802.

45. Malik R. Vitamin D and secondary hyperparathyroidism in the institutionalized elderly: a literature review. *J Nutr Elder.* 2007;26(3–4): 119–138.

46. El-Hajj Fuleihan G, Dib L, Yamout B, Sawaya R, Mikati MA. Predictors of bone density in ambulatory patients on antiepileptic drugs. *Bone.* 2008;43(1):149–155.

47. Hosseinpour F, Ellfolk M, Norlin M, Wikvall K. Phenobarbital suppresses vitamin D3 25-hydroxylase expression: a potential new mechanism for drug-induced osteomalacia. *Biochem Biophys Res Commun.* 2007;357(3):603–607.

48. Tonstad S, Knudtzon J, Sivertsen M, Refsum H, Ose L. Efficacy and safety of cholestyramine therapy in peripubertal and prepubertal children with familial hypercholesterolemia. *J Pediatr.* 1996;129(1):42–49.

49. Heaney RP. Nutritional factors in bone health in osteoporosis. In: Riggs Bl, Melton LJ, eds. *Aetiology, Diagnosis and Management.* New York: Raven Press; 1998.

50. Harris JE. Interaction of dietary factors with oral anticoagulants. *Rev Applications J Am Dietetic Ass.* 1995;95:580–584.

51. Williams KJ, Bax RP, Brown H, Mackin SJ. Antibiotic treatment and associated prolonged prothrombin time. *J Clin Pathol.* 1991;44:738.

52. Bertoli M, Battistella PA, Vergani L, et al. Carnitine deficinency induced during hemodialysis and hyperlipidemia: Effect of replacement therapy. *Am J Clin Nutr.* 1981;34(8):1496–1500.

53. De Vivo DC, Bohan TP, Coulter DL, et al. L-Carnitine supplementation in childhood epilepsy: current perspectives. *Epilepsia.* 1998;39:1216–1225.

54. Melegh B, Trombitas K. Valproate treatment induces lipid globule accumulation with ultrastructural abnormalities of mitochondria in skeletal muscle. *Neuropediatrics.* 1997;28:257–261.

55. Altunbasak S, Baytok V, Tasouji M, Herguner O, Burgut R, Kayrin L. Asymptomatic hyperamonaemia in children treated with valproic acid. *J Child Neurol.* 1997;12: 461–463.

56. Arrigoni-Martelli E, Caso V. Carnitine protects mitochondria and removes toxic acyls from xenobiotics. *Drugs Exp Clin Res.* 2001;27(1):27–49.

57. Ganapathy ME, Huang W, Rajan DP, et al. Beta-lactam antibiotics as substrates for OCTN2, an organic cation/carnitine transporter. *J Biol Chem.* 2000;275(3):1699–1707.

58. Klein GL. Aluminium in parenteral solutions revisited—again. *Am J Clin Nutr.* 1995;61(3):449–456.

59. Ittel TH, Gladziwa U, Muck W, Sieberth HG. Hyperaluminaemia in critically ill patients: role of antacid therapy and impaired renal function. *Eur J Clin Invest.* 1991;21(1): 96–102.

60. Milanino R, Frigo A, Bambara LM, et al. Copper and zinc status in rheumatoid arthritis—studies of plasma, erythrocytes, and urine, and their relationship to disease-activity markers and pharmacological treatment. *Clin Exp Rheumatol.* 1993;11(3):271–281.

61. Fiske DN, McCoy HE, Kitchens CS. Zinc-induced sideroblastic anemia: report of a case, review of the literature, and description of the hematologic syndrome. *Am J Hematol.* 1994;46:147.

62. O'Dell BL. Mineral interactions relevant to nutrient requirements. *J Nutr.* 1989;119:1832–1838.

63. Hurd RW, Van Rinsvelt HA, Wilder RJ, Karas B, Maenhaut W, De Reu L. Selenium, zinc, and copper changes with valproic acid: possible relation to drug side effects. *Neurology.* 1984;34(10): 1393–1395.

64. Graf WD, Oleinik OE, Glauser TA, Maertens P, Eder DN, Pippenger CE. Altered antioxidant enzyme activities in children with a serious adverse experience related to valproic acid therapy. *Neuropediatrics.* 1998;29(4):195–201.

65. Wester PO. Zinc during diuretic treatment. *Lancet.* 1975;I:578.

66. Peretz A, Nere T, Famaly IP. Effects of chronic and acute corticosteroid therapy on zinc and copper status in rheumatoid arthritis patients. *J Trace Elem Electrolytes Health Dis.* 1989;3:103.

67. Sweeney JD, Ziegler P, Pruet C, Spaulding MB. Hyperzincuria and hypozincemia in patients treated with cisplatin. *Cancer.* 1989; 2093:63.

68. Peczkowska M, Kabat M, Janaszek-Sitkowska H, Mirocha M, Pulawska M, Sznajderman M. Zinc metabolism in essential hypertension and during angiotensin-converting enzyme inhibitor therapy—preliminary report. *J Trace Elem Electrolytes Health Dis.* 1997;14:82.

69. Ackerman BH, Kasbekar N. Disturbances of taste and smell induced by drugs. *Pharmacotherapy.* 1997;17:482.

70. Solomons NW. Competitive interaction of iron and zinc in the diet. Consequences for human nutrition. *J Nutr.* 1986;116:927–935.

71. Taylor A. Detection and monitoring of disorders of essential trace elements. *Ann Clin Biochem.* 1996;33:486.

72. Abu-Hamdan DK, Mahajan SK, Migdal SD, Prasad AS, McDonald FD. Zinc tolerance test in uremia. Effect of ferrous sulphate and aluminium hydroxide. *Ann Intern Med.* 1986;104:50.

73. Shek CC, Natkunam A, Tsang V, Cockram CS, Swaminathan R. Incidence, causes and mechanism of hypercalcaemia in a hospital population in Hong Kong. *Q J Med.* 1990;77(284):1277–1285.

74. Jones DP, Cesney RW. Renal toxicity of cancer chemotherapeutic agents in children: ifosfamide and cisplatin. *Curr Opin Pediatr.* 1995;7:208.

75. Barton CH, Pahl M, Vaziri ND, Cesario T. Renal magnesium wasting associated with amphotericin B therapy. *Am J Med.* 1984;77:471.

76. Brown GR, Greenwood JK. Drug- and nutrition-induced hypophosphatemia: mechanisms and relevance in the critically ill. *Ann Pharmacother.* 1994;28:626.

77. Widmer P, Maibach R, Künzi UP, et al. Diuretic-related hypokalaemia: the role of diuretics, potassium supplements, glucocorticoids and beta 2-adrenoreceptor agonists. Results from the comprehensive hospital drug monitoring programme, Berne (CHDM). *Eur J Clin Pharmacol.* 1995;49:31.

78. DuBose TD, Codina J. H,K-ATPase. *Curr Opin Nephrol Hypertens.* 1996;5(5):411–416.

79. Boton R, Gaviria M, Batlle DC. Prevalence, pathogenesis, and treatment of renal dysfunction associated with chronic lithium therapy. *Am J Kidney Dis.* 1987;10(5):329–345.

80. Robertson JL. Dietary salt and essential hypertension. *Lancet.* 1996;348(9038):690–691.

81. Liamis G, Milionis H, Elisaf M. A review of drug-induced hyponatremia. *Am J Kidney Dis.* 2008;52(1):144–153.

82. Sonnenblick M, Friedlander Y, Rosin AJ. Diuretic-induced severe hyponatremia. Review and analysis of 129 reported patients. *Chest.* 1993;103(2):601–606.

83. Leppik IE. Metabolism of antiepileptic medication: newborn to elderly. *Epilepsia.* 1992;33(suppl 4):S32–S40.

84. Ames RP. The effects of antihypertensive drugs on serum lipids and lipoproteins. I Diuretics. *Drugs.* 1986;32(3):260–278.

85. Lehren P. Comparison of effects on lipid metabolism of antihypertensive drugs with alpha- and beta-adrenergic antagonistic properties. *Am J Med.* 1987;82(suppl 1A):31.

86. Fogari R, Zopi A, Pascotti C, et al. Plasma lipids during chronic antihypertensive therapy with different betablockers. *J Cardiovasc Pharmacol.* 1989;14(suppl 7):S28.

87. Herrmann JH, Bischof F, Von Heymann F, Freischuetz G, Burghagen H. Effects of celiprolol on serum lipids in systemic hypertension. *Am J Cardiol.* 1988;61(5):41C–44C.

88. Ames RP. The effects of antihypertensive drugs on serum lipids and lipoproteins. II. Nondiuretic drugs. *Drugs.* 1986;32:335.

89. Jefferys DB, Lessof MH, Mattock MB. Corticosteroid treatment, serum lipids and coronary artery disease. *Postgrad Med J.* 1980;56:491.

90. *Neoral Summary of Product Characteristics.* Novartis Pharmaceuticals; 2008.

91. Yarchoan R, Pluda JM, Thomas RV, et al. Long-term toxicity/activity profile of 2,3-dideoxyinosine in AIDS or AIDS-related complex. *Lancet.* 1990;336:526–529.

92. Notelovitz M, Feldman EB, Gillespy M. Lipid and lipoprotein changes in women taking low dose triphasic oral contraceptives: a controlled comparative 12-month clinical trial. *Am J Obstet Gynecol.* 1989;160:1269.

93. Chait A, Brunzell JD. Acquired hyperlipidemia. *Endocrinol Metab Clin North Am.* 1990;19(2):259–278.

94. Nikolaos T, Stylianos G, Chryssoula N, et al. The effect of long-term antiepileptic treatment on serum cholesterol (TC, HDL, LDL) and triglyceride levels in adult epileptic patients on monotherapy. *Med Sci Monit.* 2004;10(4):MT50–2.

95. Markowitz M, Saag M, Powderly WG, et al. A preliminary study of ritonavir, an inhibitor of HIV-1 protease, to treat HIV-1 infection. *N Engl J Med.* 1995;333(23):1534–1539.

96. Tucker RM, Haq Y, Denning DW, Stevens DA. Adverse events associated with itraconazole in 189 patients on chronic therapy. *J Antimicrob Chemother.* 1990;26(4):561–566.

97. Rosenblatt HM, Byrne W, Ament ME, Graybill J, Stiehm ER. Successful treatment of chronic mucocutaneous candidiasis with ketoconazole. *J Pediatr.* 1980;97(4):657–660.

98. Rollman O, Jameson S, Lithell H. Effects of long-term ketoconazole therapy on serum lipid levels. *Eur J Clin Pharmacol.* 1985;29(2):241–245.

99. Stanley CA. Hypoglycemia in the neonate. *Pediatr Endocrinol Rev.* 2006;4(suppl 1):76–81.

100. Jung D. Pharmacokinetics of theophylline in protein calorie malnutrition. *Biopharm Drug Dispos.* 1985;6(3):291–299.

101. Krishnaswamy K, Kalamegham R, Naidu NA. Dietary influences on the kinetics of antipyrine and aminopyrine in human subjects. *Br J Clin Pharmacol.* 1984;17(2):139–146.

102. Anderson KE, McCleery RB, Vesell ES, Vickers FF, Kappas A. Diet and cimetidine induce comparable changes in theophylline metabolism in normal subjects. *Hepatology*. 1991;13(5):941–946.

103. Neuvonen PJ, Kivisto KT, Lehto P. Interference of diary products with the absorption of ciprofloxacin. *Clin Pharmacol Ther*. 1991; 50(5 pt 1):498–502.

104. Jung H, Peregrine AA, Rodriguez JM, Moreno-Esparza R. The influence of coffee with milk and tea with milk on the bioavailability of tetracycline. *Biopharm Drug Dispos*. 1997; 18(5):459–463.

105. Sadowski DC. Drug interactions with antacids. Mechanisms and clinical significance. *Drug Saf*. 1994;11(6):395–407.

106. Bailey DG, Spence JD, Edgar B, Bayliff CD, Arnold JMO. Ethanol enhances the haemodynamic effects of felodipine. *Clin Investig Med*. 1989;12:357–362.

107. Bailey DG, Arnold JMO, Spence JD. Grapefruit juice–drug interactions. *Br J Clin Pharmacol*. 1998;46:101–110.

108. Greenblatt DJ, Patki KC, von Moltke LL, Shader RI. Drug interactions with grapefruit juice: an update. *J Clin Psychopharmacol*. 2001;21(4):357–359.

109. Edgar B, Bailey DG, Bergstrand R, Johnsson G, Regardh CG. Acute effects of drinking grapefruit juice on the pharmacokinetics and pharmacodynamics of felodipine— and its potential clinical relevance. *Eur J Clin Pharmacol*. 1992;42: 313–317.

110. Lilja JJ, Kivisto KT, Backman JT, Neuvonen PJ. Effect of grapefruit juice dose on grapefruit juice-triazolam interaction: repeated consumption prolongs triazolam half-life. *Eur J Clin Pharmacol*. 2000;56:411–415.

111. Michalets EL, Williams CR. Drug interactions with cisapride; clinical implications. *Clin Pharmacokinet*. 2000;39(10):49–75.

112. Kantola T, Kivisto KT, Neuvonen PJ. Grapefruit juice greatly increases serum concentrations of lovastatin and lovastatin acid. *Clin Pharmacol Ther*. 1998;63:397–402.

113. Lilja JJ, Kivisto KT, Neuvonen PJ. Grapefruit juice-simvastatin interaction: effect on serum concentrations of simvastatin, simvastatin acid, and HMG-CoA reductase inhibitors. *Clin Pharmacol Ther*. 1998;64:477–483.

114. Lilja JJ, Kivisto KT, Neuvonen PJ. Grapefruit juice increases serum concentrations of atorvastatin and has no effect on pravastatin. *Clin Pharmacol Ther*. 1999;66:118–127.

115. Bistrup C, Nielson FT, Jeppesen VE, Diepenink H. Effect of grapefruit juice on sandimmun neoral absorption among stable renal allograft recipients. *Nephrol Dial Transplant*. 2001;16(2): 373–377.

116. Griffiths AP, Beddall A, Pegler S. Fatal haemopericardium and gastrointestinal haemorrhage due to possible interaction of cranberry juice with warfarin. *J R Soc Promot Health*. 2008;128(6):324–326.

117. Mergenhagen KA, Sherman O. Elevated international normalised ratio after concurrent ingestion of cranberry sauce and warfarin. *Am J Health Syst Pharm*. 2008;65(22): 213–216.

118. Li Z, Seenam NP, Carpenter CL, Thames G, Minutti C, Bowerman S. Cranberry does not affect prothrombin time in male subjects on warfarin. *J Am Diet Assoc*. 2006;106(12):2057–2061.

119. Lilja JJ, Backman JT, Neuvonen PJ. Effects of daily ingestion of cranberry juice on the pharmacokinetics of warfarin, tizanidine, and midazolam—probes of CYP2C9, CYP1A2 and CYP3A4. *Clin Pharmacol Ther*. 2007;81(6):833–839.

120. Nagata M, Hidaka M, Sekiya H, et al. Effects of pomegranate juice on human cytochrome P4502C9 and tolbutamide pharmacokinetics in rats. *Drug Metab Dispos*. 2007;35(2):302–305.

121. Antal EJ, Hendershot PE, Batts DH, Shen WP, Hopkins NK, Donaldson KM. Linezolid, a novel oxazolidinone antibiotic: assessment of monomine oxidase inhibition using pressor response to oral tyramine. *J Clin Pharmacol*. 2001;41:552–562.

122. Cantarini MV, Painter CJ, Glimore EM, Bolger C, Watkins CL, Hughes AM. Effect of oral linezolid on pressor response to intravenous tyramine. *Br J Clin Pharmacol*. 2004;58(5):470–475.

123. Schulz R, Antonin KH, Hoffman E, et al. Tyramine kinetics and pressor sensitivity during monoamine oxidase inhibition by selegiline. *Clin Pharmacol Ther*. 1989;46(5): 528–536.

124. Patker AA, Pae CU, Zarzar M. Selegiline. *Drugs Today*. 2007;43(6):361–377.

125. Maxwell MB. Reexamining the dietary restrictions with procarbazine (an MAOI). *Cancer Nurs*. 1980;3(6):451–457.

126. DiMartini A. Isoniazid, tricyclics and the 'cheese reaction'. *Int Clin Psychopharmacol*. 1995;10(3): 197–198.

127. Walker SE, Shulman KI, Tailor SA, Gardner D. Tyramine content of previously restricted foods in monoamine oxidase inhibitor diets. *J Clin Psychopharmacol*. 1996; 16(5):383–388.

128. Cremer SA, Gelfand DW. Esophageal bezoar resulting from enteral feedings. *JPEN J Parenter Enteral Nutr*. 1996;20(5): 371–373.

129. Wright DH, Pietz SL, Konstantinides FN, Rotschefer JC. Decreased in vitro fluoroquinolone concentrations after admixture with an enteral feeding formulation. *JPEN J Parenter Enteral Nutr*. 2000;24(1):42–48.

130. Cook MC, Taren DL. Nutritional implications of medication use and misuse in the elderly. *J Fla Med Assoc*. 1990;77:606–613.

131. Lewis CW, Frongillo EA, Roe DA. Drug-nutrient interactions in three long term care facilities. *J Am Dietetic Assoc*. 1995;95:309–315.

Food hypersensitivity—allergy and intolerance

7

Isabel Skypala

Introduction

Definition

Adverse food reactions can be classified into toxic and non-toxic;[1] toxic reactions occur in any individual exposed to a sufficient dose of a substance, but non-toxic ones only occur in an individual susceptible to certain foods. Non-toxic reactions are classified as food hypersensitivity (FHS) reactions, with reactions to foods involving immunologic mechanisms defined as food allergy (FA), and divided into IgE and non-IgE mediated reactions (see Figure 7.1).[2,3]

FHS reactions not known to involve the immune system are classified as non-allergic FHS, but may also be referred to as non-toxic, non-immunologic reactions.[3,4] These reactions include enzymatic reactions such as lactose intolerance and carbohydrate malabsorption, and pharmacological reactions related to the ingestion of foods containing vasoactive amines or salicylates. Conditions such as food-dependant, exercise-induced anaphylaxis (FDEIA) and reactions to food additives may involve the immune system, but the aetiology and pathogenic mechanisms are uncertain.[4]

Epidemiology and prevalence

About 20% of the population alter their diet because they believe they react to a food or food component; however, perceived prevalence is usually much greater than actual prevalence.[5–7] The prevalence of allergic disorders is associated with age and commonly referred to as the 'allergic march' with food allergy and atopic dermatitis predominating in early years and asthma and allergic rhinitis peaking in teenage and adult years.[8] Most IgE-mediated FA is acquired in the first 1–2 years of life, but it is still unknown whether most FA in adults represents a persistence of childhood symptoms or is a response primarily initiated in adulthood.[9] Up to 4% of adults may have an IgE-mediated FA, with prevalence often linked to aero-allergen sensitisation.[10–13] The most prevalent non-IgE mediated FA is coeliac disease, common in Europe, southern Asia, the Middle East, Africa and South America and thought to affect 1% of the UK population.[14,15]

The prevalence of non-immune mediated FHS is variable. Lactose intolerance affects on average 6–12% of Caucasians, but the range is very wide with 2% of Scandinavians and 70% of Sicilians being intolerant, and as many as 80–100% of Africans and Asians.[16] About 70% of people with irritable bowel

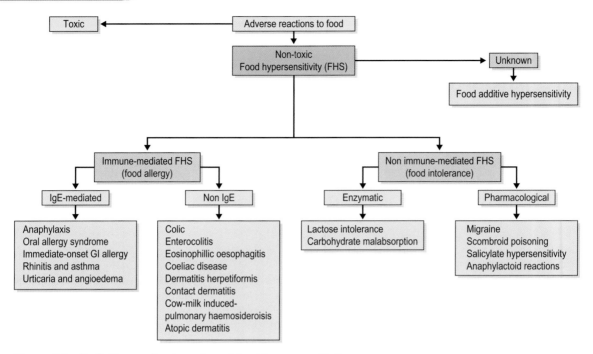

Figure 7.1 • Definition and categories of food hypersensitivity.

disorder feel they have a problem with food and often link the consumption of milk and wheat to their symptoms. In one study, 42% of subjects perceived milk to cause their symptoms, and about 15% felt wheat in the form of bread or flour caused intolerance.[17]

Physiology and pathophysiology

Mechanisms of response

Food allergic reactions are mediated by the immune system. There are two types of immunity, innate and adaptive. The main cells involved in adaptive immunity, the T and B lymphocytes, can recognise substances produced by microbes and non-infectious molecules known as antigens.[18] Sometimes antigens from pollens, animal dander or food proteins elicit immune responses known as hypersensitivity reactions; when this happens the antigens are known as allergens.[19] B lymphocytes (B cells) produce the antibodies immunoglobulin M (IgM), IgG, IgA and IgE; IgE is the main antibody involved in food allergy.[20] T lymphocytes (T cells) can be either

cytotoxic T cells or T helper (Th) cells, and it is the latter that are involved in FHS reactions. When activated by the antigen, Th cells develop into either Th1 cells or Th2 cells, depending on the type of mediator proteins (cytokines) the antigen-presenting cell (APC) is secreting.[18] When a Th2 cell is activated, it produces cytokines which make B cells produce IgE antibodies specific to the antigen presented to the T cell.[21] This antigen-specific IgE does not circulate freely but attaches itself to surfaces of mast cells and blood basophils.[22] Re-exposure enables the antigen to bind onto the specific antibody and when several IgE antibodies on the mast cell bind to the antigen, the mast cell degranulates and releases preformed mediators which cause the symptoms of food allergy (see Figure 7.2).

This response is immediate hypersensitivity or type I hypersensitivity and is the response that predominates in FHS. There are three other types of hypersensitivity reactions; types II and III are not thought to be involved in food allergy, but non-IgE-mediated food allergy may involve a type IV hypersensitivity which is cell-mediated and generally involves Th1 cells. Whereas type I hypersensitivity is immediate, type IV reactions are delayed; examples of type IV hypersensitivity include contact dermatitis and food-protein-induced enterocolitis. In coeliac

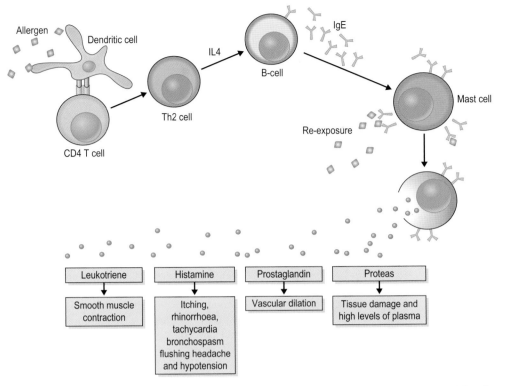

Figure 7.2 • Mechanism of a Type I allergic response responsible for IgE-mediated food allergy. [Adapted from Abbas and Lichtmann 2001].[18]

disease, a response to allergens found in cereals promotes an inflammatory reaction which involves both innate and adaptive immunity.

For non-immune-mediated FHS, the pathogenic mechanisms underlying the reactions are diverse and often unknown. There is evidence that in IBS patients, the anti-inflammatory response in respect to cytokine production may be suboptimal and also that there are increased levels of food-specific IgG antibodies.[23] Lactose intolerance is caused by lactase activity decreasing after weaning, and this occurs in 70% of adults worldwide, mainly from non-Caucasian races.[16]

Food allergens

Food allergen nomenclature is composed of the first three letters of the genus, the first letter of the species name followed by an Arabic number (http://www.allergen.org).[24] For example, the botanical name for peanut is *Arachis* (genus) *hypogaea* (species)

so the allergens are labeled Ara h 1, Ara h 2, etc. Food allergens are graded as either class 1 or class 2 allergens, and one food may have both class 1 and class 2 allergens.[25] Class 1 allergens are large water-soluble glycoproteins, stable to heat, acids and proteases, which allows them to sensitise during ingestion, breaching the normal immune tolerance to foods.[5,26] Class 2 allergens are usually heat labile, difficult to isolate and susceptible to enzymatic degradation, and so cannot sensitise upon ingestion.[25]

An allergen will have one or more sequences of amino acids known as epitopes, which are recognised by the antibody, thus enabling the allergen to bind with the antibody. There are two types of epitopes; sequential (linear) epitopes are composed of single segments of sequential amino acids along the polypeptide chain. Conformational epitopes are composed of amino acids from different parts of the protein sequence, brought together by folding. Conformational epitopes can be destroyed when the protein is altered due to heating or proteolysis, whereas sequential epitopes are not affected. Epitopes on different allergens can have a degree of amino acid sequence similarity, known as homology, which enables an antibody specific to one allergen to bind with another structurally similar allergen epitope. Homologous epitopes are common in food allergy, and account for the cross-reactivity between different foods and also between foods and pollens.

A wide range of foods and food additives are implicated in the spectrum of FHS; however, cow milk, eggs, fish, shellfish, soy, wheat, peanuts, tree nuts and seeds account for 90% of IgE-mediated food reactions.[27] Adults are most likely to have IgE-mediated allergy to fruits, fish, shellfish, peanuts and tree nuts.[5]

Diagnosis

Clinical history

One of the most important steps in the diagnostic process is establishing a good clinical history.[4] The history should uncover facts about the likely foods causing the reaction, quantity associated with a reaction, speed of onset of symptoms, duration of symptoms and other factors such as whether the reaction is concurrent with exercise, medications or alcohol.[5] The history can help determine whether the FHS is likely to be immune-mediated and therefore likely to involve specific IgE antibodies. IgE-mediated reactions are usually immediate, and involve allergic symptoms such as pruritis (itching), which may be accompanied by flushing, angiooedema (swelling) and hives or urticaria. These symptoms may be localised or systemic and accompanied by a fall in blood pressure, tachycardia and broncho-spasm. A reaction characterised by severe systemic symptoms is known as anaphylaxis and can be fatal. Other symptoms accompanying the reaction or appearing later on are nasal symptoms such as rhinorrhoea, sneeze, blockage or sinus involvement, and respiratory symptoms such as wheeze, cough and reduced lung capacity.

The symptoms of non-IgE-mediated FA may include atopic dermatitis (eczema) or non-specific GI symptoms which may appear some hours after the food has been eaten. Non-immune-mediated FHS reactions also can be delayed, although for some triggers such as histamine- or sulphite-containing foods, the symptoms can occur within 30 minutes of ingestion. The difference between FA and non-immune-mediated FHS is that the latter is often not obviously connected to just one food.

Poor dietary recall or concern about nutritional adequacy can be remedied by asking the patient to complete a diet diary. However, the clinical history can be inaccurate due to cross-reactions, or because the food has been contaminated or infested with parasites due to which the allergy is occurring. In most cases, the history should therefore be confirmed or refuted through the undertaking of different tests.

Diagnostic tests

Skin prick testing

Providing the subject has been avoiding antihistamines for 48 hours, skin prick testing (SPT) is a fast and relatively accurate way to confirm clinical history if an IgE-mediated FA is suspected.[5,28,29] A drop of allergen solution is placed on the forearm and pricked through with a sterile lancet using a separate one for each drop.[30] Positive (histamine) and negative (diluent) controls are used to evaluate the reactivity of SPT, with a positive test usually being one where the wheal diameter is $\geq$ 3 mm the negative control (see Figure 7.3).[4,30–32]

A positive test is not conclusive evidence of a food allergy; many people can be sensitised to an allergen without experiencing clinical symptoms. The positive predictive value (PPV) of SPT is only 50–60%, compared to a negative predictive value (NPV) of 95%.[25,33,34] This poor PPV underlines the importance of only testing those foods to which symptoms are reported rather than using a standard panel for screening.[4,9] However, even a 95% NPV still requires interpretation within the context of the clinical history. A negative test may be due to the destruction of heat-labile allergens during manufacture or variability of allergen extracts, so some advocate the use of fresh foods for testing.[35–37] When using fresh foods, the prick-by-prick method (PPT) is normally used; solid food is pricked and then the same lancet is used to prick the forearm, or a drop of liquid food is placed on the skin and the skin pricked through this. This form of testing is superior when investigating allergy to fruits and vegetables due to the many class 2 allergens present.[34]

The size of the SPT wheal does not correlate with severity of reported symptoms, but can help to predict the likelihood of reaction if challenged with that food. Several studies have provided predictive values for SPT wheal diameters, but none of these are for

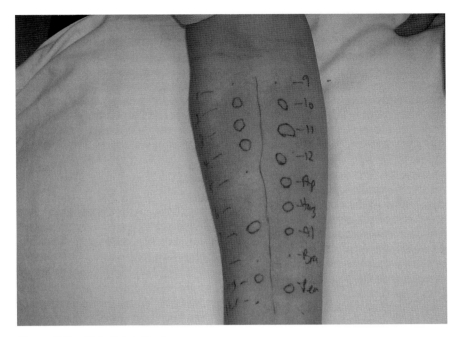

Figure 7.3 • Skin Prick Test.

adults and the variability of the results makes it difficult to extrapolate the findings to other geographical population groups (see Table 7.1).[34,38–41]

Serum-specific IgE (sIgE) antibody estimation

The measurement of sIgE antibodies is a useful alternative to SPT, when SPT are not available, or when patient has taken antihistamines, has dermographism (sensitive skin which responds by producing a wheal to a pen mark on the skin) or a severe skin condition such as eczema, or is at risk of a severe response. Guidelines suggest that SPT and sIgE estimation are interchangeable; either can be used to good effect with clinical history, but both may be required if there is a discord between the clinical history and the test result.[31] A variety of different manufacturers provide sIgE tests using different substrates and reporting results differently; some use a system of classes from 0 to 6 and others report in kilo units of allergen/litre (kU_A/L) or as 'graded' levels (grade 1–6) where

Grade 0 = < 0.35 kU_A/L
Grade 1 = 0.37–0.7 kU_A/L
Grade 2 = 0.7–3.5 kU_A/L
Grade 3 = 3.5–17.5 kU_A/L

Table 7.1 Predictive values for SPT wheal diameters

Food	PPV%	SPT (mm)	Reference:
Milk		5	Eigenmann and Sampson 1998[34]
	100	≥ 8	Hill et al 2004[38]
		≥ 8	Sporik et al 2000[39]
	95	12.5	Verstege et al 2005[40]
	99	17.3	Verstege et al 2005[40]
Egg		4	Eigenmann and Sampson 1998[34]
	100	≥ 7	Hill et al 2004[38]
		≥ 7	Sporik et al 2000[39]
	95	13.0	Verstege et al 2005[40]
	99	17.8	Verstege et al 2005[40]
Peanut		6	Eigenmann and Sampson 1998[34]
	100	≥ 8	Hill et al 2004[38]
		≥ 8	Sporik et al 2000[39]
	100	≥ 16	Rancé et al. 2002[41]

Grade 4 = 17.5–50 kU_A/L
Grade 5 = 50–100 kU_A/L
Grade 6 = > 100 kU_A/L

Generally, level 2 and above is considered as positive in clinical practice, although this is not evidence-based and those patients who have very low levels of positivity to foods should have a SPT to confirm the result. Specific IgE has a similar negative predictive value to SPT but undetectable serum food-specific IgE levels might occur in 10–25% of clinical reactions depending on the food involved.[28] Research has also been carried out to try to quantify the amount of sIgE predictive of a positive challenge for different foods. Published predictive values are summarised in Table 7.2, but again this work has only been carried out in children.[41–46]

Atopy patch test (APT)

This test is principally recommended for use in the diagnosis of delayed non-IgE-mediated FA such as atopic dermatitis, identifying cell-mediated reactions to foods.[31] APT needs an experienced evaluator and does not substantially affect the number of oral food challenges required for diagnosis.[29,47]

Table 7.2 Predictive values for sIgE levels

Food	PPV%	Specific IgE (kU/L)	Reference
Milk	95	32	Sampson 1997[42]
	95	15	Sampson 2001[43]
	95	5	Garcia-Ara et al. 2001[44]
Egg	95	6	Sampson 1997[42]
	95	7	Sampson 2001[43]
	95	13	Celik-Bilgili 2005[45]
Fish	100	20	Sampson 2001[43]
Peanut	95	15	Sampson 1997[42]
	95	14	Sampson 2001[43]
	100	57	Rancé et al. 2002[41]
Tree nut	95	15	Clark 2003[46]
Soy	73	30	Sampson 2001[43]
Wheat	74	26	Sampson 2001[43]

Serum food-specific IgG

IgG antibodies to foods are found commonly in healthy adults, independently of the presence or absence of food-related symptoms, and reflect the level of food exposure.[29,48] A high total IgE can also stimulate production of IgG antibodies.[4,49] It has been proposed that there is evidence of low grade inflammation in people with IBS that may impair the ability to mount an adequate immune response and two studies have suggested that the measurement of food IgG antibodies might be a useful way of identifying foods which could improve the symptoms of IBS if eliminated from the diet.[23,50,51] However, the role of IgG or its subclasses has not yet been substantiated in the diagnosis of clinical allergy.[4,52]

Coeliac disease

A first-line test for coeliac disease will usually be the use of serological antibody tests, which evaluate levels of the IgA class of anti-tissue transglutaminase (TTG) and/or endomysial antibody (EMA).[53] They have a sensitivity and specificity of > 90%, although test accuracy depends on there being no damage to the small intestine and normal levels of IgA antibody in the blood.[54,55] Patients with low or negative total IgA will need to have the IgG class of TTG/EMA evaluated instead.[56] It is recommended that a positive test be confirmed with a small bowel biopsy, the gold standard of diagnosis, which requires the consumption of a gluten-containing diet for at least 6 weeks prior to the test.[57–59]

Lactose intolerance

The lactose tolerance test requires a fasting blood sample, followed by an oral dose of lactose and further sequential blood samples to determine the level of lactose.[16] Another test is the breath hydrogen test; a fairly reliable method for the diagnosis of lactose malabsorption where the amount of hydrogen in the exhaled breath correlates with the amount of malabsorbed lactose.[60] Undigested lactose is fermented in the lower bowel and creates lactic acid, so lactose intolerance can also be diagnosed by checking the stool pH, or looking for faecal-reducing substances.[16]

Non-validated tests

There are a variety of other tests including the leukocyte cytotoxic test, hair analysis, bio resonance diagnostics, auto homologous immune therapy, kinesiology, iridology, sublingual provocative food testing, homeopathic remedies and electrodermal testing including electroacupuncture and Vega testing. However, few have been scientifically investigated and none validated for the accurate diagnosis of FHS.[61]

Diagnostic diets

An important clue to the role of a food causing problems can be derived from the resolution of symptoms upon removal of that food.[62] Diagnostic diets involve the supervised exclusion of a suspected food, followed by its reintroduction in the form of an oral food challenge. All patients should keep a symptom diary, to record symptoms related to the exclusion and subsequent reintroduction of foods, and also to check that foods are actually being reintroduced in a systematic way. Where there is strongly positive specific IgE to a known food trigger which elicits immediate symptoms, there is no requirement for a diagnostic diet; the patient should be advised to avoid that food.[63] Where there is discordance between the specific IgE tests and the clinical history, a 4- to 6-week avoidance of a food or food group may be helpful; if symptoms improve, then an oral food challenge should be carried out.[64] Patients waiting for a diagnosis are often already avoiding suspect food(s); however, their dietary intake should be checked as they may be ingesting small amounts of the suspect food allergen without realising.

Where there is no obvious food trigger, or non-IgE-mediated FA or non-immune-mediated FHS is suspected, then a multiple exclusion diet or oligoantigenic might be useful.[64] Such diets normally exclude foods most frequently implicated in allergic responses such as milk, grains, eggs and often citrus fruits, nuts, coffee and chocolate.[27] This diet is followed for 2–3 weeks and then foods are reintroduced singly and gradually at intervals of a few days. However, for those who report severe symptoms, or where psychological factors including food aversion may be involved, the reintroduction of food should be viewed as a food challenge and carried out under controlled conditions. A total exclusion diet is used when other avenues fail, or when extreme self-imposed restrictions need to be assessed. The diet usually consists of one meat (e.g. turkey, rabbit or lamb), two to three vegetables such as carrots, broccoli or cauliflower, two fruits (excluding citrus fruits), and two starchy foods such as rice, sago, tapioca or buckwheat.[65] The diet should be followed for a maximum of three weeks, and key foods reintroduced singly, two or three per week.

Food challenge

The aim of the oral food challenge (OFC) is to confirm or refute the involvement of a food, food additive or food component in triggering the individual's clinical symptoms.[66] Only 30-50% reported reactions to food are confirmed by an OFC, and since food allergy has a significant impact on the quality of life for the sufferer, challenges are essential in order to avoid unnecessary food restriction or misdiagnosis.[27,67,68] European Guidelines suggest that OFC should be used for everyone with a history of adverse foods reactions in order to establish or exclude a diagnosis of FHS.[69] The two main types of OFC are the open challenge (OC), where the food is not disguised, and the double-blind placebo-controlled food challenge (DBPCFC), where the food is disguised so that neither the subject nor the person administering the challenge is blinded as to the challenge dose.[27]

An OC is most suitable for immediate-onset IgE-mediated food allergy with objective symptoms that can be seen and recorded independently, or when a negative outcome is expected. For standard clinical practice, the OC is the most practical option and guidance suggests it can precede DBPCFC; a negative result negating the need for DBPCFC.[69] Some protocols commence with a labial challenge; the suspect food is rubbed on the outer lip and then exposed to the oral mucosa without being swallowed. For some types of allergy to fruits and vegetables, good contact with the oral mucosa is vital and a portion of the food may be sucked/chewed and disgorged as a starting dose prior to ingestion.[37,70] The starting dose of the suspect food should be half that reported to cause a reaction, with subsequent doses increased incrementally (usually double the preceding dose) (see Figure 7.4) given every 15 minutes, depending on the reported speed of onset of symptoms.[64] The total amount of the suspect food given during the whole challenge should equal 8–10 g of dry food or 100 ml liquid or 200 g solid 'wet' food.[64] European guidelines recommend that the final dose should equate to a standard portion of that food.[69]

For DBPCFC, the suspected food is hidden inside a carrier such as a biscuit, custard, fruit puree or

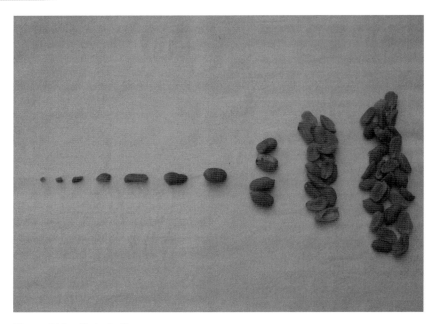

Figure 7.4 • Nut challenge.

even a hamburger. Coffee powder, cocoa powder or peppermint syrup can be used to disguise the taste of foods, and blackcurrants can disguise both taste and colour. Peel and pips may need to be removed from fruits although this does remove some of the allergen, making blinded challenges with fruits and vegetables difficult. It is recommended that fresh rather than dried food should be used, unless the dried food has been specially formulated for use in DBPCFC and its allergenicity tested prior to use.[71,72] DBPCFC are best performed using two placebo and one active challenges, randomised and given sequentially, with each challenge being given as a titrated dose as with the open challenges. Best practice recommends these challenges be given on 3 separate days but if not possible then the patient needs to be symptom free before the next challenge may commence.[73,74] Challenges for delayed reactions will need also to be given over several days, but it may be possible to complete these at home, depending on the severity of symptoms. Augmentation factors also need to be considered, such as exercise,[75] aspirin, infection, hormonal and multiple food combinations as these may all affect the final outcome of challenge.[4,66]

The difficulties experienced when undertaking challenges lead some to suggest they may not be necessary for most patients.[66,76] Predictive values for SPT and sIgE, together with better allergen

reagents, may reduce the number of challenges needed, but some IgE-mediated hypersensitivity responses are so localised that they are undetected by IgE testing and can only be confirmed by food challenge.[77]

Management

Allergen avoidance

The main management of any FHS will be to avoid known food triggers; this is greatly facilitated by EU labelling regulations,[78] which require specified allergens to be declared on prepackaged foods if they have been added deliberately, however small the amount. The foods covered include cereals containing gluten, crustaceans, eggs, fish, peanuts, soybeans, milk, nuts, celery, mustard, sesame seed and sulphur dioxide and sulphites at more than 10 mg/L/kg. The directive was updated in 2007 to include lupin and molluscs.[79]

Thus dietary exclusion can be straightforward although it is important to review the patient's current diet to assess inadvertent consumption of allergens. It is also important to give advice which will minimise accidental allergen exposure, such as occurring through inhalation of aerosolised allergens, transfer of allergens during cooking, touch and absorption through the skin, traces in foods and even kissing.[4] The Food Standards Agency has issued guidance for industry on risk assessment, although there is as yet no legislation for unwrapped foods or foods consumed in restaurants,[80] which is unfortunate since many reactions occur when eating out of the home.[81]

Food avoidance can affect quality of life,[68] and social life is improved after the reintroduction of foods following a negative challenge.[82] Children, teenagers and adults with FA experience problems associated with their FA irrespective of age.[83] Adolescents and young adults with food allergy may indulge in risk-taking behaviour, knowingly and purposefully ingesting potentially unsafe foods.[84] It is important to discuss any concerns and anxieties the patients have to help them live with a high degree of confidence and a feeling of being in control of their life.[85]

Specific foods

Milk and egg allergy

Milk and eggs are the most common causes of allergy of FA in children worldwide but this often resolves in childhood. Teenagers and adults on milk- or egg-free diets since childhood should be assessed for resolution of the allergy. Even where egg allergy has not resolved, it may be possible to allow the diet to be more relaxed since over 70% of those with a persistent egg allergy may tolerate cooked egg.[86] Both cow's milk and hen's egg are highly cross-reactive to milk and eggs from other animals, and all such relevant associated foods should also be avoided. Milk or egg allergies are rarely diagnosed in adulthood although egg allergy can occur in adults with allergy to bird feathers, through a cross-reacting allergen in the egg yolk.

Lactose intolerance is probably the most well-characterised non-immune-mediated hypersensitivity reaction to milk. Not all milk products contain lactose; hard cheeses such as cheddar and stilton have negligible lactose content, although soft cheeses such as cream cheese will need to be avoided. Some people with lactose intolerance can tolerate yoghurt. There are commercial enzyme preparations, which can be added to foods to enable them to be digested; also, milk treated with such enzymes can often be purchased in supermarkets, especially in areas with a large non-Caucasian population.

Over 40% of food-related symptoms in IBS are thought by sufferers to be caused by milk. Milk consumption has also been linked with respiratory conditions, and an increased mucous or phlegm production. Milk avoidance is therefore common in those with IBS and asthma and this can have a deleterious effect on nutritional status. For women, especially if they are taking regular corticosteroids, an optimal calcium intake is important to safeguard bone density. A milk substitute should be recommended and if one is already being taken, it needs to be checked in order to ascertain whether it is fortified. A dietary assessment is essential to ascertain whether supplements are required. For those with an egg allergy, nutritional issues are less common but it is important to review awareness of loosely cooked egg dishes such as meringue, omelettes and egg custards which can be tolerated by some egg allergic individuals but not all.

Seafood

Fish and shellfish are common causes of FA; one study suggests shellfish is the most common cause of anaphylaxis in Americans over the age of 6 years.[87] Fish and shellfish do not usually cause non-IgE-mediated FA, but a reaction due to increased levels of histamine in certain fish may occur. This is known as scombroid poisoning and may be confused with fish allergy due to the typical symptoms of flushing, sweating, urticaria, GI symptoms, palpitations and occasional bronchospasm.[88] Allergy to seafood does not usually resolve, although there have been case reports suggesting this may occur occasionally.[89]

There is strong cross-reactivity between fresh and saltwater fish, although a fish-allergic individual may not always have clinical symptoms to other cross-reacting fish.[90] The cod is the most allergenic fish, together with salmon and herring; there is strong cross-reactivity between cod, mackerel, herring and plaice;[90] also between salmon, trout and tuna; and mackerel and anchovy.[91] Crustaceans share a common allergenic protein called invertebrate tropomyosin. The main shrimp allergen Pen a 1 is similar to other allergens both in other crustaceans, such as crab, lobster and crayfish, and in molluscs, house dust mite and cockroaches.[92] There is no cross-reactivity reported between crustaceans and finned fish.[4,92]

Seafood-specific IgE tests are very reliable and so a positive test, together with a convincing history, is usually sufficient to make a diagnosis. However, due to the often very severe reported symptoms, and the possibility of a differential diagnosis, a negative specific IgE screen needs confirmation by OFC. Unless other species are tried through oral challenge, it is probably safer to advise avoidance of all fish due to cross-reactivity. Fish allergens are heat labile and so there are people who will be able to consume canned salmon or tuna but not raw, smoked or lightly cooked fish.[93] For crustacean allergy, all crustaceans and molluscs should be avoided due to unknown cross-reactivity. Also shrimp allergens are very robust and may be found in oil used to cook prawns and so contamination can be a major problem, especially when eating out.[94]

Avoidance of seafood does not normally cause any major nutritional problems, although those who are taking omega 3 fatty acid supplements in the form of fish oil will need to find an alternative source such as linseed (flax seed) or algae oil (Food Standards Agency website).

Plant foods (peanuts, tree nuts, seeds, fruits and vegetables)

Allergy to nuts, fruits and vegetables are very significant in the adult population. Many plant foods from unrelated botanical families have homologous allergens leading to extensive cross-reactivity between plant foods from different botanical families, and between plant foods and pollens. The plant food allergens are classified by their different allergen types, rather than botanical families and one food may have allergens in several different families.[95,96]

Peanuts

Peanut allergy usually presents in early childhood,[97] but unlike milk and egg allergy, only 20% of cases will resolve, with 8% of these cases likely to have a reoccurrence.[98–100] Most peanut allergy in adults will be unresolved childhood allergy; for those with newly diagnosed with peanut allergy, it unknown whether this is a primary sensitisation to peanuts or cross-reactivity reaction to other foods or aero allergens.

Many of the peanut allergens are resistant to heat and proteolysis and hard to eradicate. For example, it is known that one of the peanut allergens, Ara h 1, can remain in the saliva for up to an hour after eating,[101] requires detergent or soap to be removed from surfaces,[102] and increases in allergenicity if roasted rather than being boiled or fried.[103] Most people are sensitised to Ara h 2,[104] but only those with severe symptoms are co-sensitised to Ara h 1.[105] Not all peanut allergens are so robust; Ara

h 5 and Ara h 8 may be fully or partially destroyed on heating.[106,107]

A good clinical history and matching positive SPT or specific IgE is sufficient to make a diagnosis of peanut allergy. However, if SPT or blood tests are negative, it is very important to confirm or refute the diagnosis by undertaking OFC as a diagnosis of peanut allergy can severely restrict the diet, mainly due to the level of nut trace warnings on foods. Most people with a peanut allergy will be advised to avoid all tree nuts in addition to peanuts, partly because they are at increased risk of having reactions to tree nuts, but also because of the issue of contamination. There are no major nutritional risks for those on peanut-free diets, unless they are also avoiding other major food groups or are vegetarian or vegan.

Other legumes

People with a peanut allergy are often co-sensitised to other legumes but this rarely manifests itself as a clinical issue.[108] Soy, chickpea and lentil allergy are mostly seen in children, and although legume allergy can occur in adults the incidence is unknown.[109] However, severe reactions to lupin, a legume added to bread and flour in Europe in the form of lupin flour, have been reported. French pastry, apple flan, battered onion rings and gluten-free pasta have all been involved in reported reactions. Lupin allergy can occur independently of peanut allergy and can be very severe,[110] hence its inclusion in the EU food allergen labelling scheme in 2007.

Tree nut allergy

There is cross-reactivity between tree nuts and peanuts; up to half of those allergic to peanuts could also be allergic to tree nuts.[111–113] About 0.5–1% of people are likely to develop a tree nut allergy, with resolution in about 9% of cases.[114] In the UK, the commonest tree nuts involved are Brazil nut, hazelnut, walnut and almond, although cashew nut allergy is increasingly prevalent, often causing severe reactions on first exposure.[115,116] Most tree nut allergy is thought to develop in childhood; in adults it may be a primary allergy but more often is associated with cross-reactivity to tree pollen. Although tree nut allergy is usually diagnosed through the combination of a good clinical history and specific IgE evaluation, some test reagents do not give good results for nuts, and so a convincing history and negative tests should be followed up with PPT using fresh nuts, followed by OFC.

Seeds

Sesame and mustard seed are the two seeds most commonly involved in FA. The major allergens in sesame are oleosins, found in the oil fraction of the seed,[117] so whole seeds may not cause reactions whereas a sesame oil might. Mustard seed has been reported to cause severe reactions and is a common allergen in France.[118] SPT and specific IgE estimations are not always reliable, so a careful history is essential. Allergy to sesame and/or mustard should be excluded in people presenting with reported reactions to a variety of seemingly unconnected foods.

Fruit and vegetables

Allergy to fruits and vegetables is probably the most common form of FA in adults, affecting an estimated 5% of the population.[5] Although symptoms can be mild, severe reactions are not uncommon; fruit was cited as causing 12% of all anaphylaxis reactions in North America.[87] Allergy to fruits and vegetables is either a primary sensitisation to a plant allergen or a secondary reaction caused by cross-reactions between a plant food allergen and an antibody to pollen or latex. Primary fruit or vegetable allergy is thought to involve a group of allergens known collectively as non-specific lipid transfer proteins (nsLTP). These robust heat and proteolysis-resistant allergens have been identified in a wide range of plant foods; sensitisation will occur in the gastrointestinal tract and the symptoms can be as severe as those involved in other primary food allergies.[119] Allergy to nsLTP are much more prevalent in southern Europe; studies suggest that most apple allergy in Spain is due to sensitisation to the nsLTP.[120] The commonest foods involved in primary fruit or vegetable allergy are apples, peaches, grapes, kiwi fruit, celery and carrots.

The most common plant food allergy falls into a group of conditions known collectively as oral allergy syndrome (OAS). OAS is an umbrella term but it is most often used to describe symptoms caused by pollen–plant food cross-reactions.[121] Latex also cross-reacts with plant food allergens, in particular those found in chestnuts, avocado, banana and kiwi fruit.

The commonest manifestation of OAS involves foods which cross-react to allergens from the silver birch tree (*Betula verrucosa*), although grass and weed pollens can also cause OAS.[122] It is thought that 50–93% of birch pollen allergic patients could have OAS, due to the high cross-reactivity between the plant food allergens, the PR10 proteins and the main birch pollen allergen Bet v 1.[122–124] The other plant food allergens involved, the profilins, are found in many plant foods and cross-react to the second birch pollen allergen Bet v 2, also a profilin.[95,125] Foods commonly causing OAS include apples, stone fruits and tree nuts, but OAS can also involve kiwi fruit, peanuts, soy, bean sprouts, tomatoes, avocado pear, pears, strawberry, carrots, grapes, peppers and itching of the hands when peeling potatoes or parsnips. Up to 70% of birch-sensitised patients can also be sensitised to celery, although it is not commonly reported as an allergen in the UK.[126]

Herbs and spices can also be involved in both primary and secondary reactions to plant foods. Celery root retains its allergenicity after heat treatment and therefore celery spice is allergenic for patients with an allergy to raw celery.[127] There have been case reports of reactions involving basil, fennel, parsley and coriander and reactions to curry powder could be linked to coriander, caraway, cayenne, fenugreek, celery seed or mustard.

People with OAS generally have mild symptoms very localised to the mouth and throat, characterised by numbness or itching, especially the lips, palate and ears, and also local swelling of the lips, tongue or occasionally throat. These symptoms usually only occur when the raw food is eaten, with immediate onset and rapid dissipation. Cooking or even peeling the raw food may be sufficient allergen removal to enable the sufferer to eat the food.[128] Storage of the food and the variety may also affect the amount of allergen the food contains.[129,130] It is common for people with OAS to report reactions to more than one food. Those with primary plant food allergy will report severe symptoms to a plant food, usually within 30 minutes of consumption. They too may report some symptom relief if the fruit is peeled as most nsLTP are associated with the peels of fruits and vegetables. However, they are usually symptomatic to the food whether raw, cooked, juiced or processed. Those with an allergy to one nsLTP may cross-react to other botanically unrelated foods, e.g. a peach-allergic individual may also report symptoms to corn, apples and barley.[131]

Many of the test reagents to estimate specific IgE may not contain all of the allergens, as both PR10 proteins and profilins are heat labile. Therefore it is recommended that clinical history is confirmed or refuted with PPT with the fresh fruits and vegetables reported to cause symptoms. It may be assumed that avoidance of plant foods will not affect nutritional intake; however, some will experience

OAS symptoms to a wide range of fruits and vegetables and may be at risk of nutritional deficiencies arising from extreme dietary restrictions.[132]

Wheat and other grains

Wheat can cause sensitisation by ingestion, inhalation (baker's asthma), and skin contact.[133] Wheat allergy in adults is much less common than in children and may be associated with a condition called food-dependent exercise-induced anaphylaxis, which is mediated by a specific allergen, omega-5 gliadin.[134,135] Levels of this allergen may also be higher in those who have more severe symptoms including anaphylaxis.[136] SPT and specific IgE tests for wheat have poor predictive values, but the measurement of specific IgE antibodies to omega-5 gliadin are a useful predictor of the presence or absence of wheat-dependent, exercise-induced anaphylaxis (WDEIA).[137] It is important to assess whether the patient is also grass sensitised as 80% of positive specific IgE tests to wheat in grass-sensitised individuals have no clinical significance. Symptoms involving other cereals such as barley (malt) or corn may be triggered by an nsLTP.

The alcohol-soluble gliadins in the wheat protein gluten are the main cause of coeliac disease. Similar gluten subfractions are also found in barley and rye. People presenting with symptoms to wheat and other cereals are not stereotypically malnourished and many adults with undiagnosed coeliac disease may be normal or even overweight. Coeliac disease may be misdiagnosed commonly as IBS, and therefore rigorous diagnosis of reported symptoms to wheat must include antibody tests (TTG/EMA) and specific IgA levels to confirm or refute a diagnosis of coeliac disease before other differential diagnoses such as IBS can be considered.[138,139] Those with a confirmed diagnosis of coeliac disease require life-long exclusion of all gluten in wheat, rye and barley. Oats may not precipitate reactions but often need to be avoided as they may be contaminated with wheat. Cereals which can be consumed include rice, millet and maize/corn and wheat starch is also permitted. Those with medically diagnosed coeliac disease are eligible for gluten-free products on prescription, but not those with a wheat allergy. Apart from the obvious gluten-containing foods, other foods which need to be avoided include foods with high barley malt or barley flour content such as malted drinks or barley waters. People with dermatitis herpetiformis also gain symptom relief through dietary exclusion of gluten, and IBS sufferers and others may also benefit from excluding wheat, which is often reported to cause bloating and fatigue.

People avoiding wheat and other cereals need to be advised on suitable substitutes, and also have a dietary assessment to evaluate the adequacy of energy, iron, calcium, folic acid and vitamin B_{12} intakes. People with coeliac disease may suffer from osteoporosis or osteopenia and so will require assessment and possibly supplements of calcium and vitamin D.

Food additives

In adults, food additives such as naturally derived colourings can be involved in IgE-mediated reactions to foods.[140] However, synthetic colourings such as tartrazine (E102) and sunset yellow (E110) and benzoates (cinnamon, cloves, tea, prunes, raspberry, cranberry and E210–219) have also been linked to food hypersensitivity in adults, often anectdotally to urticaria or angio-oedema. The few studies undertaken to consider this have concluded that rigorous testing shows only 1–2% of those with reported symptoms to benzoates or colourings have the hypersensitivity confirmed on challenge.[141,142] Monosodium glutamate (MSG) and sodium metabisulphite are the two additives with the most convincing evidence of involvement in food hypersensitivity reactions. Sulphites (E220–227) have been reported to cause wheeze, bronchospasm, rhinitis and sinusitis in affected individuals, and could affect up to 5% of asthmatics.[143] High sulphite foods include cider, dried fruit, wine, lager, dried onions, horseradish, lemon and lime juice, frozen or tinned potatoes and frozen beef burgers. MSG is a flavour enhancer reported to cause sweating, tachycardia and other immediate symptoms on ingestion of large amounts in sensitive individuals.[144] It is found naturally in tomatoes, parmesan cheese, yeast extract, hydrolysed vegetable protein and soy sauce, but about one-third of intake comes from added MSG, used widely in food manufacturing and restaurants.

Naturally occurring compounds causing pharmacologic reactions

Salicin, the chemical precursor of aspirin (acetylsalicylic acid), is also found naturally in many plant foods. There are several published sources of the salicylate content of foods, which vary due to the different chemical methodologies used for analysis.[145,146] Scotter et al found apples, lemons and bananas contained significant amounts of salicylate,[146] whereas Swain et al considered them to be low salicylate foods.[145] Concordant results from both studies showed that coffee, tea, herbs and spices, black pepper, mint, yeast spreads, and tomatoes and grapes are all high salicylate foods. Evidence supporting the efficacy of dietary salicylate avoidance is scarce, but it may be useful for people with aspirin sensitivity, particularly those with concomitant nasal polyps and/or asthma, to undergo a trial avoidance of high salicylate foods.

Vasoactive amines such as histamine and tyramine affect sensitive individuals. Histamine-containing foods include parmesan, blue cheese, Roquefort cheese, red wine, spinach, aubergines, yeast extract and scombroid fish such as tuna and mackerel. Tyramine is often found in fermented foods such as cheese, yeast extract, red wine (especially Chianti), chicken liver, fermented beans such as soy and miso soup, and pickled roll mop herring.

Key points

- Correct classification of FHS assists with diagnosis, and removes the stigma associated with a diagnosis label of food intolerance.
- The immune mechanisms of IgE-mediated FA are well characterised but other FHS mechanisms are less well known or unknown.
- Clinical history involves assessing suspected foods, speed of onset of symptoms, symptom type and augmentation factors.
- Confirmation of clinical history with appropriate tests is necessary for every patient reporting FHS.
- SPT and specific IgE tests are useful for IgE-mediated FA and diagnostic if supported by a good clinical history.
- Oral food challenge is the gold standard of diagnosis and should be undertaken when test results do not concord with clinical history.
- Foods causing most of the IgE-mediated FA in adults are tree nuts, peanuts, seafood, fruits and vegetables; milk and wheat are the two commonest causes of other types of FHS.
- Reported reactions to wheat or milk, which are not IgE-mediated, need to be followed up with tests for coeliac disease or lactose intolerance.
- FHS to seeds, herbs, spices, additives, salicylate or vasoactive amines should be considered when no obvious food is involved or the reaction is to a wide range of different foods.
- Avoidance of known triggers is currently the only treatment for most types of FHS.
- Nutritional issues can be relevant for adults, especially if avoiding key staple foods such as milk and wheat, or avoiding multiple food groups.

Developing issues

Risk factors for the development of IgE-mediated food allergy

The development of FA in infancy is related to exposure to foods during weaning and the eating habits of the population. The maternal and infant diet could both therefore affect the development of allergic disease. A review of the effects of dietary magnesium, omega-3 and omega-6 fatty acids, sodium, antioxidants and milk intake concluded that not enough evidence was available to make firm recommendations, and large multicentre trials were needed.[147]

There is good evidence to support exclusive breastfeeding up to the age of 4–6 months,[147] but prolonged breastfeeding and delayed weaning of allergenic foods may not be protective.[148–151] The optimal timing of the introduction of solid food is particularly contentious; however, the British Dietetic Association guidance on weaning for high-risk infants is now supported by two definitive publications.[152] They suggest at-risk infants should be exclusively breastfed for 4–6 months, or given formula milk with documented reduced allergenicity for the first 4 months,[153] with weaning not commenced before 17 weeks and foods added one at a time to allow for detection of reactions.[154]

Novel diagnostic methods

Many allergens have been characterised using recombinant DNA technology to produce allergen extracts containing individual allergens.[155] These purified recombinant allergen extracts are highly effective in the diagnosis of allergy to some foods, especially where this involves labile.[104,122] The development of individual allergens for testing will improve specificity and sensitivity of specific IgE tests; for example all peanut allergic individuals are sensitised to Ara h 2, compared to less than 10% of those tolerant to peanuts.[104,105,156] Knowledge of the epitope-blinding capacity of some allergens may help characterise individual allergies and enable more specific advice to be given. It has been demonstrated that children who do not outgrow egg allergy have IgE antibodies to sequential epitopes in contrast to those with resolved egg allergy who make IgE antibodies to conformational epitopes;[157] a similar picture has emerged with regard to milk allergy.[158] The egg allergen Gal d 1 (ovomucoid) is resistant to heat and contains linear epitopes; one study showed that the presence of serum-specific IgE antibodies to Gal d 1 could be used as a marker of persistent egg allergy.[159] The epitope-binding domains of the wheat gliadins may also differ depending on the type of symptoms elicited by wheat. Those with WDEIA, anaphylaxis and urticarial reactions to wheat recognise sequential epitopes on gliadins, whereas those suffering from wheat-induced atopic dermatitis recognise conformational epitopes.[160]

Case study

A 46-year-old man was referred following a reported systemic reaction 15 minutes after consuming several handfuls of raw peanuts. He developed periorbital swelling, nasal congestion and a sense of impending doom, but his airway, respiratory tract and gastrointestinal tract were not affected. He was admitted to his local hospital, given intravenous hydrocortisone, intramuscular adrenaline, a saline drip, oxygen, oral prednisolone and antihistamines, and discharged home 48 hours later with two epinephrine auto-injector pens. Since that reaction he has eaten Brazil nuts, walnuts and almonds with no ill effects, but is avoiding both raw and roasted peanuts and foods with peanut trace warnings. He had no family history of allergy or allergies as a child, no allergies to drugs or latex, but did report hay fever symptoms from March to late July/August. He had no previous reactions to foods although on questioning reported mild tingling of the lips when eating raw carrots, and strange sensations in his hands when peeling potatoes/parsnips and facial swelling if he then touched his face. He ate milk, eggs, fish and tree nuts without a problem and had consumed large quantities of roasted peanuts daily without ill effect prior to the reaction.

Blood tests for full blood count, thyroid function, liver function, renal function and ESR were all normal. SPT were positive to grass (12 mm), mugwort (4 mm), three trees (birch, alder and hazel) (7 mm), silver birch (5 mm) and horse (4 mm), with a negative control of 0 mm and positive control of 9 mm. House dust mite, cat, dog and moulds were all negative. Specific IgE blood tests for peanut, hazel nut, almond, walnut, Brazil nut, cashew nut, pistachio nut and coconut were also negative ($< 0.35\,kU_A/L$).

These results confirmed that, consistent with his history, the seasonal rhinitis was due to both tree and grass pollen. The pollen sensitivity, together with the reactions to carrots, potatoes and parsnips, also suggested he had mild OAS. The negative specific IgE tests for nuts did not concord with his history and so for clarification it was agreed that an open oral challenge to peanuts should be performed. Prior to commencing the challenge, SPT undertaken using the prick-by-prick test method (PPT) with fresh nuts were positive for both raw (12 mm) and roasted (5 mm) peanuts. This result suggested an oral food challenge to raw peanuts was inappropriate. However, since the patient was very keen to eat roasted peanuts again, an open challenge with the roasted peanuts was performed with caution. By the end of the challenge, the patient had consumed the equivalent of a whole bag of roasted peanuts (50 g) without any ill effect.

QUESTIONS

1. Why were the blood tests negative but the skin prick tests positive?
2. Why, if the PPT with roasted peanuts was positive, did the challenge go ahead?
3. Does the positive PPT to raw peanuts mean he has a peanut allergy?
4. Which peanut allergens would it have been useful to test for individually?
5. Would this challenge have been safe to perform at home and if not why not?
6. Are there any quality of life or nutritional issues in this case?
7. Does this man need to avoid other legumes and tree nuts?

ANSWERS

1. Why were the blood tests negative but the skin prick tests positive?

   The negative blood tests suggest that the allergen causing the symptoms is likely to be one which is destroyed on heating and therefore only available in the native food. An example would be either Ara h 5 or Ara h 8, both of which are homologous to tree and grass pollens.
2. Why, if the PPT with roasted peanuts was positive, did the challenge go ahead?

   The challenge with roasted peanuts went ahead because he gave a very good history of not reacting to

Case study (Continued)

roasted nuts, and also wanted to eat roasted nuts again.

3. Does the positive PPT to raw peanuts mean he has a peanut allergy?

The positive PPT to raw nuts is an indicator that his symptoms are due to oral allergy syndrome rather than a primary peanut allergy. Most peanut allergy starts in childhood and so it would be unusual for a man of his age to develop a primary peanut allergy. Reported symptoms to raw plant foods only is a very good predictor that the person has OAS rather than a primary allergy.

4. Which peanut allergens would it have been useful to test for individually?

It would be useful to test for Ara h 5 and Ara h 8, the allergens in peanuts most likely to be linked to OAS.

5. Would this challenge have been safe to perform at home and if not why not?

The challenge would not have been safe to perform at home as we could not be 100% sure he did not have a

peanut allergy and also he had severe symptoms on exposure to raw nuts.

6. Are there any quality of life or nutritional issues in this case?

There are no nutritional issues in this case, but this patient's quality of life was severely affected by being on a nut-free diet, not only because he had been advised by his local hospital to avoid all nuts and traces of nuts, but also because he wanted to eat roasted peanuts again.

7. Does this man need to avoid other legumes and tree nuts?

There is no evidence that this man needs to avoid tree nuts or other legumes. People with OAS only need to avoid the foods which cause symptoms. Also, even if he had a peanut allergy, he would not have been advised to avoid legumes unless there was evidence that they were causing symptoms. It is very rare for peanut allergic individuals to develop symptoms to other legumes, although people with a legume allergy can develop symptoms to peanuts.

References

1. Bruijnzeel-Koomen C, Ortolani C, Aas K, et al. Adverse reactions to foods. *Allergy*. 1995;50:623–635.

2. Johansson SGO, Bieber T, Dhal R, et al. Revised nomenclature for allergy for global use: report of the nomenclature review committee of the World Allergy Organisation, October 2003. *J Allergy Clin Immunol*. 2004;113(5):832–836.

3. Johansson SGO, Hourihane JO'B, Bousquet J, et al. A revised nomenclature for allergy. An EAACI position statement from the EAACI nomenclature task force. *Allergy*. 2001;56:813–874.

4. Chapman JA, Bernstein IL, Lee RE, et al. Food allergy: a practice parameter. *Ann Allergy Asthma Immunol*. 2006;96:S1–S68.

5. Sicherer SH, Sampson HA. Food allergy. *J Allergy Clin Immunol*. 2006;117(2):S470–475.

6. Young E, Stoneham MD, Petuckevitch A, Barton J, Rana R. A population study of food

intolerance. *Lancet*. 1994;343: 1127–1130.

7. Pereira B, Venter C, Grundy J, Clayton CB, Arshad SH, Dean T. Prevalence of sensitisation to food allergens, reported adverse reaction to foods, food avoidance, and food hypersensitivity among teenagers. *J Allergy Clin Immunol*. 2005; 116(4):884–892.

8. Durham SR, Church MK. Principals of allergy diagnosis. In: Holgate ST, Church MK, Lichtenstein LM, eds. *Allergy*. Edinburgh: Elseveir Science; 2002:3–16.

9. Crespo JF, Rodriguez J. Food allergy in adulthood. *Allergy*. 2003;58:98–113.

10. Jansen JJ, Kardinaal AF, Huijbers G, et al. Prevalence of food allergy and intolerance in the adult Dutch populations. *J Allergy Clin Immunol*. 1994;93:446–456.

11. Zuberbier T, Edenharter G, Worm M, et al. Prevalence of adverse reactions to food in

Germany—a population study. *Allergy*. 2004;59:338–345.

12. Osterballe M, Hansen TK, Mortz CG, Høst A, Bindslev-Jensen C. The prevalence of food hypersensitivity in an unselected population of children and adults. *Pediatr Allergy Immunol*. 2005;16: 567–573.

13. Woods RKA, Thien F, Raven J, Walters EH, Abramson M. Prevalence of food allergies in young adults and their relationship to asthma, nasal allergies and eczema. *Ann Allergy Asthma Immunol*. 2002;88(2):183–189.

14. West J, Logan RF, Hill PG, et al. Seroprevalence, correlates and characteristics of undetected coeliac disease in England. *Gut*. 2003;52:960–965.

15. Cataldo F, Montalto G. Celiac disease in the developing countries: a new and challenging public health problem. *World J Gastroenterol*. 2007;13(15):2153–2159.

16. Vesa TH, Marteau P, Korpela R. Lactose intolerance. *J Am Coll Nutr.* 2000;19(suppl 2): 165S–175S.

17. Monsbakken KW, Vandvik PO, Farup PG. Perceived food intolerance in subjects with irritable bowel syndrome – aetiology, prevalence and consequences. *Eur J Clin Nutr.* 2006;60:667–672.

18. Abbas AK, Lichtman AH. *Basic Immunology: Functions and Disorders of the Immune System.* Philadelphia: WB Saunders; 2001.

19. Chaplin DD. Overview of the human immune response. *J Allergy Clin Immunol.* 2006;117(S2): S430–S435.

20. deFranco AL, Locksley RM, Robertson M. *Immunity: The Immune Response in Infectious and Inflammatory Disease.* Oxford: Oxford University Press; 2007.

21. Maggi I, Parronchi P, Manetti R, et al. Reciprocal regulatory effects of IFNγ and IL-4 on the in vitro development of human Th1 and Th2 clones. *J Immunol.* 1992;148: 2142–2147.

22. Sutton BJ, Gould HJ. The human IgE network. *Nature.* 1993;366: 421–428.

23. Whorwell PJ. The growing case for an immunological component to irritable bowel syndrome. *Clin Exp Allergy.* 2007;27:805–807.

24. IUIS/WHO Allergen Nomenclature Subcommittee Bulletin. *World Health Organ.* 1994;72:797–806.

25. Sampson HA. Update on food allergy. *J Allergy Clin Immunol.* 2004;113(5):805–819.

26. Lack G. New developments in food allergy—old questions remain. *J Allergy Clin Immunol.* 2004; 114(1):127–130.

27. Bock SA, Sampson HA, Atkins FM, et al. Double-blind, placebo-controlled food challenge (DBPCFC) as an office procedure. *J Allergy Clin Immunol.* 1988; 82(6): 986–997.

28. Ives AJ, Hourihane JO'B. Evidence-based diagnosis of food allergy. *Current Paed.* 2002;12:357–364.

29. Allen KJ, Hill DJ, Heine RG. Food allergy in childhood. *Med J Aust.* 2006;185:394–400.

30. Rusznak C, Davies RJ. Diagnosing allergy. *Br Med J.* 1998;316: 686–689.

31. Høst A, Andrae S, Charkin S, et al. Allergy testing in children: why, who, when and how? *Allergy.* 2003;58:1–11.

32. Bernstein IL, Storms WW. Practice parameters for allergy diagnostic testing. Joint Task Force on Practice Parameters for the Diagnosis and Treatment of Asthma. The American Academy of Allergy, Asthma and Immunology and the American College of Allergy, Asthma and Immunology. *Ann Allergy Asthma Immunol.* 1995;75:543–625.

33. Bock SA, Buckley J, Hölst A, May CD. Proper use of skin tests with food extracts in diagnosis of hypersensitivity to food in children. *Clin Allergy.* 1977;7:375–383.

34. Eigenmann PA, Sampson HA. Interpreting skin prick tests in the evaluation of food allergy in children. *Pediatr Allergy Immunol.* 1998;9(4):186–191.

35. Akkerdaas JH, Wensing M, Knulst AC, et al. How accurate and safe is the diagnosis of hazelnut allergy by means of commercial skin prick test reagents? *Int Arch Allergy Immunol.* 2003;132:132–140.

36. Rancé F, Juchet A, Brémont F, Dutau G. Correlations between skin prick tests using commercial extracts and fresh foods, specific IgE, and food challenges. *Allergy.* 1997;32: 1031–1035.

37. Anhøj C, Backer V, Nolte H. Diagnostic evaluation of grass- and birch-allergic patients with oral allergy syndrome. *Allergy.* 2001; 56:548–552.

38. Hill DJ, Heine-Ralf G, Hosking CS. The diagnostic value of skin prick testing in children with food allergy. *Pediatr Allergy Immunol.* 2004; 15(5):435–441.

39. Sporik R, Hill DJ, Hosking CS. Specificity of allergen skin testing in predicting positive open food challenges to milk, egg and peanut in children. *Clin Exp Allergy.* 2000;30:1540–1546.

40. Verstege A, Mehl A, Rolinck-Werninghaus C, et al. The predictive value of the skin prick test weal size for the outcome of oral food challenges. *Clin Exp Allergy.* 2005;35:1220–1226.

41. Rancé F, Abbal M, Lauwers-Cancès V. Improved screening for peanut allergy by the combined use of skin prick tests and specific IgE assays. *J Allergy Clin Immunol.* 2002;109:1027–1033.

42. Sampson HA. Food allergy. *J Am Med Assoc.* 1997;276(22): 1888–1894.

43. Sampson HA. Utility of food-specific IgE concentrations in predicting symptomatic food allergy. *J Allergy Clin Immunol.* 2001;107(5):891–896.

44. Garcia-Ara C, Boyano-Matrinez T, Diaz-Pena JM, Martin-Munoz F, Reche-Frutos M, Martin-Esteban M. Specific IgE levels in the diagnosis of immediate hypersensitivity to cows' milk protein in the infant. *J Allergy Clin Immunol.* 2001;107:185–190.

45. Celik-Bilgili S, Mehl A, Verstege A, et al. The predictive value of specific immunoglobulin E levels in serum for the outcome of oral food challenges. *Clin Exp Allergy.* 2005;35:268–273.

46. Clark AT, Ewan PW. Interpretation of tests for nut allergy in one thousand patients, in relation to allergy or tolerance. *Clin Exp Allergy.* 2003;33:1041–1045.

47. Niggemann B, Rolinck-Werninghaus C, Mehl A, Binder C, Zeigert M, Beyer K. Controlled oral food challenges in children – when indicated, when superfluous? *Allergy.* 2005;60:865–870.

48. Spickett G. *Oxford Handbook of Clinical Immunology and Allergy.* Oxford: Oxford University Press; 2006.

49. Bahna SL. The diagnosis of food allergy. *Ann Allergy Asthma Immunol.* 2003;90:80.

50. Atkinson W, Sheldon TA, Shaath N, Whorwell PJ. Food elimination based on IgG antibodies in irritable bowel syndrome: a randomised controlled trial. *Gut.* 2004;53:1459–1464.

51. Zuo XL, Li YQ, Li WJ, et al. Alterations of food antigen-specific serum immunoglobulins G and E antibodies in patients with irritable-bowel syndrome and functional

dyspepsia. *Clin Exp Allergy*. 2007;37:823–830.

52. Stapel SO, Asero R, Ballmer-Weber BK, et al. Testing for IgG4 against foods is not recommended as a diagnostic tool: EAACI Task Force Report. *Allergy*. 2008;63: 793–796.

53. Fasono A, Catassi C. Current approaches to diagnosis and treatment of celiac disease: an evolving spectrum. *Gastroenterology*. 2001;120:636–651.

54. Rostom A, Dubé C, Cranney A, et al. The diagnostic accuracy of serologic tests for celiac disease: a systematic review. *Gastroenterology*. 2005;128:S38–S46.

55. Abrams JA, Diamond B, Rotterdam H, Green PH. Seronegative celiac disease: increased prevalence with lesser degrees of villous atrophy. *Dig Dis Sci*. 2004;49:546–550.

56. *Clinical Resource Efficiency Support Team (Northern Ireland)*. Guidelines for the diagnosis and management of coeliac disease in adults. Available at http://www.crestni.org.uk; 2006.

57. *British Society of Gastroenterology (BSG)*. Guidelines for the management of patients with coeliac disease. Available at http://www.bsg.org.uk; 2002.

58. Hopper AD, Cross SS, Hurlstone DP, et al. Pre-endoscopy serological testing for coeliac disease: evaluation of a clinical decision tool. *BMJ*. 2007; 334(7596):729.

59. Coeliac Working Group of British Society of Paediatric Gastroenterology Hepatology and Nutrition (BSPGHAN). Guideline for the diagnosis and management of coeliac disease in children. Available at http://www.bspghan.org.uk; 2006.

60. Bond JH, Levitt MD. Use of breath hydrogen (H_2) in the study of carbohydrate absorption. *Am J Dig Dis*. 1977;22(4):379–382.

61. Niggemann B, Grüber C. Unproven diagnostic procedures in IgE-mediated allergic diseases. *Allergy*. 2004;59:806–808.

62. Committee on Toxicity of Chemicals in Food, Consumer Products and the Environment. *Adverse Reactions to Food and Food Ingredients*. London: Food Standards Agency; 2000.

63. Sampson HA. Food allergy. *J Allergy Clin Immunol*. 2003;111: S540–S547.

64. Sicherer SH, Teuber SS. Academy practice paper: current approaches to the diagnosis and management of adverse food reactions. *J Allergy Clin Immunol*. 2004;114: 1146–1150.

65. Minford AMB, MacDonald A, Littlewood JM. Food intolerance and food allergy in children: a review of 68 cases. *Arch Dis Child*. 1982;67: 474–477.

66. Niggemann B, Beyer K. Diagnostic pitfalls in food allergy in children. *Allergy*. 2005;60:104–107.

67. Sicherer SH. In vivo diagnosis: skin testing and challenge procedures. In: Metcalfe DD, Sampson HJ, Simon RA, eds. *Food Allergy: Adverse Reactions to Foods and Food Additives*. Oxford: Blackwell; 2003:104–117.

68. Sicherer SH, Noone SA, Muñoz-Furlong A. The impact of childhood food allergy on quality of life. *Ann Allergy Asthma Immunol*. 2001;87: 461–464.

69. Bindslev-Jensen C, Ballmer-Webber BK, Bengtsson U, et al. Standardisation of food challenges in patients with immediate reactions to foods—position paper from the European Academy of Allergology and Clinical Immunology. *Allergy*. 2004;59(7): 690–697.

70. Ballmer-Weber BK, Vieths S, Luttkopf D, Heuschmann P, Wüthrich B. Celery allergy confirmed by double-blind, placebo-controlled food challenge. *J Allergy Clin Immunol*. 2000;106(2):373–378.

71. Vlieg-Boerstra BJ, Bijleveld CM, van der Heide S, et al. Development and validation of challenge materials for double-blind, placebo-controlled food challenges in children. *J Allergy Clin Immunol*. 2004;113:341–346.

72. Noè D, Bartemucci L, Mariani N, Cantari D. Practical Aspects of preparation of foods for double-blind, placebo-controlled food challenge. *Allergy*. 1998;53(suppl 46):75–77.

73. Sicherer SH. Food allergy: when and how to perform oral food challenges. *Pediatr Allergy Immunol*. 1999;10:226–234.

74. Niggemann B. Role of oral food challenges in the diagnostic work-up of food allergy in atopic eczema dermatitis syndrome. *Allergy*. 2004;59(suppl 78):32–34.

75. Chong S, Worm M, Zuberbier T. Role of adverse reaction to food in urticaria and exercise-induced anaphylaxis. *Int Arch Allergy Immunol*. 2002;129:19–26.

76. Ewan PW, Clark AT. IgE mediated food allergy: when is food challenge needed? *Arch Dis Child*. 2005;90: 555–556.

77. Lin XP, Magnusson J, Ahlstedt S, et al. Local allergic reaction in food-hypersensitive adults despite a lack of systemic food-specific IgE. *J Allergy Clin Immunol*. 2002;109: 879–887.

78. Directive 2003/89/EC of the European Parliament and of the Council of 10 November 2003 amending Directive 2000/13/EC as regards indication of the ingredients present in foodstuffs. *OJ L*. 2003; 308:15–18.

79. Commission Directive 2006/142/EC of 22 December 2006 amending Annex IIIa of Directive 2000/13/EC of the European Parliament and of the Council listing the ingredients which must under all circumstances appear on the labelling of foodstuffs. *OJ L*. 2006;368:110–111.

80. Food Standards Agency. *Nut Allergy Labelling—Report of Research into the Consumer Response*. Food Standards Agency; 2002.

81. Pumphrey RSH. Lessons for management of anaphylaxis from a study of fatal reactions. *Clin Exp Allergy*. 2000;30:1144–1150.

82. Eigenmann PA, Caubert JC, Zamora SA. Continuing food-avoidance diets after negative food challenges. *Pediatr Allergy Immunol*. 2006;17:601–605.

83. De Blok BMJ, Vlieg-Boerstra BJ, Oude Elberink JN, et al. A framework for measuring the social impact of food allergy across Europe: a EuroPrevall state of the art paper. *Allergy*. 2007;62(7): 733–737.

84. Sampson MA, Munoz-Furlong Anne, Sicherer SH.

Risk-taking and coping strategies of adolescents and young adults with food allergy. *J Allergy Clin Immunol.* 2006; 117(6):1440–1445.

85. Walker S, Sheikh A. Managing anaphylaxis: effective emergency and long-term care are necessary. *Clin Exp Allergy.* 2003;33: 1015–1018.

86. Boyano-Martínez T, García-Ara C, Díaz-Pena JM, Esteban MM. Prediction of tolerance on the basis of quantification of egg white-specific IgE antibodies in children with egg allergy. *J Allergy Clin Immunol.* 2002;110:304–309.

87. Ross MP, Ferguson M, Street D, Klontz K, Schroeder T, Luccioli S. Analysis of food-allergic and anaphylactic events in the National Electronic Injury Surveillance System. *J Allergy Clin Immunol.* 2008;121:166–171.

88. Attaran RR, Probst F. Histamine fish poisoning: a common but frequently misdiagnosed condition. *Emerg Med J.* 2002;19:474–475.

89. Solensky R. Resolution of fish allergy: a case report. *Ann Allergy Asthma Immunol.* 2003;91: 411–412.

90. Helbling A, Haydel R, McCants ML, Musmand JJ, El Dhar J, Lehrer SB. Fish allergy: is cross-reactivity among fish species relevant? Double-blind placebo-controlled food challenge studies of fish allergic adults. *Ann Allergy Asthma Immunol.* 1999;83: 517–523.

91. Van Do, Elsayed S, Florvaag E, Hordvik I, Endresen C. Allergy to fish parvalbumins: studies on the cross-reactivity of allergens from 9 commonly consumed fish. *J Allergy Clin Immunol.* 2005;116: 1314–1320.

92. Reese G, Ayuso R, Lehrer SB. Tropomyosin: an invertebrate pan-allergen. *Int Arch Allergy Immunol.* 1999;119(4):247–258.

93. Bernhisel-Broadbent J, Strause D, Sampson HA. Fish hypersensitivity. II: Clinical relevance of altered fish allergenicity caused by various preparation methods. *J Allergy Clin Immunol.* 1992;90:622–629.

94. Lehrer SB, Kim L, Rice T, Saidu J, Bell J, Martin R. Transfer of shrimp

allergens to other foods through cooking oil. *J Allergy Clin Immunol.* 2007;119(S1):S112.

95. Breiteneder H, Radauer C. A classification of plant food allergens. *J Allergy Clin Immunol.* 2004; 113(5):821–830.

96. Radauer C, Breiteneder H. Evolutionary biology of plant food allergens. *J Allergy Clin Immunol.* 2007;120:518–525.

97. Lack G, Fox D, Northstone K, Golding J. Factors associated with the development of peanut allergy in childhood. *N Engl J Med.* 2003;348(11):977–985.

98. Skolnick HS, Conover-Walker MK, Barnes Koerner C, Sampson HA, Burks W, Wood RA. The natural history of peanut allergy. *J Allergy Clin Immunol.* 2001;107:367–374.

99. Fleischer DM, Conover-Walker MK, Christie L, Burks AW, Wood RA. The natural progression of peanut allergy: resolution and the possibility of recurrence. *J Allergy Clin Immunol.* 2003; 112(1):183–189.

100. Fleischer DM. The natural history of peanut and tree nut allergy. *Curr Allergy Asthma Rep.* 2007;7(3): 175–181.

101. Maloney JM, Chapman MD, Sicherer SH. Peanut allergen exposure through saliva: assessment and intervention to reduce exposure. *J Allergy Clin Immunol.* 2006;118(3): 719–724.

102. Perry TT, Conover-Walker MK, Pomés A, Chapman MD, Wood RA. Distribution of peanut allergen in the environment. *J Allergy Clin Immunol.* 2004;113: 973–976.

103. Pomés A, Butts CL, Chapman MD. Quantification of Ara h 1 in peanuts: why roasting makes a difference. *Clin Exp Allergy.* 2006;36:824–830.

104. Astier C, Morisset M, Roitel O, et al. Predictive value of skin prick tests using recombinant allergens for diagnosis of peanut allergy. *J Allergy Clin Immunol.* 2006; 118(1):250–256.

105. Peeters KABM, Kopplemann SJ, van Hoffen E, et al. Does skin prick test reactivity to purified allergens correlate with clinical severity of

peanut allergy? *Clin Exp Allergy.* 2007;37:108–115.

106. Kleiber-Janke T, Crameri R, Scheurer S, Veiths S, Becker WM. Patient -tailored cloning of allergens by phage display: peanut (Arachis hypogaea) profilin, a food allergen derived from a rare mRNA. *J Chromatogr B Biomed Sci Appl.* 2001;756:295–305.

107. Mittag D, Akkerdass J, Ballmer-Weber B, et al. Ara h 8, a Bet v 1-homologous allergen from peanut, is a major allergen in patients with combined birch pollen and peanut allergy. *J Allergy Clin Immunol.* 2004;114(6):1410–1417.

108. Bock SA, Atkins FM. The natural history of peanut allergy. *J Allergy Clin Immunol.* 1989;83:900–904.

109. Ibáñez MD, Martínez M, Sánchez JJ, Fernández-Caldas E. Legume cross-reactivity. *Allergol Immunopathol (Madr).* 2003;31: 151–161.

110. Peeters KABM, Nordlee JA, Penninks AH, et al. Lupine allergy: not simply cross-reactivity with peanut or soy. *J Allergy Clin Immunol.* 2007;120:647–653.

111. Ewan PW. Clinical study of peanut and nut allergy in 62 consecutive patients: new features and associations. *BMJ.* 1996;312: 1074–1078.

112. Hourihane JO, Kilburn SA, Dean P, Warner JO. Clinical characteristics of peanut allergy. *Clin Exp Allergy.* 1997;27:634–639.

113. Sicherer SH, Furlong TJ, Munoz-Furlong A, Burks AW, Sampson HA. Prevalence of peanut and tree nut allergy in the United States determined by means of a random digit dial telephone survey: a 5-year follow-up study. *J Allergy Clin Immunol.* 2003;112: 1203–1207.

114. Fleischer D, Conover-Walker M, Matsui E, Wood R. The natural history of tree nut allergy. *J Allergy Clin Immunol.* 2005;116: 1087–1093.

115. Clark AT, Ewan PW. The development and progression of allergy to multiple nuts at different ages. *Pediatr Allergy Immunol.* 2005;16:507–511.

116. Clarke AT. Cashew nut causes more severe reactions than peanut: case matched comparison in 141

children. *Allergy*. 2007;62: 913–916.

117. Leduc V, Moneret-Vautrin DA, Tzen JTC, Morisset M, Guerin L, Kanny G. Identification of oleosins as major allergens in sesame seed allergic patients. *Allergy*. 2006;61: 349–356.

118. Morisset M, Moneret-Vautrin DA, Maadi F, et al. Prospective study of mustard allergy: first study with double-blind placebo-controlled food challenge trials (24 cases). *Allergy*. 2003;58:295–299.

119. Breiteneder H, Clare Mills EN. Molecular properties of food allergens. *J Allergy Clin Immunol*. 2006;115:14–23.

120. Fernández-Rivas M, Bolhaar S, González-Moncebo E, et al. Apple allergy across Europe: how allergen sensitisation profiles determine the clinical expression of allergies to plant foods. *J Allergy Clin Immunol*. 2006;118(2):481–488.

121. Pastorello EA, Ortalani C. Oral allergy syndrome. In: Metcalfe DD, Sampson HJ, Simon RA, eds. *Food Allergy: Adverse Reactions to Foods and Food Additives*. Oxford: Blackwell; 2003:425–437.

122. Mari A, Ballmer-Weber BK, Veiths S. The oral allergy syndrome: improved diagnostic and treatment methods. *Curr Opin Allergy Clin Immunol*. 2005;5: 267–273.

123. Veiths S, Scheurer S, Ballmer-Weber B. Current understanding of cross-reactivity of food allergens and pollen. *Ann N Y Acad Sci*. 2002;964:47–68.

124. Hoffmann-Sommergruber K, Radauer C. Bet v 1-homologous allergens. In: Clare Mills EN, Shrewy PR, eds. *Plant Food Allergens*. Oxford: Blackwell Science; 2004.

125. Radauer, Hoffmann-Sommergruber K. Profilins. In: Clare Mills EN, Shrewy PR, eds. *Plant Food Allergens*. Oxford: Blackwell Science; 2004.

126. Ballmer-Weber BK, Veiths S, Luttkopf D, Heuschmann P, Wüthrich B. Celery allergy confirmed by double-blind, placebo-controlled food challenge. *J Allergy Clin Immunol*. 2000; 106(2):373–378.

127. Ballmer-Weber BK, Hoffmann A, Wüthrich B, et al. Influence of food processing on the allergenicity of celery: DBPCFC with celery spice and cooked celery in patients with celery allergy. *Allergy*. 2002;57: 228–235.

128. Fernandez-Rivas M, Cuevas M. Peels of Rosaceae fruits have a higher allergenicity than pulps. *Clin Exp Allergy*. 1999;29:1239–1247.

129. Sancho AL, Foxall R, Browne T, et al. Effect of post harvest storage on the expression of the apple allergen Mal d 1. *J Agric Food Chem*. 2006;54:5917–5923.

130. Veiths S, Jankiewicz A, Schoning B, Aulepp H. Apple allergy: the IgE-binding potency of apple strains is related to the occurrence of the 18-kDa allergen. *Allergy*. 1994;49: 262–271.

131. Salcedo G, Sanchez-Monge R, Diaz-Perales A, Garcia-Casado G, Barber D. Plant non-specific lipid transfer proteins as food and pollen allergens. *Clin Exp Allergy*. 2004;34:1336–1341.

132. des Roches A, Paradis L, Paradis J, Singer S. Food allergy as a new risk factor for scurvy. *Allergy*. 2006;61: 1487–1488.

133. Weichal M, Vergoossen NJ, Bonomi S, et al. Screening the allergenic repertoires of wheat and maize with sera from double-blind, placebo-controlled food challenge positive patients. *Allergy*. 2006; 61:128–135.

134. Matsuo H, Morita E, Tatham AS, et al. Identification of the IgE-binding epitope in omega-5 gliadin, a major allergen in wheat-dependent exercise-induced anaphylaxis. *J Bio Chem*. 2003; 279:12135–12140.

135. Palosuo K. Update on wheat hypersensitivity. *Curr Opin Allergy Clin Immun*. 2003;3(3):185–188.

136. Shibata R, Nishima S, Kohno K, Morita E, Matsuo H, Tanaka A. Specific IgE antibodies to omega-5 gliadin-indicator of what anaphylaxis and its tolerance in wheat sensitised children. *J Allergy Clin Immunol*. 2007;119(1, suppl 1): S120.

137. Matsuo H, Dahlström J, Tanaka A, et al. Sensitivity and specificity of recombinant omega-5 gliadin-

specific IgE measurement for the diagnosis of wheat-dependent exercise-induced anaphylaxis. *Allergy*. 2008;63:233–236.

138. Shahbazkhani B, Forootan M, Merat S, et al. Coeliac disease presenting with symptoms of irritable bowel syndrome. *Aliment Pharmacol Ther*. 2003;18:231–235.

139. National Institute for Health and Clinical Excellence. Irritable bowel syndrome in adults: diagnosis and management of irritable bowel syndrome in primary care. NICE Clinical Guideline 61. 2008.

140. Lucas CD, Hallagan JB, Taylor SL. The role of natural color additives in food allergy. *Adv Food Nutr Res*. 2001;43:195–216.

141. Nettis E, Colanardi MC, Ferrannini A, Tursi A. Suspected tartrazine-induced acute urticaria/angioedema is only rarely reproducible by oral challenge. *Clin Exp Allergy*. 2003;33(12): 1725–1730.

142. Nettis E, Colanardi MC, Ferrannini A, Tursi A. Sodium benzoate-induced repeated episodes of acute urticaria/angio-oedema: randomized controlled trial. *Br J Dermatol*. 2004;151: 898–902.

143. Simon RA. Update on sulfite sensitivity. *Allergy*. 1998;53:72–74.

144. Geha RS, Beiser A, Ren C, et al. Multicenter, double-blind, placebo-controlled, multiple-challenge evaluation of reported reactions to monosodium glutamate. *J Allergy Clin Immunol*. 2000;106:973–980.

145. Swain AR, Dutton SP, Truswell AS. Salicylates in foods. *J Am Diet Assoc*. 1985;85(8):950–960.

146. Scotter MJ, Roberts DPT, Wilson LA, Howard FAC, Davis J, Mansell N. Free salicylic acid and acetyl salicylic acid content of foods using gas chromatography-mass spectrometry. *Food Chem*. 2007; 105:273–279.

147. Tricon S, Willers S, Smit HA, et al. Nutrition and allergic disease. *Clin Exp Allergy Rev*. 2006;6:117–188.

148. Mazer BD, Matush L, Platt R, Vanilovitch I, Kramer M. Does breastfeeding prevent allergic

sensitisation? Results of Probit II. *J Allergy Clin Immunol*. 2007; 119(1, suppl 1):S126.

149. Pesonen M, Kallio MTJ, Ranki A, Simes MA. Prolonged exclusive breastfeeding is associated with increased atopic dermatitis: a prospective follow-up study of unselected healthy newborns from birth to age 20 years. *Clin Exp Allergy*. 2006;36: 1011–1018.

150. Kull I, Bergstrom A, Lilja G, Pershagen G, Wickman M. Fish consumption during the first year of life and development of allergic diseases during childhood. *Allergy*. 2006;61:1009–1015.

151. Poole JA, Barriga K, Leung DYM, et al. Timing of initial exposure to cereal grains and the risk of wheat allergy. *Pediatrics*. 2006;117(6): 2175–2182.

152. Food Allergy and Intolerance Interest group: BDA. Position statement: practical dietary prevention strategies for infants at risk of developing allergic diseases. 2004.

153. Høst A, Halken S, Muraro A, et al. Dietary prevention of allergic diseases in infants and small children. *Pediatr Allergy Immunol*. 2008;19:1–4.

154. Agostoni C, Decsi T, Fewtrell M, et al. Complementary feeding: a commentary by the ESPGHAN Committee on Nutrition. *J Pediatr Gastroenterol Nutr*. 2008;46: 99–110.

155. Bischoff S, Crowe SE. Food allergy and the gastrointestinal tract. *Curr Opin Gastroenterol*. 2004;20: 156–167.

156. Beyer KB, Ellman-Grunther L, Jarvinen KM, Wood RA, Hourihane JO'B, Sampson HA. Measurement of peptide-specific IgE as an additional tool in identifying patients with clinical reactivity to peanuts. *J Allergy Clin Immunol*. 2003;112(1):202–207.

157. Cooke SK, Sampson HA. Allergenic properties of ovomucoid. *J Immunol*. 1997;159:2026–2032.

158. Vila L, Beyer K, Jarvinen KM, Chatchate P, Bardina L, Sampson HA. Role of conformational and linear epitopes in the achievement of tolerance in cow's milk allergy. *Clin Exp Allergy*. 2001;31:1599–1606.

159. Jarvinen KM, Beyer K, Vila L, Bardina L, Mishoe M, Sampson HA. Specificity of IgE antibodies to sequential epitopes of hen's egg ovomucoid as a marker for persistence of egg allergy. *Allergy*. 2007;62:758–765.

160. Battais F, Mothes T, Moneret-Vautrin DA, et al. Identification of IgE-binding epitopes on gliadins for patients with food allergy to wheat. *Allergy*. 2005;60:815–821.

Inflammatory bowel disease (IBD) and colorectal cancer

8

Anne Payne

LEARNING OBJECTIVES

By the end of this chapter the reader will be able to:

- Differentiate between the pathology of Crohn's disease (CD) and ulcerative colitis (UC);
- Discuss the influence of IBD on nutritional status;
- Critically reflect on the rationale for nutritional support in both CD and UC;
- Identify risk factors for colorectal cancer;
- Explain the influence of colorectal cancer on nutritional status; and
- Consider effective dietary strategies for the nutritional management of patients with colorectal cancer.

Inflammatory bowel disease (IBD)

Ulcerative colitis (UC) and Crohn's disease (CD) are chronic inflammatory conditions of the GI tract. UC was described 150 years ago in 1859 by Wilks and CD was first described by Crohn in 1932. Both are painful, debilitating conditions that follow a relapsing–remitting pattern. Despite decades of research, we cannot yet define the exact cause of either form of IBD. Current opinion favours a complex aetiology that predominantly involves genes and the gut microbiology, though other environmental risk factors, including the presence or absence of smoking in CD and UC respectively and a stressful lifestyle, are still of consideration in IBD.[1] It has been postulated that several genetic polymorphisms may contribute to risk of IBD and that these may influence the immune response of the gut to normal microflora. Thus in genetically susceptible individuals, microflora that is normally harmless may induce an abnormal immune response with the production of inflammatory cytokines, including tumour necrosis factor-alfa (TNF-α).[2] TNF-α is known to have a major role in the pathogenesis of CD and may have an influence on the permeability of the mucosa to antigens.[1]

Diagnosis of CD and UC

While UC only affects the colon, CD may occur at any site in the GI tract and though infrequent, can also affect proximal parts of the GI tract including the mouth. Investigation to establish a diagnosis includes endoscopy and haematological tests of inflammation such as C-reactive protein (CRP). In the colon, it can be difficult to distinguish between CD and UC. In the case of UC, endoscopy of the colon reveals a continuous area of lesion that affects the superficial layers of mucosa with no fistulas and very few or no fissures.[3] In UC the rectum is always affected, unlike CD.[4] In CD, inflammation is patchy, often described as having a cobblestone appearance. The inflammation is deep, with fissures and fistulas present. Abscesses and strictures occur in advanced disease. Granulomas, a collection of monocyte/macrophage cells within the lamina propria, are a reliable feature of CD.[5] Active involvement of the ileum occurs in 40% of patients with CD and this is often the feature that differentiates between UC and CD in distal disease. In 25% of patients with CD, the disease is confined to the colon and in 30% the disease is confined to the small intestine.[3]

Both conditions may occur at any age in either sex and their incidence is high in early adulthood. The prevalence of IBD in Europe is approximately 50 per 100,000 with little evidence of a recent increase in incidence. There are wide geographic and racial variations in the incidence of IBD, with a particularly high incidence of CD in American and European Jewish populations while the incidence in Asia and Africa is low.[6]

Influence of IBD on nutritional status

Diarrhoea, abdominal pain and weight loss are the most frequent presenting symptoms of CD. Loss of blood in stools is a feature of UC and may be severe. Blood loss occurs less frequently in CD unless there is active involvement of the colon. Poor oral intake is often regarded as the most likely cause of weight loss and malnutrition in IBD, occurring in up to 80% of patients with CD.[3] The cause of malnutrition in active CD includes inflammation leading to malabsorption and diarrhoea. Inflammation reduces the available surface area for absorption of fluid and nutrients and there is decreased hydrolysis of disaccharides, including lactose which may lead to lactose intolerance.

Active inflammation of the terminal ileum decreases the availability of bile salts for recycling via the liver leading to steatorrhoea and reduced absorption of triglycerides and fat soluble vitamins. Inflammation of the terminal ileum also reduces the absorption of vitamin B_{12} leading to macrocytic anaemia. Abdominal cramps and diarrhoea reduce appetite and there may be associated nausea and vomiting. In both CD and UC patients may associate abdominal pain and diarrhoea with consumption of specific food and so food avoidance may contribute to weight loss and malnutrition. This is of particular concern when food avoidance occurs without dietetic support. Hypoproteinaemia, subclinical serum levels of vitamin A, D, K, C and B group, may occur and low serum levels of minerals such as iron, zinc, magnesium and selenium all contribute to poor wound healing and reduced immune-competence, thus increasing the risk of infection.[7,8]

Both microcytic and macrocytic anaemia are common in CD, related to a combination of poor oral intake, bleeding from the inflamed mucosa and malabsorption of iron, vitamin B_{12} and folate.

A recent Canadian study found subclinical iron deficiency anaemia in 40% of subjects while only 13% had a poor oral intake.[9] The side effects of drug treatment of IBD with sulfasalazine and methotrexate can compound macrocytic anaemia caused by poor absorption of folate (see Chapter 6, Drug–Nutrient Interactions).

Definition of disease severity

There is no standard system to define the severity of disease in IBD and a variety of activity indices are in use. The European Crohn's and Colitis Organisation (ECCO) defines the severity of Crohn's disease in terms of the Crohn's disease activity index (CDAI).[5]

In mild disease, with a CDAI of 150–200, there is < 10% weight loss, with no obstruction, fever, dehydration, abdominal mass or tenderness. The acute phase protein CRP activity may be increased above normal. In moderate disease with a CDAI of 220–450, weight loss may be > 10%, with vomiting. There is no obstruction but CRP is raised above normal.

In severe disease with a CDAI > 450, there may be either advanced cachexia with a BMI < 18 or evidence of obstruction or abscess. Symptoms are persistent and CRP is raised. In contrast, during a period of remission the activity index is usually taken to be < 150.[5]

The extent of weight loss is related to disease activity. The degree of inflammation influences the acute phase stress response, provoking an elevated resting metabolic rate and increased energy requirement. Simultaneously, abdominal pain, diarrhoea and poor appetite conspire to reduce oral intake, increasing risk of weight loss.

The acute phase response may also inhibit the production of nutrient transport proteins in the mucosa and this may indirectly reduce the absorption of nutrients from the gut and influence the immune competence of the gut mucosa. For example, a reduced circulating level of retinol binding protein is related to the acute phase response in CD.[7] In a recent nutritional assessment of patients with IBD, low serum carotene levels were reported in 23% of subjects and there was an inadequate intake of vitamin A in 26% of subjects.[9] Deficiency of vitamin A is known to impair mucosal function in the GI tract through loss of microvilli and through loss of mucin and goblet cells.[8] This leads to an impaired immune response to pathogens and antigens.

When IBD affects the colon, more so than the small intestine, the immune response may not only be confined to the GI tract. Systemic features of inflammation thought to be related to the activity of proinflammatory cytokines may present. These include arthritis, skin ulceration, inflammation of the eye and hepatitis. The influence of proinflammatory cytokines on bone metabolism may increase risk of osteoporosis.[7] Malabsorption of calcium and 25-hydroxycholecalciferol (vitamin D) from the small intestine may also contribute to an increased risk of osteoporosis, compounded by poor dietary intake of calcium and treatment with corticosteroids.[9,10]

Management of Crohn's disease

The management of Crohn's disease requires a coordinated multidisciplinary team (MDT) approach including medical, dietetic, nursing and pharmacology practitioners in tandem with the patient. The disease activity, site and extraintestinal symptoms influence the choice of clinical treatment. The aim of treatment in CD is to reduce inflammation, induce remission and maintain optimal nutritional status. The role of the dietitian as part of the MDT is to assess and monitor nutritional status, to promote nutritional support as an important adjunct to pharmacological treatment, to improve or maintain nutritional status and where indicated, to facilitate nutritional support as a primary therapy in CD.

Drug treatment

In mild CD the corticosteroid budesonide is the preferred pharmacological treatment, achieving remission in 51–60% over 8–10 weeks. Antibiotics are not recommended in mild disease due to side effects that include nausea, metallic taste and polyneuropathy.[10] Prednisolone is very effective and the preferred corticosteroid for moderately active ileocaecal CD, but is associated with more side effects than budesonide.[10]

Extensive disease, affecting more than 100 cm of the small intestine, has a severe impact on nutritional status and so medical treatment involves both corticosteroids and immunomodulators to reduce inflammation and so limit the debilitating consequences of disease on nutritional status. Prednisolone or intravenous hydrocortisone is the initial treatment of choice for severely active ileocaecal CD. Following this, the thiopurine immunomodulators, azathioprine or mercaptopurine, are effective at maintaining remission. However, the side effects of thiopurines include bone marrow toxicity and hepatitis and so blood count and liver function must be monitored every 2–3 months.[4]

When severe ileocaecal disease is resistant to medical treatment, surgery may be considered as a management strategy[10] (please see Chapter 9, Short Bowel Syndrome). In severe disease that is managed conservatively with medication, the potent anti-inflammatory drug infliximab may be considered. This is a chimeric anti-TNF-α monoclonal antibody that binds with this proinflammatory cytokine.[11] Despite the risk of side effects of antibiotics causing nausea and altered taste acuity, thus reducing food intake, they may be necessary when a fever or abscess is present.[10]

Nutritional support

Nutritional support is recommended by the ECCO, in addition to medical treatment, to minimise deterioration in nutritional status due to disease and also prior to surgical intervention to reduce the nutritional risk associated with short bowel syndrome.[10]

ECCO recommend that we distinguish between:

- The role of nutritional support as a primary therapy in CD; and
- The role of nutritional support as an important adjunct to improve or maintain nutritional status.

Liquid diets

The use of liquid diets for nutritional support, as a primary therapy in CD to induce remission, is a well-established treatment. It was introduced during the 1970s to help manage active disease and it may be the treatment of choice for some patients as it reduces exposure to the harmful effect of corticosteroid treatment.[12] Studies have compared the efficacy of elemental, semi-elemental and whole protein liquid preparations to both induce and maintain remission and there is no clear evidence of benefit of one over the other.[13] While the exact nature of the action of nutritional therapy is unclear, its efficacy is thought to transcend improvement in nutritional status and gut rest. It has been suggested that nutritional therapy may influence the inflammatory response of the gut and have a direct immunomodulatory effect by influencing the production of cytokines that act on the microflora of the gut.[2]

A recent Cochrane systematic review suggests that the corticosteroid prednisolone is a more effective treatment for inducing remission than nutritional therapy.[14] For this reason ECCO does not recommend nutrition as a primary therapy in CD, other than in mild disease or in patients who decline drug therapy. They recommend that nutritional therapy is not appropriate as a sole therapy for inducing remission in corticosteroid refractory or corticosteroid-dependent disease, but it may be taken as an adjunct to improve nutritional status.[10]

However, in a recent review of the use of liquid diets in CD, it is argued that if clinical trials were to take account of the issue of compliance, liquid diets would be as effective a means of inducing remission as corticosteroids. It was identified that the ECCO guidance excludes patients with active disease who may benefit from it and discourages consideration of nutritional therapy by gastroenterologists, especially as clinics tend to have poor dietetic support.[15] Many patients do not complete treatment due to a dislike of the taste of products, taste fatigue, boredom on liquid diets or poor support and lack of regular dietetic contact. However, in patients who do comply and complete the treatment, the remission rate in studies has been shown to be as high as 85%.[15]

Practical considerations of liquid diets

When it is decided to offer a patient nutritional therapy to induce remission as a primary treatment, practical considerations include:

- Patient comprehension;
- Motivation;
- Taste preference;
- Composition of available formula; and
- Toleration of formula.

On the basis of taste, whole protein formulas such as Modulen IBD (Nestlé) or Alicalm (Nutricia) are usually the liquid treatments of choice and preferred if taken orally. Semi-elemental products, such as Elemental 028 (SHS International), may be best tolerated if taken via the nasogastric route. The quantity of feed and total fluid should aim to provide adequate energy, nitrogen and micronutrient requirements to maintain nutritional status and fluid balance.

- When the feed commences, all normal food should be withdrawn.
- The liquid feed should be sipped slowly and gradually increased in volume over 3–4 days to maximise toleration.
- Permitted oral fluids, such as water and other clear fluids, may also be sipped to maintain an adequate fluid intake until the full volume feed is taken daily.

Oral liquid feeds can be introduced and managed in the outpatient setting; otherwise a short admission period is required to establish nasogastric feeding. Not surprisingly, tiredness, hunger, diarrhoea and weight loss are frequently experienced and may limit compliance.[16] If nutritional therapy is tolerated with good compliance there are usually signs of improvement in symptoms within 2 weeks and remission is achieved within 4 weeks.

The LOFFLEX diet

Protocols for return to normal eating vary between gastroenterology units and for many years have been based on the possibility that specific foods may have a precipitating role in the aetiology of CD. While there is no evidence that food intolerance per se is a causative agent in CD, an elimination diet has been shown to be effective in prolonging remission, relative to treatment with steroids.[12] The LOFFLEX diet is a well-established low fat, low fibre diet based on a modified elimination regimen.[17] This includes foods normally well tolerated in CD, such as rice, potato, chicken and fish for up to 4 weeks. The addition of supplementary nutritional sip feeds ensure nutritional adequacy. Other foods are then introduced at 4-day intervals over a period of 3–4 weeks until a full normal diet is resumed.

While the mode of action of the LOFFLEX regime is not known, it has been found to be as effective as an elimination diet in maintaining remission in CD. In a recent Cochrane review of enteral nutrition for the maintenance of remission in Crohn's disease, two small studies were evaluated.[13] In one Japanese study, 26 subjects received half of their nutritional requirements by normal diet and half by nutritional support, in comparison to the control group of 25 subjects who followed a normal diet. After almost

12 months only 9 subjects receiving nutritional support had relapsed (35%), compared to 16 on full normal diet (64%). The second study undertaken in the UK evaluated 33 adults with CD who received their energy and nutritional requirements as 35–50% normal diet, supplemented with either a semi-elemental sip feed or whole protein sip feed. This study found no difference in relapse rate between the two sip feeds. However, it did not compare them to normal diet alone. The Cochrane review concludes that these studies suggest that supplementary enteral nutrition with either semi-elemental or whole protein formula may be effective for maintaining remission in CD. While the above studies are small and larger trials are needed, this conclusion supports the use of nutritional support for all patients with CD whether experiencing active CD or during remission, to both enhance nutritional status and as an adjunctive primary therapy for CD. It is feasible that the LOFFLEX diet is effective, not because it reduces intake of poorly tolerated food substances during inflammation, such as fibre or because it may eliminate food allergens, but because it encourages the continuation of nutritional support during a further period of 2–4 weeks of remission.

Omega-3 fatty acids

The role of other forms of nutritional therapy has been studied in Crohn's disease, including the efficacy of omega-3 fatty acids as fish oil capsules (omega-3 therapy) for maintenance of remission, due to their anti-inflammatory properties. The omega-3 fatty acid eicosapentaenoic acid (EPA) may act by reducing the production of the leukotriene B_4.[10] A recent Cochrane review of four studies, involving 166 patients, found a non-statistically significant benefit of omega-3 therapy, taken as capsules, for maintenance of remission. The authors conclude that the evidence does not merit recommending the routine use of omega-3 therapy in CD, but taken as enteric coated capsules, is safe and may be an effective adjunct for the maintenance of remission in CD.[18]

Probiotics and prebiotics

The role of probiotics in the management of IBD has been investigated in recent years, in parallel with studies to investigate the role of the gut microflora in IBD. In a recent study of 15 people with CD and 5 with UC, the anti-inflammatory effect of probiotic yoghurt was investigated and the results compared to 20 healthy control subjects.[19] All subjects consumed probiotic yoghurt for 30 days and a significant increase in protective T cells in the peripheral blood of IBD patients was found and an improved anti-inflammatory profile including a decrease in serum TNF-α. However, it is suggested that further studies are required to confirm the immunosuppressive action of probiotic yoghurt in IBD. Whether prebiotics, in the form of inulin and oligofrucose, have a protective role in inflammatory disease has also been reviewed as they are known to support growth of the colonic bacteria lactobacilli and bifidobacteria, to promote homeostatis of the gut ecosystem. Early clinical trials suggest that these prebiotics may be effective to treat colonic inflammation in CD and UC.[20]

Management of ulcerative colitis

The management of UC also requires a coordinated multidisciplinary approach in tandem with the patient, including medical, dietetic, nursing and pharmacology practitioners. The aim of treatment in UC is to reduce inflammation of the colon, induce remission, support the management of bowel function and maintain optimal nutritional status.

Drug treatment

In UC the most frequent pharmacological treatment is the anti-inflammatory drug aminosalicylate (5-ASA), indicated for UC of mild to moderate severity and during periods of remission. This drug is available in several forms, as enemas, suppositories or oral form and choice will depend on the site and severity of disease. Though usually well tolerated, a range of side effects from mild, such as headache, to severe, such as renal involvement, necessitates close medical monitoring.[4]

As with CD, corticosteroids such as prednisolone may be prescribed for more severe disease. Total colitis requires hospital admission and treatment with IV hydrocortisone and oral 5-ASA. Enteral nutrition support and IV fluids are usually required in preference to parenteral nutrition (see Chapters 10 and 11, Enteral Nutrition and Parenteral Nutrition, respectively).

Nutritional support

The role of the dietitian as part of the MDT is to assess and monitor nutritional status and to facilitate nutritional support when indicated, to improve or maintain nutritional status. Unlike CD, there is no indication for use of nutritional support as a primary therapy in UC. Weight loss may occur due to chronic abdominal cramp, diarrhoea and poor appetite during periods of relapse and anaemia is common due to poor oral intake and blood loss in stools. Patients should undergo nutritional screening with an appropriate nutritional screening tool, such as MUST, in an outpatient clinic or on admission to hospital and referred for nutritional support, as indicated.[21]

The rationale for nutritional support in patients at risk of malnutrition is outlined in the 2006 NICE Clinical Guideline 32, Nutrition Support in Adults.[22] This include a review of the physical and psycho-social side effects of malnutrition and the following are of particular relevance in IBD: impaired immune response, impaired wound healing, reduced muscle strength and fatigue, water and electrolyte disturbance, vitamin and mineral deficiencies and impaired psycho-social function. In patients requiring oral nutrition support who are not at risk of re-feeding syndrome, aim to provide:

- 25–35 kcal/kg/day total energy;
- 0.8–1.5 g protein (0.13–0.24 g nitrogen/kg/day);
- 30–35 mL fluid/kg; and
- Adequate electrolytes, micronutrients and fibre, as appropriate.

Unfortunately there is a lack of clinical evidence to underpin the efficacy of nutritional support for management of malnutrition in IBD. A recent Cochrane review, entitled 'Dietary Advice for Illness-Related Malnutrition in Adults', included only one study of patients with CD and none with UC.[23] This report examines dietary advice as food products, oral nutritional supplements or both, in 36 studies involving 2714 people with disease-related malnutrition, often cancer. Pooled results from four studies suggest that dietary supplements are more effective than food advice to improve weight and energy intake. From examination of five studies they report a significantly greater weight gain in groups receiving dietary advice plus supplements than either dietary advice or supplements alone. These were small short-term studies and did not include patients with UC; however, the authors conclude that there is insufficient information to suggest that nutritional intervention should vary according to the underlying condition.[23]

Food intolerance

Many patients follow self-imposed dietary restrictions because they associate their symptoms with certain foods. Fruit and vegetables with a high content of dietary fibre may be poorly tolerated and so patients tend to choose a low fibre diet. They often also avoid fried foods and spicy foods. Although lactose intolerance is rare in UC, dairy foods are often perceived to exacerbate symptoms. While maintaining respect for the patient's view, acceptable alternative sources of calcium and vitamin D should be discussed and encouraged and small quantities of dairy foods included as tolerated. Adequacy of intake of energy, protein, micronutrient and fluid must be considered, as outlined above.[22]

The use of probiotics in UC to induce remission

A recent Cochrane report has reviewed studies comparing the use of probiotics in combination with placebo or standard medical treatment (5-ASAs, sulfasalazine or corticosteroids) for induction of remission in ulcerative colitis.[24] A meta-analysis was not performed due to the differences in methodology between the trials considered. The authors conclude that there is limited evidence that probiotics may reduce disease activity in mild to moderate UC when taken with standard treatment, but they do not improve overall remission rates. Their effect in severe UC is unknown.[23] Larger randomised control trials are required.

Surgery in UC

Surgery may be indicated in UC if the patient does not respond to treatment as indicated by a raised temperature, falling Hb, potassium and albumen, raised white cell count and bloody diarrhoea, or if toxic dilation of the colon occurs in advanced disease.[11] Surgery of the colon can take the form of total colectomy with the formation of a permanent ileostomy or of a partial colectomy. In acute disease, a partial colectomy may be performed with the formation of a temporary ileostomy and retention of the rectum. This permits reversal of the ileostomy at a later date, by formation of an ileoanal anastomosis. For further information see Chapter 9, Short Bowel Syndrome.

Colorectal cancer

Colorectal cancer is also strongly associated with IBD and risk is related to duration of disease in both UC and CD with an 18% incidence of carcinoma after 30 years duration of IBD.[25] Tumours may occur anywhere in the colon but are most frequently present in the caecum, sigmoid colon or rectum. While most cases of colorectal cancer are sporadic about 20% of patients probably have a component of familial risk.[25] It most frequently occurs in people over 50 years but a family history of bowel cancer in first degree relatives under 45 years indicates a high risk factor for disease. The two main hereditary types of colorectal cancer are hereditary non-polyposis colorectal cancer (HNPCC) and familial adenomatous polyposis (FAP). Both are caused by an autosomal-dominant mutation of genes.

On a global scale, the 5-year survival rate from colorectal cancer mirrors access to specialist care and the availability of modern drug therapy. It is the world's fourth most frequent cause of cancer death.[25] In the USA the 5-year survival rate is over 60% but it is only 40% in less developed countries.[25] It is more common in men than women and the average age at diagnosis is 65 years, with age being the greatest risk factor for sporadic colorectal cancer.[26] In women in the UK it is second only to breast cancer in prevalence and in men, after prostate or lung cancer, the third most common cancer, with an average lifetime risk of 5% and an incidence rate of 44.3 per 100,000 population.[26] Surprisingly, 5-year survival rates are lower in the UK compared to the European average of 50% and this is thought to be related to a greater delay in presentation to medical services rather than poor medical care.[26]

Other identified risk factors for colorectal cancer include:

- Diet;
- Smoking; and
- Low physical activity level.

The use of hormone replacement therapy and non-steroidal anti-inflammatory medication (NSAIDs), such as aspirin, may be protective of colorectal cancer.

The relationship between diet and risk of colorectal cancer

World cancer research fund (WRCF) report

In 2007, the World Cancer Research Fund (WRCF) in partnership with the American Institute for Cancer Research published an extensive global review of the relationship between food, nutrition, physical activity and the prevention of cancer.[27] Their findings on red meat and processed meat, fruit, vegetables, dairy foods and alcohol are of particular interest. This report advises that there is a substantial amount of evidence to indicate that red meat and processed meat are a convincing cause of colorectal cancer. It found that the available evidence for fruit and non-starchy vegetables was inconsistent, providing limited evidence to suggest that they are protective for colorectal cancer.

Fruit and vegetables

More recent evidence from two large studies provides greater support for a protective association of fruit and vegetables with colorectal cancer.[28,29] The Prostate, Lung, Colorectal and Ovarian (PLCO) Cancer Screening Trial included over 30,000 participants aged 55–74 years who provided dietary information by Food Frequency Questionnaire (FFQ), to compare with the results of histological screening for adenoma in the distal colon.[28] Men and women in the highest quintile consumed 5.7 portions of fruit daily, compared to 1.2 in the lowest quintile and had a statistically significant decrease in risk of adenoma in the colon (not rectum) that remained after adjustment for non-dietary risk factors.[28] A significant protective effect was also found for deep-yellow vegetables, onion and garlic but the relationship with green vegetables was weaker.

The results of the National Institute of Health–AARP Diet and Health Study were published in 2008.[29] This study of over 500,000 men and women strengthens the evidence of a relationship between colorectal cancer and intake of fruit and vegetables, but gender differences emerged. Data were collected by FFQ and fruit and vegetables were combined for data analysis. A high intake of fruit and vegetables was associated with reduced colorectal incidence in men and was found to offer protection in women but this was not significant in women on multivariate statistical analysis.[29] It is of note that this study found no relationship between red and processed meats and colorectal cancer. FFQ methodology incurs a high risk of measurement error, lifestyle bias and unknown risk factors that the authors stress could readily confound the relationship between food intake and disease risk.

Dietary fibre, sugar and the glycaemic load

The relationship between dietary carbohydrate and colorectal cancer risk has also been extensively studied; this includes the role of dietary fibre, sugar and the glycaemic load (GL).[30] It was proposed by Burkitt over 30 years ago that dietary fibre may reduce risk of colorectal cancer. The mechanism is unclear but may be related to decreased transit time of rate of flow of the food stream through the colon or reduced absorption of bile acids. While the prevailing opinion is that dietary fibre possibly reduces risk, the results of prospective clinical trials do not consistently support this hypothesis, when adjusted for diet and lifestyle confounding variables.[31]

There is insufficient evidence available in relation to sugar and the glycaemic load to draw any conclusion in relations to risk of colorectal cancer.[31] In an interesting multiethnic cohort study involving over 200,000 people in the US aged 45–75 years, followed up for 8 years, total carbohydrate intake and food with a high glycaemic load, as measured by FFQ, appeared to be protective of colorectal cancer in women, but not men.[31] This is contrary to the outcome of earlier studies that suggest greater risk is associated with high GL and the authors propose that the source of carbohydrate may be of relevance to risk, as women in this study were largely eating white rice.

Soy and soy products

The relationship between soy and health has been extensively studied over the past decade. As soy is a rich source of many nutrients including protein, dietary fibre, carbohydrate and isoflavones, it potentially has a complex relationship with bowel health. A comprehensive recent study, the Shanghai Women's Health Study, has investigated the relationship

between soy intake and risk of colorectal cancer in almost 75,000 women age 40–70 years. Soy intake was assessed using a validated FFQ with 11 soy items including, for example, soy milk, tofu, and fresh and dried soy beans. This study found that each 5 g/day increment of dry soy food, equivalent to 28 g/1 oz of tofu per day, was associated with an 8% reduction in risk in postmenopausal women, suggesting that soy food may reduce the risk of colorectal cancer in postmenopausal women.[32]

Calcium and dairy foods

Intake of calcium and dairy foods has also been linked to risk of colorectal cancer. Gender differences in pattern of risk appear to be emerging.[33–35] A Swedish study of 45,000 men age 45–79 years, by FFQ, found that both dietary calcium intake and consuming upwards of seven portions of dairy foods daily, compared to those taking less than two portions daily, was associated with a lower risk of colorectal cancer.[33] A further Japanese study including almost 75,000 men and women also found a significant decrease in risk of colorectal cancer with high intakes of dietary calcium in men.[34] No clear association was observed in women.[34] While dietary calcium has been the main focus of research investigating the link between dairy foods and colorectal cancer, other nutrients may have a chemo-protective role including vitamin D, conjugated linoleic acid (CLA) and probiotics but evidence in humans remains inconclusive.[35] Evidence from animal studies suggests that the production of lactic acid by probiotic bacteria may protect against tumour development in the colon but further research in humans is required to more clearly identify possible protective mechanisms and relevant strains of probiotic bacteria.[36]

Fat intake and *trans* fatty acids

The WCRF report of 2007 advises that there is a limited amount of fairly consistent evidence to suggest that consumption of foods containing animal fats is a cause of colorectal cancer.[27] The National Institute of Health–AARP Diet and Health Study also reports that a fat-reduced food pattern of eating was associated with a reduced cancer incidence in men, but the association was not significant in women.[29] A small number of studies in both humans and animals have specifically examined intake of *trans* fatty acids in relation to colon cancer. *Trans* fatty acids are predominantly found in spreads and commercial baked goods containing hydrogenated vegetable fats. These studies provide inadequate evidence to draw any conclusion on whether *trans* fatty acids enhance the development of colorectal tumours.[37]

Obesity and body mass index

Nutritional status is of relevance to colorectal cancer as a risk factor for cause and a risk factor for recovery. Body Mass Index (BMI) is known to be associated with greater cancer risk, including risk of colon cancer and breast cancer in women, and the extent of risk is now known to be age related. A UK study of 1.3 million women between 1996 and 2001 aged 50–64 years found the effect of BMI on risk was significantly related to menopausal status and concludes that 5% of all cancers in postmenopausal women are attributable to being overweight or obese.[38] A recent meta-analysis of prospective studies for risk of obesity in colorectal cancer of both men and women found a significant association with colon cancer in both sexes, but the relationship was stronger in men.[39] It is proposed that hormonal status is relevant to both men and women with oestrogen being protective in women and testosterone protective in men.[39] BMI was found to be positively associated with rectal cancer in men but not women.[39]

Symptoms of colorectal cancer

Symptoms of colorectal cancer are highly varied, depending on the site of the tumour and the severity of disease activity. These typically include:

- Change in bowel habit: either persistent diarrhoea or constipation may occur;
- Blood in stools;
- Rectal bleeding;
- Abdominal pain in some cases;
- Anaemia;
- Weight loss;
- Faecal incontinence;
- Intestinal obstruction; and
- Mass in rectum on physical examination.

Iron deficiency anaemia in men and postmenopausal women is an indication for urgent investigation of cause as 10% of patients will have colorectal cancer, most likely on the right side of the colon.[26] A change in bowel habit may indicate a left-sided cancer caused by narrowing of the lumen with diarrhoea, progressing to bowel obstruction.[26]

Diagnosis of colorectal cancer

There are advantages and disadvantages to the three methods for the diagnosis of colorectal cancer: traditional colonoscopy, computed tomography and flexible sigmoidoscopy. They all ideally require patients to undergo bowel preparation regimes to cleanse the bowel prior to examination and so maximise sensitivity of detection of colon cancer to 97%. The method of choice for the majority of patients is colonoscopy, regarded as the gold standard though it has the highest risk of perforation, at 2:1000. Flexible sigmoidoscopy has a lower risk of perforation but can only examine the left colon. In the frail elderly who often poorly tolerate bowel preparation regimes, radiological examination by plain computed tomography, without the need for bowel preparation, has a sensitivity of 88–94%.[26] In addition to colonoscopy, abdominal ultrasound, chest radiography and a physical examination are also performed.[25]

Early diagnosis of disease greatly improves the 5-year survival rate. However, patients often tolerate the symptoms of disease for many months, either unaware or reluctant to accept they may have a serious condition that requires investigation. The patients prognosis and medical treatment regimen depends on the site, size, nature of tumour and whether lymph node involvement is identified on examination. The traditional Dukes system of classification of colorectal tumours is currently used in tandem with a relatively new diagnostic scale termed the TNM classification.[26]

Table 8.1 indicates that the 5-year survival rate at stage 1 (Dukes A) is high, at 80–95% when the tumour is confined to the submucosa and muscularis propria. However, in stage 4 (Dukes D), 5-year survival is as little as 5–7%, if distant metastases are identified. These may occur, for example, in the liver or the lungs.[25]

Treatment of colorectal cancer

Only complete removal of the tumour by surgery can lead to complete recovery from colorectal cancer; hence this is the treatment of choice for over 80% of patients. This is often followed by chemotherapy to destroy any remaining cancerous cells. For patients

Table 8.1 Staging and survival of colorectal cancers

TNM classification		Modified Dukes classification		5-year survival (%)
Stage I (N0, M0)	Tumours invade submucosa	T1	A	80–95
	Tumours invade muscularis propria	T2		
Stage IIA (N0, M0)	Tumours invade into subserosa	T3	B	72–85
IIB	Tumours invade directly into other organs	T4		65–66
Stage III (M0)	T1, T2 + 1–3 regional lymph nodes involved	N1	C	55–65
IIIB	T3, T4 + 1–3 regional lymph nodes involved	N1		35–42
IIIC	Any T + 4 or more regional lymph nodes	N2		25–27
Stage IV	Any T, any N + distant metastases	M1	D	5–7

From: Kumar P and Clark M (eds), *Clinical Medicine*, 6th edn. Edinburgh: Elsevier Saunders, 2005, p 331, Table 6.17.

with rectal cancer, radiotherapy is also indicated to reduce recurrence and improve survival rate. The evidence to support the use of adjunct radiotherapy for the post-surgical treatment of colon cancer is weak; however, radiotherapy may be used as a treatment to inhibit the spread of a tumour in preference to surgery.[25]

Surgical resection of liver or pulmonary metastases can also increase the 5-year survival rate to 35–58% and palliative chemotherapy with a new generation of cytotoxic drugs also aim to improve long-term survival and quality of life.[25]

The influence of disease on nutritional status

Weight loss occurs in the majority of patients with colorectal cancer. It is an early indicator of malnutrition and together with anaemia influences both functional ability and quality of life.[40] Early symptoms of disease, such as persistent diarrhoea, can reduce appetite and inhibit oral intake. This may be compounded by anxiety, intestinal obstruction, abdominal pain, nausea, malabsorption and fatigue as the disease progresses. The term cancer cachexia refers to loss of body fat and skeletal muscle leading to weight loss, muscle atrophy, muscle weakness and both physical and mental fatigue and has its roots in the early stages of disease. It is associated with alteration in protein, lipid and carbohydrate metabolism, impaired immune response to infection and impaired wound healing and may shorten survival.[41,42]

The relationship between weight loss, disease and fatigue is complex. Fatigue is reported to affect 70% of patients and is a common symptom of cancer.[40] Its psychological symptoms include pain, depression and sleep disorders. Weight loss is due in part to poor oral intake but may also be influenced by the systemic inflammatory response to disease, progressive tumour growth and the catabolic side effects of conventional therapy for cancer, causing a reduction in food intake and altered metabolism.[41,42] While the inflammatory effects of the tumour tend to enhance metabolism, the influence of fatigue is to reduce physical activity; thus energy expenditure does not necessarily increase.[41] Proinflammatory cytokines such as TNF are believed to play a key role as mediators in cancer cachexia. Interleukin-6 (IL-6) has been associated with weight loss and the acute phase inflammatory response in colorectal cancer.[41]

A recent investigation of the relationship between anaemia, unintentional weight loss and inflammatory status on cancer-related fatigue in 164 patients, where one-third of patients had colon cancer found that 32% were anaemic and 47% had lost more than 5% of body weight prior to treatment.[40] Weight loss and anaemia were significantly correlated with both fatigue and quality of life. Unintentional weight loss was also significantly correlated with inflammatory status, as measured by levels of CRP.[40] Because of its sensitivity, specificity and relative ease of measurement, CRP is frequently used to assess the level of systemic inflammatory response in cancer. In the systemic inflammatory response, hepatocytes preferentially synthesize acute phase proteins such as CRP and reduce synthesis of albumen. The magnitude of this inverse relationship between CRP and albumin level is independent of tumour stage and is a predictor of survival.[43] There is evidence that elevated CRP, in combination with hypoalbuminaemia, can be used as an independent indicator of prognosis in primary operable colorectal cancer.[43]

Treatment for cancer tends to have an inhibitory effect on appetite, with altered taste perception and early satiety. This may be caused by opiates following surgery, chemotherapy or radiotherapy. Appetite stimulants, such as the steroid prednisolone, may be taken as a treatment for anorexia but their side effects, such as fluid retention and insulin resistance, limit their use. It has been found that in colorectal cancer patients, levels of acute phase proteins, IL-6 and cortisol can be reduced with the NSAID ibuprofen, but this drug can be poorly tolerated in the gut, limiting its application.[41]

There is currently interest in the manipulation of appetite by hormones to treat cachexia. It has been proposed that the gut hormone ghrelin could be of potential future benefit as an appetite stimulant.[44] It acts on the hypothalamus to stimulate the release of neuropeptides, stimulating appetite. It is also thought to have an anti-inflammatory effect that may be of therapeutic benefit in cachexia.[44] However, further research in this field is required.

Nutritional care in colorectal cancer

Nutritional screening on admission to a surgical unit will identify those who have experienced weight loss and are at risk of malnutrition, to enable presurgical nutritional support to commence. Weight loss prior to surgery has been identified as a risk factor for complications. Periods of fasting in preparation for colonoscopy and surgery add to this risk. Nutritional care in bowel surgery is considered in Chapter 9, Short Bowel Syndrome.

If treatment involves radiotherapy then abdominal pain, malabsorption, diarrhoea and a poor appetite may cause further weight loss for up to 4 weeks following a period of treatment. Antidiarrhoeal medication may be required to reduce the motility of the remaining colon. Nutritional care should aim to maintain a good fluid and electrolyte intake. Oral nutritional support is usually required to ensure an adequate energy intake.[45] This should focus on:

- Small frequent meals and snacks;
- Fortification of food;
- Nourishing drinks; and
- Proprietary sip feeds, if indicated and if tolerated.

As outlined in the NICE Clinical Guideline 32, Nutrition Support in Adults (2006),[22] nutritional care should aim to provide:

- 25–35 kcal/kg/day total energy;
- 0.8–1.5 g protein (0.13–0.24 g nitrogen/kg/day);
- 30–35 mL fluid/kg;
- Adequate electrolytes and micronutrients; and
- Dietary fibre, as tolerated.

If chemotherapy is indicated, the side effects of diarrhoea and anorexia can be anticipated during the treatment period. Nausea may occur, exacerbated by rich fatty foods and the odour of cooking, so cold snacks may be preferred. Mucositis is a painful side effect of chemotherapy caused by the anti-mitotic effect of treatment on the mucosa. Antibiotic therapy and an antiseptic mouthwash may be required and supplementary enteral feeds or fluids indicated, if pain causes difficulty with swallowing. The sipping of sharp-flavoured drinks can help to stimulate saliva and so promote a better oral intake. The strong flavour of pineapple chunks or fruit juice may help a dry mouth.[46]

In all stages of the patient's care pathway, the dietitian has a key role to play in promoting optimal health and well being. While nutritional screening will identify patients for referral to the dietitian, a dietetic care plan requires a full nutritional assessment of the patient, including weight history, BMI, influences on food intake (anorexia/appetite, nausea, abdominal pain, bowel habits, food preferences), fluid intake, cooking skills, social influences, carer support and mood/psychological support. A well-considered care plan with ongoing support can greatly ease the nutritional burden of disease. The dietitian is part of a multidisciplinary team involving nursing staff, occupational therapists, physiotherapists, pharmacists and medical practitioners. Each team member has a role to play in promoting and supporting the patient's nutritional care and thus their response to treatment.[45,46]

Conclusions

Inflammatory bowel disease is a chronic debilitating condition that has a profound effect on health and quality of life. The influence of disease on nutritional status is related to the site of inflammation in the GI tract. Extensive disease of the ileum may have a severe consequence on the absorption of nutrients and fluid, leading to malnutrition. Many patients can be managed conservatively by diet or drug treatment but surgical intervention may be the treatment of choice. Extensive surgical resection at this site incurs a high risk of short bowel syndrome.

IBD is a risk factor for colorectal cancer. Both IBD and colorectal cancer have a complex aetiology with familial involvement. Risk of colorectal cancer has been linked to diet. Current evidence suggests that fruit and vegetables may have a protective role along with calcium-rich dairy products in men and soy products in postmenopausal women. Colorectal cancer is most frequently managed by surgical intervention.

Both IBD and colorectal cancer may have a detrimental effect on nutritional status. Nutritional management of both conditions should involve nutritional screening on admission and nutritional support to maintain an optimal intake of energy, nutrients and fluid to minimise disease-related weight loss and malnutrition.

Key points

- The cause of IBD remains obscure. Current theory favours a complex aetiology that links genetic polymorphisms with toleration of the gut microflora and production of proinflammatory cytokines, including TNF-α.
- CD exhibits deep patchy fissures that can occur anywhere in the GI tract, with granuloma present in the lamina propria. UC occurs only in the colon with a continuous lesion affecting the superficial layers of mucosa, extending to the rectum.
- Diarrhoea, abdominal pain, nausea and vomiting are common in IBD. These contribute to poor oral intake, weight loss and malnutrition, occurring in up to 80% of patients with CD. Active inflammation reduces the absorption of nutrients, exacerbating malnutrition. Iron deficiency anaemia is common in CD.
- In CD, ECCO recommends that we distinguish between nutritional support as a primary therapy and nutritional support as an adjunct to improve or maintain nutritional status. Liquid diets have been used as a primary therapy to induce remission in CD since the 1970s but their mode of action is unclear. In both UC and CD nutritional support is frequently indicated to treat weight loss and malnutrition.
- Risk of colorectal cancer is related to duration of disease in IBD. Other risk factors include diet, smoking and low physical activity. The relationship with diet is complex. There is some evidence to suggest that fruit and vegetables may reduce risk while male–female differences have been observed in the outcome of studies looking at dairy foods, soy and body mass index.
- Weight loss and anaemia are early indicators of malnutrition in colorectal cancer. Cachexia is associated with altered metabolism, increased risk of infection, poor wound healing and reduced survival. All forms of treatment incur risk of malnutrition due to poor appetite, altered taste perception and early satiety. Appetite stimulants and anti-inflammatory drugs are of limited value to promote intake due to their side effects.
- Oral nutritional support should aim to promote energy balance and maintain an adequate fluid and electrolyte intake. A personalised patient care plan will take into consideration the stage of illness, symptoms, side effects of treatment, social circumstances, personal preferences and the patient's psychological well being.

Case study

A 64-year-old lady presented to her GP with a 3-month history of abdominal pain, fatigue and diarrhoea with an unintentional weight loss of 6 kg. She was referred to a gastroenterology clinic for colonoscopy and this revealed a diagnosis of Dukes B carcinoma of the sigmoid colon with lymph node involvement. She is normally fit and 'active' and enjoys cooking. She has an unremarkable past medical history, other than ongoing treatment for low back pain. She is a recently retired clerical officer and lives alone with little family support. She was referred for nutritional support and on assessment weighed 59 kg. At a height of 164 cm she has a BMI of 22.

USUAL DIET

Breakfast

Cornflakes with milk, no sugar
1 slice toast with butter and marmalade
Tea with milk, no sugar

Mid-morning

Coffee (no sugar) and chocolate biscuit

Lunch

Home-made sandwich (various fillings)
Low fat yoghurt

Mid afternoon

Fruit or cake

Evening meal

Home cooked meat, chicken or fish
Rice, potato or pasta
Fresh vegetables
Occasional pudding or cake or ice cream

During evening

Glass of wine, crisps

QUESTIONS

1. Outline possible risk factors for this case of colorectal cancer.
2. Discuss the likely reasons for weight loss prior to active treatment.
3. What is the probable effect of treatment for carcinoma on her nutritional status?
4. What are the short- and long-term aims of nutritional care for this lady?
5. Consider a possible strategy to meet the patient's short-term aim of care.

ANSWERS

1. Outline possible risk factors for this case of colorectal cancer.

   This is unlikely to be an inherited familial type of colorectal cancer as the patient is now in her 60s. She has no past medical history of IBD to link to it either. Risk factors for sporadic colorectal cancer relevant to this case include age, low physical activity and low intake of fruit and vegetables.

2. Discuss the likely reasons for weight loss prior to active treatment.

   In the early stage persistent diarrhoea may inhibit appetite. Abdominal pain, nausea and fatigue may compound a poor appetite, leading to weight loss and malnutrition. The systemic inflammatory response to disease causes a production of proinflammatory cytokines such as TNF and IL-6; this may enhance metabolism, increasing energy requirements. On diagnosis, anxiety, fear and uncertainty may also have a profound effect on appetite and motivation for shopping and cooking.

3. What is the probable effect of treatment for carcinoma on her nutritional status?

   Surgical intervention is the primary treatment for colorectal cancer. Periods of fasting prior to colonoscopy and surgery will reduce energy intake. Energy intake will be low in the immediate recovery period and the use of opiates as pain killers will further inhibit energy intake in the recovery phase as they inhibit appetite. Further weight loss is therefore inevitable and may continue for up to four weeks following surgery. As the rectum is not affected radiotherapy is an unlikely treatment choice, but chemotherapy may incur further weight loss as this is a frequent cause of nausea, change in taste perception and fatigue. Mucositis, if it occurs, exacerbates weight loss. With a recent history of 10% weight loss this patient is at high risk of malnutrition prior to treatment and added to this is a strong probability that BMI will fall below 20 in the postsurgical period.

4. What are the short- and long-term aims of nutritional care for this lady?

   The short-term aim is to minimise the degree of treatment-induced malnutrition by establishing:
   - Patient-centred goals to promote energy intake;
   - Maintenance of an adequate fluid and electrolyte intake; and
   - Anti-emetic medication if indicated during chemotherapy.

Continued

Case study (Continued)

The long-term aim is to restore optimal nutritional status. In particular:
- Restore and sustain BMI at 20–25 kg/m; and
- Increase fruit and vegetables to five portions daily.

5. Consider a possible strategy to meet the patient's short-term aim of care.
  - Small frequent meals and snacks: the usual diet provides a template for discussion of between meal snacks such as creamy yoghurt, jellies, full-fat ice-cream, sponge cake, crackers, individual cheese portions, bread and butter. Small cold snacks may be better tolerated than hot cooked meals. Support

with shopping and meal preparation may be required or an five alternative such as a frozen meal delivery service.
  - Fortification of food: extra butter and cream, if tolerated.
  - Nourishing drinks: milky drinks, such as milky coffee and fruit juice. Commercially available sip feeds may be suggested if oral intake remains poor.
  - Proprietary sip feeds: these are unlikely to be required, in this case, if the above strategy is implemented.

References

1. Bengmark S. Bioecological control of inflammatory bowel disease. *Clin Nutr.* 2007;26:169–181.
2. Ferguson RL, Shelling AN, Lauren D. Nutrigenomics and gut health. *Mutat Res.* 2007;622(1–2):1–6.
3. Mpofu C, Ireland A. Inflammatory bowel disease: the disease and its diagnosis. *Hospital Pharmacist.* 2006;13:153–158.
4. Nightingale A. Diagnosis and management of inflammatory bowel disease. *Nurse Prescribing.* 2007;5(7):289–296.
5. Stange EF, Travis SPL, Vermeire S, et al. European evidence based consensus on the diagnosis and management of Crohn's disease: definitions and diagnosis. *Gut.* 2006;55:1–5.
6. Loftus Jr EV. Clinical epidemiology of inflammatory bowel disease: incidence, prevalence and environmental influences. *Gastroenterology.* 2004;126:1504–1517.
7. Geissler C, Powers H, eds. *Human Nutrition.* 11th edn. London: Elsevier Churchill Livingstone; 2005.
8. Calder PC, Field CJ, Gill HS. *Nutrition and Immune Function.* Wallingford: CABI; 2002.
9. Vagianos K, Bector S, McConnell J, Bernstein CN. Nutrition assessment of patients with inflammatory bowel disease. *J Parenter Enteral Nutr.* 2007;31(4):311–319.
10. Travis SPL, Stange EF, Lemann M, et al. European evidence based consensus on the diagnosis and management of Crohn's disease: current management. *Gut.* 2006;55(suppl 1):i16–i35.
11. Kumar P, Clark M, eds. *Kumar & Clark: Clinical Medicine.* 6th edn. London: Elsevier Saunders; 2005.
12. Riordan AM, Hunter JO, Cowan RF, et al. Treatment of active Crohn's disease by exclusion diet: East Anglia multi-centre controlled trial. *Lancet.* 1993;342:1131–1134.
13. Akobeng AK, Thomas AG. Enteral nutrition for maintenance of remission in Crohn's disease (Review). *Cochrane Database Syst Rev.* 2007;(3):CD005984.
14. Zachos M, Tondeur M, Griffiths AM. Enteral nutritional therapy for inducing remission of Crohn's disease. *Cochrane Library.* 2001;(3):CD000542.
15. Lee J, McGeeney L. Liquid diets and adult Crohn's disease: what is current practice? *Complete Nutrition.* 2008;8(2):15–17.
16. Thomas B, Bishop J, eds. *Manual of Dietetic Practice.* 4th edn. Oxford: Blackwell; 2007.
17. Woolner JT, Parker TJ, Kirby GA, Huner JO. The development and evaluation of a diet for maintaining remission in Crohn's disease. *J Hum Nutr Diet.* 1998;11:1–11.
18. Turner D, Zlotkin SH, Shah PD, Griffiths AM. Omega 3 fatty acids (fish oil) for maintenance of remission in Crohn's disease. *Cochrane Database Syst Rev.* 2007;(2):CD006320.
19. Baroja ML, Kirjavainen PV, Hekmat S, Reid G. Anti-inflammatory effects of probiotic yoghurt in inflammatory bowel disease. *Clin Exp Immunol.* 2007;149:470–479.
20. Guarner F. Prebiotics in inflammatory bowel diseases. *Br J Nutr.* 2007;98(suppl 1):S85–S89.
21. Stratton RJ, Hackston AJ, Longmore D, et al. Malnutrition in hospital outpatients and inpatients: prevalence, concurrent validity and ease of use of the malnutrition universal screening tool (MUST) for adults. *Br J Nutr.* 2004;92(5):799–808.
22. National Institute for Health and Clinical Excellence NICE. *Nutrition support in adults: oral nutrition support, enteral tube feeding and parenteral nutrition.* Clinical Guideline 32. UK: DOH; 2006.
23. Baldwin C, Weeks CE. Dietary advice for illness related malnutrition in adults. *Cochrane Database Syst Rev.* 2008;(1):CD002008.
24. Mallon PT, McKay D, Kirk SJ, Gardiner K. Probiotics for induction of remission in ulcerative colitis.

Cochrane Database Syst Rev. 2007;(4):CD005573.

25. Weitz J, Koch M, Debus J, et al. Colorectal cancer. *Lancet.* 2005;365:153–165.

26. Ballinger AB, Anggiansah C. Colorectal cancer. *Br Med J.* 2007;335:715–718.

27. World Cancer Research Fund/ American Institute for Cancer Research. *Food, Nutrition, Physical Activity and the Prevention of Cancer: A Global Perspective.* Washington, DC: AICR; 2007.

28. Millen AE, Subar AF, Graubard BI, et al. Fruit and vegetable intake and prevalence of colorectal adenoma in a cancer screening trial. *Am J Clin Nutr.* 2007;86:1752–1764.

29. Wirfalt E, Midthune D, Reedy J, et al. Associations between food patterns defined by cluster analysis and colorectal cancer incidence in the NIH-AARP diet and health study. *Euro J Clin Nutr.* 2009;63(6):707–717.

30. Key TJ, Spencer EA. Carbohydrate and cancer: an overview of the epidemiological evidence. *Euro J Clin Nutr.* 2007;61(suppl 1): S112–S121.

31. Howarth NC, Murphy SP, Wilkens LR, et al. The association of glycaemic load and carbohydrate intake with colorectal cancer risk in the Multiethnic Cohort Study. *Am J Clin Nutr.* 2008;88:1074–1082.

32. Yang G, Shu X-O, Li H, Chow W-H, et al. Prospective cohort study of soy food intake and colorectal cancer risk in women. *Am J Clin Nutr.* 2009;89:577–583.

33. Larsson SC, Bergkvist L, Rutegard J, et al. Calcium and dairy food intakes are inversely associated with colorectal cancer risk in the cohort of Swedish men. *Am J Clin Nutr.* 2006;83:667–673.

34. Ishihara J, Inoue M, Iwasaki M, et al. Dietary calcium, vitamin D and the risk of colorectal cancer. *Am J Clin Nutr.* 2008;88:1576–1583.

35. Pufulete M. Intake of dairy products and risk of colorectal neoplasia. *Nutr Res Rev.* 2008;21:56–67.

36. Rafter J. The effects of probiotics on colon cancer development. *Nutr Res Rev.* 2004;17:277–284.

37. Thomson AK, Shaw DI, Minihane AM, Williams CM. Trans-fatty acids and cancer: the evidence reviewed. *Nutr Res Rev.* 2008; 21:174–188.

38. Reeves GK, Pirie K, Beral V, et al. Cancer index and mortality in relation to body mass index in the Million Women Study: cohort study. *Br Med J.* 2007;335:1134.

39. Larsson SC, Wolk A. Obesity and colon and rectal cancer risk: a meta- analysis of prospective studies. *Am J Clin Nutr.* 2007;86:556–565.

40. Capuano G, Pavese I, Satta F, et al. Correlation between anemia, unintentional weight loss and inflammatory status on cancer- related fatigue and quality of life before chemo and radiotherapy. *e-SPEN, the Euro e-J Clin Nutr and Metabol.* 2008;3:e147–e151. doi:20.2026/j.eclnm.2008.04.008.

41. Fearon CH, Moses AGW. Cancer cachexia. *Int J Cardiol.* 2002;85: 73–81.

42. Argiles JM, Moore-Carrasco R, Fuster G, Busquets S, Lopez-Soriano FJ. Cancer cachexia: the molecular mechanisms. *Int J Biochem Cell Biol.* 2003;35:405–409.

43. McMillan DC. An inflammation-based prognostic score and its role in the nutrition-based management of patients with cancer. *Proc Nutr Soc.* 2008;67:257–262.

44. Ashby D, Choi P, Bloom S. Gut hormones and the treatment of disease cachexia. *Proc Nutr Soc.* 2008;67:263–269.

45. Crilly M. Nutrition in colorectal cancer. *Complete Nutrition.* 2004;4:8–10.

46. Lewis S. Nutrition and cancer: everybody's business. *Complete Nutrition.* 2007;7:29–31.

Short bowel syndrome

Kirstine Farrer   Lindsay Harper

LEARNING OBJECTIVES

By the end of this chapter the reader will be able to:

- Define intestinal failure and state the main nutritional consequences of short bowel syndrome in relation to the site of bowel resection;
- Describe the nutritional management for a patient with a high output enterostomy and how to monitor this type of patient;
- State the pharmacological action of medicinal agents used to treat short bowel syndrome and oral rehydration solutions;
- Identify appropriate extended roles for dietitians in gastrointestinal disease; and
- Demonstrate awareness of the current legal situation regarding non medical prescribing including patient group directions.

Historical context

This chapter aims to focus on the dietetic and pharmacological management of patients with intestinal failure and short bowel syndrome (SBS). Patients with type 1 intestinal failure, i.e. patients who require some parenteral support (perhaps only replacement of electrolyte fluids), may, with intensive dietetic and pharmacological intervention, obviate the need for long-term parenteral nutrition (PN).

In England there are two designated national centres for the management of acute intestinal failure (IF): one at Salford Royal NHS Foundation Trust, Manchester, and the other at St Marks Hospital, London. Patients presenting with acute IF are relatively rare in the UK, and their management is complex. Fleming and Remington defined IF as follows:

A reduction in the functioning gut mass below the minimal amount necessary for adequate digestion and absorption of food.[1]

Intestinal failure is caused by underlying conditions, e.g. Crohn's disease, due to nonfunctioning absorptive surface, radiation enteritis or chronic intestinal obstruction, e.g. malignant disease; by dysmotility disorders; or by extensive removal of the small bowel, e.g. following mesenteric artery occlusion, or trauma. Recently, Lal et al reported that there are varying degrees of intestinal failure[2]:

- **Type 1 intestinal failure**—occurs following abdominal surgery and requires short-term fluid or nutritional support.
- **Type 2 intestinal failure**—characterised by sepsis and metabolic and complex nutritional needs, e.g. mesenteric vascular disease or a small bowel resection for Crohn's disease. This requires resolution of sepsis before repletion of lean body mass can be achieved. A multiprofessional approach is required and reconstructive surgery may be an option in the long term.
- **Type 3 intestinal failure**—associated with the long-term need for PN, potentially in the home setting.

Patients who have SBS can be divided in to two groups, absorbers and secretors. In patients who are absorbers the stoma output is less than the oral intake, whereas in secretors the output is greater than the input. Absorbers tend to have more than 100 cm of small intestine and the stoma output is 2 L or less. In secretors the length of small intestine is usually less than 100 cm and the stoma output is 3 L or greater.[3] When deciding on appropriate drug therapy for short bowel it is important to know which group the patient falls into, as different drugs are more effective in either absorbers or secretors.

SBS leads to the loss of the absorptive capacity of the intestine, causing a variety of symptoms. The patient is unable to absorb water and electrolytes, leading to diarrhoea or high output from a stoma, depending on the anatomy of the patient. In severe cases the patient may become dehydrated and develop electrolyte deficiencies. The patient may also develop bacterial overgrowth, which may further worsen the diarrhoea or the output from the stoma.[4] The absorption of nutrients may also be affected and the patient may become malnourished and nutritional support may be required. The enteral route is the preferred route but in severe cases the parenteral route will be required. All patients are encouraged to eat and drink even if receiving parenteral nutrition, in order to maintain the integrity of the intestine and prevent hepatic cholestasis.[5] Enteral nutrition also prevents atrophy of the intestine and encourages the adaptation of the remaining intestine.[5]

The dietitian and pharmacist working within this speciality aim to optimise the nutritional status of the patient, safely and effectively, taking into account the risks associated with refeeding syndrome and assisting in monitoring the metabolic and nutritional efficacy of the parenteral and enteral regimen, which can be challenging when the surgical team needs to stabilise a septic, catabolic patient. The pharmacist has an extensive knowledge of drug–nutrient interactions, PN formulation and the correction of abnormal electrolytes appropriately.

Physiology and pathophysiology

Site of the resection

In the normal human intestine most nutrients are absorbed and digested in the duodenum, jejunum and ileum with fluid being absorbed in the large bowel. The total length of small bowel from the duodeno-jejunal flexure to the ileocaecal valve has been reported to be between 275 and 850 cm.[6] Following a small bowel resection the ileum adapts to assume a more absorptive function. From a surgical and medical perspective loss of the ileum is more

detrimental than that of the jejunum; hence surgeons will always attempt to salvage this section of small bowel if at all feasible. Intestinal transit is rapid in the jejunum, but slows down in the ileum. An ileum resection results in fast transit time, and therefore exposure and contact time between nutrients, chyme and absorptive surface area is also reduced.[7] Loss of more than 50 cm of terminal ileum also results in malabsorption of vitamin B_{12} and fat soluble vitamins.[7] The terminal ileum also plays an important role in absorbing bile acids; more than 90% are reabsorbed in the terminal ileum, and therefore if more than 25% of the terminal ileum has been resected, bile acids in the colon impede the absorption of sodium and water, resulting in diarrhoea.[7]

Oxalate kidney stones

The absorption of oxalate from the gut is enhanced following jejuno-ileal bypass or jejuno-colonic anastomosis. Risk factors for oxalate stone formation include decreased urinary volume and urinary pH, hyperuricosuria, hyperoxaluria and hypocitraturia.[8] Normal healthy individuals only absorb a fraction of dietary oxalate; however, following restoration of continuity between the ileum and colon, patients frequently experience fat malabsorption and oxalate absorption is increased. One study reported the formation of calcium oxalate renal stones in 25% of patients with less than 200 cm of jejunum anastomosed to colon.[9] The restriction of dietary fat and oxalate have been demonstrated as being effective in reducing urinary oxalate excretion.[10] Calcium can precipitate with fatty acid to form soaps, hence oxalate is available for rapid absorption in the colon. Patients should be advised to avoid spinach, rhubarb, beetroot, nuts, chocolate, tea, wheat bran and strawberries.[10]

Intestinal adaptation

The remaining length and type of residual bowel is only one factor in predicting the clinical and nutritional outcome of the patient. A diseased bowel, as in the case of Crohn's disease, will have a reduced absorptive capacity. Structural and functional adaptation following a resection can occur over a two-year period in the healthy remaining bowel; however, the main adaptive process will occur in the first few months.[11] An enterectomy will facilitate enhanced epithelial proliferation, and increased crypt and villous height, which is associated with dilation and elongation of the remaining intestine. Luminal nutrients have the greatest trophic effect on the adaptation process and some papers advocate the use of glutamine and short chain fatty acids; however, this has yet to be proven.[12] The preservation of the colon may have an important role to play in adaption. This concurs with clinical experience, whereby patients with an intact section of ileum and colon demonstrate an improvement of absorption over time, whilst patients with a jejunostomy do not and are frequently dependent on PN unless access to the distal small bowel is possible.

Nutritional therapy and dietetic application

Dietetic knowledge and confidence to treat these patients can be limited; it is clear that improved postgraduate education for dietitians is required on the management of intestinal failure and HPN.[13] The most common queries dietitians receive from colleagues are outlined in Table 9.1.

Assessment and monitoring of nutritional status

Assessment of nutritional status should include anthropometric measurements: weight, height, body mass index (BMI), mid-arm circumference and tricep skinfold measurements. Body weight is still

the gold standard objective tool used in nutritional assessment, as it is simple and calibrated scales are readily available. Caution is required in patients with high output stomas resulting in precarious fluid balance as rapid fluctuations in weight are likely to reflect changes in hydration, rather than lean body mass. Weight is often expressed as an index of height to give a measure of body mass index (BMI), where a BMI of 20–25 kg/m^2 is considered desirable. A BMI of < 18.5 kg/m^2 is used to define undernutrition.[14] It is generally accepted that a loss of body weight greater than 10% in the preceding 3 months (and non-intentional) is considered significant in terms of clinical outcome and that 20% recent weight loss is evidence of protein energy malnutrition.[15,16] Patients should be weighed on admission and on a weekly basis.[17] Some patients present with psychological issues due to altered body image related to rapid weight loss as a consequence of malabsorption and loss of functional status which has a negative impact on quality of life. By measuring weight and mid-arm anthropometry it can provide a baseline and subsequent measure of improvement in nutritional status for the patient.[18] Measurement of upper arm anthropometry by the same dietitian in order to avoid interobserver error can be compared to standardized tables but consideration must be given to the demographics of the original populations recruited to compile the reference tables, the sample size and whether these reference tables apply to a the patient population.[19–21]

Biochemical monitoring of serum and urinary electrolytes provide an essential adjunct when assessing fluid balance and the efficacy of the nutrition support. Regular monitoring of patients receiving PN is essential to ensure safe and effective nutritional therapy. Monitoring must include clinical, nutritional and biochemical parameters. The information in Table 9.2 can to be used as a guide but each practitioner should follow local practice guidelines.

Changes in nutritional status often occur because of non-nutritional factors. Failure to improve nutritional status may be due to sepsis/acute disease state, rather than the inadequate provision of nutrition. Monitoring and noting the trend view of markers of the inflammatory response, such as C-reactive protein (CRP), white blood cell count (WCC) and platelets, are useful in indicating sepsis and when the patient is entering the anabolic phase. Albumin levels are considered to reflect disease severity rather than nutritional status, as levels can fall following

Table 9.1 Summary of dietetic queries received over a 12-month period

Theme	Total number of queries
Management of short bowel syndrome	37
Fistuloclysis/distal feeding and other enteral feeding in IF	25
HPN—indications and regimens	24
HPN—monitoring, vitamins + minerals (policies and protocols)	13
Management of other causes of IF	5

Table 9.2 Summary of biochemical monitoring[22]

Parameter	Frequency	Notes
Sodium	Daily Once stable twice weekly, then weekly	• Increased sodium: usually dehydration, rarely sodium excess. Often associated with increased urea. Check fluid balance and consider increased fluid input • Decreased sodium: usually fluid overload rather than depletion. Check for losses. Check fluid balance and consider decreased fluid input
Potassium	Daily Once stable twice weekly, then weekly	• Increased potassium: consider sample haemolysis, lipaemia or contaminated sample • Decreased potassium: check for increased gastrointestinal losses Check for hypomagnesaemia if resistant to treatment
Urea	Daily Once stable twice weekly, then weekly	• Increased urea: occurs in renal failure, suggestive of dehydration Consider increased fluid input • Decreased urea: suggestive of fluid overload or poor nutritional status. Consider decreased fluid input
Creatinine	Daily Once stable twice weekly, then weekly	• Elevated in renal failure
Phosphate	Daily Once stable twice weekly, then weekly	• Increased phosphate: occurs in renal failure • Decreased phosphate: may be a result of refeeding syndrome or existing alcohol abuse
Calcium	Daily Once stable twice weekly, then weekly	• Increased calcium: occurs in renal failure • Decreased calcium: may be result of refeeding syndrome or phosphate supplementation
Magnesium	Daily Once stable twice weekly, then weekly	• Increased magnesium: occurs in renal failure • Decreased magnesium: may be result of refeeding syndrome or existing alcohol abuse. May get hypomagnesium from increased GI losses
Glucose	Three to four times daily until stable, then daily, then weekly	• Elevated glucose: may need to start insulin • Hypoglycaemia: may occur in PN if stopped abruptly. Consider reducing rate of PN over last 1–2 hours
Liver function tests	Twice weekly, then monthly when stable	• May be elevated as a result of underlying or pre-existing hepatic disease, drug therapy, sepsis, long-term PN, overfeeding • Treat accordingly
Albumin	Twice weekly, then monthly when stable	• Poor marker of nutritional status. An indicator of the severity of disease • Treat appropriately
FBC, PT	Weekly, then monthly	• Low Hb result may be associated with lack of iron in PN • WCC rises in infection
Triglycerides	Weekly, then three monthly	• If elevated review fat intake
Trace elements	Monthly	• Long-term PN patients only • Treat appropriately
Zinc	Monthly	• Characteristic rash occurs in deficiency, often associated with poor wound healing. Increased loss in fistula/diarrhoea
Urinary electrolytes	Weekly, then monthly	• Urinary sodium is particularly useful in patients with complex fluid balance

surgery, with inflammatory markers, and can be normal in cases of severe malnutrition, such as anorexia nervosa.[23–25] However, albumin may be a predictive factor for anastomic leak; it is common practice that surgeons will aim for a patient's albumin to be within the normal range prior to reconstructive surgery.[26]

Long-term provision of PN is associated with hepatobiliary complications from mild elevation of LFTs to hepatic steatosis and intrahepatic cholestasis.[27] By actively encouraging oral diet this results in the stimulation of biliary and chyme secretions. Therefore oral intake should be encouraged, unless it is contraindicated, e.g. bowel perforation with intra-abdominal cavities, abscesses, or fistula. Lumen and Shaffer reported an inverse relationship between raised alkaline phosphatase and remaining length of small bowel, especially patients with < 100 cm of small bowel.[27]

Most patients with SBS can be managed by oral enteral nutrition and may require PN, depending on the absorptive capacity of the remaining bowel (Table 9.3).

Eating is associated with many cultural, behavioural, social and psychological factors as well as a means of providing the body with macro- and micronutrients. Patients may have experienced many adverse side effects of malabsorption, e.g. abdominal pain, cramps and diarrhoea, and may be apprehensive to eat.

Short bowel—end jejunostomy

In this group of patients the main challenge is achieving electrolyte and fluid balance. Additional sodium may need to be added to the diet at an optimal concentration of 120 mmol/L or consumed as oral rehydration solution, although compliance with the rehydration solutions can be an issue due to limited palatability.[29] Patients should be educated to:

- Recognise the symptoms of dehydration: dizziness, thirst and reduced/concentrated urine;
- Restrict hypotonic fluids, e.g. water, tea, coffee, squash to 1000–1500 mL/day;

Table 9.3 Summary of clinical and anthropometric monitoring[28]

Parameter	Frequency	Notes
Clinical condition of patient	Minimum of daily	• Observe closely for changes, e.g. pyrexia, vomiting, diarrhoea, increased gastrointestinal losses. Inform senior clinician if necessary
Weight	Weekly	• Plot on weight chart • Inform consultant/nutrition team if weight decreases over 2 or more weeks
Height	On admission	• Record in notes
Mid-arm muscle circumference	Monthly	• Record in notes
Temperature	Daily	• Pyrexia could be associated with catheter-related sepsis. Patient requires urgent review by clinician
Fluid balance	Daily	• Record fluid input/output over 24 hours to indicate fluid overload/dehydration
Total energy intake	Daily	• Calculate PN administered versus PN prescribed. Inform PN pharmacist if less than 90% administered • For patients receiving a combination of PN with enteral nutrition or food, ensure an accurate record of intake is maintained and reviewed twice weekly
Catheter entry site	Daily	• Follow local practice when handling catheter • Inform clinician if any problems, e.g. phlebitis, extravasation observed
Cardiac monitoring	Continuous	• Consider for patients receiving PN with potassium concentration in excess of 40 mmol/L

- Take additional fluids as an oral glucose-electrolyte rehydration solution, with a sodium content > 90 mmol/L, as outlined below;[30] and
- Take medications to reduce stoma losses in relation to meal times.

Nutritional requirements for fluid, electrolytes and nutrients are not likely to change over time, which is in contrast to patients with a colon in continuity with small bowel.[31]

Oral rehydration mixtures

These mixtures contain water, electrolytes and glucose to aid the active transport of sodium. Care must be taken to ensure that hypotonic solutions are not used as this will increase the gastrointestinal output.[32] The patient may also develop bacterial overgrowth, which may further worsen the diarrhoea or the output from the stoma.[32] Patients with a stoma output of greater than 1200 mL may gain benefit from sipping up to a litre of these solutions throughout the day. There are a number of different solutions available for use but they must contain at least 90 mmol/L to prevent sodium loss in the gut. Concentrations of greater that 90 mmol/L of sodium may aid sodium absorption.[32] There are a number of measures which can be instituted to increase the palatability of the solutions such as adding flavourings and keeping the solution chilled. There is evidence that swapping the sodium bicarbonate for sodium citrate or using glucose polymers in the solution may further increase palatability of the solutions.[33]

Pharmacological treatments for short bowel syndrome

There are a number of pharmacological treatments which may be used to reduce stoma/fistula output in patients with SBS.[32] In many cases a combination of agents will be used to control the output. If these agents are used correctly it may prevent a patient requiring long-term parenteral support.[32] The choice of pharmacological agent used to reduce the diarrhoea or the output from the stoma will depend on the length and type of bowel remaining. The most common classes of drug used are the antimotility and antisecretory agents.

If the patient has any coexisting diseases the drug therapy should be reviewed as the absorption of drugs may be reduced. The dose may need to be increased or syrup used to increase the surface area to improve the absorption. In some cases a different route may need to be employed to ensure effective therapy, e.g. topical patches for hormone replacement therapy, or pain control.[34] It is common practice to administer antibiotics parenterally to ensure the minimum inhibitory concentration is achieved.

Antimotility agents

The most commonly used antimotility agents are loperamide and codeine phosphate.[35,36]

Loperamide acts on opiate receptors in the gut wall to increase the tone of the small and large intestine lengthening bowel transit time. This reduces intestinal motility and enhances the absorption of fluid, so reducing the intestinal output.[36] Codeine phosphate acts directly on the intestinal smooth muscle to improve absorption from the gastrointestinal tract; the maximum dose used is 60 mg qds, as above this, side effects are seen.[35] Loperamide has a high first-pass metabolism so very little reaches the systemic circulation; thus doses of up to 16 mg a day have been used with few side effects seen.[36] The antimotility agents are most effective when given 30–60 minutes before food. There has been debate about the benefit of using codeine and loperamide together as their actions are similar. In one study both were used together and patients reported improved symptoms and reduced output.[32] From experience at Salford Royal Hospital patients do get benefit from using the two together. It is the patients who fall into the 'absorbers' category that have been shown to benefit most from antimotility agents.

Antisecretory agents

The agents which fall into this category are the H_2 antagonists, proton pump inhibitors and octreotide.

Proton pump inhibitors

In patients with short bowel an increase in the production of gastric acid is seen. The exact mechanism is unknown but high-circulating levels of gastrin may be the cause. The increased volume of acid passes through into the small intestine and increases the output.[32,37] It has been suggested that increased gastrin levels is a transient effect which may only last for around three months but often this is not seen in practice.[32] Proton pump inhibitors reduce the output by inhibiting the secretion of acid in the stomach and in some centres the dose is triturated according to the stoma/fistula pH. In practice, our aim is to have the pH of the stoma at least above 5. Doses of omeprazole 80 mg orally twice a day have been used.[37] In patients with very short bowel, long-term intravenous omeprazole may be required; it has been suggested that patients with less than 50 cm of jejunum will require intravenous omeprazole.[32] The use of H_2 antagonists to reduce stoma output has largely been replaced by proton pump inhibitors but there is evidence to suggest that using a H_2 antagonist in combination with a proton pump inhibitor may be beneficial in patients with high outputs not controlled by proton pump inhibitors alone.[38]

Octreotide

Octreotide reduces salivary, gastric and pancreaticobiliary secretions and increases the bowel transit time.[39,40] By reducing the transit time and secretions octreotide encourages sodium and water absorption and reduces stoma output. The reduction in stoma output produced by octreotide is similar to that of omeprazole, which has led some investigators to suggest that the main mechanism of action for octreotide is the reduction in gastric acid secretion.[41]

The first case report about the use of octreotide in short bowel syndrome was published in 1984.[32] There have been several studies in which octreotide has been shown to reduce the stoma output of high-output jejunostomy patients. The best results were seen in patients who were secretors and many of the patients were able to reduce the amount of parenteral fluids they required. The average reduction in stoma output was 0.8–1.3 L/day.[40]

The recommended starting dose is 50 mcg by subcutaneous injection twice a day increased to a maximum of 100 mcg twice a day. One study has shown that 50 mcg twice a day was as effective as 100 mcg tds, suggesting a ceiling effect.[41] Tolerance to the effects of octreotide dose does not occur over time so patients will continue to get benefit in long-term treatment.[40]

Potential side effects of octreotide are pain at the site of injection and the development of gallstones. Some patients will experience hypoglycaemia but do not develop diabetes.

Therefore octreotide is a potentially useful therapy for reducing stoma output SBS. It has a similar effect on the stoma output as omeprazole. As it must be given by injection, in practice octreotide is used second line to omeprazole to reduce stoma. Octreotide is useful to add in to the therapy of patients on maximal therapy but who still have troublesome symptoms. Depot injections of octreotide are available and patients may be successfully swapped to this treatment. There is some limited evidence that octreotide therapy may aid the closure of fistulas but the trials were small so further evidence is required in this area.[42] Octreotide is unlicensed for this indication in the UK and is an expensive therapy. Therefore it is often difficult to get funding for this therapy once the patient leaves hospital.

Magnesium supplements

Hypomagnesaemia is common in patients with short bowel syndrome. This may be caused by secondary hyperaldosteronism, so it is important to first ensure the patient is adequately hydrated.[32] As a rule magnesium supplements are poorly absorbed and may worsen stoma/fistula output or cause diarrhoea. The most commonly used salts for oral magnesium replacement are the oxide and glycerophosphate.[32] There is evidence to support the use of both products but from personal experience the magnesium oxide is better tolerated and effective at correcting magnesium levels.[43] The suggested starting dose is two magnesium oxide capsules (4 mmol/cap) twice a day increased to three times a day after a week. It should be noted that both the oxide and glycerophosphate products are unlicensed so the supply of the products is often continued long term from secondary care. In 2006 a new product was launched, Magnaspartate sachets, which contains the magnesium aspartate salt in a dispersable sachet (10 mmol/sachet).[44] This is a licensed product which can easily be administered down enteral feeding tubes. Patients seem to prefer the sachets to the older magnesium products and the sachets can easily be sourced in the community. If the magnesium remains low after supplementation it is worth checking the vitamin D levels and replacing vitamin D if necessary. This may be achieved orally by giving alfacalcidol drops or ergocalciferol injection intramuscularly. It is important to monitor serum calcium levels in patients receiving vitamin D supplementation.[32]

Dietary modification for high output jejunostomy

Studies comparing different proportions of long chain triglycerides and carbohydrate have shown no differences in energy balance, total stoma output or absorption of electrolytes.[45–47] Clinical practice would suggest increasing fibre-rich foods may block the stoma, or cause obstruction or abdominal bloating and pain. A constant proportion of fat is absorbed, so as fat intake increases there is an increased amount of fat in the stoma effluent. Although increased fat excretion may reduce the absorption of calcium and magnesium high fat diets have the benefit of increasing energy intake and palatability, and achieving the necessary energy and protein intake.[46] Based on these studies a low fat diet is not advocated in terms of energy, fluid or monovalent electrolyte absorption in patients with a jejunostomy. Studies comparing dietary supplements have also shown no beneficial effects of elemental diets in absorptive capacity.[45] Elemental and semi-elemental feeds have the disadvantage of both being hyperosmolar and containing a minimal amount of sodium, which will exacerbate fluid, magnesium and sodium losses.[45]

There is no published evidence to support the avoidance of fluids or drinks at meal times with regard to improvement of energy or fluid balance; however, anecdotal evidence would warrant further investigation in this area.

Dietary management of jejunocolic anastomosis

Dietary modification is key in the management of patients with a jejuno-colic anastomosis. Energy absorption is significantly greater when high carbohydrate, low fat diets are consumed, and there is an increased jejunal absorption of macronutrients, water and electrolytes over time.[48,49] Fermentation of carbohydrate to short chain fatty acid in the colon may provide up to 1000 kcal/day.[48] Unabsorbed fatty acids and bile salts reduce water and sodium absorption,[50] bind calcium and magnesium,[51] and contribute to the formation of calcium oxalate renal stones; see earlier section in chapter.

There needs to be a pragmatic approach with dietary advice for these patients. It can be difficult to achieve a balance between an ideal dietary composition and palatability/tolerance. High carbohydrate diets are bulky and cause bloating, abdominal discomfort and flatulence. Patients should be encouraged to take sufficient carbohydrate and find a balance between reducing fat and maintaining palatability/adequate energy. MCT supplements and oils may be a useful way of fortifying the diet.

Cholestyramine sachets (Questran)

If bile acids are not absorbed in the small intestine they pass through to the colon where they cause secretion of fluid, which will increase the intestinal output. Cholestyramine binds the bile acids and helps to reduce the output only in patient with a colon in continuity. The patients should be advised to take the sachets with food and avoid taking any medications at the same time. In 2007 Colesevelam, which has a similar action to cholestyramine, was launched in the UK. At present there is only one case report to support its use in bile acid diarrhoea but it may be a useful alternative in patients unable to tolerate cholestyramine.[52]

Developing issues— fistuloclysis and distal feeding

The nutritional management of patients with high output enterocutanous fistulae with mucotaneous continuity (i.e. fistulae which will not close spontaneously with conservative management of total parenteral nutrition (TPN) and keeping the patient nil by mouth) or high output proximal loop enterostomies usually require PN. Studies have demonstrated TPN can be avoided in selected patients by administering enteral feed or saline distally via an anatomical or surgically created mucous fistula.

Patients should be carefully selected and their consent obtained for initiation of this type of enteral tube feeding: sepsis free, haemodynamically and nutritionally stable with a proximal output of between 0.5 and 2.5 L. Distal bowel should be radiologically demonstrated to show that the distal bowel is intact and not dilated. Feeding is achieved by inserting a gastrostomy feeding tube into the intestine distal to the fistula or loop stoma. Infusion of enteral feeding is increased slowly, without the reinfusion of chyme, until the patient can tolerate their nutritional and fluid requirements by a combination fistuloclysis/distal feeding and oral diet, following which TPN can be withdrawn. Teubner et al reported fistuloclysis was attempted in 12 patients with jejunocutaneous or ileocutaneous fistulas with mucocutaneous continuity.[53] Fistuloclysis replaced TPN entirely in 11 of 12 patients. Nutritional status was maintained for a median of 155 days (range 19–422), until reconstructive surgery could be safely undertaken in nine patients. One patient resumed TPN, one died of ischaemic heart disease and one was not suitable for reconstructive surgery due to medical comorbidity. Fistuloclysis and distal tube feeding are safe methods for providing effective nutritional support in selected patients with enterocutaneous fistulae or a high output loop stoma.[54] To date the intestinal failure unit in Salford has discharged 34 patients home on this new indication for home enteral tube feeding, which equates to nearly 12,000 patient days of distal enteral tube feeding.

Extended scope—prescribing rights for dietitians

There has been considerable controversy regarding the development of extended prescribing roles for nurses and pharmacists.[55] At present, pharmacists who have obtained the supplementary/independent prescribing certificate can prescribe certain drugs, in partnership with an independent prescriber, using a patient-specific clinical management plan and from May 2006 could prescribe independently.[56] Since May 2004, dietitians have been added to the list of allied health professionals who are allowed to supply and administer medicines under Patient Group Directions, and it is envisaged that dietitians will be able to participate in supplementary prescribing on the same basis in the future, under the supervision of the Health Professions Council.[57] At present some dietitians are using patient group directions to 'prescribe' or adjust doses of medications, but this is not recommended as the Patient Group Directions legal framework does not support this and therefore the dietitian is not covered legally. At present the British Dietetic Association is preparing a consultation document to argue the case for dietitian prescribing to send to the Department of Health. As a result it is envisaged that dietitians will be given supplementary prescribing rights by the Department of Health.

Key points

- Type 1 intestinal failure patients can be managed with dietetic and pharmacological support, provided sufficient functioning small bowel is available.
- It is important to optimise pharmacological therapy in short bowel patients as this may reduce the amount of parenteral support the patient may need.
- Nonmedical prescribing may be an option for dietitians in the future which will aid the extension of the dietitian's role and improve patient care.
- The regular monitoring of patients with short bowel is essential to ensuring patients receive optimal care.

Case study

Mrs Cooper, a 57-year-old school teacher, was diagnosed with Dukes B carcinoma a month ago. She has been admitted to your hospital for a bowel resection and now has a high output ileostomy, which is producing a variable output every day. Her operation notes state she has 150 cm of proximal small bowel to the ileostomy.

A week ago she was commenced on TPN and the surgeons are keen to wean her off PN; she has commenced eating and drinking, but continues to get dehydrated and complains of feeling thirsty.

She is receiving 2.4 L of a standard PN off-the-shelf regimen and an additional 1.0 L of Hartmann's solution. This is administered via a sterile Venflon peripherally.

The TPN regimen provides 3400 mL, 1500 non-protein kcal, 9 gN, 184 mmol sodium, 45 mmol potassium, 3.3 mmol Ca, 6.7 mmol Mg, 18 mmol PO_4 and vitamins + trace elements.

Her weight is 66 kg, height 1.66 m, MAC 29 cm, TSF 16 mm. She reports she usually weighs 70 kg and was considering losing some weight before her diagnosis.

She is mobile on the ward.

The food record chart reveals she is eating approx half of the normal hospital diet (800 kcal + 30 g protein), fizzy drinks, tea, coffee.

Her medication is omeprazole 20 mg bd, loperamide 2 mg tds and Dioralyte 5 sachets dissolved in 1000 mL of water.

Her biochemistry results are illustrated in Table 9.4.

The dietitian and pharmacist are asked to go to the surgical ward with a view to stopping her TPN and advising the medical team on how to reduce her output from the ileostomy.

Continued

Table 9.4 Case study: biochemistry results

	Normal range	Day 4 TPN	Day 5 TPN	Day 6 surgeons tried to stop TPN
Sodium (mmol/L)	135–150	135	133	128
Potassium (mmol/L)	3.5–5.3	3.5	3.4	3.5
Urea (mmol/L)	2.5–7.5	6.1	8.8	15.3
Creatinine (mmol/L)	50–110	102	114	119
Calcium c (mmol/L)	2.1–2.6	2.10	2.13	2.16
Phosphate (mmol/L)	0.8–1.6	0.77	0.85	1.0
Albumin (g/L)	35–50	30	28	34
Total protein(g/L)	60–80	48	50	54
Alkaline phosphatase (U/L)	30–130	71	72	71
ALT(U/L)	2–50	19	18	20
CRP	<10	40	44	48
Hb (g/L)	115–165	115	115	122
Zn (umol/L)	10–21	-	12	11
Mg (mmol/L)	0.7–1.0	0.6	0.53	0.5
PH stoma		Not recorded	3.8	3.4
Ileostomy output		1800	2500	3000
Urine ouptput/24 hr		1200	1000	450

Case study (Continued)

QUESTIONS

1. Comment on her nutritional status and biochemistry. Calculate BMI and MAMC.
2. What are your aims and objectives for nutritional support with this patient?
3. Calculate this patient's nutritional requirements.
4. What advice would the dietitian and pharmacist give regarding her diet, fluid intake and medications?
5. Which other member of the team would you liaise with regarding this lady and how would you monitor her progress?

ANSWERS

1. Comment on her nutritional status and biochemistry. Calculate BMI and MAMC.
   Weight   66 kg BMI 24 kg/m^2
   MAC   29 cm (between 25th and 50th centile)
   TSF   16 mm (between 10th and 25th centile)
   MAMC   29 cm – (3.14 × 1.6 cm) = 24 cm (between 50th and 75th centile)

Only lost 4 kg, which equates to 6% weight loss. Nutritionally this lady is not malnourished, but owing to her underlying condition and dependency on PN she is at high risk of dehydration and electrolyte depletion. Her biochemistry reflects this with initial borderline results for Na, K and low Mg. This will be due to the high output from the ileostomy and thus losses of Na and Mg. Her urea and creatinine levels start to climb as the output increases from the ileostomy. The more fluid she drinks the more her stoma output increases. Her albumin is low, reflecting postoperative stress. CRP is raised.

Her urinary electrolytes levels should be checked as she may be at risk of Na depletion. Note that every litre of ileal output contains 140 mmol of Na, which needs to be replaced.

Case study (Continued)

Fluid balance is an issue. Even with 3.4 L of PN and IV Hartmann's solution her urinary output is borderline, just over 1 L, and when PN is stopped her urinary output drops below 1 L to a worrying 450 mL/day.

2. What are your aims and objectives for nutritional support with this patient?

Aims

- To stabilise fluid and electrolyte requirements via the enteral route and meet nutritional requirements and obviate the need for PN.
- Reduce incidence of metabolic, electrolyte and nutritional complications.
- Educate on an appropriate enteral and fluid regimen in order to wean off PN.
- Pharmacist to undertake a full medication review and make recommendations about appropriate pharmacological therapy and counsel on medications.

Objectives

- Liaise with doctors regarding fluid balance.
- Assess nutritional status using appropriate anthropometric techniques.
- Calculate energy, nitrogen and electrolyte and micronutrient requirements.
- Quantify the oral intake and contribution this will make to the patient's nutritional requirements.
- Educate re low-fibre diet, limiting hypotonic fluids and liaising with pharmacy to address timely administration of medications in relation to meals.

3. Calculate this patient's nutritional requirements.

Energy
BMR $8.3 \times 66 + 846 = 1394$ kcal (Schofield)
+ 10% stress = 139 kcal, based on CRP 40 and has undergone surgery in the last week
+ 25% mobility = 348 kcal
Total = 1881 kcal (i.e. 1900 kcal is her estimated energy requirement)

Nitrogen
$0.2 \times 66 = 13$ g

Protein
$13 \times 6.25 = 81$ g protein

Fluid
$66 \times 35 = 2310$ mL maintenance requirements
+ 1800 mL (based on ileostomy output recorded on day 4 of TPN)
Total = 4110 mL
Note fluid balance will need to be reviewed on a daily basis.

Sodium
Baseline Na requirement = 66 mmol
Based on 1800 mL ileostomy output = additional 250 mmol Na
Total Na requirement = 316 mmol Na

Potassium
Baseline potassium requirement 1 mmol/kg = 66 mmol
Based on ileostomy output of 1.8 L = additional 20 mmol
Total potassium requirement = 86 mmol

Calcium
Baseline calcium requirement 0.1 mmol/kg = 6.6 mmol
Total calcium requirement = 7 mmol/day

Phosphate
Baseline phosphate requirement 0.5 mmol/kg = 33 mmol
Total phosphate requirement = 33 mmol/day

Magnesium
Baseline magnesium requirement 0.1 mmol/kg = 6.6 mmol
Total magnesium requirement = 7 mmol/day

4. What advice would the dietitian and pharmacist give regarding her diet, fluid intake and medications?

At present she is not following any dietary or fluid restrictions and she is drinking the Dioralyte at normal strength, not double strength.

She should be restricting hypotonic fluids, i.e. water, tea, coffee, squash, to 1 L per day and dissolving 10 sachets of Dioralyte in 1000 mL of water. This mixture should be sipped slowly throughout the day to prevent sodium depletion – note this will also contain additional potassium (20 mmol/L). If the patient does not tolerate double-strength Dioralyte, or this is contraindicated, there are alternative solutions available, e.g. St Mark's solution or WHO formulation.

In order to prevent the stoma blocking she would be commenced on a low fibre diet and advised to avoid pips, seeds, skins, wholegrain cereals, pithy fruit such as tangerines, pineapples, oranges, mushrooms, leeks, sweetcorn, pulses and beans.

This patient may require additional high energy snacks, such as cheese and biscuits, toast, sandwiches, yogurts or crumpets, as because of the limitations in the route of administration of the PN (at present it is being given peripherally) it will be impossible to meet her estimated energy and nitrogen requirements. If suggesting sip feeds, advise on a polymeric feed rather than elemental as the osmolality will be too high and may exacerbate her output.

The pharmacist may suggest increasing her dose of loperamide; this needs to be titrated slowly in order to avoid intestinal obstruction. The patient would also need to be counselled regarding her medication as she is not taking the loperamide half an hour before meals. Doses of loperamide of up to 80 mg/day are commonly used; it should also be noted that codeine phosphate could be added to further reduce the output from the ileostomy if required.

Continued

Case study (Continued)

The pharmacist may also request checking the pH of the ileostomy output as the dose of omeprazole may not be sufficient to suppress the production of acid. In this case, on day 6 the pH of the ileostomy output is 3.4 and Mrs Cooper is on 20 mg omeprazole b.d; the pharmacist would recommend increasing the dose to 40 mg omeprazole b.d and monitoring the pH of the ileostomy output 7 days later.

5. Which other member of the team would you liaise with regarding this lady and how would you monitor her progress?

Liaise with the stoma care therapist, to ensure the lady is coping with her stoma, and the named nurse, to stress the importance of accurate fluid balance.

The doctor would be present on the nutrition support team round to address fluid balance issues.

Close liaison with the nutrition nurse specialist is needed to ensure the Venflon is still a viable option to administer the PN or IV fluids.

Monitor this lady closely, primarily to stabilise fluid balance and biochemistry. She will need to maintain her urinary output over 1 L/day and be able to maintain Mg levels within the normal limit. If her Mg level is persistently low remember to check vitamin D status as this may be low and need to be corrected by prescribing 1-alpha-cholecalciferol or intramuscular vitamin D. It may be necessary to commence Mrs Cooper on oral Mg supplements, e.g. magnesium oxide.

Nutritionally monitor her weight twice a week and anthropometry (MAC and TSF) on a monthly basis. Once she is stable, she will need to be reviewed in dietetic outpatient clinic.

References

1. Fleming CR, Remington M. Intestinal failure. In: Hill GL, ed. *Nutrition in the Surgical Patient*. Edinburgh: Churchill Livingstone; 1981:219–235.

2. Lal S, Teubner A, Shaffer JL. Review article: intestinal failure. *Aliment Pharmacol Ther*. 2006;24:19–31.

3. Nightingale JMD, Lennard-Jones JE, Walker ER, Farthing MJG. Jejunal efflux in short bowel syndrome. *Lancet*. 1990;336:765–768.

4. Pereira SP, Dowling RH. Small bowel bacterial overgrowth. In: *Oxford Textbook of Medicine*, 3rd edn. Oxford: Oxford University Press; 1996:ii.1911–ii.1916.

5. Gugliemli FW, Moran Penco JM, Gentile A, et al. Hepatobiliary complications of long term parenteral nutrition. *Clin Nutr*. 2001;20(suppl 2): 51–56.

6. Nightingale JMD, Spiller RC. Normal intestinal anatomy and physiology. In: Nightingale JMD, ed. *Intestinal Failure*. London: Greenwich Medical Media; 2001:15–38.

7. Nightingale JMD. The short bowel. In: Nightingale JMD, ed. *Intestinal Failure*. London: Greenwich Medical Media; 2001:177–200.

8. Bambach CP, Robertson WG, Peacock M, Hill GL. Effect of intestinal surgery on the risk of urinary stone formation. *Gut*. 1981;22:257–263.

9. Nightingale JMD, Lennard-Jones JE, Gertner DJ, Wood SR, Bartum CI. Colonic preservation reduces need for parenteral therapy, increases incidence of renal stones, but does not change high prevalence of gall stones in patients with a short bowel. *Gut*. 1992;33:1493–1497.

10. Jeppesen PB, Mortensen PB. The dietary treatment of patients with a short bowel. In: Nightingale JMD, ed. *Intestinal Failure*. London: Greenwich Medical Media; 2001:393–406.

11. Pullan JM. Massive intestinal resection. *Proc R Soc Med*. 1959;52:31–37.

12. Levine GM, Deren JD, Yezdimir E. Small bowel resection: oral intake is the stimulus for hyperplasia. *Digestive Disorders*. 1976;21: 542–546.

13. Farrer K, Culkin A. What do health care professionals want to know about intestinal failure and home parenteral nutrition? *Proc Nutr Soc*. 2008;67(OCE):E102.

14. Roche AF. Grading body fatness from limited anthropometric data. *Am J Clin Nutr*. 1981;34: 2831–2838.

15. Dewys WD, Begg C, Lavin PT, et al. Prognostic effect of weight loss prior to chemotherapy in cancer patients. *Am J Med*. 1980;69:491–497.

16. Kinney JM. The influence of calorie and nitrogen balance on weight loss. *Br J Clin Prac*. 1988;63(suppl 12): 114–120.

17. NICE. *Clinical Guideline 32 Nutritional Support for Adult Patients*. London: Department of Health; 2006.

18. Hall JC, O'Quigley J, Giles GR, Appleton N, Stocks H. Upper limb anthropometry: the value of measurements variance studies. *Am J Clin Nutr*. 1980;33:1846–1851.

19. Blackburn GL, Bristrian BR, Maini BS. Nutritional and metabolic assessment of the hospitalised patient. *J Parenter Enteral Nutr*. 1977;1:11–22.

20. Jelliffe DB. *The Assessment of the Nutritional Status of the Community: With Specific Reference to Field Surveys in Developing Regions of the World*. WHO monograph. Geneva: World Health Organization; 1966.

21. Frisancho AR. New norms of upper limb fat and muscle areas for assessment of nutritional status. *Am J Clin Nutr.* 1981;34:2540–2545.

22. Bowling T, ed. *Extracted from Nutritional Support for Adults and Children: A Handbook for Hospital Practice.* Oxford: Radcliffe Medical Press; 2003.

23. Cuthbertson DP, Tompsett SL. Note on the effect of injury on the level of plasma proteins. *Br J Exper Pathol.* 1935;16:471–475.

24. Fleck A, Colley CM, Myers MA. Liver export proteins and trauma. *Br Med Bull.* 1985;41:265–273.

25. McClain CJ, Humphries LL, Hill KK, Nickl NJ. Gastrointestinal and nutritional aspects of eating disorders. *J Am Coll Nutr.* 1993;12(4):466–474.

26. Yamamoto T, et al. Reference risk factors for intra-abdominal sepsis after surgery in Crohn's Disease. *Dus Colon Rectum.* 2000;43(8):1141–1145.

27. Lumen W, Shaffer JL. Prevalence, outcome and associated factors of deranged liver function tests in patients on home parenteral nutrition. *Clin Nutr.* 2002;21(4):337–343.

28. Todorovic V, Micklewright A. *A Pocket guide to Clinical Nutrition on behalf of the PENG of the BDA.* Birmingham, UK; 2006.

29. Nightingale JMD, Lennard-Jones JE, Walker ER, Farthing MJG. Jejunal efflux in short bowel syndrome. *Lancet.* 1990;336:765–768.

30. Nightingale JMD, Lennard-Jones JE, Walker ER, Farthing MJG. Oral salt supplements to compensate for jejunostomy losses: comparison of sodium chloride capsules, glucose electrolyte solution and glucose polymer electrolyte solution (Maxijul). *Gut.* 1992;33:759–761.

31. Hill GL, Mair WSJ, Goligher JC. Impairment of 'ileostomy adaptation' in patients after ileal resection. *Gut.* 1974;15:982–987.

32. Nightingale JM, Woodward JM; Small Bowel and Nutrition Committee of the British Society of Gastroenterology. Guidelines for management of patients with a short bowel. *Gut.* 2006;55:iv1–iv12.

33. Dias JA. Improving the palatability of oral rehydration solutions has implications for salt and water transport: a study in animal models.

J Pediatr Gastroenterol Nutr. 1996;23(3):275–279.

34. White R, Bradnam V. *Handbook of Drug Administration via Enteral Feeding Tubes.* London: Pharmaceutical Press; 2006.

35. King RFJL, Norton T, Hill GL. A double-blind crossover study of the effect of loperamide HCl and codeine phosphate on ileostomy output. *Aust N Z J Surg.* 1982;52:121–124.

36. Tytgat GN, Huibregtse K. Loperamide and ileostomy output—placebo-controlled double-blind crossover study. *Br Med J.* 1975;2:667–668.

37. Nightingale JM, Walker ER, Farthing MJ, Lennard-Jones JE. Effect of omeprazole on intestinal output in the short bowel syndrome. *Aliment Pharmacol Ther.* 1991;5:405–412.

38. Nightingale JM. Management of patients with a short bowel. *World J Gastroenterol.* 2001;7(6):741–751.

39. Kusuhara K, Kusunoki M, Okamoto T, Sakanoue Y, Utsunomiya J. Reduction of the effluent volume in high-output ileostomy patients by a somatostatin analogue. *Int J Colorect Dis.* 1992;7:202–205.

40. Nightingale JM, Walker ER, Burnham WR, Farthing MJ, Lennard-Jones JE. Octreotide improves the quality of life in some patients with a short intestine. *Aliment Pharmacol Ther.* 1989;3:367–373.

41. Shaffer JL, et al. Does somatostatin analogue reduce high output stoma effulent? A controlled trial. *Gut.* 1988;29(A1):1432–1433.

42. Alvarez C, McFadden DW, Reber HA. Complicated enterocutaneous fistulas: failure of octreotide to improve healing. *World J Surg.* 2000;24(5):533–537.

43. Lennard-Jones JE. Review article: practical management of the short bowel. *Aliment Pharmacol. Ther.* 1994;8(6):563–577.

44. *Magnaspartate Product Information.* London: British National Formulary for Children; 2008.

45. McIntyre PB, Fitchew M, Lennard-Jones JE. Patients with a high jejunostomy do not need a special diet. *Gastronenterology.* 1986;91:25–33.

46. Ovesen L, Chu R, Howard I. The influence of dietary fat on jejunostomy output in patients with severe short bowel syndrome. *Am J Clin Nutr.* 1983;38:270–277.

47. Newton CR, Gonvers JJ, McIntyrre PB, Preston DM, Lennard-Jones JE. Effect of different drinks on fluid and electrolyte losses from a jejunostomy. *J R Soc Med.* 1985;78:27–34.

48. Nordgaard I, Hansen BS, Mortensen PB. Importance of colonic support for energy absorption as short-bowel failure proceeds. *Am J Clin Nutr.* 1996;64:222–231.

49. Weinstein LD, Shoemaker CP, Hersh T, Wright HK. Enhanced intestinal absorption after small bowel resection in man. *Arch Surg.* 1969;99:560–562.

50. Ammon HV, Philips SF. Inhibition of colonic water and electrolyte absorption by fatty acids in man. *J Clin Invest.* 1973;65:744–749.

51. Hessov I, Andersson H, Isaksson B. The use of low-fat diet on mineral absorption in small-bowel disease. *Scand J Gastroenterol.* 1982;18:551–554.

52. Puleston J, Morgan H, Andreyev J. New treatment for bile salt malabsorption. *Gut.* 2005;54:441–442.

53. Teubner A, Morrison K, Ravishankar HR, Anderson ID, Scott NA, Carlson GL. Fistuloclysis can successfully replace parenteral feeding in the nutrition support of patients with enterocutaneous fistula. *Br J Surg.* 2004;91:625–631.

54. Shetty V, Teubner A, Morrison K, Scott NA. Proximal loop jejunostomy is a useful adjunct in the management of multiple intestinal suture lines in the septic abdomen. *Br J Surg.* 2006;93:1247–1250.

55. Silverman J. Opposition to pharmacist prescribing. (Policy and Practice.). *Family Practice News.* 2002.

56. Department of Health. *Improving Patients' Access to Medicines: A Guide to Implementing Nurse and Pharmacist Independent Prescribing within the NHS in England.* 2006.

57. Department of Health. *HSC 2000/26: Patient Group Directions (England only).* 2000.

Enteral nutrition

Paula Murphy

LEARNING OBJECTIVES

By the end of this chapter the reader will be able to:

- Gain an insight into the evidence base for enteral nutrition;
- Understand the different routes by which enteral nutrition can be delivered, the indications for each route and their associated complications;
- Understand the role of some special substrates used in enteral feeding and examine the evidence base for their use; and
- Understand the principles of medical ethics and how these affect enteral tube feeding decisions.

Introduction

The term enteral nutrition includes all nutrients delivered via the gastrointestinal tract. For the purpose of this chapter, enteral nutrition will refer to the administration of nutrients *by tube* to the gastrointestinal tract. In the mid-1970s the techniques of enteral nutrition became established following Dobbie and Hoffineister's successful administration of a liquid diet by tube via a pump.[1] Emphasis is now placed on enteral over parenteral provision of nutrients because of general consensus that the gut should be used whenever possible and parenteral nutrition reserved for when the gut is nonfunctional or where enteral access is not feasible.

Enteral tube feeding (ETF): the evidence

Before reaching any conclusions on the effectiveness of ETF, the *quality* of available evidence must be considered. In a climate where resources are limited there is a need for established proof of efficacy from large, well-designed, high-quality randomised controlled trials. Good quality research in nutrition support is difficult to achieve as frequently it is not feasible or ethical to have 'no nutrition' as a control. Randomised placebo-controlled trials, although considered the gold standard for establishing clinical efficacy,[2] are not always possible for some groups of patients, e.g. patients who are likely to recover from prolonged unconscious state in an ICU setting or CVA patients with an unsafe swallow. In such patient groups a randomised controlled trial could not be performed as it would be unethical to withhold feeding.

An extensive systematic review and meta-analysis of enteral tube feeding concluded that ETF can increase nutritional intake, attenuate loss of body weight and lean tissue, improve functional outcomes and reduce mortality and complications in some patient groups.[3] This review included 74 trials (2769 patients) of ETF in the hospital setting. Most of the trials (80%) had a Jadad score of 2 or less (the higher the score, the better the study design; highest score is 5). This was largely due to the fact that for completeness both randomised ($n = 33$) and non-randomised controlled trials ($n = 41$) were examined and few of the studies were placebo controlled or blinded.

Many studies examine the impact of nutrition support on surrogate end points such as body weight, nitrogen balance and immunological parameters. Demonstration of improvement in these parameters does not translate into improved clinical outcome. A review of randomised controlled trials that examined the ability of enteral nutrition to influence morbidity and mortality failed to find any high-quality evidence that enteral nutrition has any beneficial effect on clinical outcome.[4] Data from low-quality randomised controlled trials suggest potential benefit to postoperative infectious complications, reduced infection rates in ICUs and improved mortality in chronic liver disease.[4] Low-quality evidence tends to show larger treatment effects, suggesting that artificial nutrition may be even less effective than the data suggest.

The NICE Nutrition Support Guideline (2006) provides recommendations for clinical practice.[5] These guidelines are the result of examination of systematic reviews, meta-analyses and randomised controlled trials of ETF. They do not include observational studies because of the potential bias associated with observational study designs. They conclude: 'although enteral tube feeding does increase nutritional intakes the evidence that this benefits outcomes such as length of hospital stay or mortality is not clear'. Consequently it is recommended that 'enteral tube feeding should not be given to people unless they are malnourished or at risk of malnutrition and have inadequate or unsafe oral intake and a functional accessible gastrointestinal tract'.[5]

When making a decision on the need for artificial nutrition support, factors such as the patient's current nutritional status, medical condition, duration of inadequate oral intake, methods of nutrition support available and whether nutrition support is in the patients' best interest must be considered.[5] Artificial nutrition support is a medical intervention with associated costs and morbidity. There is little doubt of the value of artificial feeding in patients with swallowing difficulties or patients requiring prolonged ventilation who are expected to recover. In these situations it would be unethical to withhold feeding. The controversy exists in the intermediate group of patients who are unable to meet their requirements from oral intake alone.

Enteral feeding access routes

Gastric feeding

Orogastric (OG)

May be used in patients with basal skull fractures requiring enteral feeding. A tube is passed orogastrically as if placed blindly by the nasal route, it may be malpositioned and enter the brain.

Nasogastric (NG)

This is the route of choice for short-term nutrition support (though it can be used for longer term nutrition support) in the absence of vomiting, gastro-oesophageal reflux, ileus or intestinal obstruction. Small-bore feeding tubes provide access to the gastrointestinal tract. These are inexpensive, can be inserted at the bedside and easily removed if no longer needed. Although useful, tubes are not without complications and morbidity associated with tube placement is now being appreciated. On the release of Patient Safety Alert 05,[6] the NPSA was aware of 11 deaths and one case of serious harm in the UK due to misplaced nasogastric feeding tubes over a two-year period. This alert required immediate action by NHS acute trusts, primary care organisations and local health boards in England and Wales to:

- Provide staff, carers and patients with information on correct and incorrect testing methods. The use of pH indicator paper for measuring aspirate is recommended. Radiography is also recommended but not for routine use;
- Carry out individual risk assessment prior to nasogastric tube feeding; and
- Report misplacement incidents via local risk management reporting systems.[6]

Complications continue to be reported. It is important to note that the standard confirmatory methods recommended by the NPSA may be unreliable with the use of 24-hour feeding or proton pump inhibitors. The 'gold standard' may be endoscopic or radiologic placement of feeding tubes but this is not cost effective for routine tube placement in most hospitals and not always feasible in unwell patients. There is a need for institutional protocols for safe tube placement as well as the development and adoption of new technology for safe insertion. One example of such technology is an electromagnetic sensing device that tracks and displays the path of feeding tubes during the placement procedure. There are also reports of technologies in which feeding tubes are coupled with a CO_2 sensor.[7] Regardless of the placement technique, inadvertent displacement can occur even in cooperative patients in the course of routine nursing care, in movement of patients during washing or dressing, transport through the hospital or if the patient changes position and the tube becomes caught on extraneous devices. A 'nasal bridle', first described in 1980 in the context of head and neck cancer patients,[8] has since been found to be a safe and effective method for preventing the accidental removal of nasoenteric feeding tubes.[9]

Gastrostomy

Gastrostomy feeding tubes pass through the abdominal wall directly into the stomach and can be placed endoscopically (PEG), surgically (PG) or radiologically (RIG). Patients selected for gastrostomy tube feeding should be at high risk of malnutrition and unlikely to recover their ability to feed orally in the short term. The concept of gastrostomy feeding must be acceptable to the patient and their family or carers before tubes are placed. It has the advantage over NG feeding in that patients should receive more of their feed as there is less interruption from tube displacement.[10] Ethical considerations should be taken into account prior to placement, which should always be for medical reasons and not for administrative convenience (saving money, time or manpower).[11] Common indications for gastrostomy placement are outlined in Table 10.1.

Gastrostomy tube placement options

Surgery
Surgical placement of feeding tubes is associated with higher morbidity and mortality and tends to be used only when endoscopic or radiologic placement is not possible or an adjunctive procedure if the patient is undergoing surgery.

Endoscopy (PEG)
Endoscopic placement has now largely replaced surgical placement. Patients should be fasted for at least 8 hours prior to the procedure, and given appropriate sedation and routine antibiotic prophylaxis. Techniques used for placement include the pull-through method ('pull' technique), the Seldinger technique ('push' technique), or direct puncture.

Contraindications to PEG placement include serious coagulation disorders, severe ascites, peritonitis, severe psychosis, a limited life expectancy and interposed organs, e.g. liver, colon.[11] Endoscopic placement may fail in obese patients and patients with a high stomach or large hiatus hernia, oropharyngeal cancer or oesophageal strictures.

Feeding is not without complications (Box 10.1). Complication rates are similar irrespective of the placement technique used. Major complications have been reported to arise in 3% of cases and minor complications in 20%.[12] Direct procedure-related mortality rates vary between 0.7% and 2.0%. Thirty-day mortality rates of 10-28% have been reported.[12] Such high death rates may reflect inappropriate patient selection. The FOOD trial collaboration demonstrated a benefit from early nasogastric tube feeding after a CVA but an increase in mortality in those patients randomised to early PEG placement.[13] Pre-assessment has been identified as the dominant factor responsible for a reduction in 1-week post PEG mortality. There is an increasing view that patient selection should be a function of a multidisciplinary nutrition team. The 2005 National Confidential Enquiry into Patient Outcome and Death (NCEPOD) report, 'Scoping our Practice'[14] pertaining to deaths after therapeutic endoscopy, contains three main considerations relating to PEG placement.

1. The decision to place a PEG feeding tube requires an in-depth assessment of the potential benefits to the individual.
2. All patients referred for PEG placement should be reviewed by a multidisciplinary team.

Table 10.1 Common indications for gastrostomy tube placement

Indication	Example
Neurological disorders of swallowing	CVA, Parkinson's disease, motor neurone disease
Long-term partial failure of intestinal function requiring supplementary nutrition support	Cystic fibrosis, Crohn's disease
Cognitive impairment and decreased consciousness	Head injury
Oncology disorders	Upper GI tumours: tubes may be placed for palliative care in nonoperable cases or may be placed prior to treatment and removed when the patient has recovered adequate oral intake

Box 10.1

PEG complications

1. Immediate (arising from the procedure itself)
   - Respiratory, e.g. aspiration, respiratory depression, airway obstruction
   - Bleeding, e.g. bleeding from the abdominal wall, inadvertent puncture of another intra-abdominal structure during needle passage
   - Peritonitis
2. Early (occurring within the first 4 weeks)
   - Infection, e.g. peristomal infection, abdominal wall abscess
   - Displacement: if the internal retention disc becomes displaced before the gastrocutaneous fistulous tract becomes established
   - Peritoneal leakage without displacement
   - Aspiration pneumonia: patient may aspirate oral secretions
3. Late (4 weeks or beyond)
   - Displacement
   - Leakage
   - Hypergranulation
   - Tube dysfunction, e.g. blockage or splitting of tube
   - Buried bumper. This is a particular problem in tubes with a silicone internal retention disc. The disc embeds within the gastric mucosa which then overgrows the bumper and eventually obstructs the passage of feed
   - Obstruction. This can be a problem with detachment of the internal bumper or detachment of the external fixation device
   - Tumour implantation. This has been reported when tubes are placed preoperatively in patients with oropharyngeal cancer[15]

3. There is a need for more comprehensive national guidelines for the use of PEG feeding including issues of patient selection.

Radiologically inserted gastrostomy (RIG)

Most involved in enteral nutrition are familiar with the PEG but many are less familiar with the RIG. In fact the main difference between a PEG and a RIG is simply the method of placement.

RIG placement. As with all invasive procedures fully informed consent is obtained. A fine bore nasogastric or orogastric tube is then passed under screening guidance. Because of the very fine nature of this tube and the use of X-ray control it is virtually always possible to pass the tube, even in the presence of obstructing tumours of the oropharynx or

oesophagus. The stomach can then be inflated with air or carbon dioxide. Using an aseptic technique and with local anaesthesia to the abdominal wall, the inflated stomach can then be punctured with a needle under X-ray guidance. Depending on the type of tube being inserted, the stomach may be fixed to the anterior abdominal wall at this stage with the use of stay sutures. The stomach is then re-punctured and a wire inserted. The tract can then be dilated over the wire to the size required by the selected tube. The tube is usually held in position by an inflatable balloon within the stomach.

There have been some modifications to this technique to allow the insertion of the typical PEG type tube with an internal 'mushroom', rather than a balloon.[16] This type of tube is often preferable because the aftercare is simpler and the same as for a standard PEG. The main disadvantage of the technique is that it is more fiddly and time-consuming to insert. In addition the tube is usually inserted via the mouth and most would consider this a contra-indication with head and neck cancers, due to the risk of seeding tumour in the gastrostomy track.[15] Therefore for this latter group of patients a traditional RIG is usually the method of choice, unless a gastrostomy is placed at the time of surgery.

Due to the differences in the methods of insertion, a RIG is often possible when PEG is not. This may be due to variations in the position of the stomach or difficulty intubating the patient with an endoscope. It is only on very rare occasions that RIG is not feasible. If a PEG insertion has failed, speak to a radiologist before a surgeon.

In summary, a RIG is simply an alternative method of inserting a gastrostomy. It is indicated for patients with oropharyngeal cancer; when PEG has been unsuccessful; if endoscopic skills are not readily available or on an individual patient basis when a specific tube may be required. Most radiology departments in the UK will have an interventional or gastrointestinal radiologist who will be happy to advise.

Gastrostomy tube types

Table 10.2 provides an overview of different types of gastrostomy tubes.

Standard gastrostomy tubes

These are held in place with an external fixation plate and internal retention disc (Figure 10.1). The traditional method of removing these tubes is by endoscopy. Another method for removal involves cutting

Table 10.2 Gastrostomy tube types

	Standard gastrostomy	Traction removable device	Balloon device	LPGD
Initial placement	Endoscopy or surgery	Endoscopy or radiology or surgery	Radiology or surgery	Surgery or radiology but usually after initial percutaneous gastrostomy placement
Held in place by:	External fixation plate and internal retention disc	Deforming device (flexible end)	Balloon inflated with 5–20 mL water	Balloon inflated with 5 mL water or cage design
Replacement	Suitable for long-term use	Suitable for long-term use	3–4 months	3–4 months
Possible indication	Post CVA, Parkinson's disease, MND	Post CVA, nutrition support pre chemo- or radiotherapy for head and neck carcinoma	Nutrition support pre chemo- or radiotherapy for head and neck carcinoma	Nutrition support in cystic fibrosis
Removal	Endoscopy	Bedside	Bedside (deflate balloon and apply gentle traction)	Bedside (balloon device: deflate balloon and apply gentle traction, cage device: removal with obturator)
Example	Freka PEG (Fresenius Kabi), Flocare PEG (Nutricia Advanced Medical Nutrition)	Corflo PEG (Merck Serono), Vygon MIC PEG	Vygon MIC gastrostomy tube, Corflo G tube (Merck Serono), Flocare gastrostomy tube (Nutricia Advanced Medical Nutrition)	Corflo CuBBY (Merck Serono), MIC-KEY (Vygon), Freka Button (Fresenius Kabi), Kangaroo Skin Level Cage Gastrostomy

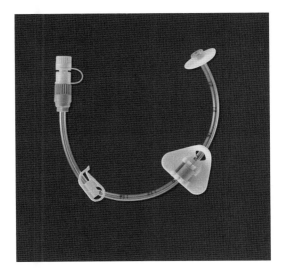

Figure 10.1 • Standard gastrostomy tube. Reproduced with kind permission of Fresenius Kabi.

the tube at skin level and allowing the inner components to be eliminated intestinally.[17] This method has advantages in terms of time and resources but is not without risk and has been associated with perforation and peritonitis.[18,19] It is not recommended by manufacturers.

Routine removal and replacement of these tubes is not necessary and with careful handling they can stay in situ for many years. Tubes are removed if they are no longer required, when broken, when deteriorating or when complications occur such as infection or erosion into the abdominal wall. Patients can take oral diet and fluids immediately after removal and the puncture canal heals rapidly when covered externally with a sterile compress.[11] Percutaneous gastrostomy tubes should not be removed for at least 14 days after insertion to ensure that a fibrous tract is established that will prevent intraperitoneal leakage. If a gastrostomy tube is inadvertently removed, a urethral catheter can be inserted through the tract and feeding recommenced until the tube is replaced.

Gastrostomy tubes with balloons or flexible ends

Those with flexible ends are designed to be removed by external traction (Figure 10.2). Balloon gastrostomy tubes are held in place by a balloon inflated with 5–20 mL water (Figure 10.3). These are particularly suitable where it can be anticipated that there will only be a temporary requirement for enteral tube feeding or if further endoscopy is not possible. Both removal and replacement can take place at the bedside. Replacement is recommended approximately every 3–4 months.

Low profile gastrostomy devices (LPGDs)

These devices are held in position by a balloon inflated with 5 mL water (Figure 10.4). In general it is recommended that LPGDs be placed secondarily after initial percutaneous gastrostomy tube placement with a mature established stoma canal (minimum 4 weeks post initial placement). It is

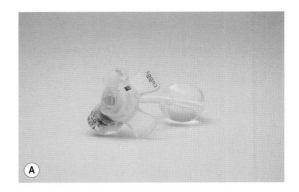

(A)

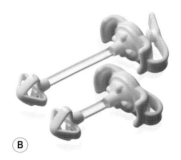

(B)

Figure 10.4 • (a) Low profile gastrostomy tube with balloon. Reproduced with kind permission of Merck Serono. **(b) Low profile gastrostomy device (cage design).** Reproduced with kind permission of Covidien plc.

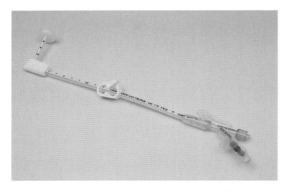

Figure 10.2 • Gastrostomy tube with flexible end. Reproduced with kind permission of Merck Serono.

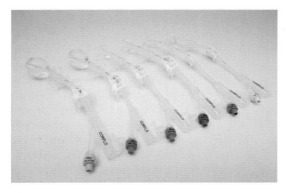

Figure 10.3 • Gastrostomy tube with balloon. Reproduced with kind permission of Merck Serono.

recommended that tubes are replaced every 3–4 months. They require an extension tube for feeding that needs to be replaced every 2 weeks. LPGDs are cosmetically appealing to patients and tend to be used more in younger patients.[11] They are composed of an internal stabilizer, a shaft, an external stabilizer, a connecting tube and an antireflux valve to prevent gastric contents from leaking onto the skin. The shaft must be of appropriate length for if too short, patients may develop pressure necrosis of the skin or the internal stabilizer may become embedded in the wall of the stomach. If an adult patient gains or loses 4 kg the shaft length should be re-evaluated.

Postpyloric feeding—the evidence

The postpyloric route may be considered where there is upper GI dysfunction, e.g. delayed gastric emptying, an increased risk of aspiration or reflux, or to facilitate early postoperative enteral feeding. Feed should always be delivered beyond the ligament of Treitz as there are no medical reasons for any kind of duodenal feeding.[11]

Aspiration and reflux

Postpyloric feeding has frequently been the route of choice in patients at risk of aspiration and reflux; however, there is conflict in the literature as to whether it definitely reduces the rate of either. Poor tube position and continued aspiration of oropharyngeal secretions have been identified as possible factors in recurrent aspiration in PEG-J and PEJ patients. Usually the nasogastric route is technically simpler and has been shown in most circumstances to achieve similar nutrient delivery. No significant differences have been reported for mortality, length of stay in intensive care or hospital, incidence of pneumonia, vomiting or diarrhoea in patients fed by the nasogastric compared with the nasojejunal route.[5] Consequently it has been recommended that postpyloric feeding may be considered in patients at *high* risk of aspiration, in malnourished patients undergoing major intra abdominal surgery, and in patients intolerant of gastric feeding despite the use of promotility agents.[5]

Early postoperative enteral tube feeding

Studies on early postoperative enteral tube feeding, compared to standard practice of 'nil by mouth' until return of gastrointestinal function, do not support the use of early enteral tube feeding.[5] However, the studies examined did not focus on very malnourished patients who might benefit from this approach. One such group is upper GI cancer patients. In a large multicentre trial, more than 300 malnourished patients with GI cancer were randomly assigned to receive enteral or parenteral isocaloric and isonitrogenous feeding regimens.[20] Postoperative complications were significantly lower at 34% in the enterally fed patients compared with 49% in those parenterally fed and postoperative stay was also reduced in the enterally fed group. Further benefits of postoperative enteral feeding with an immune-enhancing formula in this patient group on reduction in postoperative infectious complications have been reported.[21,22] More recently a randomised controlled trial involving 121 upper GI cancer patients randomised to receive early enteral nutrition via a needle catheter jejunostomy or conventional management, remaining nil by mouth until deemed safe to commence oral fluids, found a significant reduction in length of hospital stay and major complications in the early enteral nutrition group.[23]

Nasojejunal

This route is appropriate if postpyloric feeding is likely to be needed short term. Single and double lumen tubes are available, the latter enabling gastric aspiration and jejunal feeding, and are appropriate for postoperative feeding or for patients with gastric stasis (Table 10.3).

Table 10.3 Jejunal feeding tube types

		Placement	Indication	Example
Nasojejunal (NJ)	Single lumen	Bedside (self-propelling if gastric motility is normal)	Pancreatitis, risk of aspiration	Flocare Bengmark (Nutricia Advanced Medical Nutrition)
	Single lumen	Endoscopy, radiology, surgery	As above	COMPAT STAY PUT (Fresenius Kabi)
	Double lumen	Endoscopy, radiology, surgery	Postoperative, gastroparesis	Freka Easy In (Fresenius Kabi), NJ feeding tube (DOBBHOFF)
	Triple lumen	Endoscopy, radiology, surgery	Postoperative, gastroparesis	Freka Trelumina (Fresenius Kabi)
DPEJ/PEG-J		Endoscopy, radiology	As for NJ but where feeding is needed longer term	Freka PEG combination with intestinal tube (Fresenius Kabi), Jejunostomy tube via PEG (Merck Serono)
Needle catheter jejunostomy (NCJ)		Surgery	Postoperative	Freka Surgical Jejunostomy Set (Fresenius Kabi), Vygon MIC jejunostomy tube

Tube placement

The placement of a fine bore feeding tube beyond the pylorus can be difficult and a number of approaches have been described including placement at surgery, by endoscopy, under fluoroscopic guidance and blind introduction at the bedside. Fluoroscopy and endoscopy are highly effective for placement of small bowel tubes but these methods are expensive, require expertise not readily available 24 hours a day and require patient transfer to specialised areas of the hospital where the procedures are performed. Placement of small bowel feeding tubes by the blind nasoenteric approach is technically challenging with most studies showing a success rate of 15–30%.[24] Success with placement is influenced by the technique and degree of expertise of the clinician. The Bengmark tube (Nutricia Advanced Medical Nutrition, UK) is designed to pass spontaneously into the duodenum but in the absence of normal gastric motility trans pyloric passage cannot be relied upon.

In order to improve the success rate at postpyloric placement, modifications have been made to the feeding tubes including lengthening of the tube, altering the profile of the tip and adding various types of weights. Weights added to the distal end of tubes have not been found to have any advantage over unweighted tubes in terms of ability to pass into the jejunum or ability to keep the tube in place for longer. Prokinetic agents have been used to improve the likelihood of passage but are only recommended in patients with high gastric residuals for economic reasons as well as to avoid potential side effects.[24] Blind 'active' placement techniques have been described with 88–90% success.[25] One such technique is the Corpak 10-10-10 protocol that uses a fine bore 8F tube (originally called a Corpak tube), placed 10 minutes after administration of 10 mg metoclopramide and all but 10 cm of the 109-cm tube is inserted. After blind placement, tube position must be confirmed by abdominal X-ray.

Electromagnetic sensing devices that can track and display the path of feeding tubes during the placement procedure have also been used for both nasogastric and nasojejunal tube placement.

Jejunostomy

Jejunostomy tubes are appropriate for patients requiring longer term feeding and at risk of oesophageal reflux or aspiration (though the risk is not eliminated) or to facilitate early postoperative feeding following abdominal surgery.

Jejunostomy tube placement options

Open surgery

Surgical placement of jejunostomy tubes has been performed for over 100 years. Tubes pass through the abdominal wall into the jejunum. A variety of techniques can be used, e.g. Witzel jejunostomy, roux-en-y-jejunostomy, needle catheter jejunostomy and laparoscopic jejunostomy. Witzel jejunostomy involves formation of a serosal tunnel and is more likely to become infected. A number of cases of small bowel necrosis have been reported with this technique of placement.[26] Needle catheter jejunostomy is more frequently used nowadays and generally performed at the time of gastrointestinal surgery to enable postoperative enteral feeding. The tube is inserted immediately before the laparotomy wound is closed. The technique involves inserting a needle obliquely through the mesenteric border of the jejunum and a Seldringer technique is then used to insert the feeding tube through the abdominal wall. The catheter is secured to the abdominal wall with a purse string suture. The intestinal loop is fixed by 2–3 stitches to the parietal peritoneum and finally a small silicone plate preventing the catheter from slipping is fixed with two stitches to the skin at the site of the tube exit.[27]

Tubes require diligent nursing care as they are easily occluded and difficult if not impossible to replace unless a mature tract has developed. They should be flushed with water (as per local policy) before and after every feed or medication given. Any drugs given via the tube should be elixirs or suspensions rather than syrups. Minor technical complications have been reported (catheter luminal obstruction, local cellulitis) but these may be reduced by a good insertion technique and careful postoperative management. Major, life-threatening complications are rare but have been reported.[28,29]

Percutaneous endoscopic jejunostomy

A jejunal feeding tube may be passed over a guidewire into the small bowel through an existing gastrostomy tube (also known as a JET-PEG or PEG-J). Alternatively the jejunostomy tube can be placed as the initial procedure (tube placed with the PEG technique directly into the small intestine), direct PEJ (DPEJ). DPEJ should be the route of choice if long-term jejunal feeding (nonsurgical patients) is indicated as it is associated with lower rates of tube dysfunction and the need for reinterventions.[11] This method is technically difficult but is being performed more frequently. It can be used in patients who have had a gastrectomy or patients with unsuitable stomach access. Post insertion tube-related complications similar to those related to gastrostomy tubes can occur. Jejunal tubes can migrate back to the stomach (especially if there is persistent vomiting) or become disconnected with the whole tube passing through the PEG and into the gut.[10]

Radiologic gastrojejunostomy

Radiologists can insert a small feeding tube through the stomach and fluoroscopically guide it through the pylorus to the duodenojejunal flexure.

Complications of enteral tube feeding

Protocols should be in place for care and monitoring of enteral tube feeding to reduce the incidence of complications. Common problems associated with enteral feeding are listed in Table 10.4.

Gastrointestinal complications

Diarrhoea

Diarrhoea is a frequently reported complication of enteral tube feeding, causing distress for the patient and carer and increasing the risk of infection of surgical or pressure wounds and fluid and electrolyte abnormalities. The actual incidence is difficult to establish due to varying definitions used in studies, some investigators considering one single loose or non-formed stool evidence of diarrhoea, others requiring four or more liquid stools per day. An extensive review reported the existence of at least 14 definitions of diarrhoea with the incidence of diarrhoea ranging from 21 to 72%, depending on the definition used.[31]

Diarrhoea associated with enteral feeding is often multifactorial and most often caused by factors indirectly related to tube feeding, although the feed is frequently unjustly blamed. Only when causes not related to the feed itself have been eliminated should the feed be reduced, changed or discontinued. Antibiotics that have a deleterious effect on the colonic microflora, clostridium difficile infection, sorbitol or magnesium hydroxide containing antacids, hypoalbuminaemia, have all been implicated. Mechanisms related to the feed include bacterial contamination of the feed due to non-sterile handling of the feeding system and abnormal secretion of fluid into the lumen of the intestine due to intragastric infusion of feed.

Constipation

Any bowel pathology should be ruled out. Usually constipation results from inadequate fibre or fluid intake, inactivity, reduced bowel motility causing impaction, or drugs, e.g. opiates. A fibre-containing feed may help and adequate fluid replacement or laxatives may be required. A meta-analysis of the effect of fibre supplementation on the incidence of constipation found a non-significant trend for fibre to reduce the percentage of patients reporting constipation.[32] The explanation offered for failure to demonstrate statistical significance is the great variation in the definitions of constipation used in the studies.

Vomiting and aspiration

The cause of vomiting is multifactorial, although delayed gastric emptying is the most common cause. Prokinetic agents, e.g. metoclopramide, can be given to promote gastric emptying if gastrointestinal obstruction is not suspected and any pharmacological cause has been eliminated. Vomiting will increase the risk of pulmonary aspiration, but aspiration can occur without vomiting subsequent to gastric and/or small bowel reflux. Gastric feeding should only be performed when the head of the patient's bed is elevated to 30°–45° for prophylaxis of aspiration. Major risk factors for aspiration include decreased levels of consciousness, neuromuscular disease,

Table 10.4 Common complications associated with enteral tube feeding

Gastrointestinal	Diarrhoea Constipation Abdominal distension Vomiting Aspiration
Mechanical	Tube misplacement Tube displacement Tube occlusion Local complications, e.g. oesophageal erosions
Metabolic	Overfeeding Refeeding syndrome[a]
Other	Microbiological contamination[a]

[a]This topic is covered in detail elsewhere.[30]

vomiting or regurgitation, a need for prolonged supine position and persistently high gastric residual volumes.[33] Strategies for modifying risk include the use of prokinetic agents, the optimisation of oral care and elevation of the bed to 30°–45°. In high-risk patients jejunal feeding should be considered.[5]

Mechanical complications

Tube occlusion

Occlusion rates of 23–25% have been reported and are usually due to internal lumen obstruction.[34,35] Narrow tubes and long tubes are more likely to become blocked. Common reasons for obstruction are outlined in Table 10.5.

Unblocking tubes

First line of treatment is to prevent the tube blocking in the first place; there is general agreement that prevention is better than cure. It is important that protocols be put in place for flushing and drug administration. Enteral feeding pumps that can be programmed to administer water at intervals as required are now available. Water, sodium bicarbonate, carbonated drinks, e.g. coca cola, have all been used to clear blocked tubes but little evidence exists to support their use. Coca-cola may worsen the situation as its low pH 2.5 may coagulate the protein in the feed. If pancreatic enzymes are used they must first be brought to the correct pH and delivered close to the occlusion, which is not always practical in the clinical setting.

Many tubes can be unblocked with water, a 50-mL syringe and patience.[36] Smaller syringes may cause tube rupture due to high intraluminal pressure. Water in a 50-mL syringe with a gentle pumping action to aspirate and plunge the tube contents has been found to be effective. If the occlusion is in a visible part of the tube, gently squeezing and rolling the tube between the fingers may be effective. An alternative solution is to use Clog Zapper (CorPak), a commercial product designed to unblock tubes. This contains a cocktail of papain, ascorbic acid, maltodextrin and cellulose within a syringe. It is activated by mixing with water and administered through a fine bore tube that is supplied with the product and is then left for 30–60 minutes. It is an expensive option but this must be balanced against the cost of tube replacement.

Incorrect administration of oral medicines via venous catheters

In response to reports of deaths and harm caused by incorrect intravenous administration of oral liquid medicines, the NPSA released a safety alert in 2007.[37] This alert required action for the NHS and the independent sector to alter the design, supply and use of oral/enteral syringes and enteral feeding systems. The alert's key recommendations include:

- Only labelled oral/enteral syringes that cannot be connected to intravenous catheters should be used to measure and administer oral liquid medicines;

Table 10.5 Tube occlusion–causes and solutions

	Precipitating factor	Recommendation
Feed precipitate	Feed in contact with gastric secretions	Minimise checking of gastric residual volumes
Stagnant feed in tube	Tube not flushed adequately	Flush tube before and after each feeding episode and before and after any drugs given with 15–50 mL water
Incorrect drug administration	Tablets inadequately crushed Drug–feed interactions Drug–drug interactions	Liase with pharmacy regarding the suitability of drug preparations. Tablet crushing must only be considered as a last resort.[a] A tablet-crushing syringe or pestle and mortar can be used. If giving multiple drugs, give each separately and flush with water between each one
Tube material	Silicone tubes	Use polyurethane tubes with larger internal diameter

[a]Crushing tablets or opening capsules and administering drugs through enteral feeding tubes usually falls outside of a drug's product licence. The practitioner is then liable for any adverse effects that may occur.

- Enteral feeding systems should not contain ports that can be connected to intravenous syringes; and
- Appropriate policies and procedures should be put in place and audits conducted to review administration of oral liquid medicines.

Metabolic complications

Overfeeding

The provision of calories in excess of requirements should be avoided as it may result in metabolic complications, hyperglycaemia and hypercapnoea. Increased CO_2 production can delay weaning from a ventilator and cause respiratory distress.

Choice of feed

Details of the commercially prepared formulas available for enteral tube feeding and their means of delivery are outlined elsewhere.[30]

Novel substrates

Prebiotics/probiotics

A prebiotic is defined as a 'non-digestible food ingredient that beneficially affects the host by selectively stimulating the growth and/or activity of one or a limited number of bacteria in the colon and thus improving host health'.[38] Fructo-oligosaccharides (FOS) are polymers of glucose and fructose monomers in varying ratios and are the most extensively studied prebiotics. They have been added to enteral feeds for their ability to increase the concentration of bifidobacteria and reduce the concentration of potentially pathogenic bacteria, e.g. Clostridia (competitive exclusion theory).[39] No prospective randomised controlled trails of the use of prebiotics to prevent or treat diarrhoea in patients receiving enteral tube feeding have yet been published.

A probiotic is defined as 'a preparation of, or a product containing, viable defined micro-organisms in sufficient numbers, which alter the microflora in a compartment of the host and by that exert beneficial effects in this host'.[40] Probiotics include various species of *Lactobacilli*, *Bifidobacteria*, *Enterococcus* and *Saccharomyces*. The impact of probiotic provision on the incidence of diarrhoea has been investigated in two randomised controlled trials.[41,42] One used *Lactobacilli* and found no effect on the incidence of diarrhoea in patients receiving enteral tube feeding; the other used *Saccharomyces boulardii* in intensive care patients and found a 25% reduction in the number of patient-days with diarrhoea. Further research is needed using other probiotic strains and different patient populations to establish the efficacy of both pre- and/or probiotics in preventing diarrhoea during enteral tube feeding.

Fibre

Published literature on the effects of fibre in enteral feeds reveal variable results. A consensus report produced by ESPEN 2004 recommended that some form of fibre should be provided to most if not all patients receiving enteral nutrition.[43] Fibre should not be used in patients requiring enteral feeding with intestinal or colonic strictures, with fistulae or in patients with gastroparesis receiving intragastric feeding, although the evidence for this advice is poor. There is evidence that fermentable fibre (e.g. partially hydrogenated guar gum (PHGG)) may be effective in reducing diarrhoea in patients after surgery and in critically ill patients. For chronic patients requiring long-term enteral nutrition both fermentable fibre and non-fermentable fibre (e.g. soy polysaccharide) may be appropriate.

A meta-analysis of the clinical and physiological effects of fibre-containing enteral formula, found fibre supplementation to have a moderating effect on bowel function.[32] The incidence of diarrhoea in hospitalised patients participating in randomised controlled trials was found to be significantly reduced with fibre administration (odds ratio 0.68 CI: 0.48–0.96; $p = 0.03$). FOS was assumed to be part of the total fibre intake which when reported ranged from 14.0 to 34.9 g/day. Beneficial effects were found to be more likely to occur when the incidence of diarrhoea was high, in both ICU and non-ICU patients. Fibre supplementation was found to decrease bowel frequency in those with high bowel frequency and increase it in those patients with low bowel frequency; thereby fibre may have a role in the treatment of both constipation and diarrhoea. The proposed mechanism for the effect of fibre in reducing diarrhoea is the stimulation of colonic water and electrolyte absorption by short chain fatty acids (SCFA) produced as a consequence of bacterial metabolism of fibre.[32] The proposed mechanism for the effect of fibre in increasing bowel frequency is the faecal bulking effect, water retaining properties and the increase in bacterial biomass resulting from fermentation.[38]

Immunonutrition

The link between nutrition and immune function is well established and a large body of evidence exists suggesting that malnutrition has detrimental effects on immune function and susceptibility to infection.[44,45] The concept of 'immunonutrition' was first introduced 10–15 years ago based on the premise that certain nutritional components may have a favourable effect on immune function and could thus lower infectious complications in patients. These nutrients were identified initially in studies in animal models and have since been used in clinical practice. The term immunonutrition refers to the use of enteral formulas that have been supplemented by some combination of glutamine, arginine, n-3-fatty acids, ribonucleic acids, antioxidant vitamins (C, E, beta carotene) or micronutrients (zinc, selenium, chromium).

Key characteristics of these components are summarised in Box 10.2. After many years of research, little has been proven and the topic remains highly controversial despite a wealth of randomised controlled trials and at least three meta-analyses.[46–48]

Immunonutrition — the evidence

When examining the published evidence on immunonutrition in hospital patients it is notable that the existing literature has considerable limitations:

1. Most of the studies have small sample sizes and may not be adequately powered to address outcomes such as mortality.
2. Few studies use control formulas equivalent in nutrient values in all but the selected immunonutrients.
3. The immunonutrition formulas used in studies provide a number of immunonutrients at the same time, so it is impossible to establish which nutrient or which nutrient combination and in what dose is needed to optimise outcome. Some nutrients may have positive effects and others negative effects. Effects might also vary depending on patient illness and/or its severity. Individual components have not generally been rigorously and independently tested in large trials.
4. The published meta-analyses combine studies that use different immunonutrition formulas and different control formulas. For example,

Box 10.2

Characteristics of 'immunonutrients'

Arginine

Classified as a conditionally essential amino acid because endogenous production may be inadequate during periods of growth, illness or injury.[49] Supplemental arginine has been shown to improve nitrogen balance, increase T-cell immune function and increase collagen deposition in wound grafts.[49]

Glutamine

Acts as an oxidative fuel for rapidly dividing cells including enterocytes and colonocytes. It is a precursor of glutathione, purines, pyrimidines, nucleotides and amino sugars,[50] and can behave as an essential amino acid in certain clinical settings. It has been studied as a single additive to enteral and parenteral nutrition as well as being included in formulas with a mixture of immune-enhancing ingredients.

Omega-3 fatty acids

The omega-3 fatty acids eicosapentanoic acid (EPA) and docosahexaenoic acid (DHA) are anti-inflammatory; by competing with arachidonic acid (omega-6) they antagonise production of proinflammatory eicosanoids.[51]

Nucleotides

Precursors of RNA and DNA, nucleotides have been found to augment cellular immune functions as well as protect structural and functional integrity of the intestinal mucosa.[52]

some formulas contain arginine, n-3 fatty acids and nucleotides (e.g. Impact, Novartis); others contain arginine, glutamine and nucleotides and no n-3 fatty acids (e.g. Immun-Aid, B. Braun). The amount of each nutrient present differs between formulas.

5. The 'dose' of immunonutrients delivered differs between studies. It has been suggested that some randomised trials may have failed to demonstrate a treatment effect due to inadequate dosing. This is likely to occur if a product is being administered enterally and there are issues with tolerance.

Immunonutrition — the evidence in selected patient groups

Surgical and septic patients are two distinctly different groups in terms of energy requirements, and metabolic and immune response. Severe sepsis is characterised by an exaggerated inflammatory response together with cellular immune dysfunction. These patients may benefit more from immunosuppression or a blunting of the systemic inflammatory response and so nutrients such as arginine that further stimulate the systemic inflammatory response may be deleterious.[53] Elective surgical patients experience less cytokine activation and some suppression of cell-mediated immunity, putting them at higher risk for acquired infectious morbidity and mortality. Consequently, it is possible that nutrients such as arginine that stimulate the cellular defence system may reduce infectious complications.[54] It seems sensible therefore to examine these groups separately.

Elective GI surgery patients

There is evidence that immunonutrition formulas may improve outcome in elective GI surgery patients. In a systematic review of immunonutrition by Heyland and colleagues,[47] a subgroup analysis of elective surgical patients found infectious complication rates were significantly lower and length of hospital stay was less in the immunonutrition groups. Postoperative immunonutrition in patients undergoing elective gastrointestinal surgery was subsequently recommended by the US Summit on Immune Enhancing Therapy.[55] Preoperative oral feeding with an immune-enhanced formula combined with postoperative jejunal feeding with the same formula in patients with GI cancer resulted in a significantly reduced incidence of postoperative infectious complications.[21,56] Another series of studies from Italy provide further evidence of the benefits of perioperative enteral feeding with immune-enhanced formulas.[22,57] In malnourished patients the greatest benefit on the reduction of complications was achieved with an immune-enhanced formula given perioperatively.[22] In well-nourished patients the provision of an immune-enhanced formula preoperatively alone was sufficient to significantly reduce infectious complications and length of postoperative stay.[57]

Critically ill patients
Studies providing evidence in septic critically ill patients.
Bower et al randomised 326 ICU patients to early enteral administration of immune-enhanced formula or control formula.[58] In a subgroup analysis of patients with sepsis the mortality rate with immunonutrition was three times the control one. This study has been criticised for using an inappropriate control formula with low protein

content. Higher mortality in the subgroup of patients with pneumonia on ICU entry given immunonutrition compared to those given control formula was subsequently reported by Dent et al, resulting in the halting of recruitment.[59] Similarly, recruitment of patients with severe sepsis and subsequent randomisation to receive an immune-enhanced formula or parenteral nutrition was stopped by Bertolini et al on finding from the interim analysis a higher mortality rate in the treatment group given an immune-enhanced enteral formula compared to that in the group receiving parenteral nutrition.[60] The study continued to randomise non-septic critically ill patients to receive the immune enhanced formula or TPN and found no effect on mortality at 28 days but a significant difference in the occurrence of severe sepsis or septic shock. In the absence of a control arm receiving a standard enteral formula it cannot be inferred that this treatment effect is due to the use of an immune-enhanced formula and not due to the route of nutrient delivery.[61]

Studies providing evidence in non-septic critically ill patients.
Conflicting with evidence that immunonutrition may be harmful is a study by Galban and colleagues in 2000.[62] They randomised 181 patients with infection (not septic) to receive an immune-enhanced formula or an isonitrogenous, isocaloric control enteral feed. Mortality was significantly reduced in the treatment group compared to that in the controls. Subgroup analysis found the treatment effect was confined to the least sick patients. Interestingly, in this positive study successful feeding (defined as > 833 mL/day) was attained in 84% patients. In the Bower study, although negative overall, a reduction in length of stay with immunonutrition compared with that in the low protein control feed was found in the group that tolerated > 821 mL/day.[58]

Studies providing evidence in heterogenous critically ill patients.
Atkinson and colleagues in 1998 randomised 398 heterogenous ICU patients to receive immune-enhanced formula or isonitrogenous, isocaloric control formula.[63] This group found on an intention-to-treat basis no significant difference in outcome measures. On examination of those patients successfully fed at least 2.5 L in the first 72 hours, there was a significant reduction in length of hospital stay and requirement for mechanical ventilation. Infectious complications were not reported. A further study in 2005, again in a heterogenous intensive care population of 597 patients, found no

significant differences in infectious complications, mortality or length of stay between immunonutrition groups and the isocaloric control group.[64] Average calorie intake was 1330 kcal/day in those that completed the protocol. Of note in this study is that the immune formula was different to the trials of Bower, Galban and Atkinson and contained less arginine.[58,62,63] There are no randomised trials of arginine supplementation in critically ill patients. Arginine is capable of promoting nitric oxide production and may have potential for harm in critically ill patients with sepsis.[65] Studies using formulas with an arginine content < 12 g/1000 kcal report no reduction in infectious complications or length of stay,[64] while those with at least 12 g arginine/1000 kcal have demonstrated improvement in outcomes.[56,62,66] Nonetheless, because of the potential for harm in patients with severe sepsis, formulas containing high levels of arginine are not recommended until its effect on inflammatory events are more fully investigated and understood.[65]

Recommendations

The Canadian Clinical Practice Guidelines attempted to isolate the effect of individual nutrients in specific homogenous critically ill patient populations.[67] This review recommends that enteral glutamine should be considered in burn and trauma patients and that products with fish oils, borage oils and antioxidants should be considered in patients with acute respiratory distress syndrome (ARDS). This is on the basis that there is no evidence that glutamine, antioxidants or fish oils are harmful to critically ill patients. On the other hand it is recommended that 'diets supplemented with arginine and other nutrients not be used for critically ill patients'.[67] Results of two meta-analyses,[46,68] two systematic reviews,[47,48] and a consensus statement from an expert panel[55] all concluded that immuonutrition may decrease the incidence of some infectious complications but does not improve mortality in critically ill patients.

Conclusion

The use of immune-enhanced formulas continues to vary between centres and is not currently routine practice in the UK. More studies are needed with adequate patient numbers that receive feed for an adequate length of time. Immunonutrients should be the only variable difference between control and experimental formula. Which immunonutrients, in what dose and what outcome will be improved needs to be established before firm conclusions can be reached.

Ethical issues and enteral tube feeding

When considering artificial nutrition support it is frequently the patient's existing nutritional intake and their ability to meet nutritional requirements that is the centre of discussions. Ethical issues are not always considered.

Medical ethics are based on four main principles that should guide decision-making for healthcare staff when faced with ethical dilemmas.[69]

Autonomy: The person's right to self-determination

Beneficence: To do good

Non-maleficence: To avoid doing harm

Justice: Fair and equal resources to all

Crucial to any treatment decision is obtaining patient consent. Food or fluid given by tube is legally a medical therapy and not basic care and requires patient consent before commencing treatment.[70] Competent adults have the absolute right to decide what treatment he receives. A competent adult can make an advance decision (similar document to advance directive or living will) to refuse care or treatment, intending that refusal take effect when they no longer have capacity to refuse procedure or treatment. In certain circumstances it can be legal to enforce nutritional treatment for an unwilling patient, e.g. severely malnourished patients with anorexia nervosa who on assessment are considered incompetent to make rational decisions regarding their care.

The situation is more difficult if the patient lacks capacity to make a decision about their care. The Mental Capacity Act (MCA) came into force in England and Wales in 2000.[71] The Act was developed to put the needs and wishes of the person lacking capacity at the centre of any decision-making. It is recommended that an assessment of capacity should be undertaken as part of the patient's overall assessment. In the absence of mental capacity any action taken must be in the patient's best interests rather than the interests or convenience of those providing care and support. Under the MCA if an advance decision has been made to refuse treatment it must refer to a specific treatment in specified circumstances. The patient's wishes should be taken into account and decisions made on their behalf should include consultation with family members. Good communication is vital. The Act requires healthcare professionals to ensure that patients and their families understand the treatment options available so that meaningful decisions can be made. Basic care involves offering food and drink and the adoption of all possible measures to ensure the comfort of the patient and provision of pain relief. There is never an ethical justification for the withdrawal of basic care.[72] Patients and relatives can interpret a decision not to commence or to continue nutritional support as abandonment. It cannot be assumed that the commencement of feeding is always in a patient's best interests.[73] If there is any doubt as to the patient's capacity or what is or is not in their best interests, there is guidance provided by BAPEN and the General Medical Council or legal advice and, if appropriate, court intervention can be sought.[74,75]

Key points

- The gut should be used whenever possible for nutrition support.

- All patients requiring artificial enteral nutrition should receive an individual assessment to identify the most appropriate route of feeding and the most appropriate enteral feeding device.
- Education of ward staff and patients on appropriate feeding tube aftercare is important to avoid complications.
- Despite many years of research and development of novel feeding substrates (including probiotics and feeds enriched with immunonutrients) little has been proven and practice continues to vary between centres.

Acknowledgements

Dr J Shirley, Consultant Radiologist, Derriford Hospital, for his contribution on radiologically placed gastrostomy tubes.

Dina Khawnekar, dietitian, for her help with literature searching.

Case study

Mrs X is a 78-year-old woman admitted to hospital with severe progressive dysphagia to solids and liquids for the previous 3 months, resulting in 15% weight loss. She is now unable to tolerate any oral diet or fluids. Advanced inoperable oesophageal carcinoma is diagnosed. Bedside and endoscopic attempts to place a nasogastric tube fail.

QUESTIONS

1. Which type of nutritional support is best for this patient?
2. What are the likely metabolic complications she may encounter on commencing enteral feeding?
3. The NG tube is inadvertently displaced overnight; Mrs X refuses attempts to replace the tube. Should Mrs X be forced to have another tube?

ANSWERS

1. Which type of nutritional support is best for this patient?

Efforts should be made to provide enteral nutrition support for this lady until her medical management is decided. Radiologic placement of a nasogastric tube is frequently successful when endoscopy fails.

2. What are the likely metabolic complications she may encounter on commencing enteral feeding?

Due to the prolonged period of negligible oral intake and 15% weight loss this lady is at high risk of developing refeeding syndrome on commencing enteral feeding.

3. The NG tube is inadvertently displaced overnight; Mrs X refuses attempts to replace the tube. Should Mrs X be forced to have another tube?

No. Food or fluid by tube is a medical therapy and not basic care and requires patient consent before commencing treatment. If the patient is competent to make the decision she has the right to decide what treatment she receives.

References

1. Dobbie RP, Hoffineister JA. Continuous pump-tube hyperalimentation. *Surg Gynecol Obstet.* 1976;143:273–276.

2. Koretz RL. Do data support nutrition support? Part I. *J Am Diet Assoc.* 2007;107:988–996.

3. Stratton RJ, Green CJ, Elia M. *Disease Related Malnutrition: An Evidence Based Approach to Treatment.* Wallingford: CABI; 2003.

4. Koretz RL. Do data support nutrition support? Part II. *J Am Diet Assoc.* 2007;107:1374–1380.

5. National Institute for Clinical Excellence. Enteral tube feeding in hospital and the community. In: *Nutrition Support for Adults, Oral Nutrition Support, Enteral Tube Feeding and Parenteral Nutrition, Methods, Evidence and Guidance.* London: 2006:115–124.

6. *Patient Safety Alert 05. Reducing the harm caused by misplaced nasogastric feeding tubes.* National Patient Safety Agency. 2005. Available at: http://www.npsa.nhs.uk/patientsafety/alerts-and-directives/alerts/nasogastric-feeding-tubes/.

7. Howes DW, Shelley ES, Pickett W. Colorimetric carbon dioxide detector to determine accidental tracheal feeding tube placement. *Can J Anaesth.* 2005;52:428–432.

8. McGuirt WF, Strout JJ. How I do it—head and neck. A targeted problem and its solution: securing of intermediate duration feeding tubes. *Laryngoscope.* 1980;90(12):2046–2048.

9. Anderson MR, O'Connor M, Mayer P, et al. The nasal loop provides an alternative to percutaneous endoscopic gastrostomy in high-risk dysphagic stroke patients. *Clin Nutr.* 2004;23:501–506.

10. Stroud M, Duncan H, Nightingale J. Guidelines for enteral feeding in adult hospital patients. *Gut.* 2003;52(Svii):vii–vii11.

11. Löser C, Aschl G, Hébuterne X, et al. ESPEN guidelines on artificial enteral nutrition-percutaneous endoscopic gastrostomy. *Clin Nutr.* 2005;24(5):848–861.

12. O' Toole P. *Complications associated with the placement of percutaneous endoscopic gastrostomy.* British Society of Gastroenterology Guidelines in Gastroenterology; 2006:26–30. Available at: http://www.bsg.org.uk/pdf_word_docs/complications.pdf. Accessed April 2008.

13. Dennis M, Walow C. The FOOD trial collaboration: effect of timing and method of enteral tube feeding for dysphagic stroke patients. *Lancet.* 2005;365:755–763.

14. National Confidential Enquiry into Patient Outcomes and Death. *Scoping Our Practice: The 2004 Report of the National Confidential Enquiry into Patient Outcomes and Death.* London: NCEPOD; 2004.

15. Sinclair JJ, Scolapio JS, Stark ME, et al. Metastasis of head and neck carcinoma to the site of percutaneous endoscopic gastrostomy: case report and literature review. *JPEN J Parenter Enteral Nutr.* 2001;25:282–285.

16. Laasch HU, Wilbraham L, Bullen K, et al. Gastrostomy insertion: comparing the options—PEG, RIG or PIG? *Clin Radiol.* 2003;58(5):398–405.

17. Karula J, Harma C. A simple and inexpensive method of removal or replacement of gastrostomy tubes. *J Am Med Assoc.* 1991;265:1426–1428.

18. Steinberg RM, Madhala O, Freud E, et al. Skin level division of percutaneous endoscopic gastrostomy retrieval: a hazardous procedure. *Eur J Paediatr Surg.* 2002;12(2):127–128.

19. Lattuneddu A, Morgagni P, Benati G, et al. Small bowel perforation after incomplete removal of percutaneous endoscopic gastrostomy catheter. *Surg Endosc.* 2003;17(12):2028–2031.

20. Bozzetti F, Braga M, Gianotti L, et al. Postoperative enteral versus parenteral nutrition in malnourished patients with gastrointestinal cancer: a randomised multicenter trial. *Lancet.* 2001;358:1487–1492.

21. Braga M, Gianotti L, Vignali A, et al. Preoperative oral arginine and n-3 fatty acid supplementation improves the immunometabolic host response and outcome after colorectal resection for cancer. *Surgery.* 2002;5:805–814.

22. Braga M, Gianotti L, Nespoli L, et al. Nutritional approach in malnourished cancer patients. *Arch Surg.* 2002;137:174–180.

23. Barlow R, Puntis M, Hunt, et al. *Randomised Controlled Trial of Early Enteral Nutrition (EEN) versus Conventional Management (CON) in Patients Undergoing Major Resection for Upper Gastrointestinal Cancer.* 2007:OC15 BAPEN.

24. Marik PE, Zaloga GP. Gastric versus post-pyloric feeding: a systematic review. *Crit Care.* 2003;7(3):46–51.

25. Lee AJ, Eve R, Bennett MJ. Evaluation of a technique for blind placement of post-pyloric feeding tubes in intensive care: application in patients with gastric ileus. *Intensive Care Med.* 2006;32:553–556.

26. Lawlor DK, Inculet RI, Malthaner RA. Small-bowel necrosis associated with jejunal tube feeding. *Can J Surg.* 1998;41(6):459–462.

27. Meier R, Harsanyi L. Enteral nutrition. In: Sobotka L, Allison SP, Furst P, et al. *Basics in Clinical Nutrition.* 3rd edn. Prague: Galen; 2004:212–213.

28. Date RS, Clements WDB, Gilliland R. Feeding jejunostomy: is there enough evidence to justify its routine use? *Dig Surg.* 2004;21:142–145.

29. Melis M, Fichera A, Ferguson MK. Bowel necrosis associated with early jejunal tube feeding: a complication of postoperative enteral nutrition. *Arch Surg.* 2006;141:701–704.

30. Thomas B, Bishop J, eds. *Manual of Dietetic Practice.* 4th edn. Oxford: Blackwell; 2007:97–107.

31. Zimmaro BD, Guenter PA, Settle RG. Defining and reporting diarrhoa in tube-fed patients-what a mess!. *Am J Clin Nutr.* 1992;55:753–759.

32. Elia M, Engfer MB, Green CJ, et al. Systematic review and meta-analysis: the clinical and physiological effects of fibre-containing enteral formulae. *Aliment Pharmacol Ther.* 2007;27(2):120–145.

33. McClave SA, DeMeo MT, DeLegge MH, et al. North American Summit on Aspiration in the Critically Ill Patient: consensus statement. *JPEN J Parenter Enteral Nutr.* 2002;26(suppl 6):S80–S85.

34. Sriram K, Jayanthi V, Lakshmi RG, et al. Prophylactic locking of enteral feeding tubes with pancreatic enzymes. *J Parenter Enteral Nutr.* 1997;21:353–356.

35. Marcuard SP, Perkins AM. Clogging of feeding tubes. *J Parenter Enteral Nutr.* 1998;12:403–405.

36. Colagiovanni L. Restoring and maintaining patency of enteral feeding tubes. In: White R, Bradnam V, eds. *Handbook of Drug Administration via Enteral Feeding Tubes.* London: RPS; 2007:13–20.

37. *Patient Safety Alert 19. Promoting Safer Measurement and Administration of Liquid Medicines via Oral and other Enteral Routes.* National Patient Safety Agency. Available at: http://www.npsa.nhs.uk/patientsafety/alerts-and-directives/alerts/liquid-medicines/; 2007.

38. Gibson GR, Roberfroid MB. Dietary modulation of the human colonic microbiota: introducing the concept of prebiotics. *J Nutr.* 1995;125(6):1401–1412.

39. Wolf BW, Chow J, Snowden MK, et al. Medical foods and fructo-oligosaccharides: a novel fermentable dietary fiber. In: *Oligosaccharides in Food.* Washington DC: American Chemical Society; 2003:118–134.

40. Schrezenmeir J, de Vrese M. Probiotics, prebiotics and synbiotics: approaching a definition. *Am J Clin Nutr.* 2001;73:S361–S364.

41. Heimburger DC, Sockwell DG, Geels WJ. Diarrhoea with enteral feeding: prospective reappraisal of putative causes. *Nutrition.* 1994;10:392–396.

42. Bleichner G, Blehaut H, Mentec H, et al. Sacchromyces boulardii prevents diarrhoea in critically ill tube fed patients. *Intensive Care Med.* 1997;23:517–523.

43. Meier R, Gassull MA. Consensus recommendations on the effects and benefits of fibre in clinical practice. *Clin Nutr Suppl.* 2004;1:73–80.

44. Bistrain BR, Blackburn GL, Scrimshaw NS. Cellular immunity in semistarved states in hospitalised adults. *Am J Clin Nutr.* 1975;28(10):1148–1155.

45. McWhirter JP, Pennington CR. Incidence and recognition of malnutrition in hospital. *Br Med J.* 1994;308(6934):945–948.

46. Beale RJ, Bryg DJ, Bihari DJ. Immunonutrition in the critically ill: a systematic review of clinical outcome. *Crit Care Med.* 1999;27(12):2799–2805.

47. Heyland DK, Novak F, Drover JW, Minto J, et al. Should immunonutrition become routine in critically ill patients? A systematic review of the evidence. *J Am Med Assoc.* 2001;286:944–953.

48. Montejo J. Immunonutrition in the intensive care unit. A systematic review and consensus statement. *Clin Nutr.* 2003;22(3):221–233.

49. Barbul A. Arginine and immune function. *Nutrition.* 1990;6(1):53–58.

50. Souba WW, Smith RJ, Wilmore DW. Glutamine metabolism by the intestinal tract. *JPEN J Parenter Enteral Nutr.* 1985;9:608–617.

51. Calder PC. Dietary modification of inflammation with lipids. *Proc Nutr Soc.* 2002;59:553–563.

52. Grimble GK, Westwood OM. Nucleotides as immunomodulators in clinical nutrition. *Curr Opin Clin Nutr Metab Care.* 2001;4:57–64.

53. Bertolini G, Luciani D, Biolo G. Immunonutrition in septic patients. A philosophical view of the current situation. *Clin Nutr.* 2007;26:25–29.

54. Heyland D, Dhaliwal R. Immunonutrition in the critically ill: from old approaches to new paradigms. *Intensive Care Med.* 2005;31(4):501–503.

55. Bozzetti F. Summit on immune-enhancing enteral therapy. *JPEN J Parenter Enteral Nutr.* 2001;25(6):356–357.

56. Braga M, Gianotti L, Radaelli G, et al. Perioperative immunonutrition in patients undergoing cancer surgery. Results of a randomised double blind phase trial. *Arch Surg.* 1999;134:428–433.

57. Gianotti L, Braga M, Nespoli L, et al. A randomised controlled trial of preoperative oral supplementation with a specialized diet in patients with gastrointestinal cancer. *Gastroenterology.* 2002;122:1763–1770.

58. Bower RH, Cerra FB, Bershadsky B, Licari J, et al. Early enteral administration of a formula (Impact Registered Trademark) supplemented with arginine, nucleotides, and fish oil in intensive care unit patients: results of a multicenter, prospective, randomized, clinical trial. *Crit Care Med.* 1995;23:436–449.

59. Dent DL, Heyland DK, Levy H. Immunonutrition may increase mortality in critically ill patients with pneumonia: results of a randomised trial. *Crit Care Med.* 2003;30:A17.

60. Bertolini G, Luciani D, Biolo G. Immunonutrition in septic patients. A philosophical view of the current situation. *Clin Nutr.* 2007;26:25–29.

61. Radrizzani D, Bertolini G, Facchini R, et al. Early enteral immunonutrition vs. parenteral nutrition in critically ill patients without severe sepsis: a randomized clinical trial. *Intensive Care Med.* 2006;32(8):1191–1198.

62. Galban C, Montejo JC, Mesejo A, et al. An immune-enhancing enteral diet reduces mortality rate and episodes of bacteremia in septic intensive care unit patients. *Crit Care Med.* 2000;28(3):643–648.

63. Atkinson S, Sieffert E, Bihari D. A prospective, randomized, double-blind, controlled clinical trial of enteral immunonutrition in the critically ill. *Crit Care Med.* 1998;26(7):1164–1172.

64. Kieft H, Roos AN, van Drunen JD, et al. Clinical outcome of immunonutrition in a heterogeneous intensive care population. *Intensive Care Med.* 2005;31(4):524–532.

65. Suchner U, Heyland DK, Peter K. Immune-modulatory actions of arginine in the critically ill. *Br J Nutr.* 2002;87S:S121–S132.

66. Kudsk KA, Minard G, Croce MA, et al. A randomized trial of isonitrogenous enteral diets after severe trauma: an immune-enhancing diet reduces septic complications. *Ann Surg.* 1996;224(4):531–543.

67. Heyland DK, Dhaliwal R, Drover JW, et al. Canadian clinical practice guidelines for nutrition support in mechanically ventilated, critically ill adult patients. *JPEN J*

Parenter Enteral Nutr. 2003;27(5): 355–373.

68. Heys SD, Walker LG, Smith I, et al. Enteral nutritional supplementation with key nutrients in patients with critical illness and cancer: a meta-analysis of randomized controlled clinical trials. *Ann Surg.* 1999; 229(4):467–477.

69. Beauchamp TL, Childress JF. *Principles of Biomedical Ethics.* 5th edn. New York: Oxford University Press; 1994.

70. Fennell P, et al. *Airdale NHS Trust v Bland Judgement of Family Division Court of Appeal (Civil Division) and House of Lords. Medico-Legal Reports: vol 12.* London: Butterworths; 1993:64–143.

71. Department for Constitutional Affairs Justice, Rights and Democracy Mental Capacity Act 2005. *Code of Practice 2007.* Available at: http://www.dca.gov. uk/legal-policy/mentalcapacity/ mca-cp.pdf. Accessed 4 April 2008.

72. Mac Fie J. Ethical implications of recognising nutritional support as a medical therapy. *Clin Nutr Update.* 2002;7(1):3–5.

73. Lyons C, Brotherton A, Stanley N, et al. The Mental Capacity Act 2005: implications for dietetic practice. *J Hum Nutr Diet.* 2007;20:302–310.

74. Jones L. *Ethical and Legal Aspects of Clinical Hydration and Nutritional Support.* Maidenhead: British Association for Parenteral and Enteral Nutrition; 1998.

75. General Medical Council. *Withholding and Withdrawing Life-Prolonging Treatments: Good Practice in Decision Making.* London: GMC; 2002.

Parenteral nutrition

Paula Murphy

LEARNING OBJECTIVES

By the end of the chapter the reader will be able to:

- Appreciate the indications for parenteral nutrition;
- Gain an insight into the parenteral nutrition solutions available and the evolution of some special substrates;
- Understand the different routes by which parenteral nutrition can be delivered and the venous access devices available;
- Understand the complications associated with parenteral nutrition delivery and how they may be avoided;
- Gain a practical understanding of how a patient receiving parenteral nutrition should be monitored; and
- Appreciate the indications, prevalence and complications associated with home parenteral nutrition.

Introduction

Parenteral nutrition (PN) refers to the provision of nutrients by the intravenous route and was introduced by Dudrick in 1967.[1] Since then it has developed as an effective feeding technique and has been widely implemented for feeding patients with both functioning and non-functioning gastrointestinal tracts. Its use in patients with functioning gastrointestinal tracts occurred for a number of reasons including its relative ease of administration, poor understanding of gut function and enteral feeding techniques, and a limited range of enteral feeding devices. PN use is now declining with recognition of its inherent risks and evidence for the superiority of enteral nutrition (EN).

Nonetheless PN is a life-saving therapy for many patients with gastrointestinal (GI) failure.

The choice of EN versus PN is no longer an issue. There are no data from randomised trials to support the use of PN in patients with an intact gastrointestinal tract,[2] and PN may be associated with increased complications when given to patients not malnourished.[3] Worthy of consideration, however, is that many of the trials comparing enteral with parenteral nutrition are not comparable in terms of energy intake. Studies reported that an increased incidence of sepsis in patients receiving PN were fed more energy compared to enterally fed patients.[4–6] Overfeeding easily occurs with PN and increases the risk of complications. Excess delivery of nutrients by the enteral route as well as the parenteral route is associated with complications and should be avoided. Notwithstanding this, where artificial nutrition support is required, it is established that enteral tube feeding is the safer, cheaper, less demanding and a more 'physiological' option.[7] Although the exact reasons for the effectiveness of enteral over parenteral nutrition in patients with functional gastrointestinal tracts are not yet fully established, results from animal and human studies clearly show parenteral formulas to be less supportive of the immune and gastrointestinal systems.

Indications for parenteral nutrition

PN is an essential adjunct to the management of patients who are unable to obtain adequate nutrition via the enteral route. It should be reserved for patients who need support but have either a non-functioning or a non-accessible gastrointestinal tract.[7] This might include patients with short bowel syndrome, intestinal ischaemia or infarction, intestinal obstruction, severe diarrhoea, motility disorders (e.g. scleroderma), acute intestinal failure, large volume fistula output and inability to access the gastrointestinal tract. It has been suggested that up to 70% of patients receiving PN may have impaired gastric emptying and reduced colonic motility but adequate small bowel function and thus could be fed by the enteral route.[2] There is a subset of patients where the GI tract is accessible but an adequate nutrient intake cannot be achieved; in these cases supplementary PN can be provided. Optimal timing and composition of PN in these cases requires further study. If individuals are well nourished there is no evidence that withholding PN for seven days is harmful; providing PN during this period would only result in an increased risk of infection.

Administration of parenteral nutrition

Factors to be considered when planning for a patient to receive PN are outlined in Box 11.1.

Nutrient solutions should be administered through a dedicated feeding line using a volumetric pump with occlusion and air-in-line alarms.[7] Administration sets should be changed every 24 hours.[8] PN can be administered continuously (over 24 hours) or cyclically (over 10–18 hours). For patients receiving peripheral PN via peripheral venous cannulae, cyclic delivery of PN should be considered with planned routine cannula change (every 1–2 days) to reduce the risk of peripheral vein thrombosis (PVT). Cyclic PN has the advantage of facilitating patient mobility,

---

> ## Box 11.1
>
> **Factors to be considered when planning for a patient to receive parenteral nutrition (PN)**
>
> 1. Nutritional requirements
> 2. Baseline metabolic parameters
> 3. Anticipated duration of PN
> 4. Accessibility of veins
> 5. Venous access device
> 6. Complications of therapy (risks should be weighted against the benefits)

---

which is particularly important for the quality of life of patients receiving home PN. It has also been suggested that cyclic PN may be helpful in the management of PN-associated liver disease.[9] For patients receiving PN centrally, there is evidence that continuous delivery may lead to better nutrient balance.[10] It should be noted that this study included major surgery patients and may not be applicable to patients requiring long-term PN where metabolic conditions are different.

Parenteral nutrition solutions

Total parenteral nutrition (TPN) implies that all macronutrient (carbohydrate, amino acid and lipid) and micronutrient (electrolytes, vitamins and trace elements) requirements are met by a solution administered into a peripheral or central vein. TPN admixtures are referred to as all-in-one (AIO) solutions containing all the required nutritional components. Standardised fixed feeding regimens or individually compounded admixtures are available. These are described in more detail elsewhere.[11] Vitamins, trace elements and electrolytes may be added to both regimens but must be done under controlled pharmaceutical conditions and not at ward level.[7] Individually compounded admixtures are manufactured under strictly controlled aseptic conditions in a suitable pharmacy manufacturing unit. There is no evidence that outcome is improved with either regimen. It is recommended that patients' nutritional requirements be established by suitably trained personnel before the PN regimen type is decided.[7,12] Patients' requirements should be balanced with standardised PN formulations to enhance patient safety and reduce both ordering and compounding errors. Ultimately a safe PN system must be in place to minimise procedural incidents and maximise the ability to meet individual requirements.

Macronutrients in parenteral nutrition

Carbohydrate

Carbohydrate in PN is provided by glucose, a cheap energy source available in a range of concentrations, 5–70%. While the inclusion of some carbohydrate is essential for Central Nervous System (CNS) function, the maximum glucose oxidation rate, 4–5 mg/kg/min/day, should not be exceeded as this may result in hyperglycaemia, hepatic steatosis and impaired respiratory function with increased CO_2 production. Glucose tolerance is impaired in patients with sepsis and concurrent insulin treatment may be necessary to prevent hyperglycaemia.

Protein

The nitrogen component of PN is supplied as a mixture of L-amino acids with essential amino acids supplying approximately 40% of the total amino acid nitrogen. Solutions enriched with certain amino acids have become available, e.g. glutamine. Glutamine, although not an essential amino acid, may become essential during metabolic stress. There are problems providing glutamine in PN solutions due to its instability and low solubility in aqueous solutions. At present there is no evidence that supplementation is harmful but further study is required to provide evidence of benefit. Large multicentre trials are ongoing and results expected within the next few years, e.g. Scottish Intensive Care Glutamine or SeleNium Evaluative Trial (SIGNET) and the Scandinavian Critical Care Trials group study. The former is a randomised trial of glutamine-supplemented PN for critically ill patients and is being carried out throughout Scotland involving intensive care and high dependency units. The latter is a large randomised double-blind placebo controlled study of IV glutamine supplementation in intensive care patients in Scandinavia.

Lipid

Lipid in PN solutions provides non-glucose energy, minimises respiratory and metabolic stress, prevents essential fatty acid deficiency and allows peripheral infusion of nutrients. Lipid can accumulate in the reticuloendothelial system, impairing its ability to remove bacteria and endotoxins and increasing susceptibility to infection; consequently it is recommended that lipid content of PN should not exceed 1.5 g/kg/day.[13] Soybean emulsions have been used as the lipid source for more than 30 years. They contain a high proportion ($> 60\%$) of polyunsaturated fatty acids (PUFA), linoleic acid (52–54%) and alpha linolenic acids (7–9%). It has been suggested that soybean oil-based emulsions represent an imbalanced fatty acid supply with an excess of n6 fatty acids, which under conditions of stress may be proinflammatory, and promote platelet aggregation and vasoconstriction.[14] The ideal lipid emulsion would supply essential fatty acids, provide easily metabolisable energy and have anti-inflammatory properties. Novel lipids

promising to modulate inflammatory responses and improve outcomes have been developed. These include emulsions containing MCT, olive oil and fish oil in various combinations as a partial replacement for soybean oil. Supplying n-3 fatty acids may have the opposite effect to fatty acids of the n6 series. Eicosanoids derived from the former tend to promote vasodilation, inhibit platelet aggregation and reduce inflammation. Consequently fat emulsions enriched with n-3 fatty acids would be expected to have a favourable impact on outcome in critically ill patients receiving PN.[15] n-3 PUFA-containing triglycerides are poorly hydrolysed by lipoprotein lipase; consequently pure fish oil-containing emulsions must be infused at a very low rate to avoid triglyceride accumulation in the circulation. MCT are excellent substrates for lipoprotein lipase-mediated hydrolysis, facilitating plasma triglyceride clearance.[16] They are not suitable as the sole lipid source as they do not include essential fatty acids and have a tendency to cause metabolic acidosis. These problems have been overcome by combining MCT and fish oil in emulsions. Lipid preparations based on olive oil can also be used to decrease the intake of PUFA. Such novel lipids have been shown to be safe and may offer some advantages over the use of soybean oil alone but there is a lack of sufficient data on immunologic and clinical endpoints.[17] More work is needed to evaluate these emulsions before recommendations can be made.

Micronutrients in parenteral nutrition

The intravenous (IV) administration of trace elements poses a risk of toxic effects as the regulatory absorptive mechanism of the intestine is bypassed. An adequate supply of micronutrients is essential for patients on PN to prevent clinical and subclinical deficiency states. Commercially prepared mixtures that provide well-balanced amounts of all essential vitamins and trace elements are available. These commercial preparations are based on guidelines for essential trace element preparations for parenteral use developed by the Nutrition Advisory Group of the Department of Foods and Nutrition, American Medical Association in 1979.[18] Requirements for parenteral trace elements will vary among patients depending on clinical and metabolic status and the need to replace any losses from the GI tract. Further supplements may be appropriate in certain circumstances. For example, starved patients may require additional thiamine as reserves would be expected to be low, pancreatic fistula fluids have a high content of micronutrients especially zinc, biliary fistula fluid is rich in copper and manganese and thus these micronutrients are lost with fluid losses. Knowledge of the stability of micronutrients when mixed with other components of the PN solution and of the effects of the type of container and conditions of storage is essential to ensure that patients actually receive the micronutrients they require. For example, certain vitamins within PN solutions may undergo degradation by sunlight, e.g. vitamin A and E. Solutions should be protected from light by a light-shielding cover. Further losses of vitamin A may be caused by adsorption of vitamin A to the plastic container.[19] Ascorbic acid is the least stable vitamin in solution reacting with oxygen to form dehydroascorbic acid, a reaction catalysed by copper and iron. The benefit of individual micronutrient provision in larger amounts, in particular those known to affect free radical scavenging mechanisms or immune function, continues to be a matter of debate. Controlled trials are required before recommendations can be made.

Parenteral nutrition access routes

Insertion of a catheter for PN should never be an emergency procedure. Patient consent should be obtained and the risks and benefits explained in advance. Administration may be via peripheral or central routes.

Peripheral parenteral nutrition (PPN)

Peripheral parenteral nutrition refers to the administration of nutrients via superficial veins. Use of these veins reduces the risks associated with central line placement.

The principal factors influencing the selection of this route of venous access are: the patient's nutritional requirements; accessibility of veins and anticipated duration of PN. PPN will not be suitable for patients with high nutrient requirements, those requiring low volume solutions or those where the anticipated duration of PN is likely to be > 14 days. It should be considered when the duration of PN is anticipated to be short and the patient does not need central venous access for other reasons.

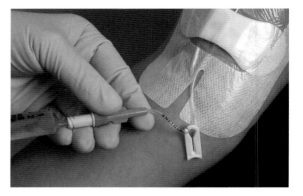

Figure 11.1 • Peripherally inserted venous access device (with kind permission from Vygon Inc).

Choice of vein

The cephalic, basilic or median cubital veins of the forearm are the veins of choice for the peripheral delivery of nutrients (Figure 11.1). Peripheral veins of the lower extremities should be avoided due to higher risks of thrombophlebitis and because of the need to confine the patient to bed.[20] The nondominant forearm should be used if possible. Frequently in practice, this route of access may not be suitable in very sick patients due to the presence of inflammation from previous cannulation, thrombosis or oedematous limbs making cannulation difficult.

Choice of device

Venous access may be obtained through a Teflon or PVC cannula (18–20 G) or an ultrafine polyurethane catheter (19–23 G). If the former is used, a short extension set should be attached to facilitate feeding. It is recommended that cannulae be covered with a sterile adhesive dressing and re-sited every 1–2 days to delay the onset of PVT.[7] This is time consuming for staff and uncomfortable for the patient. In some centres it is common practice to leave the cannula in place until the first sign of thrombophlebitis. An alternative is to use an ultrafine (19–23 G) silicone or polyurethane catheter, 10–15 cm in length that is inserted into a vein in the antecubital fossa. These are often referred to as mid-lines. Placement should only be by a competent practitioner. They have the advantage of being less thrombogenic, longer lasting and more comfortable for patients. There are a number of devices available with different dwell times recommended by the manufacturers. Blood aspirate is necessary to confirm placement. Although they are more expensive initially than cannulae, they may be longer lasting and less labour intensive for staff. Peripheral devices can be placed on the ward with a strict aseptic technique and appropriate skin preparation. Strict hand washing and an aseptic technique are important for all subsequent manipulations of the device.

Choice of nutrient solution for peripheral administration

Hyperosmotic solutions are poorly tolerated by peripheral veins, causing pain, thrombophlebitis and thrombosis. In most nutrient solutions the osmotic components are glucose, amino acids and electrolytes. The inclusion of lipid and an increase in volume of solution will reduce osmolarity. In addition, lipid emulsion-based admixtures may also have a pH better tolerated by small vessels.[7] Consideration should be given to electrolyte content, as additions of electrolytes will increase the tonicity and affect the pH. Solutions < 1200 mosm/L have been shown to be tolerated.[21] A typical PN regimen for peripheral infusion is outlined in Box 11.2.

Box 11.2

A typical all-in-one parenteral solution for peripheral administration

- 2500 mL in a 3 compartment bag (AIO) comprising:
  - 1000 mL of 5.5% amino acid solution
  - 1000 mL of 20% glucose solution
  - 500 mL of 10% lipid emulsion

The contents of the three compartments are mixed and the tertiary mixture provides:

- 9.1 g N_2
- 1520 total calories (800 glucose calories, 500 lipid calories)
- 53 mmol sodium
- 40 mmol potassium
- 5.5 mmol magnesium
- 5.0 mmol calcium
- 17.5 mmol phosphate

Osmolarity is 750 mOsm/L (this will alter with further electrolyte additions).

pH is 6.

Source: OliClinomel N4-550E 2500ml, Baxter Healthcare, UK. Reproduced with kind permission.

Care of peripheral devices

Irrespective of whether a cannula or a catheter is used, the site should be monitored daily for signs of infection or thrombophlebitis and removed if there are any early signs of inflammation. Due to the small internal diameter of devices they should be flushed on discontinuation of the infusion as the risk of occlusion is high. Staff training on peripheral cannula management is important to reduce morbidity and loss of peripheral veins.

Complications of PPN

Infectious complications

The incidence of sepsis in association with PPN can be reduced by strict aseptic technique and adherence to protocols for catheter insertion and care.

Peripheral vein thrombophlebitis

The most common complication associated with PPN is PVT (inflammation of a vein just under the skin). It is characterised by redness, pain, swelling and tenderness along a part of the vein. A myriad of factors outlined below are associated with its development. Arguably, the most important factor is mechanical trauma causing endothelial damage within the vein. Trauma may occur as a consequence of the venepuncture, as a result of the presence of the cannula within the vein or because of the irritant effects of the infusate on the vein wall. The resulting trauma may cause the release of inflammatory mediators, activation of the clotting cascade and subsequent phlebitis and thrombosis.

Factors associated with PVT

Feed composition: The incidence of thrombophlebitis is related to the osmotic content of the infused solution as well as to the osmolarity rate (product of osmolality and infusion rate).[22] The availability of lipid-based formulations enable feeds containing relatively high concentrations of solute to be administered safely.

Choice of cannula: Short Teflon cannulae such as those used to administer intravenous crystalloid are associated with phlebitis of up to 100%.[21] Use of ultrafine (22 or 23 G) polyurethane cannulae have been associated with a low incidence of PVT, approximately 15%.[23,24] The latter are narrow and flexible compared with standard Teflon cannulae and may cause less mechanical trauma to the vein. The tip of the fine bore catheter lying in a large diameter vessel may result in a greater dilution of the nutrient solution.

Timing of infusion: Over time PVT will develop in any vein in which there is an indwelling cannula.[25] It is not surprising therefore that cyclical feeding (usually a 12-hour infusion and 12-hour break) with an elective change of cannula has been found to be associated with reduced incidence of thrombophlebitis (0–18%).[26–28] These studies were small, however, and have been considered to present 'limited scientific evidence'.[29] Nonetheless, the conclusion reached by NICE was that cyclic delivery of PN should be considered when using peripheral venous cannulae with planned routine catheter change (every 1–2 days).[7] Cyclic feeding is time consuming for staff, however, and may be painful and uncomfortable for the patient.

Pharmaceuticals: Heparin and hydrocortisone added to the PN bag may have a significant and synergistic effect in reducing thrombophlebitis.[30,31] The addition of heparin to some lipid-based feeds results in the aggregation of lipid particles. Consequently it cannot be routinely recommended until stability studies have been undertaken with the prescribed formulation.[32] Glyceryl trinitrate patches or gels containing non-steroidal anti-inflammatory drugs placed over the vein distal to the insertion site have been shown to reduce thrombophlebitis in patients receiving crystalloid infusions.[33,34] This acts by venodilation and consequently increases blood flow. These drugs increase the cost of PN and necessitate additional pharmacy and nursing interventions. Although some evidence exists to support their use, it is insufficient to warrant routine use at present.

Central parenteral nutrition

Central parenteral nutrition refers to the administration of nutrients via central veins. Because of the risks associated with central vein cannulation, it should be considered only when peripheral access is not feasible or not appropriate (see section on complications of PN overleaf).[7] Central vein cannulation should be by well-trained personnel utilising ultrasound guidance and using aseptic technique under strict aseptic conditions.

Central PN is likely to be used in the following patient categories.

1. Patients with special nutrient requirements, e.g. fat free, high nutrient requirements or reduced fluid requirements;
2. Patients in whom the expected duration of PN is > 14 days;
3. Patients who do not have suitable peripheral veins; and

4. Patients who already have a central venous access device in place with a lumen that can be dedicated to feeding.

Choice of vein

Access to the superior vena cava can be gained through the internal jugular vein, the subclavian vein or through the peripheral veins in the arm (see Periphally Inserted Central Catheters below). The subclavian vein is the most commonly used access route for long-term PN. Cannulation of this vein creates higher risk of pneumothorax, requiring it to be used by experienced personnel. The tip of the catheter should be placed in the distal upper vena cava just above the right atrium. The internal and external jugular veins may also be used but the position of the catheter can be uncomfortable for the patient. Nonetheless both are clearly visible veins, easy to locate and consequently frequently used for emergency access. Another option is the femoral vein. This is used only in the absence of other suitable veins due to the high risk of infection and catheter-related venous thrombosis.

Choice of central venous access device

A central venous access device (CVAD) is defined as having its tip located in the superior vena cava.

Ideally a single lumen dedicated CVAD should be used for PN administration. In practice most acutely unwell patients requiring PN may have a previously inserted CVAD in place, placed for example during surgery, or will require other intravenous access. In this case a multilumen CVAD will be required with a lumen dedicated to PN. Device selection is based on patient factors and the anticipated duration of therapy. The ideal catheter material for long-term central venous access is chemically inert, non-thrombogenic, flexible and radio-opaque.[35] Most commonly used CVADs are silicone, polyurethane or PVC and have a diameter between 18 and 22 G. They may have single, double or triple lumens. Some devices are coated by antibiotics, which are slowly released in order to decrease the risk of infection associated with migration of bacteria over the outer surface of the catheter. CVADs are also available impregnated with chlorhexidine and silver sulfadiazine or other antimicrobial agents, and may be associated with a rate of infection lower than that of untreated devices. These are more expensive and not a substitute for good catheter care.

Central venous access devices: available options

Non-tunnelled devices

Non-tunnelled devices are the most commonly used CVADs. For the purpose of PN delivery they may be used when the duration of PN is likely to be less than 3 weeks. These are often inserted into the internal jugular vein, but can also be inserted into subclavian or femoral veins. This provides the straightest and shortest route of insertion, thereby reducing the risk of malposition. The external jugular can also be used but cannulation can be more difficult. These devices provide reliable access and as they can have up to five lumens, they are ideal for patients requiring multiple therapies (see Figure 11.2). However, they can be uncomfortable, as they are sutured in place, and patient head movements and the weight of administration sets can cause pulling on the sutures. They can also be difficult to dress, which may lead to movement of the catheter and subsequent mechanical thrombophlebitis.

Subcutaneously tunnelled devices

These are more commonly used for longer periods of therapy. The subcutaneous tunnelling of CVADs was introduced in the 1980s in an attempt to reduce the risk of catheter-related infection. It was envisaged that infection could be reduced by decreasing bacterial progression on the outer surface of the CVAD between the exit site and the intravascular part of the device. A skin-tunnelled CVAD is usually inserted via the jugular or subclavian vein and advanced into the superior vena cava so that the tip is lying at the junction of the right atrium. The technique used will depend on the type of device used and the manufacturer's recommendation. There is evidence that subcutaneous tunnelling of CVADs may reduce the risk of catheter colonisation; consequently for long-term PN (> 30 days) subcutaneous tunnelling is recommended.[7,36] Tunnelling is not a substitute for a strict aseptic technique when caring for CVADs. It has the added benefit of ensuring the line is firmly fixed in position and allows easier care of the exit site. Many devices have a Dacron cuff, which over a period of time (approximately 3 weeks) will fibrose with the subcutaneous tissue within the tunnel. The device should be secured with sutures that must remain in place until the Dacron cuff has fibrosed or the device will fall out once the sutures are removed. Most cuffed CVADs require surgical removal by blunt dissection under local anaesthetic. Gentle traction is used by some practitioners if the device has been in place for less than 14 days. Caution must be employed with this approach, as there is a risk of causing trauma to the patient if excessive force is used.

Figure 11.2 • Multiple lumen CVAD.

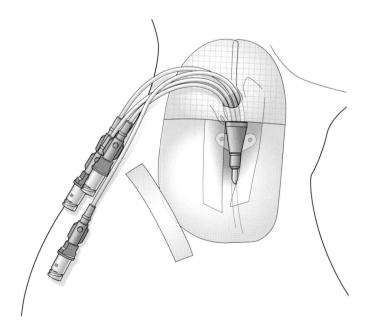

Peripherally inserted central catheters (PICCs)

An alternative means of gaining central venous access is by using a PICC. The PICC is an intermediate to long-term non-tunnelled CVAD with an average life span of 3–6 months. Catheters are silastic or polyurethane and with small diameter, 20–22 G. A PICC can be open-ended with a clamp or may have a Groshong valve at the tip. It is introduced into the basilic or cephalic veins and the tip lies in the superior vena cava. It is essential to remember that although it is inserted peripherally, the tip of a PICC is in the same position as a CVAD inserted infraclavicularly, and must therefore be cared for with the same strict aseptic protocol. The main advantage of a PICC is the avoidance of the risks of direct jugular or subclavian catheterisation and its relative ease of insertion; nurses with good cannulation skills can quickly learn the insertion technique. They can be used for short- or long-term episodes of PN and are particularly useful for patients in whom infraclavicular placement of a CVAD is not feasible, e.g. infection, thrombosis, or patients with respiratory distress. For successful placement, patients need to have good IV access in the ante-cubital fossa. Catheters have a maximum of two lumens and so are unsuitable for patients requiring simultaneous treatments.

Only one randomised controlled trial comparing the efficacy of PICC versus other directly placed CVADs has been published.[37] This study included 102 patients requiring PN and found PICCs to be associated with a greater number of difficult insertion attempts ($p < 0.05$), clinically evident thrombophlebitis ($p < 0.01$) and malposition on insertion ($p < 0.05$). PICC use is nonetheless often successful and a useful alternative to infraclavicular placement.

Totally implanted vascular access devices (TIVADs)

An implanted subcutaneous titanium or plastic port is another option and may be associated with a lower rate of infection (Figure 11.3).[38] These are suitable for patients requiring long-term intermittent venous access and are most commonly inserted in the chest or in the antecubital fossa of the arm. The port is placed by making an incision into the patient's skin, creating a subcutaneous pocket. The device is then anchored, with sutures, to the underlying muscle and the catheter tunnelled under the skin until it reaches the desired venous access point. The overlying skin is then surgically closed.

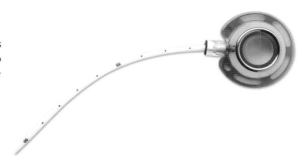

Figure 11.3 • Totally implanted vascular access device.

Only trained personnel should access the device and a non-coring angled needle should be used to pierce the skin and enter the septum of the port. The main advantage of the system is that it causes very little disturbance to daily activities. The port must be removed under local or general anaesthetic.

Choice of nutrient solution for central vein administration

The delivery of nutrient solutions into a large diameter high flow vein such as the superior or inferior vena cava enables highly concentrated nutrient solutions to be infused.

A typical all-in-one parenteral solution that may be used for patients with higher nutrient requirements and central venous access is outlined in Box 11.3. Ready made all-in-one (AIO) bags require vitamin and minerals to be added in a septic suite in pharmacy.

Central venous access device care

As catheter-related infection is the most common complication of PN, every effort should be made to avoid infection. The period of time for which a central venous access device can be used is directly related to the quality of device care.[39] The CVAD should be used for PN only and strict aseptic technique adopted for catheter site care and for accessing the system with written protocols followed. The CVAD should be flushed with 0.9% sodium chloride after each use.[36] Blood withdrawal from the catheter is not recommended, but if absolutely necessary (e.g. if catheter-related blood stream infection (CR-BSI) is suspected) it should be done aseptically and the line flushed afterwards. There has been some controversy regarding the use of dressings over the CVAD exit site and protocols vary between centres. A sterile, transparent, semipermeable polyurethane

Box 11.3

A typical all-in-one parenteral solution for central administration

- 2500 mL in a 3-compartment bag (All-in-One)
  - ○ 1000 mL of 7% amino acid solution
  - ○ 1000 mL of 25% glucose solution
  - ○ 500 mL of 20% lipid emulsion

The contents of the 3 compartments are mixed and the tertiary mixture provides:

- 11.6 g N_2
- 2280 total calories (1000 glucose calories, 1000 lipid calories)
- 80 mmol sodium
- 60 mmol potassium
- 5.0 mmol calcium
- 5.5 mmol magnesium
- 17.5 mmol phosphate

Osmolarity is 995 mOsm/L (this will alter with further electrolyte additions).

pH is 6

Source: OliClinomel N5-800E. Baxter Healthcare, UK. Reproduced with kind permission.

---

dressing is now recommended to cover the site.[8,36] These reliably anchor the CVAD, permit continuous inspection of the site, require less frequent changes than standard gauze dressings and allow patients to wash without saturating the dressing. If the insertion site is oozing or bleeding, a sterile gauze dressing is preferable and should be changed when they become damp, loosened or soiled. An alcoholic chlorhexidine gluconate solution should be used to clean the CVAD site during dressing changes and allowed to air dry.[36] Individual packages of antiseptic impregnated wipes or swabs are available which can be used to disinfect the dressing site.

The most important part of CVAD care is to avoid unnecessary accessory devices, to avoid using the line for multiple therapies, to follow a strict aseptic protocol for connecting and disconnecting the device, and catheter closure for when PN is not being infused.

Complications of parenteral nutrition

PN *can* be administered safely and effectively; however, there are associated risks and complications. Many of the complications associated with the administration of PN can be reduced with close monitoring and supervision by practitioners with specialist expertise in its use.

Complications can be classified into three categories: mechanical, infectious and metabolic.

Mechanical complications

Mechanical complications relating to CVAD placement

Pneumothorax is the most frequent complication associated with subclavian catheter placement and can be potentially life threatening.[40] It is most commonly observed in thin, elderly, cachectic and dehydrated patients. A chest X-ray must be performed immediately following catheter placement to check catheter tip location and to rule out the presence of pneumothorax. The most common symptom is pleuritic chest discomfort that may radiate to the shoulder or the back. Treatment depends on the size of the pneumothorax—if small, a chest drain will not be required. Pneumothorax can occur hours or days after subclavian catheter placement; consequently, chest X ray should be repeated.

Catheter malposition most commonly occurs due to its entrance into the internal jugular vein. If this occurs, the catheter should be repositioned from the jugular vein to the vena cava under fluoroscopic guidance under aseptic conditions.

Air embolism is a rare but serious complication that can occur any time the central venous circulation is opened to atmospheric pressure. If it occurs, the patient usually experiences shortness of breath and coughing. The majority of CVADs have either a clamp proximal to the patient or a valve at the tip of the device to prevent blood from back-flowing or air from entering.

Hydrothorax is another complication that can occur following CVAD malposition with administration of fluids into the thoracic cavity.

Perforation of the superior vena cava or atrium can occur if the CVAD is introduced too far into the right atrium. When it occurs, patients demonstrate widened mediastinum or haemothorax.

Other mechanical complications, e.g. related to poor catheter use or maintenance

CVAD occlusion

This may be due to a variety of reasons, from mechanical obstruction to thrombosis, lipid deposits or the precipitation of drugs. It can be prevented by appropriate nursing care (using a continuous infusion of PN, using appropriate protocols of flushing after use, before and after administration of medication and when the catheter is not in use). Heparin flush solutions may be useful in helping to maintain patency in catheter lumens infrequently accessed and may also be recommended by manufacturers of implantable ports. The nature of the occlusion should be established before any attempt is made to restore patency of the lumen.[41] Depending on the cause of the blockage, urokinase, sodium hydroxide or sodium bicarbonate may be used. Special repair kits are available for permanent catheters damaged in their external parts.

Venous thrombosis

Central vein thrombosis is a rare complication but is associated with high morbidity and death in severe cases. It is often asymptomatic and the first sign may be malfunction of the CVAD. An important factor in the development of thrombosis is the rigidity of the catheter and catheter tip position. The atrial caval junction is considered the optimal position of the catheter tip. Polyethylene catheters are more rigid and lead to thrombosis more often than the softer silicone and polyurethane catheters. A rigid catheter injures the venous endothelium with resulting local inflammation and formation of thrombi.[40] Patients with recurrent CR-BSI or catheter occlusions are more at risk from developing venous thrombosis. Regular antithrombotic treatment should be given to patients at high risk.

Infectious complications

CR-BSI is among the most serious complication of healthcare in clinical practice. All types of CVADs pose a risk. Approximately 3 in every 1000 patients admitted to hospital in the UK acquires a blood stream infection and nearly one-third of these are related to central venous access devices.[42] In most hospitals, risk of CR-BSI is calculated and reported as BSIs per 1000 catheter days as recommended by the CDC in the United States as this allows a more meaningful estimate of risk.[43] CR-BSI involves the presence of systemic infection and evidence implicating the CVAD as its source. It is defined as:

Bacteraemia/fungaemia in a patient with an intravascular catheter with at least one positive blood culture obtained from a peripheral vein, clinical manifestations of infection

(fever, chills and/ or hypotension) and no apparent source for the BSI except the catheter. . . . One of the following should be present: a positive semiquantitative (> 15 CFU/catheter segment) or quantitative ($> 10^3$ CFU/catheter segment) culture whereby the same organism is isolated from the catheter segment and peripheral blood, simultaneous quantitative blood cultures with a $> 5{:}1$ ratio of CVAD versus peripheral; differential period of CVAD culture versus peripheral blood culture positivity of > 2 hours.[8]

The presence of CR-BSI is suggested by signs of redness, pain, swelling or purulent fluid at the exit site and/or general signs that may be nonspecific initially, e.g. fever, chills. Catheter colonisation is defined as significant growth of a microorganism (> 15 CFU) on the catheter tip, subcutaneous segment of the catheter or catheter hub in the absence of systemic infection.[8] The microorganisms that colonise hubs and the skin adjacent to the insertion site are the source of most CR-BSI. Contamination may occur from the hands of healthcare workers during insertion or during care interventions. Infusate contamination is rarely implicated as a cause.[36]

Localised infections on the skin or surrounding tissue include infections of the exit site, pocket infections and tunnel infections. Infections of the exit site are diagnosed by the presence of erythema, tenderness, induration or purulent fluid at the exit site or along the tunnel. Pocket infections occur only with implantable ports.[40] Tunnel infections have similar symptoms but extend more than 2 cm from the exit site.

Factors influencing the development of catheter-related infections are outlined in Table 11.1.

National evidence-based guidelines for preventing healthcare-associated infections (HCAI) in NHS hospitals were commissioned by the Department of Health (England) and published in 2001.[44] The guidelines were primarily based upon an expert review of evidence-based guidelines for preventing intravascular device-related infections developed at the Centres for Disease Control and Prevention (CDC) in the USA.[45] They also involved extensive collaboration with key stakeholders in this field, especially the Infection Prevention Association (IPS), the Hospital Infection Society (HIS) and the Health Protection Agency (HPA). In 2003, complementary national guidelines for preventing HCAI in primary and community care were developed on behalf of the National Collaborating Centre for Nursing and Supportive Care (National Institute for Health and Clinical Excellence).[8] A review of

Table 11.1 Factors influencing the development of catheter related infections

Catheter placement	• Femoral or jugular veins are associated with greater risk of infection than subclavian veins • Sites with high density of skin flora are associated with greater risk • Catheters inserted over mobile joints are associated with increased risk • PICC may carry lower risk than non-tunnelled catheters • Catheter placement as emergency rather than elective procedure is associated with higher risk • Utilising ultrasound for catheter placement may be associated with reduced risk
Patient factors	• Extremes of age (< 1 year and > 60 years are at higher risk) • Immune defence: immunodeficiency and suppression of immune function • Underlying disease severity
Catheter material	• Some materials may favour collection of bacteria, e.g. polyvinyl chloride and polyethylene are associated with higher risk than polyurethane or Teflon catheters • Catheters coated or impregnated with antiseptic or antimicrobial agents may be beneficial
Catheter type	• Failure to use a dedicated catheter lumen for PN • Implanted ports and tunnelled catheters may have lower risk of infection than non-tunnelled devices
Catheter site care	Failure to adhere to strict aseptic technique when accessing the system and for changing catheter dressings
Administration sets	Failure to change sets used for PN every 24 hours
Infusate-related infection	Contamination of the PN solution with particulate matter that may subsequently enter the vascular system. Such particulate matter may be derived from additives in the solution or from reconstructed drugs

new evidence published following the last systematic reviews is represented by epic2 published in 2007.[36] These now replace the original 2001 guidelines and provide the evidence base for many elements of clinical practice essential in the prevention and control of HCAI. It is intended that they be adapted for use locally by all healthcare practitioners.

Key points from these guidelines are outlined in Box 11.4.

While awaiting confirmation of the diagnosis of infection the catheter should not be used. The use of an infected catheter can have serious implications for the patient.

Treatment of catheter-related infections

Management of catheter-related infection varies according to the type of catheter involved. When CR-BSI is confirmed in short-term non-tunnelled catheters, systemic antibiotic therapy as well as removal of the catheter is required. After CVAD removal from patients with CR-BSI, non-tunnelled catheters may be reinserted after appropriate systemic antimicrobial therapy has begun. If the catheter is intended for long-term use the decision to remove the catheter is made on an individual basis

and should be based on illness severity, documentation that the device is infected, assessment of the pathogen involved and the presence of complications, e.g. endocarditis, tunnel infection.[46] For salvage of a CVAD or TIVAD in patients with uncomplicated infections, antibiotic lock therapy should be used for 2 weeks with standard systemic antibiotic therapy. For complicated infections, tunnel infections or port abscess the CVAD or TIVAD should be removed. Reinsertion of tunnelled devices should be postponed until after the appropriate antimicrobial therapy is begun and after repeat cultures of blood samples yield negative results.[46] When the infection is restricted to the exit site of the catheter, local antiseptic treatment is provided as well as antibiotics if necessary. A protocol for the management of CR-BSI should be available.

Metabolic complications

Glucose metabolism

Hypoglycaemia and hyperglycaemia

Hypoglycaemia is most commonly caused by abruptly stopping a glucose infusion. If a high rate of glucose solution is abruptly stopped rebound

Box 11.4

Key recommendations to minimise risk of catheter-related infection

- Healthcare staff caring for a patient with a CVAD must be trained and assessed as competent in CVAD insertion and care procedures.
- A catheter should not be placed unless there is a medical indication.
- Sterility and expiry dates of devices and equipment should be checked.
- Before accessing or dressing a central venous access device, hands must be decontaminated either by washing with an antimicrobial liquid soap and water or by using an alcohol hand rub. A stringent aseptic non-touch technique should be used for site care and for accessing the system.
- A single lumen catheter should be used unless multiple ports are essential for the management of the patient. If a multiple lumen catheter is used one port should be dedicated to PN.
- If long-term PN is anticipated (> 3–4 weeks) a tunnelled or implanted CVAD should be used.
- An antimicrobial impregnated central venous access device should be considered for adult patients who require short-term (1–3 weeks) central venous catheterisation and who are at high risk for catheter-related bloodstream infection (CR-BSI) if rates of CR-BSI remain high despite implementing a comprehensive strategy to reduce rates of CR-BSI.
- Unless medically contraindicated, the subclavian site should be used in preference to the jugular or femoral sites for non-tunnelled catheter placement.
- The skin site should be decontaminated with an alcoholic chlorhexidine gluconate solution (preferably 2% chlorhexidine gluconate in 70% isopropyl alcohol) prior to the insertion of a central venous access device.
- Sterile, transparent, semi-permeable polyurethane dressings should be used where possible. They provide reliable security, allow visual inspection of the insertion site, permit patients to bathe and prevent unnecessary handling of the device. Sterile gauze dressings are required if the patient is perspiring profusely or if the insertion site is oozing or bleeding. If tape or scissors is used when securing the cannula they should be sterile.
- An alcoholic chlorhexidine gluconate solution (preferably 2% chlorhexidine gluconate in 70% isopropyl alcohol) should be used to clean the catheter insertion site during dressing changes, and allowed to air dry.
- Topical antibiotic ointments or creams on insertion sites, or systemic antimicrobial prophylaxis should not be routinely used as they may select for resistant microorganisms.
- Catheters should not be routinely replaced as a method for preventing catheter-related infection.
- Guide wire-assisted catheter exchange should be used to replace a malfunctioning catheter, or to exchange an existing catheter only if there is no evidence of infection at the catheter site or proven CR-BSI.
- If catheter-related infection is suspected but there is no evidence of infection at the catheter site, the existing catheter should be removed and a new catheter inserted over a guide wire; if tests reveal catheter-related infection, the newly inserted catheter should be removed and, if still required, a new catheter inserted at a different site.
- Guide wire-assisted catheter exchange should not be used for patients with catheter-related infection. If continued vascular access is required, the implicated catheter should be removed and replaced with another catheter at a different insertion site.
- Antibiotic lock solutions should not be used routinely to prevent CR-BSI.
- In-line filters should not be used routinely for infection prevention purposes.
- There is insufficient evidence to recommend needle-free devices to reduce the risk of CR-BSI.
- Sterile 0.9% sodium chloride for injection should be used to flush and lock catheter lumens that are in frequent use. Insertion sites should be checked daily and lines checked for patency before each use.
- Aseptic standards should be maintained when removing the device.
- Insertion, all manipulations and catheter care should be documented.

hypoglycaemia may occur, as pancreatic insulin secretion is not directly down regulated.

Hyperglycaemia is commonly caused by rapidly commencing a PN solution or the presence of sepsis.

Hypertriglyceridemia is a metabolic complication associated with PN. Its reported incidence varies considerably due to variation in the patients studied and variations in the reference values used to define hyperglyceridemia. It occurs due to alterations in lipid clearance caused by excessive supply or to a decrease in lipoprotein lipase activity.[47] It can be relatively controlled by limiting lipids provided to 0.7–1.2 g/kg/day.

Refeeding syndrome

Refeeding syndrome comprises the metabolic disturbances that can occur when feeding is commenced aggressively in malnourished patients. The topic is covered in detail elsewhere.[48]

Hepatic and biliary dysfunction

Hepatic complications are common in patients receiving PN, even in the absence of underlying liver disease. Clinical manifestations range from benign increase in liver enzymes to histologically confirmed liver disease. In adults, the predominant abnormality is steatosis and gallstones while in children it is intrahepatic cholestasis and gallstones. Cholestasis probably has a multifactorial origin. Proposed contributing factors include a lack of enteral nutrient intake, which has implications for GI hormone release, toxicity associated with PN components and the underlying disease necessitating the institution of PN. It tends to occur late (after 3 weeks of PN), may be slow to resolve and commonly gives rise to cirrhosis and hepatic failure.[49] Steatosis is more common in adults and consists of a hepatic accumulation of fat. It occurs early (within 2 weeks of starting PN), is reversible and may rarely progress to steatohepatitis and to cirrhosis. Its precise pathogenesis remains unclear. Possible causes include oxidant stress, genetic, inflammatory and nutritional factors. Nutritional factors include excess infusion of glucose or lipid and overfeeding. Glucose infusion rates of more than 5 mg/kg/min/day have been shown to result in fatty liver.[50] The infusion of fat also results in steatosis. Overfeeding is associated with increased hepatic fat synthesis and decreased mobilisation and utilization, resulting in fatty infiltration of the hepatic parenchyma, and should be avoided. An absolute or relative deficiency of carnitine is another possible contributory factor to the development of steatosis following PN but further research is needed in this area. Although studies have shown patients on long-term PN to be carnitine deficient, the prophylactic effects of carnitine supplementation on hepatic steatosis have not been well documented.[51,52]

Gallbladder stasis with sludge or stone formation is another well-recognised complication of PN. It is associated with the loss of enteric stimulation during PN that impairs gallbladder motor function. Prevention is based on stimulation of CCK secretion, gallbladder contraction and bile flow, and avoidance of drugs that may decrease gallbladder contractility and slow small bowel transit.[53] Enteral intake of even small amounts of food stimulates CCK secretion and subsequently gallbladder contraction.

Intestinal complications

PN has been associated with changes in gut morphology, intestinal blood flow and intestinal function; however, much of the research has been on animal models. Animal studies have demonstrated that lack of enteral nutrition is associated with a decrease in jejunal mass and length of villi, changes in digestive and absorptive function and changes in mucosal immunity. In adults these effects have not been clearly demonstrated though enteral tube feeding has been found to be associated with a risk of infection lower than that of PN.[54] It is claimed that even a low quantity of enteral feeding may protect the gut from PN-dependent alterations but the actual amount that constitutes 'minimal' enteral feeding is not known and requires further scientific study.

Metabolic bone disease

Osteopenia and osteomalacia have been reported in up to 50% of patients on beginning home PN.[55] It is particularly prevalent in patients with inflammatory bowel disease and short bowel syndrome. Etiological factors include immobility, acidosis, loss of parathormone rhythm, aluminium or vitamin D toxicity, excess of amino acids in PN and low calcium, magnesium, phosphate or vitamin D intake.[49] Patients likely to be receiving PN for six months or more should have a bone density measurement initially and repeated every 2 years. If there is evidence of osteopenia or osteoporosis, calcium and phosphate intake should be assessed and calcium and vitamin D supplements given. It is advisable to stop smoking, reduce alcohol consumption and optimise sunlight exposure and exercise. Drugs used to treat osteoporosis include calcitonin and bisphosphonates. Oestrogen therapy may be given to women with ovarian failure.

Monitoring and management of parenteral nutrition

A high level of knowledge and expertise is required in the management of patients receiving PN. It is a complex therapy with associated risks and complications. A multidisciplinary team approach to management has evolved since the 1990s to reduce associated morbidity. Access to a nutrition support team (NST) is not widespread with 52% of UK hospitals reporting having access to a team.[56] The composition of hospital nutrition support multidisciplinary teams varies between centres, but in general comprises a consultant, dietitian, clinical nurse specialist and pharmacist with additional support from other disciplines, e.g. biochemist, microbiologist, psychologist. The role of the team includes patient assessment for the most appropriate form of nutrition support, assessment of nutritional status and nutritional requirements and patient monitoring.

Patient monitoring is important for ensuring nutritional needs are met, for assessing the effectiveness of treatment and for enabling complications to be detected early. It should include bedside and laboratory assessment. Parameters are monitored and frequency varies between centres. Clinical and biochemical monitoring recommended by our hospital is outlined in Table 11.2. If specific abnormalities occur, more frequent monitoring may be required until stability is achieved. For patients in whom PN is likely to be required long term, zinc, copper and selenium may be measured prior to the introduction of PN. Results should be interpreted in conjunction with inflammatory markers. For example, a single test result showing low plasma zinc is of no value. Plasma zinc concentration correlates with that of plasma albumin; the zinc may be low because the albumin level is low, which is a typical result of inflammation and once the albumin recovers, the zinc level recovers as well. For patients requiring home PN, concentration of manganese should be measured every 3–6 months to assess potential toxicity. Hypermanganesemia can occur in patients with cholestatic disease because manganese is excreted in bile. If liver function deteriorates, manganese level increases, and this can be a problem in patients receiving long-term feeding.[57] Serum vitamin D and vitamin B_{12} levels should also be measured 3–6 monthly as patients on long-term PN can become deficient. Bone densitometry is recommended on starting home PN and then every 2 years.

Table 11.2 Suggested clinical, biochemical and anthropometric monitoring of patients requiring PN in hospital

Parameter	Frequency	Rationale
Clinical observations		
Respiratory and cardiovascular function	Half-hourly following initial central line placement for 4–6 h then 4–6 hourly	To detect complications post VAD placement
Temperature, pulse and respiration	Daily	To highlight early signs of sepsis, fluid overload
VAD	Daily	To detect signs of infection/thrombophlebitis
Fluid balance charts	Daily	To ensure adequate hydration To establish prescribed versus delivered feed To establish any losses from drains, diarrhoea, vomit
Body weight	Weekly, unless concerns exist regarding fluid balance	To assess change in body mass and to determine adequacy of PN prescription
Anthropometric measurements: TSF, MUAC, MAMC	Monthly	To assess body fat and muscle mass
Hand grip dynamometry	Weekly	To assess muscle function

Table 11.2 Suggested clinical, biochemical and anthropometric monitoring of patients requiring PN in hospital—Cont'd

Parameter	Frequency	Rationale
Biochemical monitoring		
Sodium, potassium, urea, creatinine	Baseline, then daily until stable, then 1–2 times a week	To detect electrolyte abnormalities and assess hydration status
Bedside glucose	Baseline, then twice daily until stable (more often if hyperglycaemia). Four hourly in diabetic patients	To detect hypo- or hyperglycaemia
Liver profile	Baseline, then twice weekly	To detect hepatic dysfunction
Calcium	Baseline, then twice weekly until stable, then weekly	To detect electrolyte abnormalities
Albumin	Baseline, then twice weekly until stable, then weekly	A prognostic indicator
Magnesium, phosphate	Baseline, then daily until stable, then weekly	To detect electrolyte abnormalities
FBC	Baseline, then twice weekly until stable, then weekly	To detect infection
Triglycerides	Within 4 hours of commencing PN	To determine lipid clearance
Ferritin, Fe	Baseline, frequency of subsequent monitoring to be decided by the NST	To assess adequacy of iron stores
Cu, Zn, Se	May be measured at baseline in particular if long-term feeding is anticipated, frequency of subsequent monitoring to be decided by the NST	To assess trace element status and establish adequacy of supplementation
Vitamin B12	Baseline, frequency of subsequent monitoring to be decided by the NST	To assess vitamin B_{12} status and establish adequacy of supplementation
Folate	Baseline, frequency of subsequent monitoring to be decided by the NST	To assess folate status and establish adequacy of supplementation

PN Monitoring Protocol used in Plymouth Hospitals NHS Trust 2009.

Home parenteral nutrition

Indications and prevalence

Data on incidence and prevalence of HPN is not available from all countries. In 2006, 746 patients were registered via British Artificial Nutrition Survey (BANS) as having received home PN in the UK (this may not capture all patients as not all centres register patients with BANS).[58] Point prevalence for the four constituent countries of the UK has shown large increases over the period 2000–2006.

New registrations were 1.7/million, point prevalence was 12/million and period prevalence was 12.5/million.[58] Since HPN was first introduced in the late 1960s[59] it has become established as the standard treatment for patients with severe intestinal failure—for these patients it is a life-saving therapy. Data collected by the BANS demonstrate short bowel syndrome to be the dominant indication for HPN followed by malabsorption and fistula representing 40.6, 18.8 and 16.8% of new registrants for 2006. Overall 1-year survival of 87% is reported. Primary disease is the chief predictor of outcome. In the UK Crohn's disease remains the predominant diagnosis for new and established HPN in the UK. There are large intercountry differences in the use of HPN with prevalence of use three to ten times greater in the USA than in Europe.[60] Within Europe percentage of use also varies considerably, probably reflecting national differences in philosophic and economic viewpoints. Indications for use also differ. For example, the top five diagnoses for patients receiving HPN in a 5-year retrospective study conducted from 1997 to 2001 in the USA were cancer, Crohn's disease, ischaemic bowel disease, motility disorders and AIDS.[61]

Discharging a patient on HPN

Patients requiring HPN will have their intravenous access and PN regimen established in hospital for home use. Permanent catheters, usually subcutaneous tunneled Broviac or Hickman catheters or totally implanted devices, are used for long-term access. Education of patients to ensure they self-manage home PN is cornerstone to minimising technical complications and improving quality of life. Training a patient or carer in the techniques to administer PN safely requires active participation of the patient/carer and multidisciplinary team (gastroenterologist, nutrition nurse specialist, dietitian, pharmacist, GP and community nurses).[62] The patient/carer must be familiar with HPN techniques, catheter care, infusion technique, delivery of equipment and methods of storage and what to do in the event of complications. Most hospitals make use of commercial companies to provide patients with all the necessary equipment to administer PN (including a refrigerator to be used exclusively for PN storage) and PN is delivered to their home weekly or fortnightly. Patients or carers should be given written instructions for all procedures and not be discharged until confident and competent. All patients should be reviewed periodically for nutritional and general status.

Complications of HPN

Infectious complications

The most frequent and serious HPN complications are infectious. Infection rates reported by European and American authors are highly variable and relate to the patient's clinical condition and the different HPN centre experience. The incidence of infectious complications is dependent on hospital-specific factors, e.g. quality of education and support, as well as patient factors, e.g. intellectual and manual skills, compliance with advice.

Quality of life and psychosocial issues

Despite the fact that it is life-saving for patients who have lost GI function, the technological and psychological burdens of HPN are significant. Studies examining the impact of HPN on quality of life have found it to be lower than the general population and lower than closely related groups, e.g. kidney transplant patients with end stage renal failure.[63,64] Negative emotions, depression, physical problems, social limitations, incapability, fatigue and sleep disorders have been found to play a central role in the daily lives of patients on HPN.[65,66] A systematic review of the literature published between 1965 and 2005 examining the implications of HPN on quality of life found reported quality of life was moderate to good but psychological problems described above were common.[67] A recognised limitation of quality of life questionnaires used in studies is the difficulty in evaluating whether the problems are a result of HPN or the underlying disease. There is a need for a standardized scientifically validated treatment-specific instrument to measure quality of life in HPN patients.[6] Patient support groups may be a useful source of support for patients receiving HPN but clearly psychosocial aspects as well as the physical aspects should be considered in the treatment plan for HPN patients.

Key points

- Parenteral nutrition is an effective feeding technique but should be reserved for patients with a non-functioning or inaccessible gastrointestinal tract due to the established superiority of enteral nutrition.
- Catheter placement for PN should never be an emergency procedure. Risks and benefits should be clearly explained to the patient.
- Nutrient solutions to meet all macronutrient and micronutrient requirements are available as fixed standardised feeding regimens or individually compounded admixtures.
- Many of the complications associated with PN administration can be reduced with close monitoring by skilled practitioners and a multidisciplinary team approach to management.

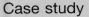
Case study

Mr X is a 79-year-old man who has undergone a limited right hemicolectomy. His preoperative BMI was 19 kg/m^2 and 15% weight loss was reported in the previous 2 months. Oral fluids are introduced day 1 postoperative. On day 3 he develops nausea and vomiting. A nasogastric tube is placed for drainage and IV fluids administered via a CVAD placed intraoperatively. For the next 5 days nasogastric output is 2–3 L; bowel sounds are absent. He is noted to have poor peripheral venous access. An abdominal X-ray reveals dilated small and large bowel loops consistent with ileus. A request is made for parenteral nutrition.

QUESTIONS

1. Is nutritional support appropriate for this patient?
2. What route should be used for PN administration?
3. What is the greatest risk posed by CVAD placement and how can this risk be reduced?

ANSWERS

1. Is nutritional support appropriate for this patient?

   Yes. His low BMI, history of weight loss and negligible intake postoperative places him at high risk of malnutrition. Duration of ileus is impossible to quantify and could be prolonged.

2. What route should be used for PN administration?

   If the existing CVAD has an unused lumen that can be dedicated for PN administration, this can be used. If not, his peripheral veins could be examined for the suitability of midline or PICC placement. If this is not possible, a single lumen CVAD should be placed for PN administration and the existing CVAD removed if not required for other infusions.

3. What is the greatest risk posed by CVAD placement and how can this risk be reduced?

   Catheter-related infection is the most common complication of PN. Ideally a CVAD dedicated to TPN shoul be used and a strict aseptic technique adopted for catheter site care and for accessing the system.

Acknowledgements

Thanks to Dr SJ Lewis, Consultant Gastroenterologist, and Julie Morley, Nutrition Specialist Nurse, Nutrition Support Team Derriford Hospital for their support with this chapter.

References

1. Dudrick SJ, Wilmore DW, Vars HM, et al. Long term parenteral nutrition with growth, development and positive nitrogen balance. *Surgery.* 1968;64:134–142.

2. Zaloga GP. Parenteral nutrition in adult inpatients with functioning gastrointestinal tracts: assessment of outcomes. *Lancet.* 2006;367: 1101–1111.

3. Koretz RL, Lipman TO, Klein S. AGA technical review on parenteral nutrition. *Gastroenterology.* 2001;121(4):970–1001.

4. Moore FA, Moore EE, Jones TN, et al. TEN versus TPN following major abdominal trauma reduced septic morbidity. *J Trauma.* 1989; 29:916–923.

5. Veterans Affairs Total Parenteral Nutrition Cooperative Study Group. Perioperative total parenteral nutrition in surgical patients. *N Engl J Med.* 1991;325(8):525–532.

6. Kudsk KA, Croce MA, Fabian TC, et al. Enteral versus parenteral feeding. *Ann Surg.* 1992;215: 503–513.

7. National Institute for Clinical Excellence. Parenteral nutrition in hospital and the community. In: *Nutrition Support for Adults, Oral Nutrition Support, Enteral Tube Feeding and Parenteral Nutrition, Methods, Evidence and Guidance.* London: 2006:125–146.

8. *NICE Infection Control. Prevention of Healthcare Associated Infection in Primary and Community Care.* London: NICE; 2003. Available at: http://www.nice.org.uk/nicemedia/ pdf/ CG2fullguidelineinfectioncontrol. pdf. Accessed September 2008.

9. Kumpf VJ. Parenteral nutrition-associated liver disease in adult and pediatric patients. *Nutr Clin Pract.* 2006;21(3):279–290.

10. Sandstrom R, Hyltander A, Korner U, et al. The effect on energy and nitrogen metabolism by continuous, bolus or sequential infusion of a defined total parenteral nutrition formulation in patients after major surgical procedures. *JPEN J Parenter Enteral Nutr.* 1995;19(5):333–340.

11. Thomas B, Bishop J, eds. *Manual of Dietetic Practice*. 4th edn. Oxford: Blackwell; 2007:113–120.

12. ASPEN. Statement on parenteral nutrition standardization. *JPEN J Parenter Enteral Nutr*. 2007;31(5): 441–448.

13. AGA American Gastroenterological Association. Medical position statement: parenteral nutrition. *Am Gastroenterol Assoc*. 2001;121: 966–969.

14. Waitzberg DL, Torrinhas RS, Jacintho TM. New parenteral lipid emulsions for clinical use. *JPEN J Parenter Enteral Nutr*. 2006;30(4): 351–367.

15. Planas M. Effects of an n3 fatty acid-enriched lipid emulsion in patients with acute respiratory distress syndrome (ARDS). *Clin Nutr Suppl*. 2007;2:7–8.

16. Carpentier YA, Portois L, Hacquebard M. Intravascular metabolism of lipid emulsions containing n3 fatty acids. *Clin Nutr Suppl*. 2007;2:3–5.

17. Wanten GJA, Calder PC. Immune modulation by parenteral lipid emulsions. *Am J Parenter Enteral Nutr*. 2007;85:1171–1184.

18. American Medical Association Department of Foods and Nutrition. Guidelines for essential trace element preparations for parenteral use—a statement by an expert panel. *J Am Med Assoc*. 1979;241: 2051–2054.

19. Shenkin A, Allwood MC. Trace elements and vitamins in adult intravenous nutrition. In: Rombeau JL, Rolandelli RH, eds. *Clinical Nutrition Parenteral Nutrition*. 3rd edn. Philadelphia: Saunders; 2001.

20. Pertkiewicz M, Dudrick SJ. Ways of delivering parenteral nutrition. In: Sobotka L, ed. *Basics in Clinical Nutrition*. 3rd edn. Prague: Galen; 2004:233–237.

21. Madan M, Alexander DJ, McMahon MJ. Influence of catheter type on occurrence of thrombophlebitis during peripheral intravenous nutrition. *Lancet*. 1992;339(8785):101–103.

22. Timmer JG, Schipper HG. Peripheral venous nutrition: the equal relevance of volume load and osmolarity in relation to phlebitis. *Clin Nutr*. 1991;10(2):71–75.

23. Everitt NJ, Wong C, McMahon MJ. Peripheral infusion as the route of choice for intravenous nutrition. A prospective two year study. *Clin Nutr*. 1996;15:69–74.

24. Plusa SM, Horsman R, Kendall-Smith S, Webster N, Primrose JN. Fine-bore cannulas for peripheral intravenous nutrition: polyurethane or silicone? *Ann R Coll Surg Engl*. 1998;80:154–156.

25. Payne-James JJ, Rogers J, Bray MJ, et al. Development of thrombophlebitis in peripheral veins with Vialon and PTEE-Teflon cannulas: a double blind, randomised controlled trial. *Ann R Coll Surg Engl*. 1991;73:322–325.

26. Kerin MJ, Pickford IR, Jaeger H, et al. A prospective and randomised study comparing the incidence of infusion phlebitis during continuous and cyclic peripheral parenteral nutrition. *Clin Nutr*. 1991;10: 315–319.

27. May J, Murchan P, Mac Fie J, et al. Prospective study of the aetiology of infusion phlebitis and line failure during peripheral parenteral nutrition. *Br J Surg*. 1996;83: 1091–1094.

28. Palmer D, Mac Fie J, Bradford IM, et al. Administration of peripheral parenteral nutrition; a prospective study comparing rotation of venous access sites with ultrafine cannulas. *Clin Nutr*. 1996;15:311–315.

29. Idvall E, Gunningberg L. Evidence for elective replacement of peripheral intravenous catheter to prevent thrombophlebitis: a systematic review. *J Adv Nurs*. 2006;55(6):715–722.

30. Makarewicz PA, Freeman JB, Fairfull-Smith R. Prevention of superficial phlebitis during peripheral parenteral nutrition. *Am J Surg*. 1986;151:126–129.

31. Messing B, Leverve X, Rigaud D, et al. Peripheral venous complications of a hyperosmolar (960mOsm) nutritive mixture: the effect of heparin and hydrocortisone. A multicentre double blinded random study in 98 patients. *Clin Nutr*. 1986;5:57–61.

32. Anderson ADG, Palmer D, Mac Fie J. Peripheral parenteral nutrition. *Br J Surg*. 2003;90:1048–1054.

33. Wright A, Hecker JF, Lewis GBH. Use of transdermal glyceryl trinitrate to reduce failure of intravenous infusions due to phlebitis and extravasation. *Lancet*. 1985; ii:1148–1150.

34. Khawaja HT, Campbell MJ, Weacwe PC. Effect of transdermal glyceryl trinitrate on the survival of peripheral intravenous infusions: a double blind prospective clinical study. *Br J Surg*. 1988;75: 1212–1215.

35. Hamilton H. Choosing the appropriate catheter for patients requiring parenteral nutrition. In: Hamilton H, ed. *Total Parenteral Nutrition A Practical Guide for Nurses*. London: Harcourt; 2000: 55–83.

36. Pratt RJ, Pellowe CM, Wilson JA, et al. epic2: National evidence-based guidelines for preventing healthcare-associated infections in NHS hospitals in England. *J Hosp Infect*. 2007;65(suppl 1):S1–S82.

37. Cowl CT, Weinstock JV, Al-Jurf A, et al. Complications and cost associated with parenteral nutrition delivered to hospitalised patients through either subclavian or peripherally inserted central catheters. *Clin Nutr*. 2000;19(4): 237–243.

38. ASPEN Board of Directors and the Clinical Guidelines Task Force. Guidelines for the use of parenteral and enteral nutrition in adult and paediatric patients. *JPEN J Parenter Enteral Nutr*. 2002;26:1S–137S.

39. Pertkiewicz M, Dudrick SJ. Central parenteral nutrition. In: Sobotka L, ed. *Basics in Clinical Nutrition*. 3rd edn. Prague: Galen; 2004: 237–246.

40. Maroulis J, Kalfarentzos F. Complications of parenteral nutrition at the end of the century. *Clin Nutr*. 2000;19(5):295–304.

41. Sherliker L. Complications. In: Hamilton H, ed. *Total Parenteral Nutrition A Practical Guide for Nurses*. London: Harcourt; 2000: 187–205.

42. Coello R, Charlett A, Ward V, et al. Device-related sources of bacteraemia in English hospitals—opportunities for the prevention of hospital-acquired bacteraemia. *J Hosp Infect*. 2003;53:46–57.

43. Centres for Disease Control and Prevention. Monitoring hospital acquired infections to promote

patient safety. United States, 1990–1999. *MMWR Morb Mortal Wkly Rep.* 2000;49:149–153.

44. Pratt RJ, Pellowe CM, Loveday HP, Robinson N, Smith GW. the *epic* guideline development team. The epic project: developing national evidence-based guidelines for preventing healthcare associated infections. *J Hosp Infect.* 2001; 47(suppl):S1–S82.

45. Centres for Disease Control and Prevention. Guidelines for the prevention of iintravascular-catheter-related infections. *MMWR Morb Mortal Wkly Rep.* 2002;51:129.

46. Mermel LA, Farr BM, Sherertz RJ, et al. Guidelines for the management of intravascular catheter-related infections. *Infect Control Hosp Epidemiol.* 2001;22:222–242.

47. Miles JM, Park Y, Harris WS. Lipoprotein lipase and triglyceride rich lipoprotein metabolism. *Nutr Clin Pract.* 2001;16:273–279.

48. Thomas B, Bishop J. *Manual of Dietetic Practice.* 4th edn. Oxford: Blackwell; 2007:97–107.

49. Nightingale JMD. Hepatobiliary, renal and bone complications of intestinal failure. *Best Pract Res Clin Gastroenterol.* 2003;17(6):907–929.

50. Burke JF, Wolfe RR, Mullany DJ, et al. Glucose requirements following burn injury. *Ann Surg.* 1979;190:274–285.

51. Hahn P, Allardyce DB, Frohlich J. Plasma carnitine levels during total parenteral nutrition of adult surgical patients. *Am J Clin Nutr.* 1982;36:569–572.

52. Bowyer BA, Fleming CR, Ilstrup D, et al. Plasma carnitine levels during total parenteral nutrition of adult surgical patients. *Am J Clin Nutr.* 1986;43:85–91.

53. Guglielmi FW, Boggio-Bertinet D, Federico A, et al. Total parenteral nutrition related gastroenterological complications. *Dig Liver Dis.* 2006; 38:623–642.

54. Braaunschweig CL, Levy P, Sheean PM, et al. Enteral compared with parenteral nutrition: a meta-analysis. *Am J Clin Nutr.* 2001;74: 534–542.

55. Epstein S, Traberg H, Levine G, et al. Bone and mineral status of patients beginning total parenteral nutrition. *JPEN J Parenter Enteral Nutr.* 1986;10:263–264.

56. Russell CA, Elia M. Nutrition screening survey in the UK 2007. A report by BAPEN. Available at: http://www.bapen.org.uk/pdfs/nsw/nsw07_report.pdf. Accessed Sept 2008.

57. Berger MM, Shenkin A. Vitamins and trace elements: practical aspects of supplementation. *Nutrition.* 2006;22:952–955.

58. Jones B, Holden C, Stratton R, et al. Annual BANS report 2007. Artificial nutrition support in the UK 2000–2006. A report by the BANS a committee of BAPEN. 2007. Available at: http://www.bapen.org.uk/pdfs/bans_reports/bans_report_07.pdf

59. Shils ME, Wright WL, Turnbull A, et al. Long term parenteral nutrition through an external arteriovenous shunt. *N Engl J Med.* 1970;283: 341–344.

60. Howard L. A global perspective of home parenteral and enteral nutrition. *Nutrition.* 2000;16(7/8): 625–628.

61. Ireton Jones C, de Legge M. Home parenteral nutrition registry: a five year retrospective evaluation of outcomes of patients receiving home parenteral nutrition support. *Nutrition.* 2005;(21):156–160.

62. Pertkiewicz M, Naber T, Dudrick SJ. Home artificial nutrition. In: Sobotka L, ed. *Basics in Clinical Nutrition.* 3rd edn. Prague: Galenn. 2004:462–467.

63. Jeppesen PB, Langholz E, Mortensen PB. Quality of life in patients receiving home parenteral nutrition. *Gut.* 1999;44:844–852.

64. Herfindal ET, Bernstein LR, Kudzia K, et al. Survey of home nutritional support patients. *JPEN J Parenter Enteral Nutr.* 1989;13: 255–261.

65. Persoon A, Huisman-de Waal G, Naber TA, et al. Impact of long-term HPN on daily life in adults. *Clin Nutr.* 2005;24:304–313.

66. Huisman de Waal G, Naber T, Schoonhoven L, et al. Problems experienced by patients receiving parenteral nutrition at home: results of an open interview study. *JPEN J Parenter Enteral Nutr.* 2006;30(3): 215–221.

67. Huisman-de Waal G, Schoonhoven L, Jansen J, et al. The impact of home parenteral nutrition on daily life—a review. *Clin Nutr.* 2007;26:275–288.

Thermal injury

12

Lynne D Hubbard

LEARNING OBJECTIVES

By the end of this chapter the reader will be able to:

- Understand the mechanism of injury that leads to the hypermetabolic response and the role of nutritional support in patient recovery
- Assess the nutritional requirements for energy, protein, vitamins, minerals and trace elements and decide on the best way to deliver these nutrients to the patient
- Monitor the effectiveness of nutritional intervention
- Recognise the dietitians role in the multidisciplinary team
- Help support and motivate the patient throughout their recovery

Introduction

The UK national burn care review in 2001 found that every year 250,000 people sustain a burn injury, 175,000 of them visit an accident and emergency department, 16,100 of those are admitted to hospital, and of these 10,200 require care in a specialist burns unit.[1] The review stated that 90% of burn injuries are preventable and a prevention strategy remains at the heart of planning in the UK. Survival has improved in the past 25 years but there are still 300 deaths per year. The majority of deaths are in people over the age of 60 years, in which there has been little improvement in survival, probably due to pre-existing medical conditions. A team approach is vital at every stage of treatment from emergency care to rehabilitation and nutritional support has played a crucial role in improving mortality and morbidity by:

- Trying to ameliorate catabolism and loss of skeletal and visceral muscle;
- Trying to understand and ameliorate hypermetabolism;
- Supporting the immune system;
- Providing the correct balance of nutrients for wound healing; and
- Providing an appropriate balance of nutrients during the anabolic phase of recovery.

The burns team sets its goals high and the national burn care review states the goal of treatment is to 'recover the individual to the pre-injury state and for them to return to their place in society with unaltered potential'. To try and achieve this goal the dietitian not only plans the dietary prescription but as part of the team plays a crucial role in motivating, supporting and encouraging the patient to help them in their road to recovery.

The structure and function of skin

Skin is the largest organ in the body comprising 15% of body weight. It has a number of key functions:[2]

- As a sensory organ for touch, pain, temperature and pressure;
- Regulation of body temperature through vasodilation and vasoconstriction of the microcirculation in the dermis and via the sweat glands; and
- As a barrier to micro-organisms from the external environment entering the body.

Histologically it is made up of two layers:[3]

- The epidermis—this outer layer of dead cells is avascular and relatively impermeable. It is produced by cells dividing at the basement membrane and migrating to the outer layer.
- The dermis—this inner layer is vascular and contains nerve fibres, hair follicles and sebaceous glands in connective tissue, composed of collagen, elastin and ground substance. Beneath this is a layer of fat.

The pathophysiology of thermal injury

Burn injury is described in relation to which layer of skin is damaged:

- A superficial burn, e.g. a sunburn involves some damage to the epidermis;
- A partial thickness burn, e.g. a scald involves destruction of the epidermis and part of the dermis;
- Deep dermal; e.g. a scald of longer duration in which more of the epidermis and dermis is destroyed including hair follicles and sweat glands; and
- Full thickness, e.g. flame burn includes the destruction of the epidermis, dermis and basement membrane. Because blood vessels and nerve endings are destroyed there is no pain.

During the first 3–6 hours and lasting for up to 36 hours the microcirculation becomes hyper-permeable.[4] The increased permeability means larger molecules such as albumin and other plasma proteins leak out into the extravascular space, producing tissue oedema and inflammation. The aim of the inflammatory response is to dilute, destroy or wall off the cause of injury, e.g. damaged cells and invading bacteria, and stimulate a series of events resulting in healing the damaged area. A variety of endogenous vasoactive mediators are thought to be involved in the development of wound oedema, including histamine, serotonin, bradykinin, catecholamines and products of arachidonic acid metabolism. The injury of cells stimulates tissue macrophages, monocytes, keratinocytes and fibroblasts to produce peptides called cytokines, particularly interleukin 1 and 6.[5] These are important in:

- Activation and increased production of neutrophils;
- Acting on the hypothalamus to produce fever; and
- Acting on the liver to reset it to synthesise acute phase proteins, e.g. C-reactive protein.

However, the activation of the macrophage-monocyte system which ensures phagocytosis produces unstable oxygen free radicals which produce lipid peroxidation. This leads to secondary damage of the cell membrane and where injury is great, this can result in the systemic inflammatory response.[4] The role of antioxidants in the body, in decreasing the damage done by oxygen free radicals, may be of vital importance (see Trace Elements below).

Metabolic response to injury

The resting energy expenditure falls during the period of fluid resuscitation, due to hypothermia, decreased cardiac output and a decrease in delivery of oxygen to the tissues, a period referred to as the ebb phase. As fluid resuscitation restores circulating volume and delivery of oxygen to tissues, the body enters the flow phase, a prolonged period of hypermetabolism. This is driven by an increase in the catabolic hormones, adrenalin and noradrenalin (catecholamines), cortisol (glucocorticoid) and glucagon.[6] The burn injury necessitates the mobilisation of large amounts of substrate from fat stores, glycogen and muscle for energy and repair. The catabolic hormones stimulate mobilisation of fat reserves, protein breakdown, glycogenolysis and gluconeogenesis. Glycogen reserves are utilised in less than 24 hours; therefore, skeletal muscle is converted to glucose via gluconeogenesis.

The effect of modern treatment on hypermetabolism and recovery

By understanding the pathogenesis of burn injury it has been possible to reduce energy expenditure:

- Occlusive dressings—Fluid is lost through the burn-injured area by evaporation. Combined with plasma exudates this can reach 300 mL/m/hour or 7 L per day at an energy cost of 580 kcal/L. The use of occlusive dressings can reduce evaporative losses by 50% and with it the energy expenditure of evaporation is reduced.[7]
- Temperature regulation—Because cytokines act on the hypothalamus to raise the internal body temperature, by controlling the environmental

temperature to 28–32°C. Arturson found patients decreased their rate of heat production and dry heat loss, thus conserving energy.[8]

- Pain control—Pain may be caused directly from the burn injury or during dressing changes and physiotherapy. Adequate pain medication reduces anxiety and energy expenditure.[9]
- Early excision and grafting—While this does not decrease hypermetabolism, it does attenuate muscle catabolism when compared to delay in surgery and result in reduced sepsis and wound colonisation.[10]
- The use of beta-blockers—Herndon used propanolol to block beta-adrenergic stimulation in children with burns of greater than 40%, resulting in a reduction in tachycardia, supraphysiologic thermogenesis, cardiac work and resting energy expenditure.[11] It was also found to increase protein synthesis with a reduction in protein catabolism. Potential risks include hypoperfusion from decreased cardiac output, decrease in blood pressure and bronchospasm.

In addition:

- The use of paralysing agents reduces measured energy expenditure by 24–33% in critically ill burns patients on mechanical ventilation.[12]
- The use of inotropic support, i.e. adrenalin and noradrenalin, common in burn injury increases the stress response.[13]

Global assessment and monitoring

In order to decide on an individual patient's requirements a thorough assessment of nutritional status, medical history and injury history must be made on admission (see Table 12.1). Each unit needs to establish a protocol for biochemical and haematological monitoring. Table 12.2 gives a guide to monitoring, which may be increased in a critically ill patient or decreased in the later stages of recovery. Monitoring of progress should include:

- Weekly weights;
- Detailed description of the healing of the burn wound, the success of skin grafting and healing of donor sites;

Table 12.1 Global assessment: risk factors in burn-injured patients

Medical history	Diabetes, renal impairment, alcoholism, gastric ulcers, epilepsy, previous diarrhoea or vomiting
Social history	Living alone, low income, elderly, physical disability, mental health problems, ethnicity, religious beliefs
Diet and weight history	Height, dry weight, BMI, physical signs of weight loss, food preferences, vegetarian, dentition, allergies, history of normal intake
History of injury	Where, when, mechanism (flame, chemical, scald, electrical), non-accidental, suicide
Total body surface area burn	Size of burn, depth and exact area plotted on a Lund-Browder chart. Note if face, hands or feet are included

Table 12.2 Biochemical and haematological monitoring

Test	Frequency
Urea, electrolytes and creatinine	Daily for first week
Liver function tests	Twice weekly
Serum phosphate, magnesium and calcium	Weekly
Serum glucose	Daily for first week
Serum albumin	Twice weekly
Haemoglobin	Twice weekly
White cell count	Twice weekly
Trace elements (copper, zinc, selenium)	On admission and weekly for first month in burns > 20%
24-hour urinary collection	Twice weekly in burns > 20%

- Information on infection and any other medical problems;
- Daily food and fluid charts;
- Bowel activity; and
- Discussion by the multidisciplinary team of the physical, social and psychological progress.

Calculating energy requirements

Whatever method of calculation is used, a useful guide is that energy expenditure does not exceed twice basic metabolic rate.[14,15] Using indirect calorimetry to measure energy expenditure is ideal but the cost of the equipment, the time to take the measurements, the skills required to take accurate measurements and the potential inaccuracies in some of the sickest patients means that currently this is not an available option in the UK in non-research settings.[16] This is problematic as it is recognised that in critically ill patients overfeeding can cause hyperglycaemia, fatty infiltration of the liver and increased production of carbon dioxide while underfeeding can affect immunocompetence, wound healing and mortality.[17,18]

Numerous predictive equations exist for calculating energy expenditure in burns patients using either predicted BMR added to a predicted stress factor or stepwise multiple regression. However, the physiological response of people with burn injury varies according to age, sex, genetics and previous medical condition, meaning:

- While Matsuda found that mean resting energy expenditure in patients with burns of 0–30% and 31–60% was significantly higher in the latter group, there is no simple linear relationship between burn size and hypermetabolism, which can vary by as much as 30–40% for burns of equal size.[19,20]
- The peak of the hypermetabolic response varies as does the length of time it continues, which can be up to 42 days.[13]
- Body weight error can easily be introduced into a calculation, as fluid resuscitation may have begun before admission or it may be difficult to weigh the patient on ITU.
- There is no agreement on the use of body weight, body surface area, surface area of burn or basic metabolic rate in different calculations.

Currently the British Dietetic Association Burns Interest Group recommends the use of the Schofield formula based on BMR plus an added stress factor related to the size of the burn.[21] However, this introduces potential error from body weight and estimated stress factor. As much care as possible should be taken in establishing the patient's dry weight at the time of injury. Taylor has suggested the use of the Toronto formula, developed from multiple regression analysis, for use in ventilated or spontaneously breathing adults.[13,22] Total energy expenditure is calculated as 120% of REE.

$$REE = -4343 + (10.5 \times \%\text{burned BSA}) \\ + (0.23 \times \text{kcal intake}) \\ + (0.84 \times \text{Harris Benedict}) \\ + (114 \times \text{temp}°C) \\ - (4.5 \times \text{post} - \text{burn day})$$

However, this is less user friendly than the Schofield equation and needs further evaluation to establish benefit. With the move towards larger and fewer burns centres in the UK, the purchase of equipment enabling the use of indirect calorimetry should be given a high priority if overfeeding or underfeeding is to be avoided.[1]

Protein requirements

The increased production of cortisol stimulates muscle breakdown and protein oxidation, resulting in an increased level of circulating amino acids. It is thought these are required for:

- Wound repair;
- The production of acute phase proteins;
- Cellular immunity; and
- Glucose production.

Increased production of glucagon drives gluconeogenesis as protein is broken down into amino acids in the liver.[23]

The burn injury therefore increases the requirement and changes the body's priorities for the type of protein that needs to be produced. At the same time protein losses increase through the wound as plasma exudate and through the urine as urea.

Research continues over the amount and type of protein that can meet the patient's requirements, reduce skeletal breakdown, maximise wound healing and the immune response. Currently the following is known:

- Although studies have shown no reduction in net protein catabolism above 0.23 g nitrogen per kilogram,[24] it seems likely that patients with large burn injuries still benefit from high protein intakes in relation to wound healing. Gore infused a radioisotope of phenyl alanine into 10 patients with burns over 40% and used it to measure the rate of protein synthesis in the wound, muscle and skin.[25] It was found that there was a net consumption of phenyl alanine by the wound but net release by the muscle. Compared with the skin the wound had a much greater rate of protein synthesis and reduced rate of protein breakdown.

- Alexander found that supplementation of protein (0.4–0.64 g nitrogen/kg, in an feed of 80 kcal to 1 g nitrogen) in severely burned children resulted in a statistically significant increased survival, opsonic index, serum total protein, C3, immunoglobulin G, nitrogen balance and decreased number of infectious episodes.[26]

- The infusion of glucose or glucose and amino acids does not reverse gluconeogenesis and nitrogen loss.[27] However, Gore looked at the effects of infusing glucose and insulin on the peripheral amino acid metabolism.[28] Isotopic tracers of phenyl alanine and alanine were used to monitor metabolic changes. When glucose was infused without insulin the result was increased efflux of amino acids. When insulin was infused there was an increased uptake of phenyl alanine into the leg. The conclusions were that hyperglycaemia increased muscle catabolism while the supply of exogenous insulin producing euglycaemia impedes muscle breakdown.

- Catabolism is driven by catecholamines and peaks around day 5–8 but muscle breakdown continues long after this. This may be due to prolonged bed rest in the burn-injured patient, which continues to cause amino acid efflux from muscle.[29]

- Early excision and grafting and aggressive enteral feeding, while not decreasing energy expenditure, decreased muscle protein catabolism and the number of infectious episodes compared with those whose excision and grafting and feeding had been delayed.[10]

- A high protein diet may well be important during the period of rehabilitation, when patients have become anabolic. Demling studied patients who were healed and free of infection who had had burn injuries of 30–50%, all involved in physiotherapy programmes that included resistance exercise.[30] The group fed a high protein diet (0.32 g nitrogen/kg) gained more weight and showed greater muscle strength and ability to do endurance exercise than those on a lower protein intake (0.2–0.24 g nitrogen/kg). Regaining muscle is slow, with the rate of muscle protein synthesis reported as 10–25 g per day (5-10 times slower than the rate of loss during catabolism) in burn-injured patients.

Oxandrolone

Oxandrolone is an anabolic steroid, a testosterone analog with ten times the anabolic activity but one-tenth of the androgenic activity of testosterone. Research into its use in burn injury for preventing loss or restoring muscle mass has been going on since the mid-1990s. Demling found that patients in the rehabilitation phase on an exercise programme, oxandrolone and a high protein diet gained more body weight than those on an exercise programme and normal or high protein diet.[31] Oxandrolone was effective in older adults, over 60 years, as well as in younger adults.[32] This is important in light of the difficulties older adults face due to loss of lean body mass. In 2000 Demling used oxandrolone (20 mg/day) in the acute phase on burn injury, beginning when patients reached a minimum of 75% of their energy and protein requirements.[33] Twenty patients were studied in a double-blind randomised controlled trial. Patients on oxandrolone had an improved net nitrogen balance, decreased weight loss, faster healing of donor sites and a shorter length of stay. Oxandrolone did not decrease metabolic rate and there were no side effects. The use of oxandralone is being considered in burns in the UK.

Glutamine

Glutamine is an amino acid that becomes essential during critical illness.[34] Its role as the main fuel source for rapidly dividing cells in the mucosa of the GI tract and for lymphocytes, its involvement in gluconeogenesis and as a precursor for other amino acids all make it of crucial importance in burn injury. Increased uptake during this period by the intestinal mucosa, dividing leukocytes, liver and kidneys cannot be met by release from skeletal muscle and plasma levels fall. The European Society for Parenteral and Enteral Nutrition has supported the supplementation of burn-injured patients with glutamine.[35] Garrel and Zhou conducted trials that found a significant improvement in wound healing and a reduction in the length of stay.[36,37] Chen and Peng found a reduction in plasma endotoxin levels and an improvement in intestinal permeability.[38,39] Windle conducted a thorough review of all published data on the clinical impact of supplementation on patients with major burn injury and concluded that supplementation is of benefit.[40] Windle recommended that a minimum period of supplementation to be of benefit was 5 days, with trials varying from 1 to 4 weeks and most RCTs lasting at least 10–14 days. While a recommended dose has not been established the majority of trials on burns have used 0.35–0.57 g/kg. Plasma glutamine levels may be of benefit initially as an indication to begin therapy; however, reports vary on the effects of supplementation on plasma levels, therefore not clearly indicating an end point. However, Windle points out that this could be due to the different levels of glutamine supplementation in different trials. Even where plasma levels did not increase, clinical benefit was still found. A study by Wischmeyer identified raised plasma ammonia levels in patients with acute renal failure and liver dysfunction;[41] otherwise, the use of glutamine in burns has reported no other side effects. Some major burns units in the UK now supplement patients with burns who are critically ill.

Calculating protein requirements

In burns of 20% or greater monitoring of nitrogen balance using 24-hour urinary urea is beneficial and the calculation simple:[42,43]

Nitrogen output = 24-hour urinary urea $\times$ 0.33
+ obligatory losses
+ any extra renal losses

Obligatory losses = $2-4$ g/day (hair, skin, faeces)

Any extra renal losses:

- pyrexia 0.6 g nitrogen/1°C with sweating
- burns exudates 0.2 g/% surface area burn
- extensive bed sores, GI fistulae or inflammatory bowel disease.

Currently the British Dietetic Association Burns Interest Group guidelines recommend the use of the Elia equation to initially calculate protein requirements (see Table 12.3).[44] While it is not possible to achieve nitrogen balance in patients with large burn injuries, high nitrogen intakes may well be beneficial in wound healing.

Table 12.3 Elia equations for calculating nitrogen requirements

	Nitrogen g/kg/day
Normal	0.17 (0.14–0.2)
Hypermetabolic	
5-25%	0.2 (0.17–0.25)
25-50%	0.25 (0.20–0.30)
> 50%	0.30 (0.25–0.35)
Depleted	0.3 (0.2–0.40)

Type of energy

Carbohydrate

During burn injury ketogenesis is partially inhibited. Glucose is the preferred source of energy as the substrate for the production of adenosine triphosphate through anaerobic glycolysis. Wolfe studied glucose metabolism in burns using radio-isotopes and found that it was raised during burn injury compared with non-burn controls.[45] Wolfe went on to find that this was due to increased levels of glucagon, converting amino acids from protein catabolism into glucose.[46] Gluconeogenesis was not reversed by the infusion of glucose or glucose and amino acids. However, somatostatin, which was used to partially block the production of glucagon, did reduce the rate of protein breakdown. Provision of exogenous insulin also reduced muscle breakdown.[30] The burn wound has up to a tenfold increase in uptake of glucose compared with non-burned tissue.[47] Gottschlich recommended the provision of 60–65% of energy as carbohydrate as long as it does not exceed 5 mg/kg per minute, the maximum oxidation rate.[48] Hyperglycaemia during critical illness also needs to be controlled as it impairs immune function by altering cytokine production from macrophages, reducing lymphocyte production and the intracellular bactericidal activity of leukocytes.[49]

Fat

Catecholamine production leads to the breakdown of adipose during burn injury, producing raised levels of free fatty acids and glycerol in the systemic circulation. Abbott found that ketone bodies are not significantly elevated, suggesting that ketogenesis is inhibited and fatty acid oxidation is not increased.[50] It appears that the majority of free fatty acids are re-esterified by the liver to triglycerides or phospholipids. Excessive amounts of dietary fat associated with high lipid levels have been associated with impaired clotting and depression of the immune system. Therefore the provision of high levels of fat as an energy source is not recommended and 10–15% of total energy from fat has been proposed by Gottschlich.[51] However, dietary fat is also important as a carrier of fat soluble vitamins, for which a minimum of 15–25 g a day is required. Essential fatty acids, namely linolenic and linoleic acid, need to be provided. They cannot be synthesised by the body and form part of the cells' phospho-lipid membrane. Evidence regarding the benefits of the provision of omega-3 fatty acids and their anti-inflammatory effects remains inconclusive and further studies are required.

Micronutrients

Trace elements

Since the 1980s it has been known that people sustaining large burn injuries could develop low serum levels of copper, zinc and selenium.[52] Trace element levels are, however, difficult to interpret during critical illness due to the redistribution around the body. Plasma zinc, iron and selenium fall while copper increases.[53] Trace elements are crucial as cofactors or as metalloenzymes in antioxidant systems (glutathione peroxidase, superoxide dismutase), wound healing (Lysyl oxidase, integrins) and protein synthesis (RNA polymerase). For more detail see Table 12.4. In 1992 Berger conducted balance studies over a 7-day period in patients with burn injuries of 20–55% TBSA, measuring trace element intake including intravenous fluids, blood products, enteral or parenteral feeding and supplementation.[54] Losses were calculated from plasma exudate, urine, faeces, gastric and bronchial aspirations. The main route of loss was found to be the plasma exudates. The mean zinc loss in the 7-day study was 190 mg (5–10% of total body zinc). The mean copper loss was 33 mg (20–40% total body copper) and the mean loss of selenium was 2.5 mg (10% of total body selenium). In 1994 Berger[55] conducted a small study of five patients (TBSA burn 30–55%) given standard (20 μmmol Cu, 0.4 μmmol Se and 100 μmmols Zn) or high dose trace elements (40.4 μmmol Cu, 2.9 μmmol Se and 406 μmmol Zn) intravenously. The high dose group showed a larger leukocyte increase and shorter hospital stay. This has been followed by two randomised controlled studies, which have shown that patients receiving trace element supplementation had lower levels of interleukin-1 and C-reactive protein, significantly lower levels of pulmonary infection and a significantly shorter stay

Table 12.4 Table showing normal levels of trace elements, their role and symptoms of deficiency

Element	Normal serum level	Metallo-enzyme or protein	Clinical symptoms of deficiency
Copper	0.7–1.7 μg/L 13–22 μmol/L	Lysyl oxidase Cytochrome oxidase Super oxide dismutase Ceruloplasmin	Hypochromic anaemia Neutropenia
Selenium	0.8–1.6 μmol/L 70–139 ng/mL	Glutathione Peroxidase	Cardiomyopathy
Zinc	0.15–0.23 mmol/L	Carbonic anhydrase Alkaline phosphatase Integrins A number of collagenases Super oxide dismutase DNA and RNA polymerases	Skin rash Diarrhoea Taste impairment Poor wound

Adapted from 'Feeding Guidelines by the Burns Interest Group of the British Dietetic Association, 2004. Reproduced with kind permission of the British Dietetic Association.

on intensive care.[56,57] The hypothesis is that these supplements are maintaining immune function, particularly in the lung which the IV supplements reach first, as well as preventing deficiency.

Vitamins

Less research exists on the role and requirements of vitamins in burn injury. Patients on sip feeds or enteral feeds may already be receiving high doses of vitamins. However, patients who are critically ill and not able to tolerate their enteral feeds not only receive an inadequate supply of macronutrients but also micronutrients. Also at risk are patients with smaller burns who are taking mainly milk and small meals, but who dislike fortified sip feeds. Both these groups may require a multivitamin supplement to reach their requirements.

B vitamins

Little research has been done specifically on burns and B vitamins, which should be given in relation to energy and protein intake. However, a significant number of patients with burn injury do have a history of alcoholism and will therefore require supplementation of vitamin B in line with hospital protocols on alcoholism.

Vitamins A, C, E

Vitamin C has long been recognised as being necessary in collagen synthesis where it is required for the hydroxylation of proline. In addition it is important in the immune system where deficiency results in the impairment of neutrophils to migrate when stimulated by a chemotactic substance. However, evidence that high doses lead to an improvement in either wound healing or immune function is lacking.

More recently interest has turned towards the role of vitamins in the body's antioxidant defence system. While enzyme systems, e.g. glutathione peroxidase, provide one aspect of defence, vitamins C and E and carotenoids are also active free radical scavengers in the plasma, helping to reduce the damaging effects of peroxidation to lipid membranes, enzymes and DNA. Rock monitored levels of beta-carotene, vitamin C and vitamin E in 26 adults with burn injuries greater than 20% for 21 days after admission.[58] Patients were fed enterally on a high protein high

vitamin feed (1 kcal/mL, 0.62 g protein/mL, 237 mg vitamin C/1000 kcal and 35.8 IU vitamin E/1000 kcal). Beta-carotene, at a dose of 30 mg/day, was administered to half the patients; the feed contained very little. Plasma levels of these vitamins were measured on admission and then twice weekly. Plasma concentrations were low immediately after burn injury; plasma levels of vitamin C, retinol and vitamin E were found to normalise over the 3-week period. This was hypothesised to be due to increased uptake of the antioxidant vitamins post injury and also due to decreased levels of plasma transporters (e.g. retinol binding protein, lipids). As the plasma transport proteins returned to normal levels and the patients received high intakes of vitamins in the enteral feed, plasma levels of vitamin C and E returned to normal. However, beta-carotene (the main precursor for vitamin A) did not return to normal in the non-supplemented group and remained very low. Those on beta-carotene supplements had normal plasma levels by the second week post injury. The levels of vitamin C were over 10 times the RDA in the UK, so it is unclear if plasma levels would have returned to normal in a non-supplemented group. It suggests beta-carotene supplementation leads to a faster return to normal levels but the clinical significance of this is unclear.

A study by Mingjian et al. found patients with large burn injuries supplemented with vitamin E had lower levels of lipid peroxides, an end product of oxidative damage, than those patients not given a supplement.[59] However, the study was small, not linked with any clinical outcome and lipid peroxide levels are affected by many things.

The evidence base for giving high doses of vitamins remains weak and further randomised controlled trials need to be conducted.

Calcium and vitamin D

Vitamin D is a steroid hormone essential for calcium and phosphorus homeostasis and skeletal bone integrity. In humans the main source is endogenous; cholecalciferol is synthesised from 7-dehydrocholesterol by ultraviolet irradiation of the skin. A smaller amount is obtained from the diet as ergocalciferol in, e.g., fatty fish. After further metabolic changes in the liver and kidney the active form of vitamin D is formed, 1,25-dihydroxycholecalciferol (1-25D). This facilitates the absorption of phosphorus and calcium from the intestine and is involved in bone re-adsorption mechanisms after they have been started by parathyroid hormone. Wray et al.[60] found that levels of vitamin D fell in children with large burns over a 6-week period, were positively correlated with hypocalcaemia (even after correction for hypoalbuminaemia) and hypophosphataemia and fell progressively with increased burn size.[60] Gottschlich also found the lowest levels of vitamin D in children with larger burns or inhalational injury as well as those treated with oxandrolone.[61] They noted that burns patients have lack of exposure to sunlight; wound losses and malabsorption may affect availability in some cases. Immobilisation has an impact on bone matrix formation. Parathyroid hormone (PTH) is also essential for renal conversion of 25-dihydroxycholecalciferol (25D) to 1-25D but PTH metabolism is disturbed in burn injury, which may effect 1-25D synthesis. When Gottschlich supplemented patients with low vitamin D levels with 25D it did not result in improvement.[61] It was postulated that either there was a problem with absorption, exacerbated by the oxandrolone therapy, or a different form of vitamin D would be more beneficial. Concerns exist as to whether there is a possible relationship between vitamin D depletion and reduced bone mineral density, with Klein documenting low levels 2–7 years after injury in children.[62] Further studies are required in adults, who could also be at risk.

Route of feeding

Oral feeding

Many adults who were well before injury can meet their nutritional requirements orally with a burn injury of up to 20% total body surface area. By considering food preferences, providing small regular meals, high protein energy snacks and supplementary drinks the dietitian can design an individualised patient prescription. Wherever possible this should be discussed with the patient to gain their full cooperation and to involve them in understanding the reasons for their treatment and the role of nutrition in their recovery. A patient will have a better chance of meeting their requirements if pain control is adequate; they are free of constipation and starvation for procedures is kept to a minimum. Intake may also be affected by antibiotic therapy, effecting taste and smell, odours from dressings and exhaustion from dressing changes, physiotherapy and other procedures.

Careful monitoring of intake using food charts is necessary to ensure goals are met. However, if patients:

- Are malnourished on admission;
- Require ventilatory support;
- Exhibit signs of confusion; and
- Have burns to the face or hands making oral feeding difficult

then these patients should be considered for a nasogastric tube immediately and reasons explained to the patient and their family.

Nasogastric feeding

In patients with burn injury of over 20–30%, a nasogastric tube should be passed as early as possible with enteral feeding commencing on a low rate and increasing every 4 hours as tolerated to final target. A nasogastric tube is safe to pass by an appropriately trained nurse, doctor or dietitian, is easy to pass (not requiring an endoscope) and is far cheaper than a nasojejunal tube. In addition gastric feeds are more beneficial in ulcer prophylaxis.[63] Therefore the majority of burn-injured patients in the UK requiring enteral feeding are fed by fine bore nasogastric tube. In patients who are not sedated oral feeding is often combined with overnight nasogastric feeding.

Nasojejunal feeding

In patients who are critically ill with a larger burn injury and septic complications and requiring ventilation, the stomach may develop delayed emptying, identified by large gastric residuals of undigested feed. Most UK burns units administer prokinetics, particularly metaclopropamide and erythromycin to try and resolve this problem. However, because small bowel motility and absorptive ability usually continue, this means that if prokinetics fail, the passage of a nasojejunal tube into the duodenum or upper jejunum using an endoscope is established practice.[64] A study by Sefton showed the success of nasojejunal feeding in burns patients in whom nasogastric feeding had failed.[65] Some units pass a nasojejunal tube in large burns (greater than 40%) irrespective of large gastric residuals as these sicker patients are more likely to develop gastric stasis. They require multiple trips to theatre in the first few weeks after injury and repeated starvation before, during and after theatre, which can compromise their nutritional intake. Nasojejunal feeding allows feeding to continue until just before theatre and begin immediately afterwards. Jenkins successfully fed burns patients during theatre and found they had a significant reduction in wound infections compared with nasogastrically fed patients, starved for theatre.[66]

Total parenteral nutrition

Studies by Herndon showed burns patients fed TPN had a significantly higher mortality than enterally fed patients.[67] However, these patients were overfed by current standards, often in excess of 8000 kcal per day. If the gut is functional there is no indication for TPN, which may have an adverse effect on the gut by increasing permeability and resulting in villous atrophy in patients fed long term.[68,69] However, it is undecided whether a place exists for giving some component of the diet such as amino acids or giving a mixture of TPN and enteral feeding if there are difficulties meeting a patient's requirements by enteral feeding alone.[70]

Early enteral feeding

McDonald demonstrated that early enteral feeding (within 6 hours) was well tolerated in burns patients.[71] It did not lead to an increase in aspiration pneumonia and resulted in the prescribed volume of feed being delivered earlier. Taylor found that patients fed early had significantly fewer infectious complications.[72] Gottschlich found that patients fed within 24 hours versus those fed after 48 hours had a reduced calorie deficit, higher serum insulin levels during the first week and a decrease in protein breakdown (measured by 3-methyl-histidine output) but no difference in infectious complications, endocrine status, mortality or morbidity.[73] Enteral feeding may improve gut perfusion but in periods of sepsis patients need to be carefully observed as high calorie enteral nutrition may lead to an imbalance between the perfusion and demand of intestinal oxygen.[74]

Maintaining the health of the gastrointestinal tract in burn injury

Even patients with small burn injuries are at risk of constipation due to the use of opiates for pain control, reduction of fibre intake, limited mobilisation and lack of fluid available to the colon during fluid resuscitation. It is important that patients on opiates are given laxatives to try and avoid constipation as the effect is to decrease appetite and tolerance of enteral feeding. Although enteral feeding has decreased the incidence of gastric ulcers, critically ill patients have a risk of other gastrointestinal complications. A review by Liolios highlighted the factors that often cause these problems to go unnoticed:[75]

- Sedated patients cannot report abdominal pain, nausea or anorexia;
- The presence of bulky dressings make abdominal examination difficult and obscures the development of abdominal distension;
- Pain control means patients may not display abdominal tenderness on physical examination; and
- An increase in temperature or white cell count can be attributed to wound or chest infection.

Acute non-occlusive mesenteric ischaemia can occur in the critically ill due to an imbalance between splanchnic oxygen delivery and demand. In burn-injured patients this seems to be a problem during septic episodes in which oxygen demand by other organs increases. Andel used an increase in the carbon dioxide gap between arterial and gastric carbon dioxide as a measure of intestinal oxygen balance.[74] In a small study of 15 nasoduodenally fed patients, it was found that the carbon dioxide gap increased in seven patients between days 6 and 13, the septic period, but fell with reduction of enteral feeding. Another possible risk is ischaemia reperfusion injury. If a patient is poorly perfused from, e.g., inadequate fluid resuscitation, tissue becomes hypoxic and is maintained on anaerobic metabolism, resulting in the production of toxic oxygen free radicals. It has been shown that two 15-minute periods of low blood flow, followed by reperfusion, results in greater tissue damage than a single 30-minute period of ischaemia.[76] Critically ill burns patients are vulnerable to such repeated episodes. Patients with a previous history of diabetes or arteriosclerosis may already have circulatory damage, compromising blood supply to the GI tract.

Peristalsis may be greatly decreased in patients on morphine and midazolam infusions for pain control and sedation. A survey found 50% of intensive care units in the UK treating major burns used morphine and midazolam.[64] Sullivan found that patients treated in 2000 were given higher levels of opiates compared with matched cases treated in the 1970s.[77] Yet evaluating pain in the sedated patient remains problematic. The survey by Hubbard in 2005 also found one-third of units increased morphine dosage for a dressing change in large burns rather than using the short-acting anaesthetic ketamine.[64] Serious constipation was a problem and did not always respond to laxatives or erythromycin. Fibre feeds were routinely used in only two centres, as the priority was to use high protein feeds, which did not contain fibre. One centre used probiotics in sick patients. Recommendations from the survey included more considered use of morphine, careful monitoring of faecal output and abdominal distension, use of fibre in feeds and evaluation of the Zassi bowel management system (based on colonic lavage).

Antibiotic therapy due to wound or chest infection is often required, altering the intestinal flora. Research is currently taking place to evaluate the benefits of a powder containing probiotics and prebiotics.

Future developments in treatment

- Reduction in the loss of skeletal and visceral muscle while avoiding increasing fat mass: Further investigation into the role of oxandrolone and insulin in reducing muscle loss and propanalol in reducing energy expenditure may be informative, as would the use of indirect calorimetry to better assess resting energy expenditure particularly during acute illness and bioimpedance to look at muscle composition.
- Improvement in the care of the gut; three key issues need exploring here:
  - The use of probiotics and prebiotics to help maintain gut integrity and reduce diarrhoea;
  - The clinical value of using tonometry to assess splanchnic perfusion and tailor our feeding regimens around this; and
  - Improved use of opiates to balance pain control without severely effecting peristalsis.

- Further clinical trials into the role of vitamins and trace elements are needed so that evidence-based recommendations can be made on supplementation.

Improve patient follow-up

Currently there is virtually no patient follow-up; yet some patients are vulnerable to weight loss after discharge and have difficulty regaining muscle mass while some become obese from increased intakes and reduced mobility. Follow-up in clinics integrated with physiotherapists and possible use of oxandrolone would help patients regain their physical strength and help restore normal body image.

Key points

- Changes in the treatment of thermal injury e.g., treating patients in a thermo-neutral environment have ameliorated the hypermetabolic response, reducing energy expenditure.
- Increased production of catecholamines from thermal injury drives muscle breakdown. Although the provision of additional protein does not prevent this research suggests it does support improved wound healing and may decrease the number of infectious episodes during the acute phase.
- During the anabolic phase a high protein diet combined with exercise leads to slow accretion of muscle mass.
- Large exudate losses containing trace elements requires intravenous supplementation to replace these losses in patients with total body surface area burns of 30% or greater. Patients with burns of 20–20% need to be monitored as they are at risk of depletion. Insufficient evidence currently exists for supplementing vitamins in large doses.
- The gut is effected by opiate use (reducing peristalsis), episodes of ischaemia (from sepsis or inadequate fluid resuscitation) and poor blood or nerve supply (secondary to diabetes or other medical conditions). Careful monitoring of the gut function, bowel action and abdominal distension is vital in critically ill patients.

Case study

Mrs Harris, a 72-year-old lady, sustained a scald of 17% (10% full thickness) from a kettle of recently boiled water. She felt dizzy and grasped the kettle as she fell to the floor. She sustained burns to her face, right arm and hand, neck and chest. Her weight on admission was 48 kg and her height from memory is 5 feet 4 inches. Although she is not normally diabetic, she had a blood glucose of 11 mmol/dL.

QUESTIONS

1. What further background information do you require to complete her global assessment?
2. Would you nasogastrically feed Mrs Harris immediately or wait and see how she did with oral diet and supplements?
3. Calculate her energy and protein requirements and suggest how this might be given. Does she need additional vitamins or trace elements?
4. Does she require insulin?
5. How will you learn from the MDT meetings and ward rounds whether her progress is satisfactory? What monitoring will you be doing and reporting on to the team?

ANSWERS

1. What further background information do you require to complete her global assessment?

   More detailed medical history especially in relation to her dizziness and a history of any weight changes. She already has a BMI of only 18.5. History of social situation as to whether she lives alone and has any help from family, neighbours or social services. What is her mood like?

2. Would you nasogastrically feed Mrs Harris immediately or wait and see how she did with oral diet and supplements?

   A nasogastric tube should be passed immediately due to her facial burns. As her face swells it may be increasingly difficult to eat, her eyes may also close temporarily and it may be impossible to pass a nasogastric tube at his stage. This should be written into the unit protocol so it occurs even when the dietitian is not present. Explanation needs to be given to her and her family about how this will help her wound healing and immune response and that the facial swelling will greatly reduce after about 48 hours.

3. Calculate her energy and protein requirements and suggest how this might be given. Does she need additional vitamins or trace elements?

   Energy requirements calculated using the Schofield equation:

$$9 \times 48 + 656 = 1088$$

$$1088 \times 1.35 = 1468 \text{ kcal (20\% for burn and}$$
$$15\% \text{ for combined activity and DIT)}$$

Protein requirements using Elia equations:

$$0.2 - 0.25 \text{ g N/kg} \times 48 = 9.6 - 12 \text{ g N } (\times 6.25$$
$$= 60 - 75 \text{ g protein})$$

Add 2 g N for insensible losses
$$= 11.6 - 14 \text{ g N } (75 - 87.5 \text{ g protein})$$

This could be given as 1000 mL of Fresubin HP Energy or 1200 mL Nutrison high protein energy fibre. Neither would give enough vitamins and a further supplement would need to be given. She is borderline for measuring trace elements but in light of her low BMI it may be advisable to measure these. She needs to be encouraged to drink and take mouthfuls of diet orally and as soon as the facial swelling resolves, her NG feed needs to be reduced in favour of diet and supplements. If she is catheterised she needs twice weekly 24-hour urinary urea measurements so you can calculate her nitrogen losses.

4. Does she require insulin?

   It is likely she will require an insulin infusion to control her blood glucose. It is vital this is not ignored as poor control will effect wound healing and accelerate muscle breakdown. It is likely this will resolve as she recovers.

5. How will you learn from the MDT meetings and ward rounds whether her progress is satisfactory? What monitoring will you be doing and reporting on to the team?

   You need to ask about her wound healing—Have her skin grafts taken, are the donor sites healing and are the areas of partial thickness burns healing? Are the wounds clean or infected? What is her clinical condition like? What plans are being made for her discharge? You need to be aware of changing biochemistry and haematology. You need to know what she is receiving orally and nasogastrically and whether she is absorbing her feeds, requires prokinetics or NJ feeding. You need to be aware of any problems in relation to her bowels and ensure she is on laxatives if she is on opiates for pain control. From discussion you need to be aware of her appetite before and during admission and whether she had been losing weight. You need to be able to assess her motivation and how well she is coping with her treatment. You need to ensure she is being weighed at dressing changes whenever possible and that she is being starved for as short a period as possible before and after theatre.

References

1. National Burn Care Review-Committee Report. *Standards and Strategy for Burn Care—A Review of Burn Care in the British Isles*. 2001.

2. Cook D. Patho-physiolgy of burns. In: Bosworth-Bousfield C, ed. *Burn Trauma Management and Nursing Care*. London: Whur; 2002.

3. Greenhalgh DG. The healing of burn wounds. *Dermatol Nurs*. 1996;8: 13–25.

4. Latha B, Babu M. The involvement of free radicals in burn injury: a review. *Burns*. 2001;27:309–317.

5. Dinarello CA. Interleukin-1 and the pathogenesis of the acute-phase response. *N Engl J Med*. 1984;311:1413–1418.

6. Pasulka PS, Wachtel TL. Nutritional considerations for the burned patient. *Surg Clin N Am*. 1987;67: 109–131.

7. Zawacki BE, Spitzer KW, Mason AO, et al. Does increased evaporative water loss cause hypermetabolism in burned patients? *Ann Surg*. 1970;171:236–240.

8. Arturson MGS. Metabolic changes following thermal injury. *World J Surg*. 1978;2:203–214.

9. Swinamer DL, Phang PT, Jones RL, et al. Effect of routine administration of analgesia on energy expenditure in critically ill patients. *Chest*. 1988;92: 4–10.

10. Hart D, Wolf S, Chinkes D, et al. Effects of early excision and aggressive enteral feeding on hypermetabolism, catabolism and sepsis after burn. *J Trauma*. 2003; 54:755–761.

11. Herndon D, Hart DW, Wolf SE, et al. Reversal of catabolism by beta-blockade after severe burn injury. *N Engl J Med*. 2001;345:1223–1229.

12. Barton RG, Craft WB, Mone MC, et al. Chemical paralysis reduces energy expenditure in patients with burns and severe respiratory failure treated with mechanical ventilation. *J Burn Care Rehabil*. 1997;18: 461–468.

13. Taylor SJ. *Energy and Nitrogen Requirements in Disease States*. London: Smith-Gordon; 2007.

14. Dickerson R, Gervasio J, Riley M, et al. Accuracy of predicted methods to estimate REE of thermally-injured patients. *JPEN J Parenter Enteral Nutr*. 2002;26:17–29.

15. Milner EA, Cioffi WG, Mason AD, et al. A longitudinal study of resting energy expenditure in thermally injured patients. *J Trauma*. 1994;37: 167–170.

16. Curreri PW. Assessing nutritional needs for the burned patient. *J Trauma*. 1990;30:20–23.

17. Burke JF, Wolfe RR, Mulaney CJ, et al. Glucose requirements following burn injury. Parameters of optimal glucose infusion and possible hepatic and respiratory abnormalities following excessive glucose intake. *Ann Surg*. 1979; 190:274–285.

18. Sheldon GF, Peterson SR, Sanders R. Hepatic dysfunction during hyperalimentation. *Arch Surg*. 1978;113:504–508.

19. Matsuda T, Kagan RJ, Hanumadass M, et al. The importance of burn wound size in determining the optimal calorie nitrogen ratio. *Surgery*. 1983;95: 562–568.

20. Noordenbos J, Hansbrough J, Gutmacher H, et al. Enteral nutritional support and wound closure do not prevent postburn hypermetabolism as measured by continued metabolic monitoring. *J Trauma*. 2000;49:667–671.

21. Burns Interest Group of the British Dietetic Association. *Feeding Guidelines for Adult Burned Patients*. 2004.

22. Allard JP, Jeejeebhoy KN, Whitwell J, et al. Factors influencing energy expenditure in patients with burns. *J Trauma*. 1988;28:199–202.

23. Hart D, Wolf S, Micak R, et al. Persistence of muscle catabolism after severe burn injury. *Surgery*. 2000;128:312–319.

24. Wolfe RR, Goodenough RD, Burke JF, et al. Response of protein and urea kinetics in burn patients to different levels of protein intake. *Ann Surg*. 1983;197:163–171.

25. Gore DC, Chinkes DL, Wolf SE, et al. Quantification of protein metabolism for skin, wound and muscle in severe burn patients. *JPEN J Parenter Enteral Nutr*. 2006;30: 331–338.

26. Alexander JW, Macmillan BG, Stinnett JD, et al. Beneficial effects of aggressive protein feeding in children. *Ann Surg*. 1980;192: 505–517.

27. Wilmore DW, Mason AD, Pruitt BA, et al. Insulin response to glucose in hypermetabolic burn patients. *Ann Surg*. 1976;183:314–320.

28. Gore DC, Wolf SE, Herndon DN, et al. Relative influence of glucose and insulin on peripheral amino acid metabolism in severely burned patients. *JPEN J Parenter Enteral Nutr*. 2002;26:271–277.

29. Ferrando AA, Stuart C, Sheffield-Moore M, et al. Inactivity amplifies the catabolic response of skeletal muscle to cortisol. *J Clin Endocrinol Metab*. 1999;275:3515–3521.

30. Demling RH, DeSanti L. Increased protein intake during the recovery phase after sever burns increases body weight gain and muscle function. *J Burn Care Rehabil*. 1998;19:161–168.

31. Demling RH, DeSanti L. Oxandrolone, an anabolic steroid significantly increases the rate of weight gain in the recovery phase after major burns. *J Trauma*. 1997;43:47–51.

32. Demling RH, DeSanti L. The rate of restoration of body weight after burn injury using the anabolic agent oxandrolone is not age dependant. *Burns*. 2001;17:46–51.

33. Demling RH, Orgill DP. The anticatabolic and wound healing effects of the testosterone analog oxandrolone after severe burn injury. *J Crit Care*. 2000;15:12–17.

34. Haji-Michael PG. Antioxidant therapy in the critically ill. *Br J Intensive Care*. 2000;May/June:88–93.

35. Kreyman KG, Berger MM, Deutz NEP, et al. ESPEN Guidelines on enteral nutrition: intensive care. *Clin Nutr*. 2006;25:210–223.

36. Garrel D, Patenaude J, Nedelec B, et al. Decreased mortality and infectious morbidity in adult burn patients given enteral glutamine supplements: a prospective, controlled randomized clinical trial. *Crit Care Med*. 2003;31: 2444–2449.

37. Zhou YP, Jiang ZM, Sun YH, et al. The effect of supplemental enteral glutamine on plasma levels, gut function and outcome in severe burns: a randomized double blind, controlled clinical trial. *JPEN J Parenter Enteral Nutr*. 2003;27: 241–245.

38. Chen G, Xie W, Jiang H. Clinical observation of the protective effect of oral feeding of glutamine granules on intestinal mucous membrane. *Zhanghua Shao Shang Za Zhi*. 2001;17:210–211.

39. Peng X, Yan H, You Z, et al. Effects of enteral supplementation with glutamine granules on intestinal mucosal barrier function in severe burned patients. *Burns*. 2004; 30135–30139.

40. Windle ME. Glutamine supplementation in critical illness: evidence recommendations and implications for clinical practice in burn care. *J Burn Care Res*. 2006;27: 764–772.

41. Wischmeyer PE, Lynch J, Liedel J, et al. Glutamine administration reduces gram-negative bacteremia in severely burned patients: a prospective, randomized double-blind trial versus isonitrogenous control. *Crit Care Med*. 2001;29: 2075–2080.

42. Lee HA, Hartley TF. A method of determining daily nitrogen requirements. *Postgrad Med J*. 1975;51:441–445.

43. Streat SJ, Beddoe AH, Hill GL. Changes in body nitrogen—comparison of direct measurement with nitrogen balance. *Aust N Z J Surg*. 1986;56:257.

44. Elia M. Artificial nutritional support. *Med Internat*. 1990;82:3392–3396.

45. Wolfe RR, Durkot MJ, Allsop JR, Burke JFl. Glucose metabolism in severely burned patients. *Metabolism*. 1979;28:1031–1039.

46. Wolfe RR, Herndon DN, Jahoor F, Miyoshi H, Wolfe M. Effect of severe burn injury on substrate cycling by glucose and fatty acids. *N Engl J Med*. 1987;317:403–408.

47. Wilmore DW, Aulick LH, Mason AD, Pruitt BA. Influence on the burn wound of local and systemic responses to injury. *Ann Surg*. 1977; 186:444–458.

48. Reinhold D, Ansorge S, Schleicher ED. Elevated glucose levels stimulate transforming growth factor-beta 1 suppress interleukin-2, IL-6 and IL-10 and DNA synthesis in peripheral blood mononuclear cells. *Hormone Metab Res*. 1996;345: 1223–1229.

49. Gottshclich M. Early and perioperative nutrition support. In: Matarese L, Gottschlich MM, eds. *Contemporary Nutrition Support Practice*. Philadelphia: Saunders; 1998.

50. Abbott WC, Schiller WR, Long CL, et al. The effect of major thermal injury on plasma ketone body levels. *JPEN J Parenter Enteral Nutr*. 1985;9:153–158.

51. Gottschlich MM, Alexander JW. Fat kinetics and recommended dietary intake in burns. *JPEN J Parenter Enteral Nutr*. 1987;11:80–85.

52. Shakespeare PG. Studies on the serum levels of iron, copper and zinc and the urinary excretion of zinc after burn injury. *Burns Incl Therm Inj*. 1982;8:358–364.

53. Shenkin A. The key role of micronutrients. *Clin Nutr*. 2006;25: 1–13.

54. Berger MM, Cavadini C, Bart A, et al. Cutaneous copper and zinc levels in burns. *Burns*. 1992;18: 373–380.

55. Berger MM, Cavadini C, Chiolero R, et al. Influence of large intakes of trace elements on recovery after major burns. *Nutrition*. 1994;10: 327–334.

56. Berger MM, Spertini F, Shenkin A, et al. Trace element supplementation modulates pulmonary infection rates after major burns; a double blind placebo-controlled trial. *Am J Clin Nutr*. 1998;68:365–371.

57. Berger MM, Eggimann P, Heyland DK, et al. Reduction of nosocomial pneumonia after major burns by trace element supplementation: aggregation of two randomised trials. *Crit Care*. 2006;10:R153.

58. Rock CL, Dechert RE, Khilnani R, et al. Carotenoid and antioxidant vitamins in patients after burn injury. *J Burn Care Rehabil*. 1997;18: 269–278.

59. Mingjian Z, Qifang W, Lanxing G, et al. Comparitive observation of the changes in serum lipid peroxides influenced by the supplementation of vitamin E and healthy controls. *Burns*. 1992;18:19–21.

60. Wray CJ, Mayes T, Khoury J, et al. Metabolic effects of vitamin D on serum calcium, magnesium and phosphorus in paediatric burn patients. *J Burn Care Rehabil*. 2002;23:416–423.

61. Gottschlich MM, Mayes T, Khoury J, et al. Hypovitaminosis D in acutely injured paediatric burn patients. *J Am Diet Assoc*. 2004;104: 931–941.

62. Klein GL, Langman CB, Herndon D. Vitamin D depletion following burns in children: A possible factor in post burn ostopenia. *J Trauma*. 2002;52: 346–350.

63. Prelack K, Dylewski M, Sheridan RL. Practical guidelines for nutritional management of burn injury and recovery. *Burns*. 2007;33:14–24.

64. Hubbard LD. Conference paper, annual meeting of the British Burn Association; 2005.

65. Sefton D. Enteral feeding inpatients with major burn injury: the use of nasojejunal feeding after the failure of nasogastric feeding. *Burns*. 2002;28:386–390.

66. Jenkins ME, Gottschlich MM. Enteral feeding during operative procedures in thermal injuries. *J Burn Care Rehabil*. 1994;15: 199–205.

67. Herndon DN, Barrow RE, Stein M, et al. Increased mortality with intravenous supplemental feeding in severely burned patients. *J Burn Care Rehabil*. 1989;10: 309–313.

68. Illig KA, Ryan CK, Hardy DJ, et al. Total parenteral nutrition-induced changes in gut mucosa function: atrophy alone is not the issue. *Surgery*. 1992;112:631–637.

69. Pironi L, Paganelli GM, Miglioli M, et al. Morphological and cytoproliferative patterns of duodenal mucosa in two patients after long term total parenteral nutrition: changes with oral feeding and relation to intestinal resection. *JPEN J Parenter Enteral Nutr*. 1994;18:351–354.

70. Wolf SE. Nutrition and metabolism in burns: state of the science, 2007. *J Burn Care Res*. 2007;28:572–576.

71. McDonald WS, Sharp CW, Deitch EA. Immediate enteral feeding in burn patients is safe and effective. *Ann Surg*. 1990;213: 177–183.

72. Taylor SJ. Early enhanced enteral nutrition in burned patients is associated with fewer infective complications and shorter hospital stay. *J Human Nutr Diet*. 1999;12: 85–91.

73. Gottschlich MM, Jenkins ME, Mayes T, et al. An evaluation of the safety of early versus delayed eneteral support and effects on clinical, nutritional and endocrine outcomes after severe burns. *J Burn Care Rehabil*. 2002;23:401–415.

74. Andel H, Rab M, Andel D, et al. Impact of duodenal feeding on the oxygen balance of the splanchnic region during different phases of severe burn injury. *Burns*. 2002;28: 60–64.

75. Liolios A, Oropello JM, Benjamin E. Gastrointestinal complications in the intensive care unit. *Clin Chest Med*. 1999;20:329–345.

76. Bassiouny HS. Nonocclusive mesenteric ischaemia. *Surg Clin N Am*. 1997;77:319–326.

77. Sullivan SR, Friedrich JB, Engrav LH, et al. Opioid creep is real and may be the cause of fluid creep. *Burns*. 2004;30:583–590.

Nutrition and liver disease

Michelle M Romano   Jaime Aranda-Michel

By the end of this chapter the reader will be able to:

- Identify the pathogenic mechanisms of malnutrition in liver disease;
- Assess nutritional status of a liver failure patient, utilising appropriate assessment tools for this population;
- Identify parameters for utilising branched-chain amino acids (BCAA); and
- List components of medical nutrition therapy in liver disease.

Physiology

The liver is the largest metabolic organ in the human body, which integrates a wide variety of complex biochemical processes that contribute to a well-nourished state (Box 13.1). These processes actively impact carbohydrate (gluconeogenesis and glycogenolysis), fat (cholesterol synthesis from acetate, triglyceride synthesis from fatty acids and secretion of both in VLDL particles, solubilisation of fats and fat-soluble vitamins in bile for uptake by enterocytes) and protein (transamination and de novo synthesis of nonessential amino acids, synthesis of various plasma proteins, including albumin, clotting factors, binding proteins, apolipoproteins, angiotensinogen and insulin-like growth factor I), vitamin storage and activation and detoxification and excretion of endogenous and exogenous waste. Liver cells have a great ability to regenerate. Severe liver injury leads to a variety of metabolic derangements that lead to the development of protein-energy malnutrition (PEM).

Pathophysiology

Liver disease can be categorised as acute or chronic, acquired or genetic.

Acute liver disease

Acute hepatitis is most commonly caused by viral infections (hepatitis A, B and less commonly C). Acute hepatitis is also sometimes caused by exposure to drugs (e.g. acetaminophen) or poisons/toxins (e.g. alcohol) and metabolic (Wilson's disease) and autoimmune diseases (autoimmune hepatitis, primary biliary cirrhosis, sclerosing cholangitis). The mechanism of liver injury is most often hepatocellular necrosis but some diseases can cause bile duct damage inducing cholestasis. The patient may be asymptomatic, have mild symptoms with anorexia, jaundice, nausea and vomiting (as in hepatitis A, B) or may present in acute liver failure (fulminant hepatitis). Acute liver failure involves massive liver necrosis leading to encephalopathy, increased intracranial pressure and metabolic derangements such as hypoglycaemia, hemodynamic changes, coagulopathy and oliguric renal failure. Malnutrition in acute liver failure may not be present at the outset, but if the disease progresses to chronic liver failure, nutrition support will be a component of care. Comorbid conditions such as diabetes and obesity are associated with poor outcomes with acute liver failure.[1,2]

Box 13.1

Functions of the normal liver

Energy metabolism and substrate interconversion

- Glucose production through gluconeogenesis and glycogenolysis
- Glucose consumption by pathways of glycogen synthesis, fatty acid synthesis, glycolysis and the tricarboxylic acid cycle
- Cholesterol synthesis from acetate, triglyceride synthesis from fatty acids and secretion of both in VLDL particles
- Cholesterol and triglyceride uptake by endocytosis of HDL and LDL particles with excretion of cholesterol in bile, beta-oxidation of fatty acids and conversion of excess acetyl-CoA to ketones
- Deamination of amino acids and conversion of ammonia to urea via the urea cycle
- Transamination and de novo synthesis of nonessential amino acids

Protein synthetic functions

- Synthesis of various plasma proteins, including albumin, clotting factors, binding proteins, apolipoproteins, angiotensinogen and insulin-like growth factor I

Solubilisation, transport, and storage functions

- Drug and poison detoxification through phase I and phase II biotransformation reactions and excretion in bile

- Solubilisation of fats and fat-soluble vitamins in bile for uptake by enterocytes
- Synthesis and secretion of VLDL and pre-HDL lipoprotein particles and clearance of HDL, LDL and chylomicron remnants
- Synthesis and secretion of various binding proteins, including transferrin, steroid hormone-binding globulin, thyroid hormone-binding globulin, ceruloplasmin and metallothionein
- Uptake and storage of vitamins A, D and B_{12} and folate

Protective and clearance functions

- Detoxification of ammonia through the urea cycle
- Detoxification of drugs through microsomal oxidases and conjugation systems
- Synthesis and export of glutathione
- Clearance of damaged cells and proteins, hormones, drugs and activated clotting factors from the portal circulation
- Clearance of bacteria and antigens from the portal circulation

Nguyen T.T., Lingappa V. Liver disease. In: McPhee S, Gangong W, eds. *Lange's Pathophysiology of Disease: An Introduction to Clinical Medicine*, 5th edn. London: McGraw Hill; 2006.

Chronic liver disease

In chronic liver disease, liver function declines due to ongoing hepatocellular damage, due to the combination of liver cell necrosis and inflammation. Laboratory abnormalities are usually present for at least six months, and can be caused by viral (especially hepatitis B or C), autoimmune, metabolic or toxic etiologies (alcohol). As fibrosis increases due to inflammation and necrosis, portal hypertension develops. Portal systemic shunting takes place when portal venous pressure exceeds systemic venous pressure. This leads to the development of oesophageal and gastric varices and portal hypertensive gastropathy. Early symptoms of chronic liver disease may include fatigue, malaise, low-grade fever, anorexia, weight loss, mild intermittent jaundice and

hepatosplenomegaly. In later stages, complications include variceal haemorrhage, coagulopathy, encephalopathy, jaundice and ascites with hyponatraemia.

A frequent complication in chronic liver disease is PEM. Initially it was thought to be to be more prevalent in alcoholic liver disease. Studies show similar prevalence of PEM in all patients with chronic liver disease regardless of aetiology.[3] In early or compensated cirrhosis PEM can be found in 20% of patients, without the easily recognised signs of muscle wasting and loss of subcutaneous fat stores.[4] A recent study found that in 46.9% of patients with Child–Pugh class A score had a reduction in total body fat and 15% reduction in body cell mass (BCM).[5] Others found the prevalence of PEM in 100% of patients at the time of liver transplantation.[6] Clinical outcomes in patients with alcoholic liver disease undergoing orthotopic liver transplantation (OLT) are worse when PEM is present.[7] High metabolic rates and low lean body weights or BCM, which are features of malnutrition in end-stage liver disease (ESLD), are associated with shorter mean survival post OLT.[8,9] Some of these factors may be modified with aggressive nutritional support. Therefore, it is crucial to identify these high-risk patients so that morbidity and mortality may improve with focused therapy. Intervention in early stages of PEM may improve short-term mortality.[10]

The aetiology of malnutrition in chronic liver disease is multifactorial and can generally be attributed to impairments in dietary intake, absorption and metabolism, and increased nutritional losses (see Box 13.2).

Oral intake is frequently reduced in patients with chronic liver disease for a variety of reasons. Their appetite can be impaired due to early satiety, side effects of medications and psychological and neurological impairment. Zinc deficiency can be associated with anosmia (lack of smell), dysguesia (altered taste) and appetite suppression.[11] Proinflammatory cytokines (TNF) and leptin, which are increased in chronic liver disease, may impose an anorexic effect.[12–14] It is not uncommon to have intermittent anorexia for episodes of gastrointestinal bleeding and portosystemic encephalopathy. The concern for precipitating encephalopathy and worsening fluid retention often leads to excessive restriction of protein and fluid intake, exacerbating general illness and negative nitrogen balance.

Malabsorption may occur with liver disease in the presence of cholestasis. Fat, fat-soluble vitamins and mineral stores may be depleted. Medications used to treat encephalopathy, such as lactulose and neomycin, can also affect absorption. Pancreatic insufficiency with alcoholic liver disease will play a role with poor absorption of vitamins and nutrients. Thiamin and magnesium deficiency are common in the setting of alcoholic liver disease.

Patients with ascites requiring large-volume paracentesis (LVP) will experience losses of protein and electrolytes, exacerbating negative nitrogen balance. The impact of frequent LVP on nutritional status is so far undefined.

Abnormal fuel metabolism is associated with chronic liver disease. As the liver is responsible for metabolism of most nutrients, liver disease alters the metabolic processes, causing changes in energy, carbohydrate, protein and lipid. These changes are similar to those seen in states of starvation.[15]

Box 13.2

Etiology of protein-energy malnutrition

Poor dietary intake
- Anorexia, hospitalisation (fasting)
- Dietary restrictions (sodium and protein)
- Hyperinsulinemia and hyperglycemia
- Ascites/encephalopathy
- Leptin levels
- Increased proinflammatory cytokines (TNF-α, IL-1)
- Increased energy expenditure
- Portosystemic encephalopathy
- Gastroparesis
- Gastrointestinal bleeding

Nutrient malabsorption/maldigestion
- Pancreatic insufficiency
- Cholestatic liver disease
- Excessive protein losses

Medications
- Neomycin, lactulose, antibiotics, diuretics, antimetabolites, cholestyramine, prednisone

Iatrogenic
- Large-volume paracentesis
- Sodium and protein restriction
- Fluid restriction

IL, interleukin; TNF, tumour necrosis factor.

Aranda-Michel J. Nutrition in hepatic failure and liver transplant. *Curr Gastroenterol Rep.* 2001;3:363
Copyright Elsevier 2001.

The respiratory quotient (RQ) of cirrhotic patients is lower than controls after an overnight fast, indicating utilisation of fat as fuel.[16]

The metabolic rate in patients with chronic liver disease has been studied using indirect calorimetry, and compared with the Harris–Benedict equation to determine basal energy expenditure (BEE) and found to be quite variable. In a recent study of 476 patients, high metabolic rate was found in 33.8%.[17] These patients could not be identified by clinical or biochemical measures of liver disease, such as Child–Pugh class or aetiology of disease. Variability based on an earlier study, in which 18% were hypermetabolic and 31% were hypometabolic, did not consistently correlate with the cause, duration or severity of cirrhosis.[16] However, BEE was found to closely relate to fat-free mass, age, gender and increased beta-adrenergic activity. Hypermetabolism has been found to be associated with decreased survival in patients with cirrhosis undergoing OLT, regardless of the aetiology.[18] In the same study it was shown that presence of ascites was not associated with changes in metabolic rate; that is, it did not contribute to hypermetabolism.

It is also important to differentiate between total body mass and body cell mass. Body cell mass is directly responsible for basal energy expenditure. Energy expenditure relative to body cell mass is more reflective of true BEE and patient physiology. Irrespective of the degree of ascites or Child–Pugh score, low body cell mass and hypermetabolism correlated with a poorer prognosis after OLT. In fact, hypermetabolism appears to persist after transplantation. This suggests that hypermetabolism may be an extrahepatic manifestation of liver disease.

Glucose intolerance, insulin resistance and hyperinsulinemia are found in a majority of liver disease patients. Glucose intolerance can occur in over 70% of cirrhotic patients with diabetes mellitus developing in up to 37% of patients.[19] Fortunately, they do not appear to be at higher risk for cardiovascular disease.[20] These patients have decreased hepatic circulation and extraction of insulin, decreased hepatic sensitivity to insulin and decreased production and storage of glycogen in muscles. Because of the decreased glycogen stores, fat is utilised as their main substrate for energy.[15,21,22] This leads to an 'accelerated starvation', in which patients with overnight fasting have biochemical evidence of increased gluconeogenesis, lipid oxidation and protein catabolism. Increased gluconeogenesis eventually leads to loss of subcutaneous fat tissue and muscle wasting.

Alterations in lipoproteins and essential fatty acid profile occur in liver disease. Hypertriglyceridemia (250–500 mg/dL) is found frequently in both alcoholic and viral liver disease and tends to resolve when the liver disease improves. Polyunsaturated and essential fatty acid levels are reduced, which may correlate for both malnutrition and liver dysfunction.[23] Arachidonic acid is necessary for prostaglandin and leukotriene synthesis, as well as cell membrane function. Supplementation with arachidonic acid in cirrhotic patients may improve platelet aggregation.[24]

Protein stores in liver disease are altered due to decreased absorption, decreased synthesis of body protein and increased degradation of body protein. Increased protein catabolism can be present in early cirrhosis. In a study of 268 patients with cirrhosis,

51% were found to have significant protein depletion.[25] Even in patients with mild liver disease (Child–Pugh A), malnutrition was observed in > 40%.[25] The group with the greatest depletion was with alcoholic liver disease. In general protein deficiency worsens as liver disease progresses. Abnormal amino acid metabolism is common, including decreased leucine oxidation. Increased proteolysis may be present, which is not suppressed with active feeding. Furthermore, patients with compensated liver disease can retain nitrogen when fed for long periods of time without developing portosystemic encephalopathy.[26,27] Protein intakes of up to 1.8 g/kg/day were well tolerated. These data indicate that protein-deficient patients with compensated liver disease have the capacity to retain nitrogen, provided that enough protein is present to reverse net protein loss. Therefore patients with chronic liver disease should avoid protein restriction, and avoid a fasting state, include frequent meals to balance protein synthesis and degradation. Hepatic encephalopathy should be aggressively managed with other treatment modalities before protein restriction is considered. Acute exacerbation of liver disease such as infections (urinary tract infections, spontaneous bacterial peritonitis and pneumonia), tense ascites, gastrointestinal bleeding and encephalopathic episodes may increase the protein requirement and affect nutritional status rapidly.

Nonalcoholic fatty liver disease (NAFLD)

Nonalcoholic fatty liver disease (NAFLD) encompasses simple fatty liver and nonalcoholic steatohepatitis (NASH), which can lead to cirrhosis. In the general population, the estimated prevalence of NAFLD is 20% (range 15–39%) and the prevalence of NASH is 2–3%, making NAFLD the most common form of liver disease in the USA.[28] The causes of NAFLD are listed in Box 13.3. Obesity is most-often associated with NAFLD. In a study of 210 healthy obese patients, 80% had fatty liver. Insulin resistance is a major risk factors predicting NAFLD.[29] Type 2 diabetes and glucose intolerance with or without obesity is also associated with NAFLD. Hyperlipidemia is also found in this population, and there is growing evidence that there is higher overall mortality and increased risk from cardiovascular disease.[30] NASH was found in 88% of patients with metabolic syndrome in a study by

Box 13.3

Aetiology of NAFLD

Chronic metabolic syndromes

- Obesity
- Diabetes mellitus
- Hyperlipidemia

Congenital metabolic diseases

- Dysbetalipoproteinemia
- Glycogen disease
- Homocystinuria, tyrosinemia, galactosemia

Metabolic syndromes

- Jejunoileal bypass
- TPN
- Mitochondrial diseases
- Rapid weight loss

Toxin and medication

- Amiodarone
- Glucocorticoids
- Nucleoside analogues (HAART)
- Tetracycline

Marchesini and colleagues,[31] and should now be considered a component of metabolic syndrome.

NAFLD is typically asymptomatic and usually discovered incidentally. Vague right upper quadrant pain, fatigue and malaise may be reported. Serum ALT and AST may be elevated two- to fourfold; serum ferritin level and alkaline phosphatase may be elevated. Bilirubin, albumin and prothrombin time typically are normal. Large prospective studies are needed to define the disease progression in this population. Those who progress to steatohepatitis with necrosis and fibrosis are at greatest risk for morbidity and mortality.

Cholestatic liver disease

Primary sclerosing cholangitis

Sclerosing cholangitis is a disease characterised by patchy inflammation, fibrosis and destruction of the intrahepatic and extrahepatic bile ducts. It is typically chronic and progressive, which leads to biliary obstruction, cholangitis and biliary cirrhosis and hepatic failure with associated complications. Primary sclerosing cholangitis (PSC) is an idiopathic

disorder usually associated with inflammatory bowel disease (IBD), but may develop independently. Common features include pruritus, jaundice, fatigue and abdominal pain. Pruritus is thought to be a result of accumulation of bile acids in plasma and tissue which causes itching. This is typically treated by oral bile acid resins such as cholestryamine. The reported frequency of cholangiocarcinoma in patients with PSC who have undergone liver transplantation has ranged from 7 to 36%.[32] Nutritional deficiencies can occur due to reduced intestinal concentrations of conjugated bile acids, causing malabsorption of fat-soluble vitamins. Concomitant diseases such as IBD, chronic pancreatitis and celiac sprue may also contribute to nutritional deficiencies. Metabolic bone disease may also be frequently found. The only treatment to halt the progress of the disease is liver transplantation.[33]

Primary biliary cirrhosis (PBC)

PBC is characterised by ongoing inflammatory destruction of the intralobular bile ducts leading to chronic cholestasis and biliary cirrhosis, and complications such as portal hypertension and liver failure. Like PSC, PBC may have an autoimmune pathogenesis. Patients are treated with ursodeoxycholic acid (UDCA) to delay or prevent disease progression. Complications of chronic cholestasis such as osteopenic bone disease, fat-soluble vitamin deficiency, hypercholesterolaemia and steatorrhoea should be recognised and treated.[34] The presence of osteoporosis in PBC patients has been reported to be 20%, which represents a 30-fold increase of developing severe bone disease compared with age- and weight-matched population.[35] Patients with low cholesterol, low serum albumin levels and advanced disease stage should be screened for fat-soluble vitamin deficiencies.[36]

Inherited disorders

Hemochromatosis is the most common genetic disorder in the Caucasian population. Due to gene mutation(s), excessive absorption of dietary iron may lead to development of life-threatening complications of cirrhosis, hepatocellular cancer, diabetes and heart disease. Treatment includes phlebotomy and avoidance of iron or vitamin C supplements.

Wilson's disease is an autosomal recessive disorder of copper metabolism characterised by the abnormal transport and storage of copper. Copper accumulates in the liver, kidney, brain and cornea (Kayser–Fleischer rings) and may have toxic effects on tissues. Symptoms include hepatic, neurological and psychiatric dysfunctions. Therapy consists of medications to remove copper or maintain balance. A low copper diet is advised.

Other

This category includes alpha-1 antitrypsin deficiency (inherited), hepatocellular carcinoma, Budd–Chiari syndrome and hepatoveno-occlusive disease. Cryptogenic cirrhosis is any cirrhosis for which the aetiology is unknown.

Hepato-renal syndrome occurs in patients with cirrhosis and ascites up to 18% within 1 year, and 35% within 5 years.[37] Renal failure occurs in the absence of intrinsic renal disease. Constriction of the renal arterial vasculature results in oliguria and sodium retention.

Nutrition therapy

Assessment

A careful diet history should be conducted with special attention to degree of anorexia, postprandial fullness, taste changes and chronic diarrhoea. Hospitalised patients have been shown to have suboptimal intake corresponding with severity of disease.[10] Therefore calorie counts for in-patients (and food diaries for outpatients) should be initiated. Many of the common nutrition assessment parameters such as BMI, weight changes and visceral proteins are not useful in this population due to excess fluid retention (ascites and oedema) and impaired protein metabolism. A combination of the following measurements will be helpful in evaluation.

Anthropometric measurements of triceps skin fold and mid-arm muscle circumference will reflect nutritional reserves. Although fluid retention can also involve the upper arms, these measurements are still a useful way of assessing subcutaneous fat and muscle mass.

Subjective global assessment (SGA) is a general nutritional evaluation based on weight, nutrition history and changes on physical examination that include oedema and ascites. Although this test has been reported to be highly specific (96%), it was also found to be very insensitive (22%) in diagnosing malnutrition in patients with alcoholic liver disease.[38]

Muscle mass is thought to be more reliable and important than fat-free mass for determining PEM. Measurement of fat-free mass is not accurate in patients with ESLD due to fluid retention.[4] BCM rather than fat-free mass should be measured, as it represents the true metabolic compartment. Several tests can be conducted to determine BCM, including 24-hour urinary creatinine excretion, total body potassium and bioelectrical impedance analysis (BIA).

A 24-hour urinary creatinine excretion has been used and validated for assessing muscle mass, as well as BCM in patients with ESLD.[39] However, the reliability of the former is significantly impaired in the setting of renal dysfunction.

Total body potassium has been found to correlate with skeletal muscle mass and BCM;[40] however, this has not been validated in adult patients with ESLD.

Bioelectrical impedance analysis is a simple, inexpensive and noninvasive test that yields immediate results in determining BCM. The test measures body electrical conductivity and resistance or impedance. In principle, fat offers resistance, while water conducts electric current. The comparison of conductivity and resistance can reflect lean body weight and fat mass. Fluid retention in ESLD may represent a major limitation of this technique; however, a recent report suggest that BIA is a reliable tool for determination of BCM in cirrhotic patients with and without ascites.[41] Further studies are needed to validate this technique in patients with varying degrees of oedema or ascites and for comparison with other techniques for measuring body composition.

Dual-energy X-ray (DEXA) can be used to measure total body bone mineral, fat and fat-free soft tissue mass. Although very accurate in assessing body composition in healthy individuals, DEXA has not been validated in patients with ESLD. This test is also influenced by fluid retention. In cirrhotic patients without overt fluid retention, DEXA has shown accuracy in assessing percentage of body fat.[42]

Energy needs

As mentioned previously, most patients with liver disease have a normal metabolic rate, but up to a third have a high metabolic rate (> 20% BEE). Various predictive equations have been used to estimate energy expenditure. Utilising these equations in the liver disease population may not be accurate due to the contribution of fluid to total body weight. In a study comparing six predictive equations (Harris-Benedict, Schofield, Mifflin, Owen, Cunningham and disease-specific Müller formulas) compared with indirect calorimetry to measure energy expenditure in cirrhotic patients, these formulas either significantly under- or overestimated REE.[43] The most accurate measure of energy expenditure in ESLD with fluid retention is indirect calorimetry. The European Society for Parenteral and Enteral Nutrition (ESPEN) published a group consensus for non-protein calorie needs. For compensated cirrhosis or encephalopathy, it is 25–35 non-protein calories/kg/day, while for inadequate intake or malnutrition it is 35–40 non-protein cal/kg/day.[44]

Protein needs

Protein restriction should not be considered routine. Basal protein requirements are approximately 0.8–1 g/kg/day; however, in periods of stress it may approach 2 g/kg/day. In the absence of renal failure, measurement of 24-hour urinary urea nitrogen could be used to assess the true catabolic rate. If the patient has severe refractory encephalopathy requiring hospitalisation only then could protein restriction be used. This should be a temporary measure, with advancement of protein provision after a few days. Use of protein restriction or branched-chain amino acids (BCAA; discussed below) in hepatic encephalopathy has not been of proven benefit.

Fat

Most patients with liver disease are able to tolerate dietary fat, and it should be used as an integral form of kilocalories in the diet. In cases of steatorrhoea (stool fat > 6 g in 24 hours), a diet restricted in dietary fat, but supplemented with medium-chain triglycerides (MCT) should be considered.

Micronutrients

- Sodium restriction is only needed in cases of fluid retention (ascites and oedema).

- A multivitamin, and other supplements as needed such as folic acid, zinc and magnesium, should be taken daily.
- Thiamin should be supplemented in alcoholic liver disease.
- Specific fat-soluble vitamin supplementation should be provided if a deficiency is present.
- Vitamin K deficiency may be encountered in both cholestatic and non-cholestatic liver disease. Supplementation with 5–10 mg/day is frequently required to treat coagulopathy. Vitamin K may also play a role in maintaining bone mineral density.
- Calcium 1500 mg/day and vitamin D 800 IU/day are recommended routinely for prevention of osteomalacia, but it does not prevent bone loss or improve lumbar mineral density in the presence of osteoporosis.[36]
- If a deficiency of vitamin D is present, 25,000–50,000 IU can be given orally 2–3 times per week, with follow-up serum levels in eight weeks.
- Serum vitamin A levels can be decreased in all types of liver disease.[45] There is no proven role for aggressive supplementation; furthermore, aggressive supplementation can potentially produce vitamin A toxicity. These patients may have impaired hepatic release versus malabsorption. Supplementation with standard formulations as multivitamins may be the best approach.

Laboratory assessment

Liver testing includes aspartate aminotransferase (AST, or serum glutamic oxaloacetic transaminase (SGOT)) and alanine aminotransferase (ALT, or serum glutamic pyruvic transaminase (SGPT)), bilirubin, prothrombin time (PT), alkaline phosphatase, gamma glutamyl-transpeptidase (GGT) and serum cholesterol levels.

Vitamin and mineral stores include retinol, vitamin D, vitamin E and zinc.

The Child–Turcotte–Pugh scoring classification (often called Child–Pugh or Child score) is used to predict prognosis after surgery (see Table 13.1). Patients are assigned an 'A', 'B' or 'C' based on the degree of disease and relative risk for poor surgical outcome. This scoring system lacks specificity in late stage of disease.

Table 13.1 Child–Turcotte–Pugh classification

Parameter	Numerical score		
	1	2	3
Ascites	None	Slight	Moderate/severe
Encephalopathy	None	Slight/moderate	Moderate/severe
Bilirubin (mg/dL)	< 2.0	2–3	>3.0
Albumin (g/dL)	> 3.5	2.8–3.5	<2.8
Prothrombin time (seconds increased)	1–3	4–6	>6.0

Total numerical score	Child–Turcotte–Pugh class
5–6	A
7–9	B
10–15	C

From Feldman M, Friedman L, Brandt L, eds. *Sleisenger & Fordtran's Gastrointestinal and Liver Disease*, 8th edn. Philadelphia, Saunders, 2006. Copyright Elsevier.

The model for end-stage liver disease (MELD) (see Box 13.4) is a scoring system devised to identify patients whose predicted survival post-TIPS procedure would be 3 months or less. It was subsequently evaluated and found to be a predictor of survival with

Box 13.4

Model for end-stage liver disease (MELD) scoring equation[a]

MELD score for TIPS = $0.957 \times \log_e$(creatinine [mg/dL]) + $0.378 \times \log_e$(bilirubin [mg/dL]) + $1.120 \times \log_e$(INR) + 0.643 (cause of liver disease)[b]

MELD score for liver transplantation[c] = $0.957 \times \log_e$(creatinine [mg/dL]) + $0.378 \times \log_e$(bilirubin [mg/dL]) + $1.120 \times \log_e$(INR) + 0.643

INR, international normalised ratio; TIPS, transjugular intrahepatic portosystemic shunt.

[a]Laboratory values less than 1.0 are set at 1.0. The maximum serum creatinine level considered in the MELD score equation is 4.0 mg/dL.

[b]0 if cholestatic or alcoholic liver disease, and 1 if other liver disease.

[c]Multiply by 10 and round to the nearest whole number.

From: Feldman M, Friedman L, Brandt L, eds. *Sleisenger & Fordtran's Gastrointestinal and Liver Disease*, 8th edn. Philadelphia, Saunders, 2006. Copyright Elsevier.

liver disease in general. This score is used with the United Network for Organ Sharing (UNOS) program in prioritising liver transplant candidates nationwide.

Treatment

Oral diet

For patients with fluid retention a 2-g sodium diet should be implemented; otherwise, a regular, unrestricted diet is recommended. A fluid restriction should not be implemented unless serum sodium is <120 mmol/L. Standard protein food sources and polymeric liquid formulas are effective and well tolerated, even in patients with advanced liver disease. Food diaries and/or prospective calorie counts should be implemented to ensure the patient is consuming their nutritional requirements. Frequent meals should be encouraged. A night-time snack is especially important for minimising the consumption of muscle tissue and fat stores during the non-prandial state.[46] An early study utilising a bedtime snack supplying 17% kcal and 20% protein needs was found to improve nitrogen balance in cirrhotic patients.[47] More recently, night-time snacks with BCAA versus standard snacks were studied in patients with hepatitis C.[48] This study group received a supplement with 210 calories, 13.5 g protein and 3.5 g of fat and they were followed for 3 months. Total energy intakes were similar in both control and BCAA groups, but the BCAA group had significantly greater protein intake. The BCAA group had improved nitrogen balance and serum albumin levels as compared with controls.

Branched-chain amino acids

BCAA have been studied as a treatment for hepatic encephalopathy and as a nutritional supplement to improve nutritional status. Although the exact mechanism is not known, one of the theories in development of hepatic encephalopathy in liver disease is derangement in the balance of amino acids, specifically imbalances in the ratio of plasma BCAA (valine, leucine, isoleucine) to aromatic amino acids (AAA) (tyrosine, phenylalanine, tryptophan). This ratio is normally 3.5 but it is decreased to 1.0 in cirrhotic patients. This change results in an increased uptake of AAA in the central nervous system. Central nervous system metabolism of AAA (especially tryptophan) leads to the formation of false neurotransmitters, which is a hypothesised mechanism of hepatic encephalopathy. Low plasma BCAA found in liver disease may be a result of increased catabolism in skeletal muscle and the kidneys. In a comprehensive meta-analysis of BCAA and hepatic encephalopathy, no evidence was found for clinical benefit or survival, when only good quality studies were considered.[49] There were limited data that suggested a benefit in encephalopathy using parenteral BCAA in acute hepatic encephalopathy and enteral BCAA in chronic hepatic encephalopathy. However, a recent prospective randomised trial comparing BCAA to standard preparation in patients with advanced cirrhosis did show an advantage in reduced rates of death and hospitalisation.[50] There was a 15% dropout rate partially due to palatability of the supplement or lost to follow-up. Those that completed the study had improvement in nutritional parameters and Child–Pugh scores. When encephalopathy is refractory, despite maximum medical efforts, BCAA can be considered. Several BCAA-enriched enteral/oral supplements and a parenteral formulation are available.

Enteral nutrition

Patients without PEM may be able to tolerate 5–7 days of inadequate intake. However, it should be assumed that patients with liver disease are malnourished until proven otherwise. Therefore, nutrition support should be instituted when patients cannot meet their nutritional requirements orally. Recent practice guidelines have been published on enteral nutrition and liver disease.[51] Whole protein formulas are recommended. For patients with ascites and/or fluid retention, a more concentrated formula should be used. As mentioned previously, BCAA-enriched formulas should be considered only in refractory encephalopathy. Enteral access using a small bore (10 French) nasogastric or nasoenteric tube is safe, even in the presence of esophageal varices. Placement of a gastrostomy tube is associated with a higher risk of complication (due to ascites or varices) and is not recommended.

Parenteral nutrition

Parenteral nutrition should only be considered in patients with contraindications for enteral feeding (i.e. ileus, bowel obstruction, short bowel syndrome). For patients with fluid retention, low-volume parenteral nutrition should be utilised. If BCAA are indicated, an IV source is available for short-term use.

NAFLD/NASH

Several Cochrane reviews addressing aspects of treatment proposed for NAFLD have been conducted. Probiotics have been suggested because of their modulating effect on gut flora that could influence hepatotoxic oxidative injury.[52] The reviewers were unable to identify any randomised trial in this population, although pilot studies appeared promising. The use of medications to lower insulin resistance was reviewed. There were three randomised studies that could be included. In two trials, metformin versus diet or vitamin E supplementation was associated with significant improvement of ALT levels. In studying pioglitazone, a statistically significant improvement of histological improvement was demonstrated.[53] Antioxidant supplements for protecting cells against oxidative stress and resulting lipid peroxidation have been suggested. Six studies were identified. Two studies were of high methodological quality. Treatment with antioxidant supplements showed a significant, although not clinically relevant reduction in AST levels, but not ALT levels. Adverse events were nonspecific. The authors concluded there were insufficient data to support or refute this therapy.[54] Other than these reviews, large trials have not been published to guide the clinician.

For now, nutrition therapy should focus on features of the metabolic syndrome, i.e. obesity, insulin resistance, dyslipidemia and hypertension.[55,56,59] Obesity may mask underlying muscle-wasting; therefore the clinician should attempt to uncover potential risk factors for malnutrition.

Liver transplantation

Immediate post-transplant goals include provision of energy and repletion of depleted nutrient stores. Patients should be encouraged to meet their nutritional needs by oral diet as soon as bowel function returns. Small frequent meals may be better tolerated. Depending on the clinical condition and degree of malnutrition prior to transplant, enteral feedings may be initiated. Enteral access with a nasoenteric tube will provide interim nutrition support. If the patient is on ventilator support, tube feedings can be infused continuously. If the patient is eating, but inadequately, night-time tube feedings can be provided to supplement needs. Calorie needs for stable post-transplant patients are 1.2 to 1.5 times the BEE or 30–35 cal/kg/day.[57] Protein needs are 1.5–2 g protein/kg/day, depending on renal function.

The long-term nutrition needs are based on the patient's activity level, and their need to gain, lose or maintain weight. Calorie needs can be based on 1.2–1.5 times the BEE. Protein needs are 0.8–1.2 g protein/kg/day. Liver transplant patients are at risk for excessive weight gain, hyperlipidaemia, diabetes and cardiovascular complications; therefore nutrition therapy should be tailored to treat these conditions. Immunosuppressive medications may result in food–drug interactions, such as cyclosporine, which may cause hypertension, hypertriglyceridaemia, hypomagnesaemia and hyperkalaemia, and tacrolimus which may cause hyperkalaemia, hyperglycaemia and hypomagnesaemia in some patients. Rapamycin can cause hypercholesterolaemia and hypertriglyceridaemia.

Key points

- Patients with ESLD have protein-energy malnutrition until proven otherwise.
- Patients with ESLD may have a high metabolic rate.
- Investigate malabsorption and maldigestion in patients with cholestatic liver disease.
- Frequent nutritional assessment, including anthropometrics, changes in body weight, 24-hour creatinine excretion and 24-hour urinary urea nitrogen in patients awaiting liver transplant, should be performed.
- BEE should be measured using indirect calorimetry in patients with decompensated liver disease, and predicted in patients with compensated liver disease.
- Small, frequent meals should be encouraged, especially bedtime snack to decrease gluconeogenesis.

- Progressive increments of protein should be given up to 1.8–2 g/kg/day as tolerated.
- Sodium restriction (2 g/day) is advised in the presence of ascites/peripheral oedema.
- All patients with ESLD should receive multivitamins; rule out deficiency of fat-soluble vitamins.
- Give aggressive oral supplementation and low threshold to place a nasoenteric feeding tube in patients awaiting Liver transplant.
- Close monitoring of patients after liver transplant is important; particular attention should be given to the development of obesity, hyperlipidaemia, osteoporosis and hypertension.

Developing issues

NAFLD: A Cochrane database protocol has been developed for review of evidenced-based studies on weight loss therapy.[58]

Leptin: Leptin is a hormone produced by the adipocyte. It appears to play a role in maintenance of body weight by regulating food intake and resting energy expenditure. Leptin is present as free and protein bound. Protein-bound leptin has a good correlation with energy expenditure and BMI.[60] Bound leptin levels have been suggested to be a surrogate marker for resting energy expenditure, and therefore may be a measure used to identify liver patients in need of nutritional intervention.

Adiponectin: In addition to leptin, another adipokine, adiponectin, is also being studied for its role in fatty accumulation of the liver, enhancement of liver inflammation and fibrogenesis.[61,62]

BCAA: Large, multicentre trials are needed to provide more definitive guidelines for the use of BCAA in ESLD.

Case study

(PART 1)

A 57-year-old Hispanic male presented to the liver transplant clinic. He had been diagnosed with end-stage liver disease secondary to alcohol one year earlier by his local physician. At that time he presented with increasing intermittent confusion and forgetfulness, increasing abdominal girth and peripheral oedema, and had been consuming 3-6 beers per night for 30 years. He was advised to stop alcohol and was started on diuretic therapy. Lactulose was begun for encephalopathy, and he received low sodium and low protein diet instructions. Later, when he presented to our clinic he was found to have ascites, peripheral oedema, malnutrition, encephalopathy and fatigue. He reported he had stopped alcohol 6 months ago. His BMI was 21.9; however, it was noted he had a positive fluid balance skewing this result. His height is 163 cm; weight is 58.3 kg. His weight history included stable weight 8 months ago at 68.2 kg, then weight fluctuations due to fluid excess. He gained 6.8 kg within 2 weeks time, and required periodic abdominal paracentesis. His TSF was 4 mm, and MAMC was 200 mm. He underwent bone mineral density testing showing osteoporosis in the spine and osteopenia in the right hip. His diet history consisted of three small meals, with snacks of high carbohydrate content such as cookies or fruit. The patient had complaints of early satiety and fear of gaining more fluid. His pertinent laboratory values are as follows: Na 125 mmol/L, glucose 94 mg/dL, albumin 2.4 g/dL, total bilirubin 4.6 mg/dL, direct bilirubin 2.3 mg/dL, alkaline phosphatase 161 u/L, ALT 56 u/L, AST 50 u/L, zinc 0.37 µg/mL (normal 0.66-1.10), total 25-dihydroxy vitamin D 6 ng/dL (normal 25-80).

QUESTIONS

1. What nutrition assessment methods should be used to evaluate nutritional status?
2. Based on the nutrition assessment methods, what are the calorie and protein needs?
3. What medical nutrition therapy should be implemented?

(PART 2)

The patient returned the following week. His weight was 63.6 kg and a paracentesis was scheduled for the following day. His food records were incomplete and he had complaints of little desire to eat. His caregiver who was present reported patient was consuming approximately one-fourth of three meals per day. He was drinking 1 can of liquid nutritional supplement daily. It is estimated he was consuming ~750 cal/day. Based on this, he was not meeting his nutritional requirements, and due to anorexia, he would not likely improve his intake.

QUESTIONS

4. Is the patient a candidate for nutrition support?
5. If so, what method should be used to meet this patient's nutritional needs?

ANSWERS

1. What nutrition assessment methods should be used to evaluate nutritional status?

There are several tools that would help with identifying nutritional status. For instance, his TSF measurement places him at the 5th percentile for age and gender. His MAMC places him at < 5th percentile. Based on these two values he has severe muscle and fat wasting. The SGA score based on physical parameters of fat and muscle loss, acites and oedema, his diet history and functional impairment places him as a 'C' rating, which refers to severely malnourished.

2. Based on the nutrition assessment methods, what are the calorie and protein needs?

Nutritional needs are difficult to estimate in this population. Based on the Harris-Benedict equation, his basal needs are 1292 cal/day. Additional factors for activity (25%) and weigh gain (plus 500 cal/day) might place his total needs at approximately 2100 cal/day. Based on ESPEN guidelines (35-40 non-protein cal/kg/day), his non-protein calories would be approximately 2000-2300 kcal/day. Protein needs of 1.5 g protein/kg/day would calculate to 87 g protein/day, and an additional 348 cal/day if using the ESPEN guidelines. An indirect calorimetry study was conducted and determined resting energy expenditure to be 1628 cal. Based on this we calculated total calories for anabolism as 2535 cal/day.

3. What medical nutrition therapy should be implemented?

The patient was instructed on 2-g sodium, high calorie and high protein diet based on his measured needs. This was divided into 6 small meals per day, emphasising importance of night-time snack. Various standard polymeric calorically dense liquid nutritional supplements were discussed and encouraged. He was started on a daily multivitamin, calcium with vitamin D (500 mg BID) and zinc sulphate supplementation 220 mg. He was instructed to keep a food diary and return the following week. The patient and family present agreed to make best efforts with intake.

Continued

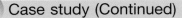

Case study (Continued)

4. Is the patient a candidate for nutrition support?

   The patient is a candidate for nasojejunal tube placement for tube feeding to supplement oral intake. Patients with liver disease have coagulopathy; therefore it is important to note platelet count and INR prior to tube placement. In patients with platelet counts less than 50,000, a platelet infusion is given prior to placement of the enteric tube. A gastrostomy or jejunostomy tube is not indicated in this patient as his ascites places him at higher risk of infection and poor stoma healing.

5. If so, what method should be used to meet this patient's nutritional needs?

Since this patient is not hospitalised, a cycling tube feeding method was initiated to run over 14 hours at night. Since the tip of his tube is placed in the jejunum, a pump would be needed to infuse the tube feedings. The cyclic method would allow him to be more mobile during the day. His supplemental calorie needs were based on his oral intake. A high calorie formula (1.5 cal/mL; however, 2 cal/mL formulas have been tolerated well) was chosen to limit volume. He was given as schedule to begin at a low rate (30 mL/hr) and advance daily to his goal rate (85 mL/hr). For hospitalised patients a 24-hour infusion would be acceptable.

References

1. El-Serag HB, Everhart JE. Diabetes increases the risk of acute hepatic failure. *Gastroenterology*. 2002;122: 1822–1828.

2. Rutherford A, Davern T, Hay JE, et al. Influence of high body mass index on outcome in acute liver failure. *Clin Gastroenterol Hepatol*. 2006;4:1544–1549.

3. McCullough JA, Bugeanesi E. Protein calorie malnutrition and the etiology of cirrhosis. *Am J Gastroenterol*. 1997;92:734–738.

4. Prijatmoko D, Strauss BJ, Lambert JR. Early detection of protein depletion in alcoholic cirrhosis: role of body composition analysis. *Gastroenterology*. 1993; 105:1839–1845.

5. Fegueiredo F, Perez R, Kondo M. Effect of liver cirrhosis on body composition: Evidence of significant depletion even in mild disease. *J Gastroenterol Hepatol*. 2005;20: 209–216.

6. DiCecco SR, Wieners EJ, Wiesner RH. Assessment of nutritional status of patients with end-stage liver disease undergoing liver transplantation. *Mayo Clin Proc*. 1989;64:95–102.

7. Mendenhall CL, Moritz TE, Rosell GA. Protein energy malnutrition in sever alcoholic hepatitis: diagnosis and response to

treatment. The VA Cooperative Study Group 275. *J Parenter Enteral Nutr*. 1995;19:258–265.

8. Selberg O, Bottcher J, Tusch G. Identification of high-and low-risk patients before liver transplantation: a prospective cohort study of nutritional and metabolic parameters in 150 patients. *Hepatology*. 1997; 25:652–657.

9. Tajka M, Kato M, Mohri H, et al. Prognostic value of energy metabolism in patients with viral liver cirrhosis. *Nutrition*. 2002; 18(3):229–234.

10. Campillo B, Richardet JP, Scherman E, Bories PN. Evaluation of nutritional practice in hospitalized cirrhotic patients: results of a prospective study. *Nutrition*. 2003;19(6):515–521.

11. Prasad AS. The role of zinc in gastrointestinal and liver disease. *Clin Gastroenterol*. 1983;12(3): 713–741.

12. Miki C, Iriyama K, Mayer AD. Energy storage and cytokine response in patients undergoing liver transplantation. *Cytokine*. 1999;11: 244–248.

13. Testa R, Franceschini R, Gianni E. Serum Leptin levels in patients with viral chronic hepatitis or liver cirrhosis. *J Hepatol*. 2000;33:33–37.

14. McCullough AJ, Bugeanesi E, Marchesini G, Kalhan SC. Gender-dependent alterations in serum letpin in alcoholic cirrhosis. *Gastroenterology*. 1998;115(4): 947–953.

15. Yamanaka H, Genjida K, Yokota K, et al. Daily pattern of energy metabolism in cirrhosis. *Nutrition*. 1999;15(10):749–754.

16. Müller MJ, Lautz HU, Plogmann B. Energy expenditure and substrate oxidation in patients with cirrhosis: the impact of cause, clinical staging and nutritional state. *Hepatology*. 1992;15:782–794.

17. Müller MJ, Bottcher J, Selberg O. Hypermetabolism in clinically stable patients with liver cirrhosis. *Am J Clin Nutr*. 1999;69:1194–1201.

18. Mathur S, Peng S, Gane EJ, et al. Hypermetabolism predicts reduced transplant-free survival independent of MELD and Child-Pugh scores in liver cirrhosis. *Nutrition*. 2007;23: 398–403.

19. Müller MJ, Pirlich M, Balks HJ, et al. A Glucose intolerance in liver cirrhosis: role of hepatic and non-hepatic influences. *Eur J Clin Chem Clin Biochem*. 1994;32:749–758.

20. Marchesini G, Ronchi M, Forlani G, et al. Cardiovascular disease in cirrhosis: a point-prevalence study in

relation to glucose tolerance. *Am J Gastroenterol*. 1999;94:655–662.

21. McCullough AJ, Tavill AS. Disordered energy and protein metabolism in liver disease. *Semin Liver Dis*. 1991;11:265–277.

22. Riggio O, Angeloni S, Ciuffa L, et al. Malnutrition is not related to alterations in energy balance in patients with stable liver cirrhosis. *Clin Nutr*. 2003;22(6):553–559.

23. Cabre E, Abad-Lacruz A, Nunez MC. The relationship of plasma polyunsaturated fatty acid deficiency with survival in advanced liver cirrhosis. Multivariate analysis. *Am J Gastroenterol*. 1993;88:718–722.

24. Pantaleo P, Marra F, Vizzutti F, et al. Effects of dietary supplementation with arachidonic acid on platelet and renal function in patients with cirrhosis. *Clin Sci (Lond)*. 2004;106(1):27–34.

25. Peng S, Plank L, McCall JL, et al. Body composition, muscle function, and energy expenditure in patients with liver cirrhosis: a comprehensive study. *Am J Clin Nutr*. 2007;85:1257–1266.

26. Kondrup J, Neilsen K, Juul A. Effect of long-term refeeding on protein metabolism in patients with cirrhosis of the liver. *Br J Nutr*. 1997;77:197–212.

27. Nielsen K, Kondrup J, Martinsen L, et al. Long-term oral refeeding of patients with cirrhosis of the liver. *Br J Nutr*. 1995;74:557–567.

28. Younossi ZM, Diehl AM, Ong JP. Nonalcoholic fatty liver disease: an agenda for research. *Hepatology*. 2002;35(4):746–753.

29. Hsiao TJ, Chen JC, Want JD. Insulin resistance and ferritin as major determinants in nonalcoholic fatty liver disease in apparently healthy obese patients. *Int J Obes Relat Metab Disord*. 2004;28:167.

30. Targher G, Arcaro G. Non-alcoholic fatty liver disease and increased risk of cardiovascular disease. *Atherosclerosis*. 2007;191:235–240.

31. Marchesini G, Bugianesi E, Forlani G, et al. Non-alcoholic fatty liver, steatohepatitis, and the metabolic syndrome. *Hepatology*. 2003;37:917.

32. Burak K, Angulo P, Pasha TM, et al. Incidence and risk factors for cholangiocarcinoma in primary sclerosing cholangitis. *Am J Gastroenterol*. 2004;99:523.

33. Tung BY, Kowdley KV. Sclerosing cholangitis and recurrent pyogenic cholangitis. In: Feldman , ed. *Sleisenger and Fordtrans Gastrointestinal and Liver Disease*. 8th ed. Philadelphia: Saunders; 2006.

34. Angulo P, Lindor KD. Primary biliary cirrhosis. In: Feldman, ed. *Sleisenger and Fordtrans Gastrointestinal and Liver Disease*. 8th ed. Philadelphia: Saunders; 2006:1985.

35. Menon K, Angulo P, Weston S, et al. Bone disease in primary biliary cirrhosis: independent indicators and rate of progression. *J Hepatol*. 2001;35(3):316–323.

36. Levy C, Lindor KD. Management of osteoporosis, fat-soluble vitamin deficiencies and hyperlipidemia in primary biliary cirrhosis. *Clin Liver Dis*. 2003;7(4):901–910.

37. Gines A, Escorsell A, Gines P, et al. Incidence predictive factors and prognosis of the hepatorenal syndrome. *Gastroenterology*. 1993;105:229–236.

38. Naveau S, Belda E, Borotta E. Comparison of clinical judgment and anthropometric parameters for evaluating nutritional status in patients with alcoholic liver disease. *J Hepatol*. 1995;23:234–235.

39. Pirlich M, Selberg O, Boker K. The creatinine approach to estimate skeletal muscle mass in patients with cirrhosis. *Hepatology*. 1996;24:1422–1427.

40. Wang Z, Zhu S, Want J, Pierson RN, Heymsfield SB. Whole-body skeletal muscle mass: development and validation of total-body potassium prediction models. *Am J Clin Nutr*. 2003;77(1):76–82.

41. Perlich M, Schutz T, Spachos T. Bioelectrical impedance and analysis is a useful bedside technique to assess malnutrition in cirrhotic patients with and without ascites. *Hepatology*. 2000;32:1208–1215.

42. Fiore P, Merli M, Andreoli A. A comparison of skin fold anthropometry and dual-energy x-ray absorptiometry for the evaluation of body fat in cirrhotic patients. *Clin Nutr*. 1999;18:349–351.

43. Madden A, Moran MY. Resting energy expenditure should be measured in patients with cirrhosis, not predicted. *Hepatology*. 1999;30:655–664.

44. Plauth M, Merli M, Kondrup J, et al. ESPEN guidelines for nutrition in liver disease and transplantation. *Clin Nutr*. 1997;16:43–55.

45. Scolapio JS, DeArment J, Hurley DL, Romano M, Harnois D, Weigand SD. Influence of tacrolimus and short-duration prednisone on bone mineral density following liver transplantation. *J Parenter Enteral Nutr*. 2003;27(6):427–432.

46. Owen OE, Trapp VE, Reichard GA, et al. Nature and quantity of fuels consumed in patients with alcoholic cirrhosis. *J Clin Invest*. 1983;72:1821–1832.

47. Swart GR, Zillikens MC, van Vuure JK, et al. Effect of a late evening meal on nitrogen balance in patients with cirrhosis of the liver. *Br Med J*. 1989;299:1202–1203.

48. Nakaya Y, Kiwamu O, Kazuyuki S, et al. BCAA-enriched snack improves nutritional state of cirrhosis. *Nutrition*. 2007;23:113–120.

49. Als-Nielsen B, Koretz RL, Kjaergard LL, Gluud C. Branched-chain amino acids for hepatic encephalopathy. *Cochrane Database Syst Rev*. 2003;(2):CD001939.

50. Marchesini G, Bianchi G, Merli M, et al. Italian BCAA Study Group. Nutritional supplementation with branch-chain amino acids in advanced cirrhosis: a double blind, randomized trial. *Gastroenterology*. 2003;124(7):1792–1801.

51. Plauth M, Cabre E, Riggio O, et al. ESPEN guidelines on enteral nutrition: liver disease. *Clin Nutr*. 2006;25:285–294.

52. Lirussi F, Mastropasqua E, Orando S, et al. Probiotics for non-alcoholic fatty liver disease and/or steatohepatitis. *Cochrane Database Syst Rev*. 2007;(1):CD005165.

53. Angelico F, Burattin M, Alessandri C, et al. Drugs improving insulin resistance for non-alcoholic fatty liver disease and/or non-alcoholic steathepatitis. *Cochrane Database Syst Rev*. 2007;(1):CD005166.

54. Lirussi F, Azzalini L, Orando S, et al. Antioxidant supplements for non-alcoholic fatty liver disease and/or steatohepatitis. *Cochrane Database Syst Rev*. 2007;(1):CD004996.

55. Sanyal AJ. American Gastroenterology Association. AGA technical review on nonalcoholic fatty liver disease. *Gastroenterology*. 2002;123:1705–1725.

56. Day CP. Non-alcoholic fatty liver disease: current concepts and management strategies. *Clin Med*. 2006;6:19–25.

57. Hasse JM. Adult Liver transplantation. In: Hasse JM, Blue LS, eds. *Comprehensive Guide to Transplant Nutrition*. American Dietetic Association; 2002:58–85.

58. Wang RT, Koretz RL, Yee HF. Weight reduction for non-alcoholic fatty liver (protocol). *Cochrane Database Syst Rev*. 2005;(4).

59. Hickman IJ, Jonsson JR, Prins JB, et al. Modest weight loss and physical activity in overweight patients with liver disease results in sustained improvements in alanine aminotransferase, fasting insulin, and quality of life. *Gut*. 2004;53:413–419.

60. Testa R, Franceshini R, Giannini E, et al. Serum leptin levels in patients with viral chronic hepatitis or liver cirrhosis. *J Hepatol*. 2000;33:33–37.

61. Tsochatzis E, Paptheodoridis GV, Archimandritis AJ. The evolving role of leptin and adiponectin in chronic liver disease. *Am J Gastroenterol*. 2006;101:2629–2640.

62. Jonson JR, Moschen RA, Hickman IJ, et al. Adiponectin and its receptors in patients with chronic hepatitis C. *J Hepatol*. 2005;43:929–936.

HIV

14

Clare Stradling

LEARNING OBJECTIVES

By the end of this chapter the reader will be able to:

- Appreciate the context, global impact and nutritional consequences of HIV infection;
- Evaluate the aetiology of the clinical manifestations of HIV infection including lipodystophy and dyslipidaemia;
- Be aware of the side effects associated with the use of antiretroviral therapies, in particular increased cardiovascular risk;
- Critically discuss the evaluation of cardiovascular risk and nutritional status in HIV-infected patients;
- Critically discuss the dietary and nonpharmacological interventions used to manage consequences of HIV infection.

Introduction

This chapter will aim to give a general overview of most aspects of HIV disease, focusing in detail on the metabolic complications. The needs of specific groups such as intravenous drug users, children and the management of coinfections are beyond the scope of this chapter and will not be covered.

A glossary and list of abbreviations is included at the end of the chapter.

Historical context

Acquired Immune Deficiency Syndrome (AIDS) was first recognised in 1981, as a strange new disease, where previously healthy homosexual men became ill with severe weight loss and developed unusual infections such as *Pneumocystis carinii* pneumonia (PCP) and Kaposi's sarcoma (KS) (see Tom Hanks in the film *Philadelphia*). In 1983 the causative agent, human immunodeficiency virus (HIV), a novel retrovirus, was identified and is thought to have resulted from a 'species jump' of nonpathogenic simian immunodeficiency virus (SIV) passed from monkeys to humans during bush meat hunting expeditions.

The early epidemic in North America and Western Europe may have been driven by sex between men, and individuals sharing drug-injecting equipment; but HIV continues its relentless global spread through heterosexual transmission. Twenty-five years on and with the advent of highly active antiretroviral therapy (HAART), HIV infection has changed from a universally fatal condition to a manageable chronic illness. Yet unfortunately this is still not the reality for the majority of the 40 million people infected with HIV worldwide living in resource-poor countries where a diagnosis of HIV is seen as a death sentence.

In the UK, 78,938 individuals have been reported with HIV infection, of whom 47,517 accessed care in the UK during 2005. The estimated figures are much higher with one in every three UK HIV infections remaining undiagnosed (see Figure 14.1).

HIV transmission

HIV is present in body fluids and is transmitted via contact with infected blood, semen or cervical secretions during unprotected sexual intercourse,

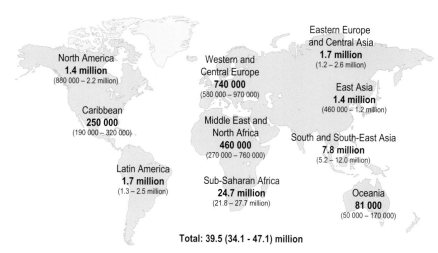

North America
1.4 million
(880 000 – 2.2 million)

Caribbean
250 000
(190 000 – 320 000)

Latin America
1.7 million
(1.3 – 2.5 million)

Western and
Central Europe
740 000
(580 000 – 970 000)

Middle East and
North Africa
460 000
(270 000 – 760 000)

Sub-Saharan Africa
24.7 million
(21.8 – 27.7 million)

Eastern Europe
and Central Asia
1.7 million
(1.2 – 2.6 million)

East Asia
1.4 million
(460 000 – 1.2 million)

South and South-East Asia
7.8 million
(5.2 – 12.0 million)

Oceania
81 000
(50 000 – 170 000)

Total: 39.5 (34.1 - 47.1) million

Figure 14.1 • Adults and children estimated to be living with HIV in 2006. Reproduced with kind permission from UNAIDS (2006).

sharing contaminated drug injecting equipment, transfusions of infected blood and mother to baby. Occupational infection from contaminated needles to healthcare workers remains exceptionally rare.

Pathogenesis of HIV infection

As a virus, HIV can only replicate by becoming part of the host cells. It does this by entering T lymphocytes, monocytes and macrophages using a primary receptor (CD4 glycoprotein) on the surface of the cells (Figure 14.2). Once inside, the HIV viral core copies its RNA into DNA using reverse transcriptase and integrates with the DNA of the host cell, hijacking the cell processes to produce many more viruses. Viral replication with reverse transcriptase is error prone and characterised by a high spontaneous mutation rate. The initial phase of very rapid virus proliferation, with 10^9 new virus particles produced per day, activates the CD4 T lymphocytes to mount an immune response from B lymphocytes, producing antibodies, phagocytes and cytotoxic T lymphocytes, all with the aim of destroying the infected CD4 cells, which clears much of the virus in the acute phase (see Figure 14.3). After some time CD4 lymphocyte production fails to keep up with their relentless destruction which leads to reduced numbers and a dysregulation of the immune system, reducing the body's ability to mount an effective immune response to the infection. Consequently the infected individual is vulnerable to a host of normally benign opportunistic infections.

Natural history of HIV progression

Immediately after HIV infection the virus replicates rapidly, causing a high viraemia and marked decrease in CD4 count (acute phase—Figure 14.3). This may be accompanied by transient flu-like symptoms of fever, rash and lymphadenopathy.

Following the acute phase:

- The CD4 cells recover, but not to previous levels, and reach equilibrium between viral replication and the host immune response approximately a year after infection (clinical latency in Figure 14.3).
- Once equilibrium is achieved CD4 cell counts and plasma HIV RNA levels (viral load) are used to monitor the progression of HIV disease.

As key prognostic indicators among untreated individuals infected with HIV, they have been likened to a steam train careering towards a fallen bridge, with the viral load (quantity of virus present in blood) representing the speed of the train and the CD4 count (measure of immune function) representing the length of remaining track. Viral load (VL) often remains fairly

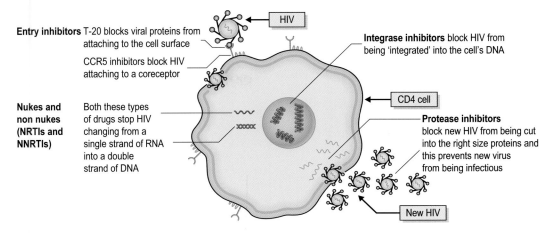

Entry inhibitors T-20 blocks viral proteins from attaching to the cell surface

CCR5 inhibitors block HIV attaching to a coreceptor

Integrase inhibitors block HIV from being 'integrated' into the cell's DNA

Nukes and non nukes (NRTIs and NNRTIs) Both these types of drugs stop HIV changing from a single strand of RNA into a double strand of DNA

CD4 cell

Protease inhibitors block new HIV from being cut into the right size proteins and this prevents new virus from being infectious

New HIV

Figure 14.2 • HIV lifecycle—how drugs work in different ways. Reproduced from Introduction to Combination Therapy, May 2009, with permission of i-Base, http://www.i-Base.info

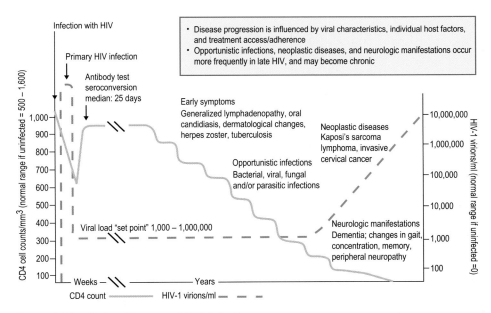

Figure 14.3 • Natural history of HIV infection.

constant during this period of clinical latency, which varies widely among individuals and is characterised by a gradual decline in CD4 cell numbers, at approximately 60–100 cells/mL blood per year.

As the CD4 count drops, the infected person becomes increasingly susceptible to infection, and in the absence of antiretroviral treatment (ARV), immune system degenerates to a point where it becomes unable to mount an effective immune response to opportunistic infections or AIDS defining illnesses present in the everyday environment (AIDS phase—Figure 14.3). Typically at this stage the CD4 count is < 200 cells/mL.

Immune function of the gut

Although this gives an overall picture of what happens to the infected person, it is important to acknowledge the key role that the gut plays in the course of HIV disease progression. During the first few weeks of infection, HIV predominantly infects and destroys CD4 memory cells, found mainly in the gut mucosal lymphoid tissue.[1] This viral replication causes inflammation with T cell and epithelial cell apoptosis in the gut mucosa, resulting in significant damage to the integrity of the mucosal barrier. Translocation of Gram-negative bacteria, as a result of this increased gut permeability, may induce the immune activation that is a hallmark of pathogenic immunodeficiency virus infection. This association has yet to be proven as cause–effect, but it is clear that events in the gut mucosa are central and pivotal to the pathogenesis of HIV.

Nutrition, HIV and the immune system

Early epidemiological studies, in developing countries, established the link between nutrition and immune function, where malnutrition was associated with increased incidence and severity of infections leading to higher mortality rates. Nonetheless, specific nutrient excess via megadosing is not the solution as this can also depress immunity and increase susceptibility to infectious disease. Both deficiency and excess of specific nutrients have been shown to have deleterious effects on the immune system in HIV disease.[2] Interactions between nutrition, infection and immunity are complex and multidirectional, illustrated by the impact of infections, such as tuberculosis, on nutritional status via the immune system. In summary, many cofactors including other viral infections, cytokines and nutrition are likely to play a role in the progression of HIV disease by altering its natural course.

Nutritional therapy in early HIV infection

Historically HIV was characterised by wasting, of both lean body mass and fat, which was associated with shortened survival and diminished quality of life.[3] HAART has now transformed HIV to a chronic condition with greatly improved survival, requiring a shift in emphasis from prevention of weight loss to consideration of conventional diseases such as diabetes and heart disease.

Nutritional therapy in early HIV infection involves nutritional assessment with monitoring of body composition and advice regarding primary cardiovascular disease (CVD) prevention, micronutrient intake and food hygiene.

Nutritional assessment

The methods utilised to monitor body composition have changed over time with the evolution of HIV disease. Historically regular monitoring of body weight was the priority in HIV care, allowing identification of acute or chronic weight loss, shown to be early indicators of underlying systemic or gastrointestinal infection respectively.[4] In conjunction with weight, bioelectrical impedance analysis or more simply, mid-arm muscle circumference was used to monitor loss of lean body mass, seen in wasting associated with AIDS-related illnesses.

With AIDS-related wasting, dual-energy X-ray absorptiometry scanning (DEXA) was adequate to distinguish fat loss from muscle wasting. But now more sophisticated cross-sectional imaging methods, such as magnetic resonance imaging (MRI) and computed tomography (CT) scans, are required to quantify changes in visceral fat (VAT) and subcutaneous fat (SAT) seen in lipodystrophy (LD) and the more subtle fatty infiltration of the liver, heart and muscle. These methods are too expensive for routine clinical use; therefore waist circumference (WC) is the surrogate marker of choice, being more closely associated with VAT and central adiposity than BMI (see Chapter 18 on obesity). Although little agreement has been found between four actual methods of measuring WC, the self-reported WC estimates correlate adequately for monitoring purposes[5] and have been found to mirror MRI results for VAT changes.[6]

Likewise anthropometric measurements of four site skinfold thicknesses (triceps, biceps, subscapular and suprailiac) with the Durnin-Womersley formula has been validated against the criterion method of whole body MRI scanning to monitor lipoatrophy (LA) in this population.[7] Alongside global subjective assessment and patient report, early signs of lipodystrophy can easily be spotted and action taken to prevent worsening.

Other assessments

Assessment of cardiovascular risk, with full lipid profile and calculation of 10-year risk, is required due to increased risk of cardiovascular disease observed in this population (see p. 183). Similarly, evaluation of insulin resistance and changes in body fat distribution are necessary, with fasting glucose levels and waist circumference, respectively, due to their likely occurrence (see p. 181). Screening of the above is recommended at baseline, before commencing ARVs, 3–6 months later, and annually thereafter.[8] Routine screening for bone and renal disease is not currently recommended, but is likely to become an integral part of metabolic management in the future.

Primary CVD prevention

HIV infection is now a recognised risk factor for CVD; therefore dietary advice for people with asymptomatic HIV infection essentially reflects current primary CVD prevention guidance (see Chapter 19):

- At least 30 minutes of moderate intensity activity daily:
- Smoking cessation;
- Alcohol consumption limited to 3 units per day;
- At least five portions of fruit and vegetables daily;
- Dietary fat to provide no more than 30% total energy intake, replacing saturated fats with monounsaturated; and
- Two servings of omega-3 fatty acid-containing fish per week.

Micronutrients

Pre-HAART, general descriptive studies associated low micronutrient serum levels (low vitamin E, B_{12}, Se, vitamin A) and variable intakes (low B, high zinc) with adverse clinical outcomes.[2] Conversely zinc and selenium levels have been associated with improved virologic control in patients taking HAART.[9]

Supplementation trials in resource-poor settings have shown some benefit on HIV-related death rates and reduced disease progression in those taking micronutrient versus placebo.[10,11] Whilst these results are encouraging it is conceded that they cannot be generalised to other HIV populations because the subjects had no access to antiretroviral therapy, and were potentially nutritionally deficient prior to supplementation. Hence a systematic review of 15 randomised controlled trials found no conclusive evidence that micronutrient supplementation effectively reduced or increased morbidity and mortality in HIV-infected adults.[12] Larger trials with sufficient duration of follow-up are required to describe the clinical benefits and adverse effects of micronutrient supplements in the long term, especially in individuals who are not yet symptomatic before we see routine prescription of micronutrients as the standard of care.[2,12]

Food and water hygiene

General guidance on food storage, preparation and cooking practices, promoted by the Food Standards Agency (http://www.food.gov.uk; http://www.eatwell.gov.uk), is recommended for all patients. As the risk of food borne infections varies according to the degree of immunosuppression, patients with CD4 < 200 need to avoid high-risk foods as recommended to all vulnerable groups. The most common causes of bacterial diarrhoea in patients with HIV infection are *Clostridium difficile*, *Shigella* and *Campylobacter jejuni*.

Common sources of infection are:[13]

- Listeria—mould-ripened soft cheese, cook chill/ready-to-eat foods from delicatessen counters;
- Salmonella—raw eggs, contact with pet reptiles;
- *Campylobacter jejuni*—cross contamination between raw and cooked food;
- *Escherichia coli*—unpasteurised dairy products, undercooked meat;
- *Clostridium perfringens*—meat dishes not reheated thoroughly;
- *Bacillus cereus*—rice dishes cooled slowly or kept warm;
- *Toxoplasmosis*—cat litter, undercooked meat;
- *Cryptosporidium*, *Giardia* and *Shigella*—changing nappies, handling pets, gardening and sexual practices (faecal–oral route).

Cryptosporidium parvum is a protozoan parasite that infects the gastrointestinal tract, causing acute enteritis, which is self-limiting when the immune system clears the infection at the mucosal surface. The course of the disease is closely linked to immunocompetence; thus when CD4 < 50 it can be a persistent and life-threatening infection with no effective treatment, highlighting the need to ensure that infection is avoided.[14] For this reason patients with CD4 cell counts < 200 are advised to boil water, from whatever source, before drinking it, as a measure for preventing water-borne cryptosporidiosis.[15] As boiling dechlorinates water, it then requires refrigeration and use within 24 hours.

Whilst bottled water and water from jug filters are unlikely to contain parasites, the lack of enforceable standards means that they may carry an increased bacterial load and should be avoided.[16] High levels of bacterial contamination were found in 40% of the 68 samples of commercially bottled mineral water tested.[16] When neither boiling nor filtering is possible, carbonated water bottled from a deep mineral source will offer some protection via the acidity reducing bacterial load.

Use of submicron filters installed to the mains water supply is the preferred method for provision of safe drinking water in hospitals, whilst provision of cooled boiled water is an alternative for older wards.

Probiotics

Small studies have supported the safety of use of probiotics containing lactobacilli or bifidobacteria in people with HIV infection with no increase in risk of opportunistic infection.[17] However, extreme caution is required in those with advanced disease where the risk of bacterial translocation is greater, evidenced by cases of bacterial sepsis from *Lactobacillus*

acidophilus and cases of fungal sepsis from *Saccharomyces boulardii*.[17]

The rationale for using probiotics for infectious diarrhoea is that they act against enteric pathogens by competing for available nutrients and binding sites, and increasing specific and nonspecific immune responses. Similarly, there may be a role in ARV-related diarrhoea, which was reduced by probiotics in combination with soluble fibre in one small study.[18]

Whilst *Lactobacilli* might appear safe, generalisation cannot be made to other probiotics, as the properties of different species are strain specific and infections have been reported from *Streptococcus*, *Enterococcus* and *Saccharomyces* yeasts.

Untreated HIV

In the absence of HAART, the CD4 declines, allowing infection from opportunistic agents. There is a multitude of AIDS-defining illnesses affecting every system in the body as seen in Table 14.1.

Patients who are unaware of their HIV status still commonly present with these illnesses in which malnutrition is a major complication and a significant prognostic factor in advanced disease.[3] HIV-related wasting is associated with poor outcomes including

Table 14.1 Nutritional consequences of AIDS-defining illnesses

System affected	Clinical manifestation of HIV disease	Issues related to nutrition
Respiratory	*Coccidiodomycosis* *Kaposi's sarcoma* *Pneumocystis carinii pneumonia* *Tuberculosis*	Pyrexia Lethargy Anorexia Rapid weight loss
Reproductive	*Cervical cancer*	Anorexia
Neurological	*Cerebral toxoplasmosis* *Cryptococcal meningitis* *Cytomegalovirus retinitis* *HIV encephalopathy* *Peripheral neuropathy* *Progressive multifocal leukoencephalopathy*	Nausea and vomiting Confusion Loss of vision Pyrexia Cognitive impairment Depression Feeding difficulty
Endocrine	Pancreatitis	Nausea
Gastrointestinal	Oral hairy leukoplakia *Candidiasis* *Herpes oesphagitis*	Sore mouth Altered taste perception Dysphagia

Table 14.1 Nutritional consequences of AIDS-defining illnesses—Cont'd

System affected	Clinical manifestation of HIV disease	Issues related to nutrition
	Salmonellosis	Abdominal pain
	Listeriosis	Diarrhoea
	Mycobacterial disease	Malabsorption
	Cryptosporidiosis	Weight loss
	Isosporiasis	
	Wasting syndrome	
Bone	*Lymphoma*	Weight loss
	Osteoporosis	Reduced mobility
Muscle	Myopathy	Muscle wasting
Renal	HIV associated nephropathy (HIVAN)	Diet restrictions
Circulatory	Anaemia	Fatigue
All of the above	Immune reconstitution inflammatory syndrome (IRIS)	All of the above

Directly or indirectly, HIV can affect every organ or system in the body. AIDS-defining illnesses, as defined by Category C of the Center for Disease Control classification system, are in italics (CDC 1993).

Centers for Disease Control. 1993 Revised classification system for HIV infection and expanded surveillance case definition for AIDS among adolescents and adults. *MMWR* 1992;41:R1-17. Available at: http://www.cdc.gov/mmwr/preview/mmwrhtml/00018871.htm

decreased muscle mass, strength, ability to function in daily living; increased mortality, infections and disease progression. The incidence of wasting has declined significantly with access to HAART, but remains a relevant phenomenon, with 5% involuntary weight loss doubling mortality risk.[19]

It is beyond the scope of this chapter to go into detail about opportunistic infections. Suffice to say that the priority is the diagnosis and treatment of the underlying infection, but nutritional support should be commenced whilst waiting for results of diagnostic tests. The multidisciplinary team will provide a supportive role offering symptomatic control, minimising drug side effects and improving functional impairment. The dietitian's role is to optimise nutritional status by:

- Meeting increased nutritional requirements;
- Optimising nutritional intake; and
- Limiting malabsorption and alleviating gastrointestinal symptoms.

Nutritional therapy is indicated when the BMI is < 18.5 kg/m^2 or when there is significant weight loss ($> 5\%$ in 3 months) or a significant loss of body cell mass ($> 5\%$ in 3 months) has occurred.[20] The application of nutritional support and utilization of skills from all other clinical areas is required in a progressive

manner for the management of patients with opportunistic infections:

- Nutritional counselling;
- Oral nutritional supplements;
- Tube feeding including PEG; and
- Parenteral nutrition.

Standard formula should be used except in cases of diarrhoea, where medium chain triglyceride formulae improve stool frequency and consistency.[20] There are many anecdotal reports of improved tolerance with peptide-based formulae and those containing soluble fibre, but these are not supported by published evidence.[21]

In the changing face of HIV disease, death from 'classical AIDS' occurs predominantly in those who are diagnosed late when already acutely ill. Conversely, those in the UK who know their status and access HIV care die from causes not directly related to HIV; most commonly cancer, liver disease due to hepatitis B or C coinfection and/or alcohol and CVD. Globally, other issues predominate such as the increasing incidence of tuberculosis in Africa due to high prevalence of HIV.

With increasing migration and the global spread of HIV infection, consideration of immigration status, financial security, housing and availability of traditional foods becomes vital in order to provide culturally relevant dietary advice. Engaging with the individual to achieve adherence to nutritional and ARV treatment requires acknowledgement of differences in health beliefs and cultural practices.

Local and regional names of African carbohydrate staples

- Yam or plantain
  - Fufu—West Africa
- Cassava
  - Banku or kenkey—West Africa
  - Gari—Nigeria
  - Manioc—Central Africa
- Green banana
  - Matoke—Uganda
- Flat bread
  - Kisera—Sudan
  - Chambo—Malawi
  - Injera—Ethiopia and Eritrea
- Maize meal
  - Asida—Sudan
  - Ugali—Uganda, Rwanda, Tanzania
  - Uji—Kenya
  - Sadza—Zimbabwe
  - Nsima—Zambia, Botswana, Malawi
  - Mealie pap—South Africa

Treated HIV and ARVs

Although the first ARV (zidovudine) was used as a treatment in 1987, it was not until protease inhibitors (PIs) were developed in 1996 that adequate suppression of viral replication could be achieved using a combination of three different ARVs or highly active antiretroviral therapy. Despite dramatic reductions in morbidity and mortality it was not without its challenges, when long-term side effects emerged (see below) and evidence that near perfect adherence was required in order to maintain viral suppression. As HAART evolves over time the ideal time to start therapy is constantly re-evaluated incorporating outcomes other than survival, such as level of immune reconstitution, risk of cancers and heart disease.

Use of ARVs has implications for dietitians, all of these are crucial to assist in adherence to drug regimens and maintenance of viral suppression:

1. Timings of drugs need to be tailored to suit the patient's daily routine and meal pattern.

Many ARVs have food restrictions to enhance their absorption and maintain adequate drug plasma levels; however, strict adherence to Summary of Product Characteristics (SPC) dosing specifications may not always be clinically indicated (see Table 14.2). This is illustrated by contradictions in licensing by different countries (see tenofovir in Table 14.2). For further advice, assistance should be sought from a specialist pharmacist.

2. Short-term side effects need managing.

General nonspecific side effects, such as nausea, fatigue and rash, are expected in the first 6–8 weeks of starting HAART so patients should be prepared for this and potential solutions that will enable them to persevere with the drugs until the side effects subside should be provided.

Other side effects tend to be drug-specific and require individual management. For example, most of the PIs list diarrhoea as a side effect that can usually be managed with loperamide before considering switching to another ARV. If drug options are limited, adverse effects may require managing using alternative methods such as supplementation with ispaghula fibre, calcium carbonate,[22] or L-glutamine.[18]

3. Long-term side effects, such as metabolic complications, require preventing, monitoring and treating.

The story of lipodystrophy

Early days

Two studies published in 1998 defined a paradigm shift in HIV management. Firstly the success of HAART was reported with a dramatic decline in HIV-related mortality. Secondly, the long-term side effects of HAART began to emerge with case reports of 'Crix belly', 'buffalo hump' (Figure 14.4a) and 'gynecomastia', detailing accumulation of visceral fat in the abdomen, upper back and breast, respectively.[23] Concurrently patients complained of sunken cheeks, and 'stick' limbs with prominent veins due to loss of surrounding subcutaneous fat

Table 14.2 Interactions between antiretrovirals and food

ARV	Effect of food	on C_{max}	on AUC	Dosing specifications	Comments
Protease inhibitors (PI)					
Tipranavir	Improves tolerability of RTV side effects	Unknown—awaiting testing		With food	Requires refrigeration
Darunavir	Similar results with all meals tested*	Overall bioavailability ↑30%		With food	*High fat, standard, protein drink, or croissant and coffee
Indinavir	Light snack comparable to fasting			Without food but with water. 1 h before or 2 h after a meal, or with low fat, light meal	Drink at least 1.5 L/day
	High fat	86% ↓	80% ↓		
Lopinavir (film-coated tablets)	High fat meal (872 kcal, 56% from fat) comparable to fasting	No significant change	No significant change	With or without food	
Lopinavir (soft capsule)	Moderate fat meal (500–682 kcal, 25% fat)	23% ↑	48% ↑	With food to enhance bioavailability and minimise variability	
	High fat meal (872 kcal, 55% fat)	43% ↑	96% ↑		
Saquinavir	Increases absorption. Meal (1000 kcal, 46 g fat)	70% ↑	70% ↑	At the same time as ritonavir and with/after food	Absolute bioavailability is 4% due to poor absorption
Atazanavir	Minimizes variability	Reduces the coefficient of variation by approx 1/2		With food	
Fosamprenavir	No effect			With or without food	
Ritonavir	Increases bioavailability	'Ingestion with food results in higher drug exposure than fasted'		With food	Requires refrigeration. Used (at low dose) to boost drug levels of all PIs above
Nucleotide reverse transcriptase inhibitors					
Tenofovir	Light meal—no effect. High fat meal (1000 kcal, 50% fat)	14% ↑	40% ↑	With food	Bioavailability is 25% when fasted. No recommendation for administration in USA.

Continued

185

Table 14.2 Interactions between antiretrovirals and food—Cont'd

ARV	Effect of food	on C_{max}	on AUC	Dosing specifications	Comments
Etravirine (TMC125)	High fat meal or snack, or standard meal	↑	↑ 50%↓ fasting	With food	Low fat, high fibre meal comparable to fasting
Nevirapine	No effect			With or without food	
Rilpivirine (TMC278)	Normal meal	71% ↑	45% ↑	With food	
Nucleoside reverse transcriptase inhibitors (NRTI)					
Zidovudine				With or without food	With food to prevent nausea
Lamivudine	Delays time to C_{max}	47% ↓	No effect	With or without food	
Emtricitabine	High fat meal		No effect	With or without food	
Abacavir	Delays absorption	↓	No effect	With or without food	
Stavudine	Prolongs time at C_{max} High fat meal	↓	No effect	On an empty stomach. At least 1 h before meals.	No clinical significance—can be taken with food
Didanosine enteric coated	Reduces drug absorption 1 h before food	15% ↓	24% ↓	On an empty stomach, at least 2 h before/after a meal, with at least 100 mL water	
	Light meal (373 kcal)	22% ↓	27% ↓		
	High fat meal (757 kcal)	46% ↓	19% ↓		
Non-nucleoside reverse transcriptase inhibitors (NNRTI)					
Efavirenz	High fat meal	79% ↑	28% ↑	On an empty stomach preferably at bedtime—improve tolerability of nervous system effects	Only necessary to avoid fat if experience side effects
	Normal meal		17% ↑		
Entry inhibitors					
Enfuvirtide	No effect			By subcutaneous injection	
Maraviroc	High fat meal	↓ 33%	↓ 33% Not tested in fasting state	With or without food	Efficacy and safety studies had no food restrictions
Integrase inhibitor					
Raltegravir	Moderate fat meal	5% ↑	13% ↑	With or without food	

Dosing specifications as per electronic Medicines Compendium; September 2007 (http://www.emc.medicines.org.uk)

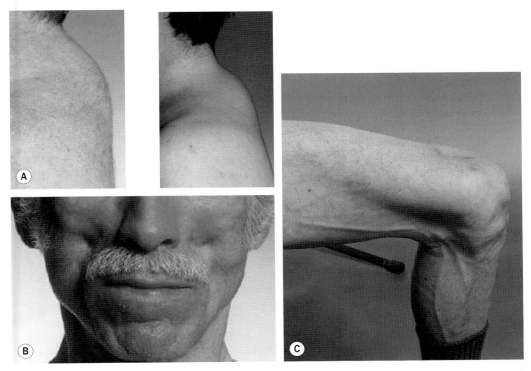

Figure 14.4 • Examples of lipodystrophy. (a) Buffalo hump, (b) facial lipoatrophy, (c) peripheral lipoatrophy. Reproduced from Dolin et al (eds), *Aids Therapy*, 3rd edn. Published by Elsevier Inc, 2008, with permission.

from face, buttocks and limbs (Figure 14.4).[23] This apparent fat redistribution coincided with metabolic changes and was termed lipodystrophy syndrome. Components included in this LD syndrome were the SAT loss of lipoatrophy (LA), the VAT gain of fat accumulation (FA), dyslipidaemia, insulin resistance (IR) and osteopenia. New manifestations continue to be reported such as fat accumulation in the axilla regions and pubic lipoma, resulting in a rather fluid characterisation of LD.

Defining lipodystrophy

Investigating the aetiology of LD proved difficult, with lack of consensus and varying definitions, so a group of experts produced a clinical case definition to provide an objective method for reporting and comparing different studies. It was based on the underlying assumption that all the metabolic abnormalities were part of a single syndrome.[24] This assumption was based on early epidemiological studies suggesting that LA occurred in tandem with FA, due to methodological reliance on self-defined LD to assess predictive values.

Multivariate analysis of large epidemiological studies elucidated multiple risk factors, suggesting complex interactions between host, disease and drug factors:

- Host (age, sex, race, BMI, diet, exercise, hormonal, genetic disposition);
- Disease (duration of infection, severity of immune depletion, magnitude of immune reconstitution); and
- Therapy (specific drugs, duration of therapy, cytokine activation, mitochondrial dysfunction).

Subsequent epidemiological exploration began to suggest that the visceral and subcutaneous fat compartments were distinct, with different pathogenic pathways affected independently by the different factors.[25]

LD as two separate issues—lipoatrophy and fat accumulation

Meanwhile, multicentre, cross-sectional trials set up to determine associations by statistical means examined all the factors of fat change separately and found that the accumulation of visceral fat and depletion of subcutaneous fat were separate entities. The Fat Redistribution and Metabolism (FRAM) study, with a cohort of 1183 HIV-infected subjects and 297 controls, demonstrated that lipoatrophy was associated with HIV infection in both men and women, but VAT was lower in HIV-infected men than in control men and higher in HIV-infected women than in control women.[6] Importantly, there was no statistical association between the amount of subcutaneous fat and visceral fat in either men or women. Similar results were obtained in the Women's Interagency HIV Study.[26] Thus LA is an HIV phenomenon, whereas FA is not. Another previously thought HIV-specific symptom, buffalo humps, were discovered at a higher incidence in uninfected controls (FRAM study) and strongly associated with insulin resistance (i.e. metabolic syndrome) rather than LA.[27]

Is fat accumulation masquerading as metabolic syndrome?

Having ascertained two distinct entities of LD, the defining features of FA were examined and found to be similar to those of the metabolic syndrome (MS). When the earlier definition of LD was validated,[24] it was found to produce results similar to scoring for metabolic syndrome (as defined by the International Diabetes Foundation 2005—see Chapter 17), indicating that the metabolic abnormalities may have been falsely attributed to the development of LD rather than MS.

Is metabolic syndrome related to HIV?

Metabolic syndrome was assumed to be more common in people with HIV infection when increased rates of individual components of MS (diabetes, dyslipidaemia, central obesity, hypertension) began to be reported in the HAART era compared to the previous pre-HAART era. However, when prospective cohorts of infected and uninfected were compared and matched for age, sex, race and smoking status the prevalence rates of MS were found to be similar (around 25%), with no link between MS and either HIV infection or ARV use.[28,29] A possible explanation is that the persistent increases in trunk fat (leading to the associated issues of obesity and metabolic

syndrome) represent a generalised 'return-to-health' phenomenon associated with viral suppression and immune reconstitution. Despite this apparent normal occurrence, the contributing factors of MS were found to be different; driven by low high density lipoprotein (HDL) and high triglycerides (TG) in those with HIV infection (synonymous with the effects of HIV infection and ARVs, respectively[28,29]) rather than increased weight and waist circumference in the general population. This incongruity highlights the potential importance of identifying and addressing MS risk factors, particularly as MS has been associated with subclinical atherosclerosis in HIV.

Causes of lipoatrophy

Returning to LA, epidemiological studies have consistently found strong associations between nucleoside reverse transcriptase inhibitor (NRTI) therapy (in particular the thymidine analogues) and LA; the effect being greater with stavudine, then didanosine, then zidovudine.[30] This has been supported by the switch studies, which demonstrated gradual reversibility of LA (see below). There are many hypotheses for the specific cause of LA: adipocyte loss via apoptosis, enhanced lipolysis, reduced lipid deposition, increasing serum free fatty acids or mitochondrial toxicity. Evidence is strongest for the latter but it is unlikely to completely explain LA development. Mitochondrial toxicity can manifest clinically as neuropathy, myopathy, hepatic steatosis, lactic acidosis, pancreatitis, pancytopenia and renal proximal tubular dysfunction in addition to LA. Toxicity results from the virus itself or adverse effects of thymidine analogues causing mitochondrial DNA depletion, which promotes LA via loss of ATP production and reduced fat deposition.

The role of ARVs in lipodystrophy aetiology

The relative contribution of the different classes of ARVs to the development of these abnormalities is not fully understood. Initial observations implicated the development of LD with protease inhibitor use probably because LD was lumped together as one syndrome and due to blurring from the combination of ARVs in the regimen.[23] Several prospective studies have now clarified that PIs may accelerate the fat wasting effects of thymidine analogues, but the risk of LA is low in PI regimens without thymidine analogues.[30] The newer PIs such as tipranavir, darunavir and fosamprenavir have actually shown increases in SAT with use. Recent trends observed in large prospective cohorts indicate that LD now occurs less frequently and this is likely to continue with the use of the newer ARVs in the future.[31]

Other metabolic complications

Insulin resistance

Another aspect of LD is the higher prevalence of diabetes mellitus and insulin resistance among HIV-infected patients, particularly in those on PI drug regimens. This may be due to a direct effect of the PIs inhibiting GLUT4 and reducing glucose uptake in adipose and muscle; or the proflammatory effect of HIV itself; or indirect effect of LD affecting adipocyte differentiation and intracellular lipid accumulation.[32]

Altered bone metabolism

Osteopenia was common in HIV patients in the pre-HAART era, but has now also been linked with ARV use. A combination of direct viral effects, disease severity and ARVs may contribute to altered bone metabolism. In addition to these HIV-specific mechanisms, some of the traditional risk factors for osteopenia are commonly found in the HIV population (such as smoking, steroid exposure, high alcohol intake, history of low body weight, low sex hormone levels) and will contribute to bone loss.

One such factor is vitamin D deficiency of which there is a high prevalence in the Caucasian HIV population, so when additional factors such as reduced skin production of vitamin D in pigmented skin are considered it means that the African population living in the northern hemisphere are at particular risk.

The role of the dietitian is to help identify those at risk of bone loss, refer for DEXA and provide nutritional advice on vitamin D, calcium and phosphorus.

Lactic acidosis

Metabolic abnormalities include lactic acidosis, a rare but life-threatening condition, usually presenting as hepatic steatosis, abdominal pain, nausea or vomiting, and caused by NRTIs. Key management involves withdrawal of the drugs and fluid resuscitation, but there is also limited evidence that large doses of thiamine, riboflavin, L-carnitine, and coenzyme Q10 improve outcomes.

Current understanding

In summary, our current understanding is that:

- Lipoatrophy is primarily caused by thymidine analogues;
- Metabolic syndrome is due to weight regain;
- Both of the above can lead to insulin resistance; and
- All of the above are risk factors for heart disease.

In general, the broad pattern of lipodystrophy following the introduction of HAART is, firstly, recovery from serious illness and weight regain in the first few months, followed by loss of SAT with the development of LA if the regimen includes thymidine analogues and/or continued gain of visceral fat and development of metabolic syndrome, but this is probably an oversimplification of the complexity and potential connections within the various metabolic issues.

Consequence of lipodystrophy

Unsurprisingly, the body shape changes of LD result in stigmatisation and subsequent reduced adherence to their HAART (with patients wanting to limit the side effects).[33] Consequently the dietitian has a pivotal role in the prevention and management of LD which is a key element of overall HIV disease management. The presence of LD undoubtedly reduces quality of life, including fear of disclosure as well as problems with self-image and self-esteem.[34]

Another consequence of LD has been the impact on prescribing patterns. In an attempt to stem the flow of patients' complaints, physicians have attempted to limit drug exposure by re-examining when to start therapy, structured treatment interruptions and variation in composition of HAART.

Management of lipodystrophy

Our understanding of LD is far from complete but as we now appreciate that changes in subcutaneous and visceral fat compartments are independent of each other, their management shall be discussed separately as LA and FA. The cornerstones for managing the various manifestations of LD are threefold: avoid, switch and treat.

Avoidance of lipoatrophy

Prospective randomised trials have found that ARV regimens containing abacavir or tenofovir result in less SAT loss than regimens containing stavudine, zidovudine and didanosine. This is reflected in the management guidelines recommending avoidance of these specific lipoatrophic agents.[8,35] Other causative agents also need to be considered, such as metformin, anabolic steroids and growth hormone.

Switching to prevent worsening lipoatrophy

For those with LA, switching from stavudine or zidovudine to abacavir in the MITOX study resulted in 0.4 kg mean gain in limb fat after 6 months. Additional analyses showed a median gain of 36% from baseline in limb fat 2 years after switching treatment, although in many cases, patients still did not notice any improvement.[36] Likewise in the RAVE study switching from either stavudine or zidovudine to either tenofovir or abacavir in patients with documented lipoatrophy resulted in a similar mean gain after 48 weeks, but median gains of 1 kg.[37] To put this into context, the baseline limb fat mass in this study was about 3 kg compared to the normal of 8 kg, so reversal was slow.

Resource-poor countries, who use ARVs according to the old WHO guidelines, may have no option but to use stavudine.[38] In this case reducing the dose to 30 mg twice daily has some beneficial effect on peripheral fat, compared with standard dosing of 40 mg twice daily.

Treatment of lipoatrophy

Surgical options for the cosmetic correction of facial and buttock lipoatrophy have been explored. 'Permanent' nonbiodegradable implants carry the risk of inflammation. With the potential recovery of fat, temporary biodegradable injections are favoured, of which polylactic acid injections are licensed for the cosmetic management of facial LA. Benefits are observed for 6–24 months before repeats are required. Autologous

fat transplant has been tried using buffalo hump fat as the donor site, but responses have been variable with reports of lumpiness.

To date the only promising pharmacological options are unusual. The unexpected outcome of significant increases in SAT (0.5 kg, larger than switching for 1 year) was discovered when pravastatin was investigated for hypercholesterolemia.[39] The other, NucleomaxX, is a supplement made from sugar cane that increases levels of uridine. After 3 months of treatment, the patients with LA had gained a significant amount of limb fat (900 g) compared to those on placebo;[40] unfortunately, they also gained VAT and HDL levels fell.

Avoidance of fat accumulation

There is no data demonstrating that an increase in visceral fat can be avoided by specific management choices. With the recent association between FA and MS, strategies to prevent the development of MS, such as diet and exercise, may be more appropriate. HIV cohort studies have observed that low fibre intake predicts insulin resistance and development of fat accumulation.[41,42]

Switching antiretroviral therapy

There is no evidence from controlled clinical trials that modification or discontinuation of PI therapy affects visceral fat content. In contrast, several studies have documented increases in trunk fat when switching from NRTIs, particularly stavudine, to PIs. Effect on TG will be discussed in the section on CVD.

Treatment of fat accumulation

Diet and exercise

Visceral fat gain in HIV patients is part of the Western epidemic of abdominal obesity but is more visually apparent when combined with concurrent lipoatrophy. Management of visceral obesity, insulin resistance and diabetes is the same as in the general population in that both diet and exercise play vital roles.

Most HIV studies have been small and focused on a combination of aerobic and resistance exercise (three times a week over 10–16 weeks). Outcomes observed were significant reductions in trunk fat, but due to use of DEXA the relative contribution of VAT could not be quantified.[43–45] Similarly, WC improved in women undertaking resistance training only,[46] whilst aerobic exercise (cycling twice a week) in 17 patients with mixed lipodystrophy found a significant reduction in visceral fat despite no weight loss.[47]

A handful of small studies in HIV patients have combined diet and exercise. A proof of principle case study led the way, demonstrating dramatic reduction in VAT for a patient with severe LD following a low glycaemic index, high fibre diet with exercise three times per week.[48] Similarly, twelve weeks of aerobic exercise and diet significantly reduced body fat and waist-to-hip ratio in 30 men with LD and WC in obese women, although the relative loss of VAT was small.[49,50]

Fitch and colleagues randomised 34 HIV-infected patients with metabolic syndrome to either lifestyle modification, consisting of National Cholesterol Education Program III (NCEP) diet including weekly consultations with a dietitian and 3 hours per week exercise, or control.[51] After 6 months, mild benefits were seen in exercise outcomes, blood pressure, waist circumference and diet.[51]

Pharmacological treatment

Various agents for treating visceral fat accumulation, such as metformin, rosiglitazone and testosterone have been explored, but whilst limited success has been seen with improvements in visceral fat and insulin resistance, it is to the detriment of subcutaneous fat and raised lipids.[52–54]

The use of recombinant human growth hormone (rhGH) as a treatment for VAT has been studied in the USA, but it is expensive and not licensed in the UK. Therefore we await further development of growth hormone releasing factor, tesamorelin, which has been found to reduce VAT by 15% after 26 weeks without the adverse effects associated with growth hormone—increased insulin resistance and subcutaneous fat loss.[55] If HAART were not causally linked to VAT accumulation then drug treatment for VAT would be purely for age-related adiposity and would be inappropriate.

Surgical options have been tried with resection or aspiration of buffalo humps but reappearance of the fat deposition is reported anecdotally as common.

Increased risk of cardiovascular disease

The epidemiological evidence from several large HIV cohorts suggests that relative rates of CVD are higher than in the general population; even after adjustment for age, sex, race, hypertension, diabetes and dyslipidaemia, the relative risk was 1.75 for HIV infection.[56] There is evidence to suggest that there are three main factors contributing to this increased risk: infection, HAART and traditional CVD risk factors associated with the non-HIV population.

Why? HIV itself

Cytokines may play a role in the altered lipid metabolism occurring in association with HIV disease itself with reduction of total, HDL and LDL cholesterol levels and increase in TG levels.[57] Excess inflammation is known to cause endothelial dysfunction and this has been found to be greater in patients with HIV than uninfected controls, when measured with surrogate markers. This theory of uncontrolled viraemia inducing an inflammatory state, accelerating atherosclerosis was recently highlighted in the SMART study where the group on intermittent ART experienced a greater rate of myocardial infarction (MIs) than the group on continuous ART.[58]

Why? HAART

The elevation of LDL associated with ARVs may represent normalisation back to preinfection levels. The observed pattern is an early increase after ARV initiation, peaking at 2–3 years and remaining high or requiring treatment thereafter.[57] Many studies have suggested that there is an association between exposure to ART (in particular PIs) and the risk of MI. This can only partly be explained by their effect on lipids.[56] The emerging picture, illustrated by the DAD cohort data, is that of the role of specific agents. Initial analysis attributed increased risk primarily to cumulative use of PIs, with relative risk of 1.16,[59] whereas further analysis has implicated recent use of didanosine (RR = 1.4) and abacavir (RR = 1.9).[60] Individual ARVs have different affects on the lipid profile, as shown by Figure 14.5. For example, some PIs (ritonavir, lopinavir, tipranavir, indinavir) are associated with substantial elevations in TG, with minor effects on other lipids, whilst other PIs (ritonavir with atazanavir or lopinavir) are also associated with a decline in HDL levels, another risk factor for CVD.

The dyslipidaemic effects of PI therapy are confirmed by a longitudinal cohort study, examining the calorie and quality of patients' diets before and after switching to PIs. Dietary intake remained

Increasing metabolic impact of drugs →		
NNRTI	NRTI	PI
Nevirapine	Tenofovir Lamivudine Emtricitabine	Unboosted fosamprenavir Unboosted atazanavir
Efavirenz	Zidovudine Abacavir	Atazanavir* Saquinavir*
	Didanosine	Lopinavir* FosAmprenavir* Darunavir*
	Stavudine	Indinavir* Tipranavir* Ritonavir*

(Left axis label: Increasing metabolic impact of drugs ↓)

* Boosted with low dose ritonavir

Limited data from use of fusion inhibitors and CCR5 inhibitors suggest these drugs to have little metabolic impact, but length of experience for some of these is limited.

Figure 14.5 • Metabolic impact of individual antiretroviral drugs. Adapted from EACS v 4, Oct 2008, p. 33, with permission of EACS, http://www.eacs.eu/Guidelines_Livret/index.htm

stable and did not contribute to changes in lipid profile.[61] However, dietary deficiencies should be considered as deficiencies of selenium and carnitine can be reversible causes of cardiomyopathy, and supplementation may improve left ventricular function.[62]

Why? traditional cardiovascular risk factors

Although these findings point to HIV treatment (and PI use in particular) as risk factors for MI, it is crucial to note that the absolute risk remains small, as the incidence of MI among patients exposed to PIs for more than 6 years was only 0.6% per year.[59] Traditional risk factors such as obesity (RR 1.7) and smoking (RR 2.83) were higher, the latter being significant as 61% of the study participants were smokers. Smoking, along with higher TG and lower HDL, were found to be the main contributors to increased CV risk in cross-sectional studies of the HIV population.[63,64] In addition, cross-sectional studies have shown that HIV patients consume higher intakes of saturated fat compared to uninfected control groups, suggesting that quality of diet may be a contributing factor to this dyslipidaemia.[65] Ethnicity is also likely to influence CV risk as black patients,

when compared with white and Hispanics, had lower TG levels overall, but the greatest increase in TG levels when exposed to PIs.[66] Other possible contributing risk factors specific to this population that need to be considered are concomitant infections (*Chlamydia* and CMV), use of cocaine, amphetamines and anabolic steroids.

In summary, although individuals face an increased risk of CVD, what proportion this excess risk is explained by higher prevalence of traditional risk factors for CVD, viral effects or HIV therapy remains unclear. With aging of the HIV-infected population, however, it is essential that prevention of CVD be incorporated into routine HIV clinical management.[64]

Management of cardiovascular risk and dyslipidaemia

Specific guidelines for the management of HIV dyslipidaemia are slowly emerging but tend to mirror those for the general population.[35,56,67] Therefore existing practice is commonly local adaptation of the US treatment guidelines using the relevant national intervention thresholds and target goals (Figure 14.6).[35,68] Thus in the UK, high risk is defined as a score of > 20% for the 10 year risk of developing CVD using the Framingham equation with targets of total cholesterol < 4 mmol/L for secondary prevention[69] although this differs from the European HIV targets seen in Figure 14.6.

CVD risk assessment

An individual's risk of developing CVD can be estimated using an equation (such as Framingham, QRISK or ASSIGN) that has been derived from longitudinal data on incidence of CVD (in USA, England and Scotland, respectively) and association with multiple risk factors. The choice of Web-based tool tends to depend on the geographical location of the cohort although modifications of the Framingham equation are most commonly used in HIV and this is reflected by UK practice.[68] When validated in the HIV population the Framingham equation was found to underpredict the risk for patients on ARVs, whilst overpredicting the risk of MI for patients not on treatment.[70] Thus existing equations may not be appropriate for the HIV population, but must be used until an HIV-specific tool is developed.[59]

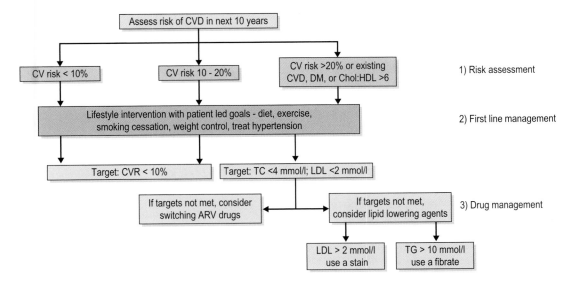

Figure 14.6 • CVD risk management in HIV.

Lifestyle intervention

Diet

A thorough trial of lifestyle intervention is favoured as first-line treatment for HIV dyslipidaemia before the instigation of drug therapies, due to the additional pill burden and complex interactions with ARVs.[8,35] The guidelines recommend consultation with a dietitian to address the competing dietary needs that frequently present with coexisting dyslipidaemia and wasting.[35]

Historically the focus of primary prevention of CVD has been reducing cholesterol levels with low saturated fat diets in both the general population and the HIV population. In the latter, studies have shown reductions of 11% in cholesterol and 21% in TG in Americans after 6 months on the low fat diet and 10% and 23%, respectively, in Spanish.[71,72] More recently the UK guidelines have expanded to include emphasis on the types of fat eaten, fish, fruit and vegetables.[69] Meanwhile other guidelines (US[35] and WHO) have included legumes and wholegrains, which in HIV studies have produced 13% reduction in cholesterol in 16 Australians.[73] However, no significant change in lipid levels was reported in a similar American study despite improvements in other cardiac risk factors: reduction in waist circumference and blood pressure.[51] In UK practice, the Mediterranean diet is commonly used and further studies are required to clarify which modifications are effective.[74]

Several randomised trials evaluating the use of lipid-lowering agents have included a placebo diet only arm, producing insignificant reductions in lipid levels.[75,76] In one study diet was equally as effective as pravastatin, in terms of achieving target lipid levels.[39]

Exploration of the actual dietary intake of HIV-infected patients revealed calorie and fat intake above national recommendations, suggesting room for improvements to minimise effects of HAART on CV risk.[61] This approach, of implementing dietary changes concurrently with HAART initialisation in an attempt to prevent worsening CVD risk, was adopted in a Brazilian randomised controlled trial. The group who commenced HAART with NCEP dietary advice reduced their calorie intake and percentage fat, generating a reduction in TG and maintenance of BMI, WHR, cholesterol and LDL, whilst the control group increased their calorie intake, causing a rise in all the parameters: BMI, WHR, cholesterol, LDL and TG. One year later 50% of the control group had developed dyslipidaemia compared to 17% of the intervention group, suggesting a role in dietary intervention to prevent ARV-related dyslipidaemia.[77] It might therefore be prudent to advise patients to enrich their diets with more vegetables, whole grains, soya, oats, wheat germ, almonds, flaxseed and plant sterols before dyslipidaemia presents rather than in response to an attempt to meet lipid targets before progressing to lipid-lowering drugs.

Smoking

Other lifestyle changes, such as smoking cessation, will improve lipid profile, increasing HDL and reducing TG and LDL. Given the much greater cardiovascular risks associated with smoking (and the high prevalence of smoking among HIV-infected patients), it has been suggested that perhaps more effort should be spent assisting patients with smoking cessation rather than focusing so intently on the dyslipidemic effects of ARV therapy.

Exercise

In the general population, physical activity is acknowledged as important in reducing the risk of CVD by 30–50%. Studies in ARV-related dyslipidaemia suggest that improvements in cholesterol are seen with aerobic exercise but not resistance exercise.[44,45,78] Both types of exercise generate reductions in TG levels and insulin resistance.[44,45,47,71,78,79] This may be due to the greater muscle mass available to remove TGs from the circulation, or as the latter study suggests, increased lipoprotein lipase expression in muscle tissue after exercise, stimulating the release of free fatty acids from plasma lipoproteins, which are used by the muscle to replenish intramuscular TG deposits, thus lowering serum TG levels.[79]

Switch ARVs to reduce lipids

Due to publicity of the copious pharmacological studies competing for the best agent with least toxicity, physicians commonly choose swapping ARVs in response to dyslipidaemia. Whilst switching agents may increase tolerability and improve lipid parameters, such as in the case of efavirenz to nevirapine, it will only improve the ARV-related aspect of the lipid derangement not that caused by traditional risk factors or the virus. Switches from PI to NNRTI do not necessarily reduce lipid levels as effects cannot be generalised across drug classes; the older PIs tend to increase TG levels, whereas newer PIs do not appear to adversely affect lipids.[80]

This practice of switching has been challenged by an Italian trial where use of pravastatin and bezafibrate proved significantly more effective in reducing LDL than switching from PI to nevirapine or efavirenz, which in contrast was more beneficial for HDL levels. Interestingly, the mean TG decline was significantly greater for nevirapine than for efavirenz.[80] On balance, consideration must also be given to additional pill burden, drug–drug interactions, cost and side effects; ultimately effective suppression of the virus must remain the primary treatment goal.

Elevated TG is the main problem for ARV-treated patients and is identified as an independent CV risk factor in the DAD study. However, there is limited evidence that correcting hypertriglyceridemia will reduce coronary events. As the level of TG is associated with glucose metabolism, targeting alcohol and sugar intake should be considered before treating with fibrates or omega-3 fatty acids.

Lipid-lowering agents

Statins are recommended for elevated LDL levels, the choice of which is determined by drug interactions. Pravastatin is the only statin not metabolised by cytochrome p450 and does not interact with ARVs. Despite limited effects on cholesterol, pravastatin showed some agreeable side effects with significant increases in subcutaneous fat.[39] Atorvastatin and rosuvastatin have been shown to be safe and effective in ARV-related hyperlipidaemia (although caution is required with dosing as interactions with PIs cause increased statin concentrations). Simvastatin is contraindicated due to drug interactions.

Since guidelines publication, other agents have been examined for safety and efficacy in HIV dyslipidaemia. Ezetimibe was shown to decrease LDL as effectively as fluvastatin, and improve lipids when added to pravastatin, or when added to patients not achieving lipid targets on maximally tolerated doses of lipid-lowering therapy with a statin and/or fibrate.[81–83] As ezetimibe blocks the intestinal absorption of dietary cholesterol and bile acid absorption, there has been concern that it would impair absorption of ARVs; however, lopinavir and nevirapine levels were found to be unchanged.[82] However, evidence that the changes in lipids achieved with ezetimibe reduce cardiovascular events, and long term safety data, are not available with this medication.

Conversely there is end-point evidence for bile acid sequestrants, which reduce LDL whilst causing increases in HDL and TG. Due to the theoretical risk of pancreatitis, they should not be used in patients with hypertriglyceridemia. Another reason for limited use is gastrointestinal side effects and requirement to take them 2 hours before or after other medications.

Likewise niacin has since been shown to improve lipids, in particular TG and HDL, safely and effectively in HIV patients without glucose intolerance.[84] Similarly, supplementation with fish oil (3 g/day) lowered ARV-elevated TG levels by 19 and 25%, respectively, but only 39 and 22% of patients achieved target levels.[85;86] In another study fish oil only achieved significant reductions in TG (65%) when used in conjunction with fenofibrate, but again only 23% normalised their TG levels.[80]

Patients with HIV-related dyslipidaemia appear to be more refractory to lipid-lowering therapy and are less likely to reach their target levels.[76,80] Whilst explanations can be offered, such as greater use of pravastatin rather than simvastatin or lack of compliance with advice, this failure to achieve targets also demonstrates the need for integrated specialist services that effectively reduce cardiovascular risk.[64,72]

Pregnancy

With over 90% of pregnant women in the UK accepting HIV testing as part of their antenatal screening, many will be referred to dietetic services following their diagnosis. Nutritional management of HIV-infected women during pregnancy follows routine care with advice regarding food safety, nausea, vomiting, glucose impairment, meeting increased requirements for calcium and iron and periconceptual folic acid supplements (of particular importance for those on PCP prophylaxis with cotrimoxazole, a folate antagonist). Additional considerations include side effect management of HAART given during the second and third trimesters to reduce mother-to-child HIV transmission from 25 to <1%.[87] Vitamin supplementation in developing countries may improve outcomes such as birth weight with vitamin A, but have failed to reduce mother-to-child transmission and may even result in harm.[11,88]

The management of paediatric HIV is beyond the scope of this chapter, but pregnant women will require counselling on their choice of infant feeding. As breastfeeding incurs an additional 14% risk of HIV transmission, avoidance is advised to HIV-infected mothers where replacement feeding is acceptable, feasible, affordable, sustainable and safe.[87,89] If these conditions cannot be met, as in many developing countries, exclusive breastfeeding up to the age of 6 months, followed by rapid cessation reduces risk of transmission threefold.[90] Whilst a 4% risk of postnatal HIV transmission remains, exclusive breastfeeding improves child survival by reducing mortality due to diarrhoeal disease.[90] Postnatal transmission can be reduced to 1% by combining exclusive breastfeeding with HAART for the mother, although adoption of this practice is slow in developing countries.

Key points

- HIV ranks fourth in cause of death worldwide, and the most common route of transmission is sex between men and women.
- HAART has substantially prolonged life expectancy for those infected with HIV living in countries with access to treatment.
- Untreated HIV infection eventually leads to wasting, malnutrition, and a succession of opportunistic infections.
- HAART is associated with a range of metabolic abnormalities that accelerate atherosclerosis and cause CVD.
- Dietitians need to monitor patients' body composition and provide advice on micronutrients, food safety, nutritional support, CVD prevention, timing of ARVs and management of adverse effects as required.
- Thymidine analogues result in lipoatrophy (loss of SAT), which is slowly reversible when the drug is withdrawn.
- Metabolic syndrome and VAT accumulation are associated with low HDL and high TG.
- LA and FA are associated with the development of insulin resistance.
- Treatment of LA and FA is limited, emphasising the importance of preventative strategies including avoidance of causative agents and lifestyle intervention.
- Some PIs are associated with dyslipidaemia, increased incidence of MIs, endothelial dysfunction and coronary artery calcification.
- Incidence of MI is higher in the HIV population due to PI use, effects of the virus and higher rate of traditional risk factors such as smoking.
- Treatment of ARV-related dyslipidaemia revolves around diet, exercise, switching ARVs and adding lipid lowering agents, but treatment targets are less likely to be achieved.

Developing issues

Given the current belief that a significant proportion of the changes in body fat distribution are a result of antiretroviral toxicity, we ought to see a considerable reduction in the frequency of these problems in several years as patients are treated with newer, and potentially less toxic, agents. However, complacency is not an option as it took many years to recognise lipoatrophy as a drug-induced toxicity and it is quite possible that other long-term problems will emerge to challenge our use of the current 'safe' regimens. In the meantime studies will continue to investigate:

- ARV switching to limit CVD;
- New markers for atherosclerosis (e.g. echocardiography to measure visceral fat around the heart);

- Micronutrient supplementation (e.g. to prevent PI inhibition of removal of excess cholesterol from the arterial wall);
- Whether diagnosis of MS is a better measure of CV risk; and
- New CV equations specific for HIV population.

Renal disease is set to become an important complication of HIV infection not simply due to long-term exposure to nephrotoxic drugs or the direct effect of the virus causing nephropathy, but the increasing prevalence of risk factors for chronic kidney failure (older age, diabetes, hypertension) in HIV patients.

Case study

In 1999, a 55-year-old man presented to A&E with confusion, headaches, nausea, vomiting and incontinence. On the ward a CT scan and lumbar puncture confirmed the diagnosis of cryptococcal meningitis. He was referred to the health advisers for an HIV test after reporting history of 2-stone weight loss, pain on swallowing and having previously lived in South Africa.

QUESTIONS

1. What are the nutritional issues for this inpatient?

   HIV infection was diagnosed with low CD4 and high VL requiring ARV treatment. Stavudine, lamivudine and nevirapine successfully reduced VL to undetectable and CD4 climbed.

   At 3-month follow-up in clinic, he had fully recovered from meningitis, regained the weight and then presented with rising lipids.

   With cholesterol 8.8 mmol/L, triglyceride 4.7 mmol/L, and as a smoker, his 10-year CVD risk was 34%.

2. What action could you take?

   Following your advice, over the next 6 months, he has lost 10 kg (BMI now 23) with reduction in cholesterol to 6 mmol/L and TG 2 mmol/L. He is happy with this but describes pain in the soles of his feet on walking.

3. Is any further action required?

   Stavudine is changed to abacavir and viral suppression maintained. Over the next year his weight, waist circumference and lipid levels escalate. Pravastatin is commenced. Glucose tolerance test is normal; fasting insulin levels are raised.

4. What are the new issues?

ANSWERS

1. What are the nutritional issues for this inpatient?
   - Weight loss and nutritionally compromised;
   - Feeding difficulties due to confusion—may need assistance;

   - Swallowing difficulties—likely to be due to oesophageal candida—needs treatment with fluconazole and soft foods; and
   - Requiring nutritional support—either supplements or tube feeding.

2. What action could you take?

   Lifestyle intervention:
   - Refer to smoking cessation clinic;
   - Increase physical activity levels;
   - Assess alcohol and sugar intake in order to advise reduction;
   - Modify fat intake from saturates to monounsaturates; and
   - Cardioprotective diet—omega-3 fats, fruit and vegetables, soya, plant stanols, soluble fibre.

3. Is any further action required?

   He has not met CVD treatment target levels; therefore he needs referring to a specialist metabolic or lipid clinic or back to HIV physicians for statin treatment and/or switching. You also need to question from where the weight loss has originated—is it subcutaneous fat, visceral fat, muscle from any specific region? With the stavudine there is a risk of lipoatrophy, so checking that there is not a disproportionate subcutaneous fat loss from limbs is advisable, with referral to the HIV physicians for switching stavudine to an alternative agent such as tenofovir or abacavir.

   Pain on walking could be caused by loss of fat pads on the soles of the feet and peripheral neuropathy, a common adverse effect from stavudine. Refer to an occupational therapist for specialist insoles.

4. What are the new issues?

   These results indicate:
   - Insulin resistance—treat with metformin; and
   - Increased visceral fat—treat with low glycaemic index foods and refer to physiotherapist for appropriate exercises.

   For further cases see Clinical Care Options website: http://www.clinicaloptions.com/HIV.aspx

Case study (Continued)

SPECIAL CONSIDERATIONS FOR THE NEEDS OF THE AGEING POPULATION

Thanks to potent anti-HIV therapy, more and more people with HIV can look forward to surviving into old age. Consideration of the needs of an ageing population is essential but also slightly a misnomer, as the population under consideration will not necessary be advanced in years, only advanced in length of time since infection with HIV, as it appears that HIV accelerates the ageing process.

As the classic AIDS-related conditions become less common with successful anti-HIV therapy, attention is now being turned to the major complications of treated HIV disease—CVD, cancer, renal, liver and bone disease, cognitive decline and dementia. Many of these are commonly associated with ageing and occur at an earlier age in the HIV-infected population.

HIV can cause cell changes in the brain that increase the risk of dementia and it also affects the brain in similar ways to Alzheimer's disease, increasing an HIV-positive individual's risk of developing this illness. The higher rate of cancer is probably caused by long-term immunosuppression. Liver disease is common due to high rates of chronic viral hepatits, alcohol misuse and long-term exposure to potentially hepatoxic drugs. The mechanism for this increased risk of age-associated disease is probably multifactorial, comprising residual immunodeficiency and inflammation, ARV toxicity and presence of other chronic comorbid conditions.[91]

HIV patients are likely to require screening and aggressive preventive care as they grow older and will need greater involvement from other specialist services.

Abbreviations and glossary

AIDS Acquired immune deficiency syndrome

ARV Antiretroviral therapy—treatment of HIV with three or more drugs that suppress viral replication, also known as HAART, highly active antiretroviral therapy.

CD4 count The number of CD4 T lymphocyte cells per cubic millimetre of blood, validated as a measure of immune function in HIV disease. A value of < 200 is indicative of immunosuppression with increased risk of opportunistic infections.

CMV Cytomegalovirus

CT Computed tomography

CVD Cardiovascular disease

DEXA Dual-energy X-ray absorptiometry scanning

FA Fat accumulation

HDL High-density lipoprotein

HIV Human immunodeficiency virus

IR Insulin resistance

Immune reconstitution When the immune system begins to recover, but then responds to a previously acquired opportunistic infection with an overwhelming inflammatory response that paradoxically makes the symptoms of infection worse.

KS Kaposi's sarcoma

LA Lipoatrophy

LD Lipodystrophy

LDL Low-density lipoprotein

MI Myocardial infarction

MRI Magnetic resonance imaging

MS Metabolic syndrome

NNRTI Non nucleoside reverse transcriptase inhibitors

NRTI Nucleoside reverse transcriptase inhibitors

PCP *Pneumocystis carinii* pneumonia

PI Protease inhibitors—antiretroviral drugs that fit exactly into the active enzyme site of the HIV protease to inhibit the enzyme and prevent it splicing the protein into its functional subunits. Developed in the early 1990s, they are powerful drugs with accompaning side effects.

SAT Subcutaneous fat

TG Triglycerides

VAT Visceral fat

Viral load the quantity of HIV in the blood measured as copies per millilitre, which when suppressed, is described as 'undetectable' and measures < 40 copies/mL.

Viral rebound When a previously suppressed virus accelerates its replication rate rapidly.

WC Waist circumference

WHO World Health Organization

WHR Waist–hip ratio

References

1. Brenchley JM, Schacker TW, Ruff LE, et al. CD4+ T cell depletion during all stages of HIV disease occurs predominantly in the gastrointestinal tract. *J Exp Med.* 2004;200:749–759.

2. Tang AM, Lanzillotti J, Hendricks K, et al. Micronutrients: current issues for HIV care providers. *AIDS.* 2005;19:847–861.

3. Kotler D, Tierney A, Wang J, et al. Magnitude of body-cell-mass depletion and the timing of death from wasting in AIDS. *Am J Clin Nutr.* 1989;50:444–447.

4. Macallan DC, Noble C, Baldwin C. Energy expenditure and wasting in HIV infection. *N Engl J Med.* 1995;333:83–88.

5. Wang J, Thornton JC, Bari S, et al. Comparison of waist circumferences measured at 4 sites. *Am J Clin Nutr.* 2003;77(2):379–384.

6. Bacchetti P, Gripshover B, Grunfeld C, et al. Fat distribution in men with HIV infection. *J Acquir Immune Defic Syndr.* 2005;40: 121–131.

7. Andrade S, Lan SJJ, Engelson ES, et al. Use of the Durnin-Womersley formulae to estimate changes in subcutaneous fat content in HIV-infected subjects. *Am J Clin Nutr.* 2002;75:587–592.

8. BHIVA. British HIV Association guidelines for the treatment of HIV-1 infected adults with antiretroviral therapy. *HIV Med.* 2008;9:563–608.

9. Jones CY, Jones CY, Tang AM, et al. Micronutrient levels and HIV disease status in HIV-infected patients on highly active antiretroviral therapy in the Nutrition for Healthy Living cohort. *J Acquir Immune Defic Syndr.* 2006;43(4):475–482.

10. Jiamton S, Pepin J, Suttent R, et al. A randomized trial of the impact of multiple micronutrient supplementation on mortality among HIV infected individuals living in Bangkok. *AIDS.* 2003;17: 2461–2469.

11. Fawzi WW, Msamanga GI, Spiegelman D, et al. A randomised trial of multivitamin supplements and HIV disease progression and mortality. *N Eng J Med.* 2004;351(1):23–32.

12. Irlam JH, Visser ME, Rollins N, et al. Micronutrient supplementation in children and adults with HIV infection. *Cochrane Database Syst Rev.* 2005;(4):CD003650.

13. USPHS/IDSA. Guidelines for prevention of opportunistic infections in persons infected with HIV. *Ann Intern Med.* 1999;131:873–908.

14. Abubakar I, Aliyu SH, Arumugam C, et al. Prevention and treatment of cryptosporidiosis in immunocompromised patients. *Cochrane Database Syst Rev.* 2007;(1):CD004932.

15. Department of the Environment, Department of Health. *Cryptosporidium in Water Supplies: Second Report of the Group of Experts.* London: HMSO; 1995.

16. Klont R, Rijs A, Warris A, et al. Bacterial and fungal contamination of commercial bottled mineral water from 16 countries. In: *Program and Abstracts of the 44th Interscience Conference of Antimicrobial Agents and Chemotherapy; October 30–November 2; 2004.* Washington, DC, Abstract K-1603.

17. Boyle RJ, Robins-Browne RM, Tang M. Probiotic use in clinical practice: what are the risks? *Am J Clin Nutr.* 2006;83:1256–1264.

18. Heiser CR, Ernst JA, Barrett JT, et al. Probiotics, soluble fiber, and L-glutamine (GLN) reduce nelfinavir (NFV)- or lopinavir/ritonavir (LPV/r)-related diarrhea. *J Int Assoc Physicians AIDS Care.* 2004;3(4): 121–129.

19. Tang AM, Forrester J, Spiegelman D, Knox TA, Tchetgen E, Gorbach SL. Weight loss and survival in HIV positive patients in the era of highly active antiretroviral therapy. *J Acquir Immune Defic Syndr.* 2002;31(2):230–236.

20. Ockenga J, Grimble R, Jonkers-Schuitema C, et al. ESPEN guidelines on enteral nutrition: wasting in HIV and other chronic infectious diseases. *Clin Nutr.* 2006;25:319–329.

21. Green CJ. Nutritional support in HIV infection and AIDS. *Clin Nutr.* 1995;14:197–212.

22. Turner MJ. The efficacy of calcium carbonate in the treatment of protease inhibitor induced persistent diarrhea in HIV infected patients. *HIV Clin Trials.* 2004;5:19–24.

23. Carr A, Samaras K, Burton S, et al. A syndrome of peripheral lipodystrophy, hyperlipidaemia and insulin resistance due to HIV protease inhibitors. *AIDS.* 1998;12: F51–F58.

24. Carr A, Emery S, Law M, et al. An objective case definition of lipodystrophy in HIV-infected adults: a case-control study. *Lancet.* 2003;361:726–735.

25. Lichtenstein KA, Ward DJ, Moorman AC, et al. Clinical assessment of HIV-associated lipodystrophy in an ambulatory population. *AIDS.* 2001;15: 1389–1398.

26. Tien PC, Cole SR, Williams CM, et al. Incidence of lipoatrophy and lipohypertrophy in the women's interagency HIV study. *J Acquir Immune Defic Syndr.* 2003;34: 461–466.

27. Mallon PW, Wand H, Law M, et al. Buffalo hump seen in HIV associated lipodystrophy is associated with hyperinsulinemia but not dyslipidaemia. *J Acquir Immune Defic Syndr.* 2005;38:156–162.

28. Jacobson DL, Tang AM, Spiegelman D, et al. Incidence of metabolic syndrome in a cohort of HIV-infected adults and prevalence relative to the US population (National Health and Nutrition Examination Survey). *J Acquir Immune Defic Syndr.* 2006;43(4): 458–466.

29. Mondy K, Overton ET, Grubb J, et al. Metabolic syndrome in HIV infected patients from an urban, midwestern US outpatient population. *Clin Infect Dis.* 2007;44:726–734.

30. Mallal SA, John M, Moore CB, et al. Contribution of nucleoside analogue reverse transcriptase inhibitors to subcutaneous fat wasting in patients with HIV infection. *AIDS.* 2000;14:1309–1316.

31. Nguyen A, Calmy A, Schiffer V, et al. Lipodystrophy and weight changes: data from the Swiss HIV

Cohort Study, 2000–2006. *4th IAS Conference; July 22–25*; 2007; Sydney, Australia.

32. Aboud M, Elgalib A, Kulasegaram R, Peters B. Insulin resistance and HIV infection: a review. *Int J Clin Pract*. 2006;61(3):463–472.

33. Duran S, Savès M, Spire B, et al. Failure to maintain long-term adherence to highly active antiretroviral therapy: the role of lipodystrophy. *AIDS*. 2001;15: 2441–2444.

34. Huang J, Lee D, Becerrra K, et al. Body image in men with HIV. *AIDS Patient Care STDs*. 2006;20: 668–677.

35. Dube MP, Stein JH, Aberg JA, et al. Guidelines for the evaluation and management of dyslipidemia in human immunodeficiency virus (HIV)-infected adults receiving antiretroviral therapy: recommendations of the HIV Medical Association of the Infectious Disease Society of America and the Adult AIDS Clinical Trials Group. *Clin Infect Dis*. 2003;37:613–627.

36. Podzamczer D, Ferrer E, Sanchez P, et al. Less lipoatrophy and better lipid profile with abacavir as compared to stavudine: 96-week results of a randomized study. *J Acquir Immune Defic Syndr*. 2007;44(2):139–147.

37. Moyle G, Sabin C, Cartledge J, et al. A randomized comparative trial of tenofovir DF or abacavir as replacement for a thymidine analogue in persons with lipoatrophy. *AIDS*. 2006;20(16):2043–2050.

38. World Health Organisation. *Antiretroviral Therapy for HIV Infection in Adults and Adolescents: Recommendations for a Public Health Approach*. Geneva: 2006. Online. Available at: http://www.who.int/hiv/pub/guidelines/adult/en/index.html.

39. Mallon PW. Effect of pravastatin on body composition and markers of cardiovascular disease in HIV-infected men—a randomized, placebo-controlled study. *AIDS*. 2006;20(7):1003–1010.

40. Sutinen J. Uridine supplementation increases subcutaneous fat in patients with HAART associated LD: a randomized placebo controlled trial. *Antivir Ther*. 2005;10:L7.

41. Hadigan C, Jeste S, Anderson EJ, et al. Modifiable dietary habits and their relation to metabolic abnormalities in men and women with human immunodeficiency virus infection and fat redistribution. *Clin Infect Dis*. 2001;33:710–717.

42. Hendricks KM, Dong KR, Tang AM, et al. High-fiber diet in HIV-positive men is associated with lower risk of developing fat deposition. *Am J Clin Nutr*. 2003;78:790–795.

43. Roubenoff R, Weiss L, McDermott A, et al. A pilot study of exercise training to reduce trunk fat in adults with HIV-associated fat redistribution. *AIDS*. 1999;13: 1373–1375.

44. Robinson FP, Quinn LT, Rimmer JH. Effects of high-intensity endurance and resistance exercise on HIV metabolic abnormalities: a pilot study. *Biol Res Nurs*. 2007;8(3): 177–185.

45. Jones SP, Doran DA, Leatt PB, et al. Short-term exercise training improves body composition and hyperlipidaemia in HIV-positive individuals with lipodystrophy. *AIDS*. 2001;15:2049–2051.

46. Dolan SE, Frontera W, Librizzi J, et al. Effects of a supervised home based aerobic and progressive resistance training regimen in women infected with HIV. *Arch Intern Med*. 2006;166:1225–1231.

47. Thoni GJ, Fedou C, Brun JF, et al. Reduction of fat accumulation and lipid disorders by individualized light aerobic training in human immunodeficiency virus infected patients with lipodystrophy and/or dyslipidemia. *Diabetes Metab*. 2002;28:397–404.

48. Roubenoff R, Schmitz H, Bairos L, et al. Reduction of abdominal obesity in lipodystrophy associated with human immunodeficiency virus infection by means of diet and exercise: case report and proof of principle. *Clin Infect Dis*. 2002;34: 390–393.

49. Terry L, Sprinz E, Stein R, et al. Exercise training in HIV-1-infected individuals with dyslipidemia and lipodystrophy. *Med Sci Sports Exerc*. 2006;38(3):411–417.

50. Engelson ES, Agin D, Kenya S, et al. Body composition and metabolic effects of a diet and exercise weight loss regimen on obese, HIV-infected women. *Metabolism*. 2006;55: 1327–1336.

51. Fitch KV, Anderson EJ, Hubbard JL, et al. Effects of a lifestyle modification program in HIV-infected patients with the metabolic syndrome. *AIDS*. 2006;20(14): 1843–1850.

52. Mulligan K, Yang Y, Wininger DA, et al. Effect of metformin and rosiglitazone in HIV-infected patients with hyperinsulinemia and elevated waist/hip ratio. *AIDS*. 2007;21:47–57.

53. Feldt T. Evaluation of safety and efficacy of rosiglitazone in the treatment of HIV-associated lipodystrophy syndrome. *Infection*. 2006;34(2):55–61.

54. Shikuma C, Parker R, Sattler F, et al. Effects of physiologic testosterone supplementation on fat mass and distribution in HIV-infected men with abdominal obesity: ACTG 5079. *Program and abstracts of the 13th Conference on Retroviruses and Opportunistic Infections; February 5–8*; 2006; Denver, Colorado. Abstract 149.

55. Falutz J, Allas S, Blot K, et al. Effects of TH9507, a growth hormone releasing factor analog, on HIV-associated abdominal fat accumulation: a multicenter, double-blind placebo-controlled trial with 412 randomized patients. *Program and abstracts of the 14th Conference on Retroviruses and Opportunistic Infections; February 25–28*; 2007; Los Angeles, California. Abstract 45LB.

56. Currier JS, Lundgren JD, Carr A, Klein D, SAbin CA, Sax PE. Epidemiological evidence for cardiovascular disease in HIV infected patients and relationship to highly active antiretroviral therapy. *Circulation*. 2008;118:e29–e35.

57. Riddler SA, Li X, Chu H, et al. Longitudinal changes in serum lipids among HIV-infected men on highly active antiretroviral therapy. *HIV Med*. 2007;8(5):280–287.

58. El-Sadr WM, Lundgren JD, Neaton JD, et al. CD4+ count-guided interruption of antiretroviral treatment. *N Engl J Med*. 2006;355:2283–2296.

59. Friis-Møller N, Reiss P, Sabin CA, et al. Class of antiretroviral drugs and the risk of myocardial infarction. *N Engl J Med.* 2007;356:1723–1735.

60. DAD Study Group. Use of nucleoside reverse transcriptase inhibitors and risk of myocardial infarction in HIV-infected patients enrolled in the DAD study: a multicohort collaboration. *Lancet.* 2008;371:1417–1426.

61. Wanke C, Gerrior J, Hendricks K, McNamara J, Schaefer E. Alterations in lipid profiles in HIV-infected patients treated with protease inhibitor therapy are not influenced by diet. *Nutr Clin Pract.* 2005;20(6):668–673.

62. Lipshultz SE, Fisher SD, Lai WW, et al. Cardiovascular risk factors, monitoring and therapy for HIV infected patients. *AIDS.* 2003;17(suppl 1):S96–S122.

63. Glass TR. Prevalence of risk factors for cardiovascular disease in HIV-infected patients over time: the Swiss HIV Cohort Study. *HIV Med.* 2006;7(6):404–410.

64. Stradling C, Roos M. Identifying patients for cardiovascular risk reduction in a specialist metabolic clinic. *HIV Med.* 2008;9(suppl 1):14.

65. Joy T, Keogh H, Hadigan C, et al. Dietary fat intake and relationship to serum lipid levels in HIV infected patients. *AIDS.* 2007;21:1591–1600.

66. Foulkes AS. Associations among race/ethnicity, ApoC-III genotypes, and lipids in HIV-1-infected individuals on antiretroviral therapy. *Plos Med.* 2006;3(3):e52.

67. Lundgren JD, Battegay M, Behrens G, et al. European AIDS Clincal Society (EACS) guidelines on the prevention and management of metabolic diseases in HIV. *HIV Med.* 2008;9:72–81.

68. Stradling C. Cardiovascular screening in HIV disease in the United Kingdom—who does it and how? In: *8th International Congress on Drug Therapy in HIV infection,* Glasgow; 2006.

69. National Institute for Health and Clinical Excellence. *Lipid Modification: Cardiovascular Risk Assessment and the Modification of Blood Lipids for the Primary and Secondary Prevention of Cardiovascular Disease.* London: NICE; 2008. Available at: http://www.nice.org.uk/CG67.

70. Law MG, Friis-Moller N, El Sadr WM, et al. The use of the Framingham equation to predict myocardial infarctions in HIV-infected patients: comparison with observed events in the DAD Study. *HIV Med.* 2006;7:218–230.

71. Henry K, Melroe H, Huebesch J, et al. Atorvastatin and gemfibrozil for protease-inhibitor-related lipid abnormalities. *Lancet.* 1998;352(9133):1031–1032.

72. Barrios AA, Blanco FA, Garcia-Benayas TA, et al. Effect of dietary intervention on highly active antiretroviral therapy-related dyslipidemia. *AIDS.* 2002;16(15):2079–2081.

73. Batterham MJ, Brown D, Workman C. Modifying dietary fat intake can reduce serum cholesterol in HIV-associated hypercholesterolemia. *AIDS.* 2003;17:1414–1416.

74. Culkin A, Stradling C. HAART to heart—where do DHIVA diets fit into BHIVA guidelines? *HIV Med.* 2005;6(suppl 1):29.

75. Moyle GJ, Lloyd M, Reynolds B, et al. Dietary advice with or without pravastatin for the management of hypercholesterolaemia associated with protease inhibitor therapy. *AIDS.* 2001;15(12):1503–1508.

76. Miller J, Brown D, Amin J, et al. A randomized, double-blind study of gemfibrozil for the treatment of protease inhibitor-associated hypertriglyceridaemia. *AIDS.* 2002;16(16):2195–2200.

77. Lazzaretti R, Pinto-Ribeiro J, Kummer R, et al. Dietary intervention when starting HAART prevents the increase in lipids independently of drug regimen: a randomized trial. *4th IAS Conference* 2007; WEAB303.

78. Yarasheski KE, Tebas P, Stanerson B, et al. Resistance exercise training reduces hypertriglyceridemia in HIV-infected men treated with antiviral therapy. *J Appl Physiol.* 2001;90:133–138.

79. Gavrila A, Tsiodras S, Doweiko J, et al. Exercise and vitamin E intake are independently associated with metabolic abnormalities in human immunodeficiency virus-positive subjects: a cross-sectional study. *Clin Infect Dis.* 2003;36:1593–1601.

80. Glesby MJ, Stein JH. *Managing Dyslipidaemia in HIV Infected Patients on Therapy.* 2008. Online. Available at http://www.clinicalcareoptions.com/HIV/TreatmentUpdates/ManagingDyslipidemia. Accessed 19 February 2009.

81. Coll B, Aragones G, Parra S, et al. Ezetimibe effectively decreases LDL-cholesterol in HIV-infected patients. *AIDS.* 2006;20:1675–1677.

82. Negredo E, Molto J, Puig J, et al. Ezetimibe, a promising lipid-lowering agent for the treatment of dyslipidaemia in HIV-infected patients with poor response to statins. *AIDS.* 2006;20:2159–2164.

83. Bennett MT, Johns KW, Bondy GP. Ezetimibe is effective when added to maximally tolerated lipid lowering therapy in patients with HIV. *Lipids Health Dis.* 2007;6:15.

84. Dube MP, Wu JW, Aberg JA, et al. Safety and efficacy of extended-release niacin for the treatment of dyslipidaemia in patients with HIV infection: a prospective, multicentre study (ACTG 5148). *Program and Abstracts of the 7th International Workshop on Adverse Drug Reactions and Lipodystrophy in HIV; November 13–16; 2005;* Dublin, Ireland. Abstract 12.

85. De Truchis P, Kirstetter M, Perier A. Reduction in triglyceride level with N-3 polyunsaturated fatty acids in HIV-infected patients taking potent antiretroviral therapy: a randomized prospective study. *J Acquir Immune Defic Syndr.* 2007;44(3):278–285.

86. Wohl DA. Randomized study of the safety and efficacy of fish oil (omega-3 fatty acid) supplementation with dietary and exercise counseling for the treatment of antiretroviral therapy-associated hypertriglyceridemia. *Clin Infect Dis.* 2005;41(10):1498–1504.

87. British HIV Association and Children's Association. *Guidelines for the Management of HIV Infection in Pregnant Women.* 2008.

88. Wiysonge CS, Shey MS, Sterne JAC, et al. Vitamin A supplementation for

reducing the risk of mother-to-child transmission of HIV infection. *Cochrane Database Syst Rev.* 2005;(4):CD003648.

89. World Health Organisation. *HIV and Infant Feeding: A Guide for Healthcare Managers and Supervisors.* Geneva: World Health Organization; 2003.

90. Iliff PJ, Piwoz EG, Tavengwa NV, et al. Early exclusive breastfeeding reduces the risk of postnatal HIV-1 transmission an d increases HIV free survival. *AIDS.* 2005;19(7): 699–708.

91. Deeks S, Phillips A. HIV infection, antiretroviral treatment, ageing, and non-AIDS related morbidity. *Br Med J.* 2009;338:a3172.

Further reading

Statistics/epidemiology. http://www. unaids.org/en/HIV_data/epi2006/; http://www.hpa.org.uk

AIDS related illnesses. http://www. hivmedicine.com

Conference reports. http://www.i-base. info/htb/index.html

Hot topics AIDS Treatment Update on. http://www.aidsmap.com

ARV side effects. http://www.i-base. info/guides/index.html

General HIV and STI. www.Sexualhealthbirmingham.co.uk

HIV in resource poor settings. http:// www.who.int/topics/hiv_aids/en/

African diets. http://www.pronutrition. org

Food safety. http://www.food.gov.uk; http://www.eatwell.gov.uk

Water safety. http://www.epa.gov/ safewater/crypto.html; http://www. nsf.org/consumer/; http://www.who. int/entity/mediacentre/factsheets/ fs256/en/

Palliative care

Cathy Payne   Max Watson

LEARNING OBJECTIVES

By the end of this chapter the reader will be able to:

- Describe the holistic principles of palliative care;
- Critically reflect on the ways in which nutritional support in the palliative care setting differs from other settings;
- Explain how patients' nutritional goals will change with disease progression;
- Recognise the need for appropriate and timely review;
- Discuss and debate the ethical issues surrounding the provision of artificial nutrition and hydration; and
- Critically reflect on the positive ways in which dietitians can help and support patients and their carers receiving palliative care.

Introduction

For many healthcare professionals the word palliative still invokes images of patients nursed in a darkened side room with a syringe driver erected for pain relief and the removal of all active forms of treatment. The term palliative is so synonymous with death and dying for some that they react very negatively to any suggestion that the patients they care for might benefit from the advice and support of palliative care input; 'It is too early to involve palliative care—we haven't given up on Mr. Jones yet..'

Since confusion often exists regarding the nature of palliative care, it is important to clearly define the terms used in connection with such care.

Palliative care is defined by the World Health Organisation as 'an approach that improves the quality of life of patients and their families facing the problem associated with life-threatening illness, through the prevention and relief of suffering by means of early identification and impeccable assessment and treatment of pain and other problems, physical, psychosocial and spiritual.'[1]

Thus palliative care is not solely related to care in the last days of life and can be provided in conjunction with active therapy also. It aims to provide comfort and to maximise quality of life. Palliative care should be considered from the point at which patients receive a life-limiting diagnosis.

Generalist palliative care is the care provided most often by the primary care team or by health professionals working within non-palliative specialities.[2] The majority of healthcare professionals working in hospitals, primary care facilities and the community regularly care for patients with palliative care needs, providing generalist palliative care and need to be able to:

- Undertake holistic interdisciplinary assessment of the patient and those who matter to them and effectively communicate treatment goals using an ethical framework to help guide decision-making;
- Use open and sensitive communication with patients and those who matter to them, to facilitate expression of needs including those of diverse cultural groups and those with special needs;
- Recognise the limitations of their own expertise and indications for onward referral to specialist palliative care or other appropriate disciplines and agencies;

- Identify the range of grief responses to appropriately assess and support those dealing with loss and bereavement;
- Participate in education and learning and contribute to audit, evaluation and research improve outcomes for patients;
- Recognise the need for support of self and others, utilising appropriate support systems.[3]

Specialist palliative care is the care provided for patients with complex needs relating to their physical, psychological, social and spiritual well being. It is underpinned by interprofessional and transdisciplinary approaches to patient care.[3] This 'whole person' or 'holistic' care requires a very flexible team approach, as no single profession can possess the skills necessary to address all areas of need. In order to be classified as a specialist palliative care service the professional team must include doctors, nurses, social workers, chaplains, physiotherapists and occupational therapists. Increasingly such teams are not only using the services of pharmacists, dietitians and speech and language therapists, but are including them as core team members.

Hospice and hospice care refer to a philosophy of care rather than a specific building or service and may encompass a programme of care and array of skills deliverable in a wide range of settings.[4] In the USA hospice care is only recognised by insurance companies when a patient is deemed to have a prognosis of less than six months. Within the UK hospice care is provided by both NHS and voluntary sector partners to anyone with advanced progressive illness requiring complex symptom management.

End-of-life care is defined in different ways in the UK and in the USA where it refers to the care of patients around the actual time of death. In the UK it is a much more embracing term including the full range of services required by patients and their families from the point of diagnosis through to bereavement care. In 2007 the UK Government initiated a three-year End-of-Life Care programme aimed at improving the care of all patients, irrespective of diagnosis, coming to the end of their lives. The three key elements of this initiative have been the Liverpool Care Pathway of the Dying, the Gold Standards Framework and the Preferred Place of Care aimed at addressing the following salient issues:[5–7]

- Given the option, most people would prefer to die at home;[8]
- The provision of effective symptom management, crisis intervention and adaptive

rehabilitation and care in the last phase of illness is crucial in enabling patients to live and die in the place of their choice;[9] and
- Emotional, practical and bereavement support for the carers is a vital need to be met by end-of-life care.[10,11]

Development of the palliative care speciality

Care of the dying has been important throughout history, though palliative care has only been fairly recently recognised as a medical specialty. The hospice movement was pioneered by Dame Cicely Saunders.[12] During her career Saunders trained and practiced as a nurse, social worker, doctor and researcher. She strongly believed that death was a process that should not be feared and should be both life-affirming and free of pain.

> You matter because you are you. You matter to the last moment of your life. We will do all we can not only to help you die peacefully, but to live until you die.[12]

In 1967 she opened the world's first purpose-built hospice, St Christopher's in south London. Patient care at St Christopher's was based on principles of combining expert pain and symptom relief with holistic care to meet the physical, social, psychological and spiritual needs of patients and their family and friends.[13]

The palliative care specialty developed with a major focus on the care of patients with cancer. More recently the concept of palliative and end-of-life care has been broadened to include care given to patients with any advanced irreversible disease and not just those with a cancer diagnosis.[11,14] It is estimated that the major causes of death by 2020 will be ischaemic heart disease, cerebrovascular disease and chronic obstructive pulmonary disease.[15] Increases in the number of old frail people with chronic cardiovascular and cerebrovascular disease is a real challenge for health services generally and palliative care services specifically.[16] It is important to recognise that different patterns of service provision may be required to address the needs of patients with non-malignant conditions, where active therapy may continue until death is imminent and where prognostication is uncertain.[17]

Over the past 10 years there have been three key documents which have helped to shape therapy services for patients with palliative care needs. These

Box 15.1

Overarching principles of palliative care

The overarching principles of palliative care are to:

- Affirm life but regard dying as a normal process;
- Neither hasten nor postpone death;
- Provide relief from pain and other distressing symptoms;
- Integrate the psychological and spiritual aspects of care;
- Offer a support system to help patients live as actively as possible until death; and
- Offer a support system to help patients' families cope during the patient's illness and in their own bereavement.[4]

are the King's Fund report on rehabilitation, 'Fulfilling Lives' and the NICE guidelines on improving supportive and palliative care for adults with cancer.[2,18,19] The overarching principles of palliative care are outlined in Box 15.1.

Nutritional challenges in the palliative care setting

Dictionary definitions of food focus on its physical attributes of providing macro- and micronutrients to sustain life. However, food has much more of a psychosocial significance than is acknowledged within these definitions. In sitting down to a family meal, people benefit from the act of gathering together socially. Sensory rewards occur from the taste, texture and smell of foods. Food is often presented as a token of affection such as preparing a favourite meal or providing a gift of confectionary.

There are many factors which may influence dietary choices.

Therapeutic diet

Does the patient need a special diet or has information been received from a professional on nutritional needs? Often dietary restrictions can be relaxed at the palliative phase of illness to increase food choice and palatability. Some restrictions are better to be retained as they may increase morbidity if relaxed such as adherence to a gluten-free diet for a patient with coeliac disease.

Religious/cultural needs

Does the patient have food restrictions or preferences associated with religion/culture and can these be better accommodated to improve dietary intake? Provision of Halal meat may significantly increase meal choice for a patient of Muslim faith who would otherwise follow a vegetarian diet within an inpatient setting.

Functional needs

Does the patient have difficulty communicating their food wishes or have they a disability which prevents them from feeding themselves without assistance that could be better managed with the provision of equipment? Use of appropriate seating and feeding aids may increase independence and limit fatigue associated with eating.

Weight change

What is the weight history of the patient and was weight loss deliberate or unintentional? Unintentional weight loss may be an indicator of disease severity and a predictor of poorer prognosis.[20]

Food intake

Compared to normal, how is the patient now eating? What was their usual eating pattern and could this be better accommodated within their current place of care to improve dietary intake, e.g. provision of between meal and late evening snacks? Are they now reliant on an artificial feeding route?

Fluid intake

Is there a restriction in fluid volume or consistency and is this still necessary? Fluid restrictions can negatively impact on nutritional intake and physical functioning.[21]

Symptoms

Are there symptoms present that could be exacerbating anorexia which are potentially responsive to treatment? Is the patient suffering from anorexia cachexia syndrome?

Psychological issues

What was the person's previous, and what is their current relationship with food? Were they a healthy eater, a strict adherer to a diet plan, a yo-yo dieter always struggling to control weight, someone who only ate when they were hungry or someone who loved to eat, with food seen as an important element of daily life? Are they facing external pressures to eat which are leading to relationship tensions? Are they depressed? Depression is common within the elderly population and particularly amongst patients with chronic medical conditions. It is important that the impact of depression upon quality of life is recognised and that depressive symptoms are adequately assessed and addressed.[22]

Patient goals

What goals does the patient have for nutritional support? Do they wish to maintain, gain or lose weight, do they wish to improve their energy levels, or is their greatest aim to regain enjoyment of food?

Determining energy requirements

Determining the nutritional needs of patients with advanced progressive illness can be a real challenge. Changes in metabolic rate and in the processing of nutrients for energy may mean that predictive equations are unrepresentative of patient need.[23] Particular caution must be taken when using predictive equations to calculate the energy requirements of elderly patients with advanced illness. Changes in body composition including a reduction in fat-free mass will significantly affect energy expenditure and macro- and micronutrient needs.[24] Most of the patients seen by specialist palliative care services will at some stage experience a loss of body weight, a decrease in appetite and a reduction in energy levels.

The syndrome of persistent weight loss in the presence of adequate nutrition as determined by predictive equations is also known as anorexia cachexia syndrome (ACS).[25,26] Weight loss from ACS is not the same as weight loss during starvation. A healthy person's body can adjust to starvation by slowing down its use of nutrients, but in patients with ACS, the body does not make this adjustment. Therefore weight loss in patients with ACS is unlikely to be reversed simply by eating more or by provision of supplementary artificial feeding.[23,26] The main symptoms of the anorexia cachexia syndrome are outlined in Box 15.2.

Box 15.2

Symptoms of anorexia cachexia syndrome

- Severe loss of weight, including loss of fat and muscle mass
- Loss of appetite
- Feeling sick (nausea)
- Feeling full after eating small amounts (early satiety)
- Anaemia (low red blood cell count)
- Weakness and fatigue[25]

Factors that may contribute to cachexia include both a reduction of nutrient intake and improper nutrient utilisation as well as activation of cytochemical processes which leads to the body moving to a predominantly catabolic state. The main causes of reduced nutrient intake in ACS are outlined in Box 15.3.

The utilisation of nutrients may be influenced by factors such as the presence of fistulae affecting the gastrointestinal tract, malabsorption of nutrients due

Box 15.3

Cause of reduced nutrient intake in anorexia cachexia

- Physical discomfort from uncontrolled pain, bloating, reflux or nausea;
- Poor appetite or early satiety due to delayed gastric emptying, slowed gastrointestinal transit or ascites;
- Oral problems including a sore or dry mouth, taste changes, infection, poor dentition or ill-fitting dentures;
- Side effects from prescribed or over-the-counter medications;
- Adherence to a therapeutic or altered consistency diet or suffering from food aversions which limit food choice;
- Reliance on others to buy or prepare food or to assist with feeding;
- Depression or anxiety caused by loss of hope, spiritual distress or loss of social status and social contact;
- Breathlessness and fatigue; and
- Mixed messages regarding optimal diet therapy and the influences of culture, family and other belief systems.[27–29]

to diarrhoea, drug–nutrient interaction or enzyme depletion and muscle atrophy as a consequence of reduced contractile work.[27–29]

Cancer ACS is often witnessed early in patients with metastatic cancers of the pancreas and lung. Cytokines released by the tumour, or by the immune response mounted against the tumour, lead to activation of metabolic and inflammatory pathways causing disproportionate depletion of lean body mass and a cascade of effects causing weight loss irrespective of food intake. Similar patterns of weight loss are seen in most advanced solid tumours, with organ failure, in progressive neurological disease and in patients with AIDS.[30]

Palliative care dietetics is a growing field with increasing need to develop a clear evidence base on which to base practice. Dietitians working with patients who have palliative care needs aim to enhance the quality of life of both patients and their families. This may be achieved by improving nutritional intake, or where this is not possible, by improving the patient and carer's ability to cope with the patient's deteriorating nutritional status.[31–36]

The role of the dietitian

Early identification of those at nutritional risk

Early identification of those at nutritional risk will enable reversible causes of malnutrition to be treated and ensure that dietetic involvement, where needed, is provided in a timely manner. Many of the most difficult to manage end-of-life issues, such as progressive weight loss, have their origins early in the course of a disease.[31] Addressing needs sooner, ensuring patient and carer's participation in treatment choices, and communicating treatment plans to colleagues may help to improve care in later stages, which may positively impact on the patient's quality of life.[37]

Nutritional screening tools which determine need for nutritional intervention by assigning a point score may fail to capture the subtleties of need within this particularly vulnerable population. Patients may also have a low priority score on a numerical screen but have a treatable nutritional symptom which significantly impacts on their quality of life. Alternatively patients may score highly but may decline the

---

> ## Box 15.4
>
> **Nutritional assessment in anorexia cachexia**
>
> Nutritional assessment in anorexia cachexia may involve the following:
>
> - Height
> - Weight
> - Body mass index
> - Anthropometry (mid-arm circumference)
> - Percentage body weight loss
> - Biochemical markers
> - Present oral intake
> - Consistency of food and fluids tolerated
> - Diagnosis and staging of disease
> - Comorbidities
> - Social circumstances

---

services of a dietitian if they have symptoms causing them greater distress which they wish to have managed first.

Parameters for consideration when undertaking a nutritional assessment are outlined in Box 15.4.

Anthropometric measurements have been used to measure decline in nutritional status when a patient is unable to be weighed.[38] However, for patients who have lost a significant amount of weight, their loose skin folds can make some anthropometric measurements questionable, such as mid-arm circumference. In an advanced state of muscle wasting with fat depletion, there may be very little change over a period of three months, making it difficult to use this measurement to meaningfully document change in nutritional status.[39] Measurements are subject to observer bias and should be consistently recorded by the same observer to demonstrate decline in muscle and fat mass.[40]

Train the healthcare team to ensure consistent dietary advice is provided

Developing a proactive structured training programme on nutrition in palliative care for all staff involved in the provision of palliative care will ensure that accurate and consistent dietary advice is provided to patients and carers. Patients with life-limiting illness are likely to receive care from many professionals throughout their illness. These professionals can come from the acute, community, statutory and/or voluntary sector and may provide services to patients with palliative care needs as a small part of their remit or as the mainstay of their work. It is important that the dietitian works closely with other members of their team to educate and support them in providing appropriate dietary advice to patients and their families, as effective management of symptoms is unlikely to be achieved in the absence of good quality communication between health professionals.[29,41] The role of dietitians in both general and specialist palliative care provision needs to be communicated better to service providers and seen as essential rather than an added extra to service provision.[28,32] A recent review of palliative services for patients with advanced cancer in the West of Scotland showed that many patients who could benefit from dietetic and other Allied Health Professional (AHP) interventions were denied these services. This was because potential referrers had a poor awareness of the role of AHPs and there was poor integration of AHP services into palliative care teams. In addition there were low AHP staffing levels and a lack of palliative care training tailored to suit the needs of specialist and non-specialist AHPs in working with these patients.[42]

Communicate appropriate and timely advice

It is important to provide appropriate and timely advice to patients and carers concerning nutritional intervention and symptom control and to also ensure that assessment of nutritional status is ongoing.[43] Communication and regular holistic assessments are the key to forward planning, as needs which are anticipated can be more easily managed. Patients receiving palliative care receive the majority of care during their last year at home and most of that care is provided by informal carers, such as family and friends. Individuals who have the greatest dependency on community palliative care services are also the most dependent on their informal carers. Poor management at home often results in inappropriate admissions to hospital.[44] Educating the patient and their family on nutritional matters enables families to build their coping resources though participation in experiences that enhance control and independence.[45-47] By actively involving the patient and family we can:

- Improve understanding of treatment goals and enable joint decision making around them;
- Better anticipate needs which can then be more readily met;

- Increase the potential for compliance with the care plan through ownership of it;
- Teach skills and techniques to improve patient functioning; and
- Give family members better access to support services as needed.[48-50]

This method challenges the traditional therapy approach which tends to rely heavily on technology and biomedical science and so disempowers patients and their families by a focus on their deficits. Traditional therapy undervalues the importance of human interactions in the healthcare experience and tends to be driven by the needs of the healthcare professionals and the system.

Provide supportive information

Information materials should be produced to support patients' care needs. Medical jargon should be avoided, keeping dietary information as concise and simple as possible and backing it up with written advice where appropriate. It is also important to review the content of written dietary advice, prior to using it with clients or providing it to other healthcare professionals to use.

Ensure appropriate nutritional support

Patients should only receive artificial nutrition support if it is deemed appropriate within their overall palliative treatment. This aims to prevent the inefficient use of resources and protect the patient from inappropriate and demanding interventions. The goal is to ensure that all interventions enhance the patient's quality of life. Eating is usually an enjoyable pastime but nutrition can become a chore for some patients with advanced disease. Despite the large number of studies that have looked at the prevalence of malnutrition in patients near the end of life there has been very little work focusing on the impact of this symptom on the patient's quality of life.[51-53] Poor appetite and weight loss are often seen in advanced disease and may be more distressing for carers than for the person exhibiting these symptoms, as carers often see weight loss as a physical reminder of the deteriorating health of a loved one.[53,54] Provision of food is inextricably linked in society to provision of care and love. When the patient refuses to eat, this can have a devastating effect on relationships within the home. Being unable to partake of food at a family gathering or a group get-together may also leave the patient feeling socially excluded. If patients feel pressurised to eat when they have no desire to do so, this can have a devastating effect on morale and on quality of life. It can also lead to family tension as further weight loss is seen by carers as their failure to provide optimally for their loved one.

Support for carers, friends and family

It is essential to ensure that carers, friends and family are looking after their own nutritional well being. Caring for a dying loved one can be both physically demanding and emotionally exhausting. It is vital that carers do not neglect their own nutritional needs and become ill themselves as a consequence of poor nutritional status. Advice from the dietitian may include:

- Accepting help from others in meal preparation, shopping and cooking;
- Use of Internet shopping to reduce time required to maintain food stocks within the house; and
- Keeping a stock of ready or convenience meals to use when cooking and preparation time is limited.

Ensure all dietary restrictions are appropriate

It is vital to ensure that any dietary restrictions, imposed by self or others, are warranted and improve life quality.[28,32,52] Since the evidence base for nutrition management in advanced disease is rapidly evolving it is important that anyone treating patients critically evaluates current research and embeds this appropriately into practice. Until disease-specific predictive equations for nutritional requirements in advanced illness are produced, then use of current equations may at least provide a starting point for estimating needs, but should not be considered as infallible in setting patient goals in this palliative population. The individual wishes of the patient must be considered alongside the effects of both the disease process and the nutritional treatment plan. Maintaining optimal quality-of-life rather than optimising nutritional intake is usually the primary goal of the dietetic intervention in this circumstance. When assessing the nutritional status of patients it is essential to use a holistic assessment covering not only the physical symptoms but also the psychological, social

and spiritual symptoms which will affect total nutritional management. In the words of the famous French philosopher Voltaire (1694-1778), 'Nothing would be more tiresome than eating and drinking if God had not made them a pleasure as well as a necessity.'

The use of complementary therapies including herbal and dietary supplements is common among patients facing a life-limiting or life-threatening diagnosis, although their use is frequently unreported to healthcare staff.[55] While there is a dearth of reliable published research on their use the Internet is full of websites where all sorts of claims are made. Since patients and their families may not volunteer the information that the patient is on any alternative or complementary therapy it is important that questions regarding their use is included routinely as part of holistic patient assessment. It can be difficult for patients and their families to have their hopes in such interventions dashed by conventional clinicians and sensitive handling of these issues is important.

Pharmacological approaches in the treatment of ACS

A number of pharmacological approaches have been trialed in the treatment of ACS with varying levels of success.

Glucocorticosteroids such as dexamethasone and prednisolone are a class of steroid hormone which have demonstrated benefits of up to 4 weeks on appetite, well being, performance status and control of nausea.[56] Glucocorticoids can produce positive effects quickly within a couple of days. Unfortunately glucocorticoids fail to elicit a gain in lean muscle weight and amongst other undesirable side effects are known to cause proximal muscle weakness, immune suppression, delirium, osteoporosis, symptomatic hyperglycaemia and gastric bleeds. In view of these side effects glucocorticosteroids should only be used to treat ACS symptoms when prognosis is limited to weeks. Their benefits are short term and they should never be prescribed 'long term' as they will end up contributing to the muscle weakness and fatigue for which they were prescribed.[57]

Progestogens such as megestrol acetate and medroxy progesterone acetate are synthetic derivatives of progesterone which have been shown to improve appetite, nutritional status and well being.[58] Crucially they also do not lead to increases in lean muscle weight. The known side effects of therapy are significant, including thromboembolism, oedema, hyperglycaemia, uterine bleeding and adrenal insufficiency. Progestogens take longer than glucocorticoids to start having effects but these effects are sustained for longer. Progestogens are recommended for use in patients as treatment for ACS who have a prognosis of months, with full benefits being seen after 3–4 weeks of treatment.[57]

Prokinetics such as metoclopramide may benefit patients with ACS by speeding up rate of intestinal transit of nutrients to counteract ACS symptoms of delayed gastric emptying, nausea, early satiety and constipation.[59]

The branched chain amino acids leucine, isoleucine and valine may help in the treatment of ACS by providing an alternative fuel source for gluconeogenesis which causes peripheral breakdown of skeletal muscle in ACS. These amino acids also help to decrease the production of serotonin, a known suppressor of appetite.[60]

Eicosapentaenoic acid (EPA) is an omega-3 fatty acid sourced primarily from polyunsaturated fish oil. EPA works as an anti-inflammatory by inhibiting lipolysis and muscle breakdown. Trials have shown some reduced levels of fatigue, decreased rate of lean body mass loss and a reduction in the inflammatory marker C-reactive protein when taken daily at therapeutic levels. Unfortunately animal trials have shown results more promising than those in humans. Reported side effects include elevation of blood glucose and cholesterol levels in some patients. Difficulty in complying with dosage regimens has been an issue due to side effects such as flatulence and problems in swallowing the large numbers of fish oil capsules or supplement drinks required.[61,62]

Cannabinoids such as dronabinol and nabilone work by inducing appetite and reducing nausea through cannabinoid receptors in the hypothalamus. However, undesirable psychotropic effects have prevented their widespread use.[63]

Melatonin is a naturally occurring hormone important in the regulation of the circadian rhythms by chemically causing drowsiness and lowering body temperature.[64] Open studies by Lissoni et al and Persson et al showed that melatonin administration led to stabilisation of weight in patients with cancer cachexia, perhaps through inhibiting cachexia-inducing cytokines, appetite promotion and the regulation of sleep patterns.[65,66]

Thalidomide is a sedative-hypnotic and a powerful antiemetic infamous for the devastating effects on foetuses when taken by pregnant women to treat morning sickness.[67] Thalidomide may have potential in reducing the symptoms of ACS by inhibiting tumour necrosis factor (TNF), one of the key cytokines involved in the cachexia process, as well as having direct effects on reducing tumour growth through inhibition of neo-angiogenesis.[68] Studies with patients affected by AIDS showed an increase in appetite and weight gain with just a 300-mg nightly dose.[69] Known side effects include birth defects, sedation and immune suppression. Strict regulatory control over prescription of thalidomide and other newer similar compounds make their wholesale prescription for ACS unlikely.

Athletes have long known the benefits of *anabolic steroids* in promoting the production of muscle mass. It is also known than nearly a quarter of patients with advanced malignancy are hypogonadal and thus at particular risk of muscle loss.[70] In studies anabolic steroids such as testosterone or fluoxymesterone have been shown to be particularly effective in producing lean muscle weight gain for patient with AIDS-associated wasting. Testosterone has also been seen to be of benefit for hypogonadal men suffering from ACS.[71] Worries about unwanted masculisation effects and fears that some anabolic agents might have a tumour promotion effect have so far limited their use, though clenbuterol in particular has had promising trials.

Ethics of artificial nutrition and hydration

Not all patients and their carers respond in the same way to the diagnosis of an incurable illness. Some adopt a 'fight it all the way' approach and others lapse into depression and do little to maintain their physical and social functioning. Consideration must be given to the patient's nutritional problems within the greater context of their illness trajectory and their combined physical, psychological, social and spiritual needs. Palliative care is an approach in which it can be categorically said that, 'one size therapy will never fit all.' By examining what helps some individuals to survive and thrive in the face of difficult or tragic life events we may develop and deepen our own understanding of appropriate support and care.[72]

Much debate has taken place concerning when and where it is appropriate to provide artificial hydration and nutrition. Most of us are taught from childhood that food and drink are essential for life. At the same time advances in technology have made artificial feeding technically possible for greater numbers of patients. Irrespective of the advances the underlying question remains, even if we are now able to provide artificial nutrition and hydration to greater numbers of people should we do so?

Ethical issues surrounding the appropriateness of artificial nutrition and hydration for patients with palliative care needs can be explored using the four main principles of healthcare ethics: respect for autonomy, nonmaleficence, beneficence and justice.[73]

Autonomy

Autonomy is the right of every individual to choose their own care independently of the views and influences of others.

Does the patient wish for artificial nutrition and fluids to be given? A small number of patients will want any intervention which offers any chance of any degree of life prolongation. Others will not. Advance directives are a way that patients can ensure that future treatments that they receive, if they were to become incompetent, comply with their preferences.[74] The Mental Capacity Act in the UK now enshrines in UK law the following key principles, which relate directly to the principle of autonomy:[75]

- A presumption of capacity—every adult has the right to make his or her own decisions and must be assumed to have capacity to do so unless it is proved otherwise;
- The right for individuals to be supported to make their own decisions—people must be given all appropriate help before anyone concludes that they cannot make their own decisions;
- That individuals must retain the right to make what might be seen as eccentric or unwise decisions;
- Best interests—anything done for or on behalf of people without capacity must be in their best interests; and
- Least restrictive intervention—anything done for or on behalf of people without capacity should be the least restrictive of their basic rights and freedoms.

The Mental Capacity Act also allows for a patient to appoint a person with lasting powers of attorney who can act on the patient's behalf if they lose capacity to make decisions in the future.

Good information needs to be provided by healthcare workers to help patients and their families make the best choice in difficult situations and with full appreciation of the consequences of their decisions. It is also necessary to consider the cultural and religious beliefs of the patient and their family as these may also significantly impact on choices concerning the use of all forms of artificial support.[76–79] If in doubt about the religious or cultural issues which may be influencing choices, always clarify these with the patient and family. Never assume that because an individual patient belongs to a particular religious group that they will automatically want particular treatment options.

Non-maleficence

Non-maleficence is the expectation that the care provided will do no harm. Many families feel that the non-provision of artificial fluid and nutrition at the end of life will contribute to quicker patient deterioration and cause suffering. Withdrawal of a drip or of NG feeding may make patients and families feel that they are being abandoned. Such interventions, which may seem futile to clinical staff, may be seen as manifestations of continuing medical support and hope.[80] Findings from studies addressing these issues show little evidence that either giving or withholding artificial nutrition and hydration impacts on the length of remaining life or that providing artificial nutrition and hydration improves patient comfort.[81]

Beneficence

Beneficence refers to intent though treatment to provide a positive therapeutic outcome for the patient. Beneficence arguments are highlighted in relation to issues such as the administration of fluids to patients in the last days of life. This practice differs considerably according to the setting of end of life care. An artificial increase in fluids at the end of life may worsen respiratory secretions, increase vomiting, raise intracranial pressure in the presence of intracerebral disease and cause an uncomfortable urinary output. On one side of the argument it is claimed that dehydration is a normal part of the dying process and to interfere with this process may in fact lead to more harm than good. Thirst is mostly due to sensations of dryness around the mouth, lips and tongue that can be appropriately treated with good oral care and a regular oral hygiene regime.[80] On the other side of the argument there are those who feel that dehydration in patients who are moribund is a significant cause of morbidity for patients due to decreased renal function leading to a build up of opioid or other active drug metabolites. This in turn will lead to deepening unconsciousness. Patients in hospitals are more likely to die with drips in situ than patients in hospices, but it is likely that the reasons behind the disparity in practices are based more on institutional cultures than an actual evidence base of what is most beneficent.

Justice

Justice is the right of the patient to receive the care that they need according to what is fair within the context of society and the moral and legal obligations of the healthcare provider. Aggressive nutritional and hydration therapy is expensive and in a system which has limited resources cost–benefit ratios cannot be ignored. For many years healthcare professionals have believed that patients with dementia have a poorer prognosis following insertion of a percutaneous endoscopic gastrostomy (PEG) tube than those without cognitive impairment.[82] Interestingly a recent article by Higaki et al proficiently challenges this belief.[83] Their retrospective cohort analysis found no statistical difference in the frequency of complications or in survival rates between those patients with or without cognitive impairment. Statistically significant risk factors for survival for both groups included a prior history of subtotal gastrectomy, hypoalbuminaemia, being over 80 years of age, having chronic heart failure and being male.

A recent systematic review of nutrition support failed to offer any strong evidence that enteral feeding provided a benefit to any cohort of patients receiving it. However, these findings must be interpreted with caution as the few studies included had poor methodological rigor due to the inherent ethical difficulties of running feeding trials.[84,85] Whilst there is insufficient evidence to support the use of PEG feeding for life prolongation in patients receiving palliative care, it would seem prudent to avoid a blanket policy of refusing to place feeding tubes in all patients who have palliative care needs, weighing up the potential for good against the potential for harm.

Families can spend precious time worrying about technical issues surrounding drips and feeding tubes instead of concentrating on quality time with the patient. Involving the family in basic comfort care including oral hygiene practice and safest consistency hand feeding techniques ensures their continued positive contribution to patient care.[86]

Conclusion

When caring for people at end of life the dietitian's role is one of education and communication, requiring the expertise, advice and support of a multiprofessional team to ensure the appropriate management of nutritional issues. It is important not to assume that as dietitians there is an obligation to correct all nutritional deficits to the detriment of any other therapy goals and irrespective of patient wishes. Provision of adequate nutrition and hydration may remain a goal of therapy but can become secondary to supportive measures such as minimising discomfort, anxiety or distress relating to food and fluid intake.

The main goals of nutritional therapy in palliative care are to:

- Limit functional decline through preservation of fat-free mass;
- Support family and other carers in making appropriate food choices;
- Increase food palatability and enjoyment using smaller plates of desired food served attractively;
- Limit food restrictions so that optimal choice is available;
- Ensure provision of feeding assistance or adaptations as required;
- Dispel food myths including the concept of good and bad foods to eat; and
- Ensure that where nutrition support is provided it is not so invasive or unacceptable that it impairs rather than improves quality of life.[33–37]

Although dietitians may not be able to provide nutritional solutions for all eventualities they can still have an active and vital role in supporting patients through their life choices. Even if patients do not wish for active nutritional support the dietitian should keep communication channels open. Simply being available for a patient and their family can be an essential element of effective palliative care provision.[87] Within palliative care, the focus of nutritional therapy is caring rather than curing.

Key points

- Palliative care is the active holistic care of patients diagnosed with noncurative illness. It aims to provide comfort and to maximise quality of life by ensuring that symptoms are identified and managed in a timely and effective manner. Patients may continue to receive active disease therapy alongside palliative care support and this is particularly true of non-malignant chronic disease where prognostication is uncertain.

- Dietitians have a central role to play in the nutritional management and support of patients with palliative care needs. As experts in interpreting and translating the science of nutrition, they must ensure that where nutrition support is provided it is not so invasive or unacceptable that it impairs rather than improves quality of life.
- Nutritional screening tools which determine need for nutritional intervention by assigning a point score may fail to capture the subtleties of need within this particularly vulnerable population and lead to inappropriate prioritisation of care.
- In advanced progressive illness the anorexia cachexia syndrome (ACS) is prevalent, with persistent weight loss occurring despite provision of conventional nutrition support. Factors that may contribute to ACS include both a reduction of nutrient intake and improper nutrient utilisation as well as activation of cytochemical processes which lead to the body moving to a predominantly catabolic state.
- Many pharmacological treatments have been used or trialled in the treatment of ACS. Whilst effective in promoting appetite and mood, glucocorticoids should not be used for ACS treatment as they contribute to muscle weakness and fatigue and do not promote lean muscle accumulation. Progestogens are less harmful than glucocorticoids with similar effects on appetite

and mood but take longer to show benefits and still do not increase lean body mass.

- Pharmacological agents which show promise in the treatment of ACS and warrant further study include prokinetics, branched chain amino acids, eicosapentaenoic acid, cannabinoids, melatonin, thalidomide and anabolic steroids.
- Within palliative care the dietitian's role is one of education and communication. Addressing needs sooner, ensuring patient and carers participate in treatment choice and communicating treatment plans to colleagues may help to improve nutritional care in the later stages, which may positively impact on the patient's quality of life.
- Dietitians caring for patients at the end of life must have a thorough understanding of disease trajectories and the ethical issues surrounding treatment goals. Consideration must be made of the patient's right to choose and the issues of non-maleficence, beneficence and justice in treatment choices. Consideration must be given to the patient's nutritional problems within the greater context of their illness trajectory and their combined physical, psychological, social and spiritual needs. By examining what helps some individuals to survive and thrive in the face of difficult or tragic life events, dietitians can develop and deepen their understanding of appropriate support and care.
- Dietitians cannot provide nutritional solutions for all eventualities. They can, however, have an active and vital role in supporting patients through their life choices until death. Within palliative care the focus of nutritional therapy is on caring rather than curing.

Case study

M was an 84-year-old gentleman with advanced dementia, living in a care home which catered for the elderly mentally infirm. During an acute hospital admission for suspected aspiration pneumonia, M had commenced artificial feeding through a PEG tube and all oral feeding was disallowed. Since insertion of the PEG tube M was repeatedly admitted to a local care of the elderly unit for management of complications arising from his repeated pulling at the tube, including tube displacement and abdominal excoriation. M became very agitated every time anyone attempted to connect his PEG tube to

the giving set or when the tube was used to administer medications. On advice of the psychogeriatrician M was commenced on a steadily increasing dose of sedative and as a consequence was rarely awake or out of bed.

M was referred to the specialist palliative care dietitian by the care home nursing staff. They were concerned that the current management of M's nutritional needs was severely impacting on his quality of life and were uncomfortable with the constant administration of medication to sedate him.

Continued

Case study (Continued)

Nursing staff described M as a man who had been pleasantly confused. Now rarely mobile, M had previously been very active and had often visited his wife who was also resident in the same care home. They had raised their concerns with M's nephew who was his closest relative, after his wife, but he had been adamant that feeding should continue, as to stop would amount to starving his uncle to death.

Following a discussion with M's key workers, a case conference was called by the specialist palliative care dietitian. In attendance were M's case manager, the nursing staff in the nursing home and M's nephew. M's general practitioner was also invited and whilst he declined attendance he gave his support to the case review.

Led by the palliative care dietitian the team sensitively discussed with M's nephew the current management of M and how it would not be in his best interests for care to continue as was. Agreement was made that PEG feeding would cease but the tube would remain in situ for administering medications until it was displaced or removed by M, or if its presence was seen to be causing M distress. An urgent review by the speech and language therapist was arranged for advice on safest consistency and appropriate positioning for feeding to allow the recommencement of oral intake for pleasure.

M's feed was discontinued along with sedation and he became brighter, returning to his previous level of pleasant confusion and ability to visit his wife and interact with care staff. Oral feeding was reestablished to the obvious delight of M, who ate his altered consistency diet with little encouragement. The PEG tube was able to be left in situ as M was no longer pulling at it, nor appeared distressed by its presence and the care staff were able to administer medications and water flushes via this route.

Following several weeks of improved health M finally developed a chest infection and died peacefully in his sleep with appropriate end of life comfort care.

QUESTIONS

1. When a patient is unable to communicate their wishes for care and treatment, legally who is able to make care decisions for them?
2. For a patient with dementia whose swallow is impaired is it appropriate to withhold food and fluids?

ANSWERS

1. When a patient is unable to communicate their wishes for care and treatment, legally who is able to make care decisions for them?

   a. A decision to withhold or withdraw life-sustaining treatment is extremely difficult for patients, families and healthcare workers but can be an important part of good medical care. The Mental Capacity Act 2005 enables people in England and Wales to draw up a 'lasting power of attorney' and appoint a friend or family member to make treatment decisions on their behalf if they become too mentally incapacitated to make such decisions.

   b. Doctors will have to be satisfied that the patient lacks capacity to make the decision and that the scope of the lasting power of attorney is broad enough to cover the particular decision. If competent and appropriately informed, a patient retains the right to make decisions about their own care, even if these decisions appear to others as eccentric or unwise.

2. For a patient with dementia whose swallow is impaired is it appropriate to withhold food and fluids?

   Oral nutrition and hydration are basic human needs and should not be withheld or withdrawn; however, at the end of life a person's desire for food and drink lessens and intake naturally declines. Speech and language therapists can enable patients to benefit from the sensory rewards and social interaction of eating whilst reducing aspiration risk.

References

1. World Health Organization. *National Cancer Control Programmes: Policies and Guidelines*. Geneva: World Health Organization; 2002.
2. National Institute for Clinical Excellence (NICE). *Guidance on Cancer Services: Improving Supportive and Palliative Care for Adults with Cancer—The Manual.* London: NICE; 2004.
3. Northern Ireland Cancer Network. *A Framework for Generalist and Specialist Palliative and End-of-Life Care Competency.* Belfast: NICaN; 2008.
4. National Council for Hospice and Specialist Palliative Care Services. *Definitions of Supportive and Palliative Care*. London: NCHSPCS; 2002. Briefing Bulletin 11.
5. Ellershaw J, Wilkinson S, eds. *Care of the Dying: A Pathway to*

Excellence. Oxford: Oxford University Press; 2003.

6. Thomas K. *The Gold Standards Framework: A Framework for Community Palliative Care*. Online. Available at: http://www.goldstandardsframework.nhs.uk Accessed 6 October 2008.

7. Department of Health. *Building on the Best: Choice, Responsiveness and Equity in the NHS*. London: HMSO; 2003.

8. Souhami R, Tobias J. *Cancer and Its Management*. 4th edn. Oxford: Blackwell; 2003.

9. National Council for Hospice and Specialist Palliative Care Services. *Dilemmas and Directions: The Future of Specialist Palliative Care*. A discussion paper. London: NCHSPCS; 1997.

10. National Council for Palliative Care. *Focus on Commissioning*. London: NCPC; 2007.

11. Northern Ireland Cancer Network. *Diagnosing Dying. Defining End of Life Care: A Position Paper*. Belfast: NICaN; 2007.

12. Saunders C. Care of the dying—1. The problem of euthanasia. *Nurs Times*. 1976;72(26):1003–1005.

13. Graham F, Clarke D. The changing model of palliative care. *Medicine*. 2007;36(2):64–66.

14. Thomas K. Palliative care. *Geriatric Med*. 2006;36(6):9–13.

15. Davies E, Higginson IJ, eds. *The Solid Facts: Palliative Care*. Copenhagen: WHO; 2004.

16. National Council for Palliative Care. *20:20 Vision: The Shape of the Future for Palliative Care*. London: NCPC; 2005.

17. Addington-Hall JM, Higginson I, eds. *Palliative Care for Non-cancer Patients*. Oxford: Oxford University Press; 2001.

18. Sinclair A, Dickinson E. *Effective Practice in Rehabilitation: The Evidence of Systematic Reviews*. London: Kings Fund Institute; 1998.

19. National Council for Hospice and Specialist Palliative Care. *Fulfilling Lives: Rehabilitation in Palliative Care*. London: NCHSPCS; 2000.

20. *Gold Standards Framework. Prognostic Indicator Guidance. NHS End of Life Care Programme*. Online. Available at: http://www.

goldstandardsframework.nhs.uk Accessed 18 September 2008.

21. Maughan RJ. Impact of mild dehydration on wellness and on exercise performance. *Eur J Clin Nutr*. 2003;57(suppl 2):S19–S23.

22. Hassall S, Gill T. Providing care to the elderly with depression: the views of aged care staff. *J Psychiatr Ment Health Nurs*. 2008;15:17–23.

23. Caro MMM, Laviano A, Pichard C. Nutritional interventions and quality of life in adult oncology patients. *Clin Nutr*. 2007;26:289–301.

24. Elmadfa I, Meyer AL. Body composition, changing physiological functions and nutrient requirements of the elderly. *Ann Nutr Metab*. 2008;52(suppl 1):2–5.

25. Carey I. Cancer cachexia. *Palliative Care Today*. 2000;19:20–22.

26. MacDonald N. Cancer cachexia and targeting chronic inflammation: a unified approach to cancer treatment and palliative/supportive care. *J Support Oncol*. 2007;5(4):157–162.

27. Alibhai SM, Greenwood C, Payette H. An approach to the management of unintentional weight loss in elderly people. *CMAJ*. 2005;172(6):773–780.

28. Richardson R, Davidson I. The contribution of the dietician and nutritionist to palliative medicine. In: Doyle D, Hanks G, Cherny N, Calman K, eds. *Oxford Textbook of Palliative Medicine*. 3rd edn. Oxford: Oxford University Press; 2004: 1047–1050.

29. Aston T. Nutrition in palliative care: effective or ineffective? *JCN Online*. 2006;20(10):41–44.

30. Davis MP, Dickerson D. Cachexia and anorexia: cancer's covert killer. *Support Care Cancer*. 2000;8: 180–187.

31. Pennington CR. Disease-associated malnutrition in the year 2000. *Postgrad Med J*. 1998;74:65–71.

32. Haylett T, Johnston J. Palliative care in the community. *Complete Nutrition*. 2006;6(1):14–16.

33. Barton AD, Beigg CL, MacDonald IA, et al. A recipe for improving food intakes in elderly hospitalized patients. *Clin Nutr*. 2000;19(6):451–454.

34. Hill D, Hart K. A practical approach to nutritional support for patients

with advanced cancer. *Int J Palliat Nurs*. 2001;7(7):317–321.

35. Holder H. Nursing management of nutrition in cancer and palliative care. *Br J Nurs*. 2003;12(11): 667–674.

36. Wallengren O, Lundholm K, Bosaeus I. Diet energy density and energy intake in palliative care cancer patients. *Clin Nutr*. 2005;24: 266–273.

37. Walton K, Williams P, Bracks J, et al. A volunteer feeding assistance program can improve dietary intakes of elderly patients—a pilot study. *Appetite*. 2008;51:244–248.

38. Powell-Tuck J, Hennessey EM. A comparison of mid upper arm circumference, body mass index and weight loss as indices of undernutrition in acutely hospitalized patients. *Clin Nutr*. 2003;22(3):307–312.

39. World Health Organization. *Physical status: the use and interpretation of anthropometry*. Report of a WHO Expert Committee. Geneva: WHO; 1995. Technical Report Series 854.

40. Bray GA, Greenway FL, Molitch ME, et al. Use of anthropometric measures to assess weight loss. *Am J Clin Nutr*. 1978; 31(5):769–773.

41. Massarotto A, Carter H, Macleod R, et al. Hospital referrals to a hospice: timing of referrals, referrers' expectations, and the nature of referral information. *J Palliat Care*. 2000;16(3):22–29.

42. Findlay L, Hourston P, Kelly A, et al. *Allied Health Professional Services for Cancer Related Palliative Care: An Assessment of Need*. Allied Health Professions Palliative Care Project Team of the Glasgow Palliative Care Information Network; 2004. Online. Available at: http://www.palliativecareglasgow.info/pdf/AHPreport.pdf.

43. Northern Ireland Cancer Network (NICaN). *AHP Integrated Care Pathways for Cancer*. Belfast: NICaN; 2007.

44. Cherny NI. The problem of suffering. In: Doyle D, Hanks G, Cherny N, Calman K, eds. *Oxford Textbook of Palliative Medicine*. 3rd edn. Oxford: Oxford University Press; 2004:7–14.

45. Shragge JE, Wismer WV, Olson KL, et al. Shifting to conscious control: psychosocial and dietary management of anorexia by patients with advanced cancer. *Palliat Med.* 2007;21:227–233.

46. Hopkinson JB, Wright DNM, McDonald JW, et al. The prevalence of concern about weight loss and change in eating habits in people with advanced cancer. *J Pain Symptom Manage.* 2006;32(4):322–331.

47. Hopkinson JB. How people with advanced cancer manage changing eating habits. *J Adv Nurs.* 2007;59(5):454–462.

48. Corben S, Rosen R. *Self-management for Long-term Conditions. Patients' Perspectives on the Way Ahead.* London: King's Fund; 2005.

49. Brooks M. Assessment in palliative care. In: Cooper J, ed. *Stepping into Palliative Care 2: Care and Practice.* Oxford: Radcliffe Medical Press; 2006.

50. Cooper J. *Occupational Therapy in Oncology and Palliative Care.* 2nd edn. Chichester: Wiley; 2006.

51. Poole K, Froggatt K. Loss of weight and loss of appetite in advanced cancer: a problem for the patient, the carer, or the health professional? *Palliat Med.* 2002;16:499–506.

52. Nourissat A, Vasson MP, Merrouche Y, et al. Relationship between nutritional status and quality of life in patients with cancer. *Eur J Cancer.* 2008;44(9):1238–1242.

53. McClement SE, Harlos M. When advanced cancer patients won't eat: family responses. *Int J Palliat Nurs.* 2008;14(4):182–188.

54. Meares CJ. Primary caregiver perceptions of intake cessation in patients who are terminally ill. *Oncol Nurs Forum.* 1997;24:1751–1757.

55. Hill FJ. Complementary and alternative medicine: the next generation of health promotion? *Health Promot Int.* 2003;18(3):265–272.

56. Mercadante S, Fulfaro F, Casuccio A. The use of corticosteroids in home palliative care. *Support Care Cancer.* 2001;9(5):386–389.

57. Loprinzi CL, Kugler JW, Sloan JA, et al. Randomized comparison of megestrol acetate versus dexamethasone versus fluoxymesterone for the treatment of cancer anorexia/cachexia. *J Clin Oncol.* 1999;17(10):3299–3306.

58. Mateen F, Jatoi A. Megestrol acetate for the palliation of anorexia in advanced, incurable cancer patients. *Clin Nutr.* 2006;25:711–715.

59. Nelson KA, Walsh TD. Metoclopramide in anorexia caused by cancer-associated dyspepsia syndrome (CADS). *J Palliat Care.* 1993;9(2):14–18.

60. Blomstrand E, Eliasson J, Karlsson HK, et al. Branched-chain amino acids activate key enzymes in protein synthesis after physical exercise. *J Nutr.* 2006;136(1 suppl):269S–273S.

61. Bauer J, Capra S, Battistutta D, et al. Compliance with nutrition prescription improves outcomes in patients with unresectable pancreatic cancer. *Clin Nutr.* 2005;24:998–1004.

62. Dewey A, Baughan C, Dean T, et al. Eicosapentaenoic acid (EPA, an omega-3 fatty acid from fish oils) for the treatment of cancer cachexia. *Cochrane Database Syst Rev.* 2007;(1):CD004597.

63. Altun A, Ugur-Altun B. Melatonin: therapeutic and clinical utilization. *Int J Clin Pract.* 2007;61(5):835–845.

64. Sanger GJ. Endocannabinoids and the gastrointestinal tract: what are the key questions? *Br J Pharmacol.* 2007;152:663–670.

65. Lissoni P, Paolorossi F, Tancini G, et al. Is there a role for melatonin in the treatment of neoplastic cachexia? *Eur J Cancer.* 1996;32A(8):1340–1343.

66. Persson C, Glimelius B, Ronnelid J, et al. Impact of fish oil and melatonin on cachexia in patients with advanced gastrointestinal cancer: a randomized pilot study. *Nutrition.* 2005;21(2):170–178.

67. Silverman WA. The schizophrenic career of a 'monster drug'. *Pediatrics.* 2002;110(2):404–406.

68. Gordon JN, Trebble TM, Ellis RD, et al. Thalidomide in the treatment of cancer cachexia: a randomised placebo controlled trial. *Gut.* 2005;54(4):540–545.

69. Klausner JD, Makonkawkeyoon S, Akarasewi P, et al. Treatment with thalidomide in AIDS patients. *Internat Conf AIDS.* 1994;10(1):221.

70. Strasser F, Palmer JL, Schover LR, et al. The impact of hypogonadism and autonomic dysfunction on fatigue, emotional function, and sexual desire in male patients with advanced cancer: a pilot study. *Cancer.* 2006;107(12):2949–2957.

71. Basaria S, Wahlstrom JT, Dobs AS. Anabolic-androgenic steroid therapy in the treatment of chronic diseases. *J Clin Endocrinol Metab.* 2001;86(11):5108–5117.

72. Monroe B, Oliviere D, eds. *Resilience and Palliative Care: Achievement in Adversity.* Oxford: Oxford University Press; 2007.

73. Beauchamp TL. The 'four principles' approach to healthcare ethics. In: Ashford R, Dawson A, Draper H, McMillan J, eds. *Principles of Healthcare Ethics.* 2nd edn. Wiley: Chichester; 2007.

74. Shaw S. Exploring the concepts behind truth-telling in palliative care. *Int J Palliat Nurs.* 2008;14(7):356–359.

75. *Mental Capacity Act.* London: HMSO.

76. Ankeny RA, Clifford R, Jordens CF, et al. Religious perspectives on the withdrawal of treatment from patients with multiple organ failure. *MJA.* 2005;183:616–621.

77. Gillick M. Artificial nutrition and hydration in the patient with advanced dementia: is withholding treatment compatible with traditional Judaism. *J Med Ethics.* 2001;27:12–15.

78. Koch T. The challenge of Terri Schiavo: lessons for bioethics. *J Med Ethics.* 2005;31:376–378.

79. Quill T, Byock IR. Responding to intractable terminal suffering: the role of terminal sedation and voluntary refusal of food and fluids: position paper. *Ann Intern Med.* 2000;132:408–414.

80. Van der Riet P, Good P, Higgins IJ, et al. Palliative care professionals' perceptions of nutrition and hydration at the end of life. *Int J Palliat Nurs.* 2008;14(3):145151.

81. National Council for Palliative Care. *Artificial Nutrition and Hydration: Guidance at the End of Life.* London: NCPC; 2007.

82. Finucane TE, Christmas C, Travis K. Tube feeding in patients with advanced dementia: a review of the evidence. *JAMA*. 1999;282: 1365–1370.

83. Higaki F, Yokota O, Ohishi M. Factors predictive of survival after percutaneous endoscopic gastrostomy in the elderly: is dementia really a risk factor? *Am J Gastroenterol*. 2008;103(4): 1018–1020.

84. Koretz RL. Do data support nutrition support? Part II. Enteral artificial nutrition. *J Am Diet Assoc*. 2007;107(8):1374–1380.

85. Koretz RL, Avenell A, Lipman TO, et al. Does enteral nutrition affect clinical outcome? A systematic review of the randomized trials. *Am J Gastroenterol*. 2007;102(2): 412–429.

86. Wijk H, Grimby A. Needs of elderly patients in palliative care. *Am J Hosp Palliat Care*. 2007;25(2):106–111.

87. Mullard E. Presencing: the unseen therapeutic relationship. In: Nyatanga B, Astley-Pepper M, eds. *Hidden Aspects of Palliative Care*. London: Quay Books; 2005.

Renal disease

16

Avril Collinson

LEARNING OBJECTIVES

By the end of this chapter the reader will be able to:

- Understand the delicate balance between the clinical chemistry and metabolic stability in renal disease;
- Assess the nutritional status of a renal patient and give appropriate intervention to optimise nutritional status; and
- Be familiar with the appropriate dietary advice for acute and chronic kidney disease.

Introduction

The optimal diet for renal disease has been the subject of much controversy in recent years. Low protein diets have been in and out of fashion for the treatment of chronic kidney disease (CKD). What is the latest advice? Markers of malnutrition are known to strongly predict morbidity and mortality rates in patients with renal failure; what nutrition interventions optimise nutritional status? Managing cardiovascular disease—what is the evidence for controlling lipid levels? The question of whether vitamin supplementation benefits renal patients is another area of much controversy, especially with the emerging importance of homocysteine.

This chapter will look at these complex and often controversial topics to piece together recommendations for the dietary management of CKD, using the latest available evidence. The five stages of CKD will be defined and the dietary recommendations for these stages will be discussed. The assessment of nutritional status in renal patients and the influence of diet on blood pressure will be reviewed. The dietary management of acute renal failure, nephrotic syndrome and renal transplantation will also be briefly outlined.

Physiology of the kidney

The kidneys, which are approximately 10 cm long and 5 cm wide, are located on the posterior wall of the abdomen at waist level. The kidney is a vital organ in the body and has a number of essential functions as shown in Table 16.1. The kidney allows a person to eat and drink as desired without causing disturbances in the composition of their intracellular and extracellular fluid compartments.

Classification of renal disease

Creatinine and urea are commonly measured as indicators of kidney function; however, both have their limitations. Creatinine is a metabolite from muscle and is excreted by the kidneys. An individual's normal creatinine level will therefore depend on their muscle mass, age and gender. Urea is a small molecule produced in the liver from dietary protein consumed and is also excreted by the kidneys. As dehydration, dietary protein intake and liver disease can significantly influence urea levels, this test is an unreliable marker of renal disease.

Each kidney consists of approximately a million filters known as glomeruli. The glomerular filtration rate (GFR) is an estimate of the filtering capacity of the kidneys and is used as a more accurate measure of

Table 16.1 Functions of the kidney

Excretion of waste products (urea, creatinine, uric acid and other nitrogenous compounds)

Regulation of fluid balance

Regulation of blood pressure (renin–angiotensin mechanism)

Acid–base balance

Activation of vitamin D (25–hydroxycholecalciferol to 1,25-dihydroxycholecalciferol)

Production of erythropoietin (EPO)

Elimination and detoxification of drugs and toxins

Regulation of metabolic processes (gluconeogenesis, lipid metabolism)

Degradation and catabolism of hormones (insulin, glucagon, growth hormone, parathyroid hormone)

Electrolyte homeostasis (sodium, potassium, phosphate)

Regulating the metabolism of calcium and phosphorus to prevent renal osteodystrophy

kidney disease. It is expressed as millilitres (mL) per minute (min) and adjusted to a 'standard' body size with a surface area of 1.73 m^2. The normal GFR range is between 90 and 130 mL/min/1.73m^2 but GFR is dependant on age, gender and body size. For example, if a GFR of 100 mL/min/1.73 m^2 is referred to as normal or 100% of kidney function, this means that a GFR of 30 mL/min/1.73m^2 represents approximately 30% of kidney function. From the age of mid-thirties a slow decrease of about 1% of GFR/year is generally seen. For example, at 70 years of age, the GFR is on average only 60–70% of the normal value.

In 1994, the Modification of Diet in Renal Disease Study Group (MDRD) published a study involving 1,628 patients that looked at the effects of dietary protein restriction and blood pressure control on kidney disease progression.[1] Using these results a formula that predicted GFR using demographic characteristics such as age, race, gender and the serum creatinine level was created. The MDRD formula was compared with the earlier Cockcroft-Gault prediction formula and found to correlate better with isotope GFR.[2] In addition it did not require the patient's weight; hence, the MDRD formula is now the recommended method for estimating GFR (eGFR).[3]

The US National Kidney Foundation-Kidney Disease Outcome Quality Initiative (NKF-K/DOQI) classification of CKD divides CKD into five stages based on GFR as shown in Table 16.2.[4] This classification, which enables the level of CKD in individual patients to be determined, has been adopted internationally. The National Institute for Health and Clinical Excellence (NICE) 2008 guidelines on CKD recommend Stage 3 CKD should be split into two subcategories as shown below and gives guidance on the management of CKD.[5] Progression of CKD is defined as a decline in eGRF of > 5 mL/min/1.73m^2 per year.

The NHS is increasingly focusing on prevention, early detection and the treatment of renal disease. It is estimated that 30% of people with advanced

Table 16.2 Stages of CKD 1-5

Stage	Description	GFR (mL/min/1.73 m²)
1	Normal kidney function (GFR) but with another abnormality[a]	> 90
2	Mild impairment of kidney function but with another abnormality[a]	60–89
3A	Moderate impairment of kidney function	45–59
3B	Moderate impairment of kidney function	30–44
4	Severe impairment of kidney function	15–29
5	Very severe or established renal failure (ERF)	< 15

[a]Already known to have proteinuria, haematuria, microalbuminurea, polycystic kidney disease or reflux nephropathy, or a biopsy-proven chronic glomerulonephritis.

kidney disease are referred late to nephrology services from both primary and secondary care and ultimately this is associated with significant cost and poor clinical outcomes.[5,6] The Quality and Outcomes Framework (QOF), a fundamental part of the new general practitioners contract, offers financial rewards for detecting CKD. As a result of the QOF, eGFR is now measured routinely in the community and more care at the earlier stages of CKD is being delivered by primary care. The NICE guidelines on CKD also promote the monitoring of kidney function in at-risk populations (individuals with hypertension, diabetes, vascular disease, urological abnormalities, family history of kidney disease or drugs affecting the kidney).[5]

In Stage 5 where established renal failure (ERF) has been reached, many patients will require renal replacement therapy (RRT) to maintain life. RRT involves regular dialysis or a kidney transplant. ERF is an irreversible, long-term condition and some people with ERF will decide on conservative management only.

At the end of 2006, 43,901 adult patients were receiving RRT in the UK, a population prevalence of 725 pmp, an increase from 694 pmp in 2005. Of these patients receiving RRT, 45% had a transplant, 43% were on centre-based haemodialysis (HD), 1% on home haemodialysis and 11% on peritoneal dialysis (PD). The median age of patients starting RRT was 65 years. The data reported here have been supplied by the UK Renal Registry of the Renal Association.[7]

As well as being a marker of the progression of CKD, eGFR is thought to be a powerful predictor of cardiovascular risk.[8] Estimated GFR should be interpreted with caution in patients where there are extremes of muscle mass, for example, in severe cases of muscle wasting or bodybuilders. In these patients a reduced muscle mass will lead to an overestimation and an increased muscle mass will lead to an underestimation of the eGFR. Ethnicity should also be considered. For example, people of Afro-Caribbean origin tend to have a greater muscle mass as compared to non Afro-Caribbeans and so it is recommended that eGRF is multiplied by 1.21 to correct for this.

Causes and incidence of renal disease

CKD is now recognised as a global public health problem.[9] Diabetes and hypertension are well-known risk factors for renal disease. Body mass index has been

Table 16.3 Common causes of established renal failure in the UK

Diabetes	22.2%
Glomerulonephritis[a]	10.4%
Pyelonephritis	7.2%
Renal vascular disease	6.8%
Polycystic kidney	6.7%
Hypertension	5.4%

[a]Biopsy proven.

found to be an independent predictor for CKD after adjustments for blood pressure level and presence or absence of diabetes mellitus.[10] Two studies in the UK have reported a higher incidence of CKD in areas with higher social deprivation scores.[11]

Current estimates suggest that 5–11% of the global population have CKD, defined as a GFR < 60 mL/min/1.73 m^2.[12,13] A figure of 8.5% has been quoted for the prevalence of stage 3–5 CKD in the UK.[14] In the UK estimates of CKD stage 3 are 4.6–4.8%; however, prevalence is associated with age, as 30.5% of men and 37.5% of women in their 80s are estimated to have CKD stage 3.[15] The question is asked as to whether a low GFR in elderly people is just a normal part of the physiological process of ageing and some question the appropriateness of applying GFR to all ages. The prevalence of CKD has been reported as higher in certain ethnic minority groups in the UK.

Table 16.3 shows the main causes of ERF as taken from the UK renal registry data 2006.[7] Worldwide these figures are known to vary considerably.

Slowing the progression of renal disease

There are many ways to slow the progression of renal disease.

Hypertension

Hypertension is a cause of CKD, but it is also a consequence of failing kidneys so the control of blood pressure is important. The use of angiotensin converting enzyme (ACE) inhibitors and/or angiotensin receptor blockers (ARBs) is considered to be the most effective in slowing the progression of CKD.[16] Proteinuria as a result of increased leakage from the glomeruli or from a decreased tubular reabsorption is a marker of CKD, and may cause progression of CKD.[17] Albumin:creatinine ratio (ACR) is the test of choice to identify proteinuria in people with diabetes and is already widely used in practice. Albumin is the predominant component of proteinuria in glomerular disease and the ACR test is considered to be a sensitive test for detecting early CKD.

NICE guidelines for recommended blood pressure (BP) targets for CKD are < 140/90 and < 130/80 mmHg in patients with diabetes or those with an ACR > 70 mg/mmol or urinary protein excretion > 1 g/24 h.[5]

Dietary management of hypertension

A consistent body of evidence from observational studies and clinical trials indicates that body weight is positively associated with BP and hypertension. A meta-analysis of randomised controlled trials (RCTs) revealed that a weight loss of approximately 5 kg led to a reduction of about 4.4 and 3.6 mmHg in systolic and diastolic BP, respectively.[18] Expressed per kilogram of weight loss this equates to a reduction of 1.05 mmHg in systolic and 0.92 mmHg in diastolic. Another high-quality systematic review in hypertensive individuals suggested that dietary measures which achieve a 3–9% reduction in body weight are likely to reduce systolic and diastolic pressure by about 3 mmHg.[19]

The relationship between salt and BP is often difficult to establish as accurate intakes of sodium intake or excretion are hard to obtain, and adherence to a salt restriction can often be poor. Some researchers believe individuals should be classified as salt-sensitive or resistant.[20] Although at present there is no way of detecting which individuals are salt sensitive, salt sensitivity appears to be more frequent amongst individuals with hypertension and/or diabetes, in black and/or older individuals.[21,22] Some believe that salt sensitivity is a transient phenomenon during the pathogenesis and development of hypertension.[23] Since the phenomenon of salt sensitivity has not been characterised it is not yet possible to identify and develop predictive markers, including genetic polymorphisms, for individuals.

This phenomenon may explain some of the variations found in the literature; however, many findings from epidemiological and intervention studies do conclude a positive relationship between salt and BP.[24–26] There is also a suggestion by some researchers that salt exposure is linked with kidney tissue injury.[27]

Several epidemiologic studies have established that dietary potassium intake is inversely related to BP.[28] An increase in potassium consumption has been shown to lower BP or reduce antihypertensive medication, especially in people who are hypertensive.[29,30] Dietary recommendations should therefore advise on an increase in fruit and vegetable consumption to help reduce BP, unless blood potassium levels are raised. This can often lead to confusion in CKD patients as they may be advised later on to reduce their intake of fruit and vegetables to help control their blood potassium levels.

For further information on hypertension please refer to the chapter on cardiovascular disease.

Diabetes

In diabetic patients, keeping glycated haemoglobin (HbA1c) levels to normal or near normal (<7.5%) has been shown to either delay the onset of diabetic nephropathy or slow the progression.[31–33] For further information on glycaemic control please refer to the chapter on diabetes.

Cardiovascular disease

The great majority of patients with early CKD will have an increased risk of cardiovascular disease (CVD).[34] It has been stated that patients with a GFR < 60 mL/min/1.73 m^2 have a higher risk of cardiovascular death, and 74% of patients on dialysis have heart damage.[35–37] The risk of CVD in patients with CKD far outweighs the risk of progression of the disease. A retrospective cohort study found that only 4% of 1,076 individuals progressed to ERF over a 5.5-year follow-up period, 69% had died at the end of follow-up and the cause of death was cardiovascular in 46% of cases.[11]

In the general population the relationship between dyslipidaemia and CVD is well known; however, in CKD patients it is still controversial. Although dyslipidemia has been associated with CKD, it is still uncertain whether lipid-lowering therapy will reduce CVD. The spectrum of dyslipidae-mia in CKD is distinct from the general population and the optimal targets for plasma lipids in people with CKD are not yet known. Lipid levels are found to vary with the stage of CKD and presence of diabetes and/or nephrotic syndrome.[38–41] Lipoprotein(a) is also influenced by CKD and the degree of proteinuria.[38,42]

Lipid-lowering therapy has been found to modestly reduce the rate of kidney function loss in patients with moderately impaired kidney function (stage 3A) with or at risk of CVD.[43] A number of other researchers have also suggested that managing risk factors for CVD may slow the rate of decline of kidney function.[44,45] Evidence for the beneficial effects of lipid therapy on reducing CVD risk in CKD is, however, scarce. A randomised, placebo-controlled, intervention trial on lipid-lowering therapy in ERF patients with diabetes showed no significant reduction in primary endpoint of cardiovascular death, nonfatal myocardial infarction or stroke by statin therapy.[46] One explanation for this could be a higher significance of structural heart disease (e.g. vascular calcification, left ventricular failure) rather than classical myocardial infarction in advanced kidney disease. Results of a larger clinical trial, the Study of Heart and Renal Protection (SHARP), which is currently investigating 9,000 CKD patients will hopefully help to answer the question of whether lipid-lowering therapy is beneficial in CKD.[47]

The NICE guidelines on CKD currently recommend that people with CKD and coronary disease should be treated according to existing guidelines and those who do not have evidence of coronary disease should be treated according to their estimated risk, using the Joint British Societies Guidelines.[5] Statins should be offered for the secondary prevention of CVD irrespective of baseline values.

Anaemia

Anaemia is very common in CKD due to a reduction in erythropoietin production. There is increasing evidence that correcting anaemia may have favourable effects on the progression of CKD.[48] Guidelines for haemoglobin targets have been developed, but there is no consistent agreement on the appropriate level. NICE recommend anaemia treatment should aim to maintain stable haemoglobin levels between 10.5 and 12.5 g/dL. One study, the Correction of Hemoglobin and

Outcomes in Renal Insufficiency (CHOIR), investigating whether achieving higher haemoglobin targets of 13.5 g/dL is beneficial was terminated as findings suggested an increased risk of CVD outcomes with these higher levels.[49]

Protein restriction

In the 1980s a number of animal studies showed that a low protein diet improved survival and slowed the progression of renal failure.[50–52] A meta-analysis in 1992 concluded that the use of low protein diets in humans also slowed the progression of renal disease.[53] In this meta-analysis 46 trials were looked at but only 6 reports of RCTs were selected. Many of the earlier human studies reporting benefits of low protein diets were flawed in their methodological approach, compliance with the prescribed protein intake was poor and little or no nutritional assessment was undertaken.

Results of two large multicentred studies were published in the 1990s. The Northern Italian Cooperative Study investigated 456 patients and found no difference in creatinine clearance when patients were randomly allocated protein intakes of either 1 g/kg or 0.6 g/kg body weight for a 2-year period. In this study the authors concluded that the underlying disease was more influential than the dietary changes but noted that compliance was poor with the 0.6 g/kg protein diet.[54]

The other study published was the MDRD study from the USA.[1] This trial operated as two concurrent studies, involving a total of 840 patients. In study 1 patients with a GFR of 25–55 mL/min/1.73 m^2 were randomly assigned to a usual protein diet (1.3 g/kg/day) or a low-protein diet (0.58 g/kg/day). Patients in study 2, with a GFR of 13–24 mL/min/1.73 m^2, were randomly assigned to the low protein diet or to a very low protein diet (0.28 g/kg/day) with a keto acid–amino acid supplement. No significant difference was found between the groups in the rate of decline of renal function in study 1. In study 2 the very low protein group had a marginally slower decline in glomerular filtration than the low protein group but there was no difference in the time to reach ERF or death.

As there were problems with compliance with the prescribed protein intake in the MDRD study, a secondary analysis was undertaken to examine the relationship between actual achieved protein intake and the rate of decline of renal function.[55] This secondary analysis pointed to a correlation between actual protein intake and a decreased rate of decline in GFR. However, as the analyses were made by correlation rather than 'intention to treat', this finding cannot be directly applied to the clinical setting.

A Cochrane review published in 2007 looked at 12 studies, including 9 RCTs, to assess the effects of protein restriction in diabetic renal patients.[56] The authors concluded that reducing protein intake appears to slightly slow progression of diabetic kidney disease but this is not statistically significant. The authors commented that individual variation existed so protein restriction may be beneficial in some individuals. No data were found on the effects of low protein diets on health-related quality of life.

Despite much research, the area of protein restriction and its possible effect of slowing the progression of CKD still remain controversial. Suggested reasons for limiting the protein intake of CKD patients include reducing uraemic symptoms, reducing acidosis and proteinuria and slowing the decline of kidney damage. Limitations over restricting protein intake have arisen, firstly, as concerns over a deterioration in nutritional status and associations between hypoalbuminaemia and increased mortality, and secondly because many patients already self-restrict their protein intake through imposed dietary restrictions or due to a loss of appetite and generally feeling unwell.[57,58] In view of the conflicting evidence, nutritional status and quality of life issues many UK units currently choose a moderate protein restriction of 0.8–1 g protein/kg ideal body weight.

Dietary advice for CKD

A number of guidelines have been published for the nutritional management of CKD.

- National Kidney Foundation–Kidney Disease Outcome Quality Initiative (NKF-K/DOQI), *Clinical Practice Guidelines for Nutrition of Chronic Renal Failure* (USA 2000).[59]
- American Dietetic Association (ADA) Medical Nutrition Therapy Evidence-Based Guides for Practice, *Chronic Kidney Disease (Non-dialysis) Medical Nutrition Therapy Protocol* (2002).[60]

- *ADA Guidelines for Nutritional Care of Renal Patients*, 3rd edn (2002).[61]
- European Dialysis and Transplantation Nurses Association/European Renal Care Association (EDTNA/ERCA), *Guidelines for the Nutritional Care of Adult Renal Patients* (2003).[62]
- Caring for Australians with Renal Impairment (CARI), *Nutrition and Growth in Kidney Disease Guidelines* (2005).[63]
- European Society for Clinical Nutrition and Metabolism (ESPEN), *Guidelines on Enteral Nutrition: Adult Renal Failure* (2006).[64]
- *Evidence Based Practice Guidelines for the Nutritional Management of CKD* (Australia/New Zealand 2006).[65]

The aims of dietary treatment for CKD are:

- To limit the build-up of waste products and help maintain fluid/electrolyte balance (urea, phosphate, potassium, fluid and salt);
- To prevent metabolic complications, e.g. renal bone disease, acidosis, anorexia, obesity;
- To attempt to delay the progression of renal failure;
- To optimise/maintain nutritional status; and
- If on dialysis, to replace nutrient losses associated with the dialysis process (nitrogen, vitamins and minerals).

Table 16.4 summarises an adapted version of the European guidelines for the nutritional care of adult renal patients. It is important to ensure that any nutritional restrictions do not compromise nutritional adequacy and quality of life. There is no agreed consensus for estimating ideal body weight (IBW) in patients outside of the normal BMI range and clinical judgement is often used. The European guidelines recommend that for a patient who is overweight (BMI > 25) IBW is calculated as the weight at a BMI of 25. Conversely if a patient is underweight (BMI < 20) IBW is calculated as the weight at a BMI of 20.

Variations do exist between the different guidelines; for example, the USA K/DOQI guidelines suggest a protein intake of 0.6–0.75 g/kg (at least 50% high biological value, HBV) for CKD stage 1–4 as compared to the Australia/New Zealand recommendation of 0.75–1 g protein (> 50% HBV) for CKD stage 3–4. For the calculation of IBW the Australia/New Zealand guidelines recommend that a modified BMI range of 23–26 should be taken as the normal range if a patient is on dialysis.[65]

Table 16.4 Adapted version of the European guidelines for the nutritional care of adult renal patients

	Pre-dialysis CKD stage 3–4	Haemodialysis CKD stage 5	Peritoneal dialysis CKD stage 5
Energy kcal	35 kcal/kg IBW[a] (30–35 kcal/kg IBW depending on age and activity)	35 kcal/kg IBW (30–35 kcal/kg IBW depending on age and activity)	35 kcal/kg IBW including calories from peritoneal absorption of glucose (30–35 kcal/kg IBW depending on age and activity)
Protein	0.6–1 g/kg IBW If < 0.8 ensure sufficient dietetic follow-up and > 55% HBV	1–1.2 g/kg IBW	1–1.2 g/kg IBW 1.5 g/kg IBW (peritonitis)
Phosphorus	600–1000 mg/day (19–32 mmol/day)	1000–1400 mg/day (32–45 mmol/day)	1000–1400 mg/day (32–45 mmol/day)
Potassium	2000–2500 mg/day (50–65 mmol/day)	2000–2500 mg/day (50–65 mmol/day)	If restricted 2000–2500 mg/day (50–65 mmol/day)
Sodium	1800–2500 mg/day (80–110 mmol/day)	1800–2500 mg/day (80–110 mmol/day)	1800–2500 mg/day (80–110 mmol/day)
Fluid	Restrict if required	500 mL plus PDUO[b]	800 mL plus PDUO

[a]IBW = Ideal body weight.
[b]PDUO = volume equal to previous day's (24 hr) urine output.
Adapted from the European Dialysis and Transplantation Nurses Association/European Renal Care Association (Dietitians Special Interest Group guidelines).[62]

CKD stages 1–4

Protein and energy

The incidence of protein energy malnutrition (PEM) increases with deteriorating kidney function and is associated with a poor outcome; therefore early dietetic intervention is important.[58] Most patients with a GFR < 30 should be referred to a dietitian. In view of the conflicting evidence around protein restriction many UK units choose a moderate protein restriction of 0.8–1 g protein/kg IBW. Renal dietitians will use protein exchanges to assess a patient's intake. Either 6 or 7 g protein exchanges are used for HBV protein and 2-g exchanges for low biological value (LBV) protein. It may not be appropriate to teach these to the patient. As patients become uraemic and symptomatic they often self-restrict protein anyway. Symptoms of uraemia can include loss of appetite, nausea and vomiting, taste changes, tiredness and itching.

An energy intake of 35 kcal/kg IBW is recommended to prevent nitrogen catabolism; however, obesity should be avoided as a BMI > 30 is associated with a variety of health problems. There are no randomised trials examining the safety and efficacy of low-fat diets in patients with CKD although dyslipidaemia is evident in a number of patients. Where possible lipid-lowering dietary measures should be advised when this is not at the detriment of the patient's nutritional status. Tight glycaemic control is essential in patients with diabetes to help slow the progression of CKD.

Potassium

The risk of developing hyperkalaemia is inversely related to renal function and it is only when at least 50% of the kidney function has been lost that the blood biochemistry is affected. Hyperkalaemia may occur as a result of impaired tubular secretion of potassium in patients with mild CKD. It is important for the dietitian to be aware that a number of other factors can contribute to hyperkalaemia: catabolism, certain medications (i.e. ACE inhibitors, potassium sparing diuretics, angiotensin receptor blockers), metabolic acidosis, blood transfusions, dehydration and constipation. Metabolic acidosis can develop with the progression of renal disease, and results in both hyperkalaemia and increased protein catabolism. Oral bicarbonate supplementation (or increasing the dialysate bicarbonate concentration if on dialysis) may be given to correct this, although this may contribute to greater sodium retention and hypertension.

Patients with serum potassium levels over 5.5 mmol/L are usually targeted for dietary advice if hyperkalaemia cannot be corrected by other means. It is important to check local guidelines for normal potassium ranges. Generally, a slow rise in serum potassium level, as seen with CKD, is tolerated better than an abrupt rise in potassium levels. Many patients with hyperkalaemia are asymptomatic, but the consequences of hyperkalaemia can be fatal as listed below:

- Paraesthesia in the extremities;
- Muscle weakness leading to possible flaccid paralysis;
- Diarrhoea due to smooth muscle hyperactivity; and
- Cardiac arrythmias and cardiac arrest.

Dietary advice for potassium restriction should be individually tailored to the patient. Advice should focus on altered cooking methods, suitable portion sizes and lower potassium food sources. As potassium is water-soluble one example of an altered cooking method is to recommend boiling potatoes and vegetables in large amounts of water instead of cooking in the microwave or steaming. The vegetable water must not be used to make gravy, soups or sauces.

If the serum potassium is slightly raised, only a few dietary changes may be advised although the patient should still be educated on which foods are high in potassium to avoid further problems. Table 16.5 gives a list of foods high in potassium which are normally limited and examples of lower potassium alternatives. The use of 4-mmol potassium exchanges can be useful for the renal dietitian and some patients may also benefit from this knowledge to allow more variety in their diet. Other patients may find this method too complex.

Potassium restrictions should only be advised if absolutely necessary as once patients have been advised to avoid certain foods they will often find it difficult to reintroduce these foods again. Remember to check the biochemistry first to see whether potassium restrictions are really required.

Table 16.5 Examples of high potassium foods (normally limited) with some lower potassium alternatives

High potassium foods	Lower potassium alternatives
Fruit juice	Squash drinks
Banana/grapes	Apple
Dried fruit	
Potatoes especially chips, sauté and jacket potato	Rice, pasta, boiled potatoes[a]
Potato crisps	Corn chips
Mushrooms	Cauliflower
Tomatoes	Carrots
Nuts	Popcorn
Chocolate	Sweets/mints
Fruit cake	Doughnut/sponge cake
Beer/wine	Spirits
Coffee	Tea
Milk[b]	
Soups	
Potassium-containing salt substitutes	

[a]Boiled potatoes usually limited to 125 g (5 oz) once/day.
[b]Milk usually limited to ½ pint/day.

Phosphorus and renal bone disease

The kidneys play a crucial role in regulating serum phosphate and calcium homeostasis, both directly and through the activation of vitamin D. Problems start to occur with the control mechanisms essential for calcium and phosphate homeostasis early in the course of CKD, before any abnormalities are seen in the biochemistry, and continue to progress as kidney function decreases.[66] As CKD advances, phosphate retention occurs and hypocalcaemia develops as the kidneys fail to activate vitamin D. Both hypocalcaemia and hyperphosphataemia stimulate an increase in the parathyroid hormone (PTH).[67,68]

Figure 16.1 • Hyperphosphataemia in chronic renal failure.

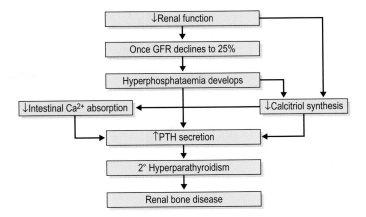

This condition shown in Figure 16.1 is known as secondary hyperparathyroidism. The excess parathyroid hormone then acts on bone to increase the release of calcium and phosphate. The blood levels of calcium and phosphate then increase, while the bones become weaker, a condition known as renal bone disease. Excess phosphate binds with calcium to form calcium phosphate which can be deposited in the heart, lungs, kidneys and other soft tissues. This is referred to as soft tissue calcification. There is evidence that poor calcium and phosphate control affect morbidity and mortality due to cardiovascular calcification.[69] Although many patients complain of itching, most are not aware of these serious developments until they experience bone pain and fractures.

Treatment for suppressing PTH levels includes a dietary phosphorus restriction, phosphate binders to limit the absorption of phosphorus and supplementation with active vitamin D and calcium-containing phosphate binders to help correct hypocalcaemia. In practice dietary phosphorus is normally referred to as phosphate to avoid confusion for patients.

Dietary phosphorus is mainly found in protein-rich foods as shown in Box 16.1. When advising on restrictions care should be taken that patients are not put at risk of PEM. Providing that the patient is not malnourished it is believed to be beneficial to consider a dietary phosphorus restriction early. PTH levels begin to rise when GFR falls below 60 mL/min/1.73 m² (CKD stage 3), even though serum phosphorus levels are normal, so levels of PTH are believed to be a better indicator of when to begin a dietary phosphorus restriction. K/DOQI clinical practice guidelines on bone metabolism and disease in CKD recommend that dietary phosphorus

Box 16.1

List of foods high in phosphorus

Cheese
Milk
Yoghurt
Poultry
Meat, particularly offal
Fish, particularly oily fish
Seafood
Eggs
Nuts
Chocolate

restrictions should be initiated when blood PTH levels begin to rise and/or when serum phosphate levels are elevated at any stage of CKD (normally > 1.4 mmol/L).[70]

Often a dietary phosphorus restriction is not sufficient to control phosphate levels so phosphate binders are required. Phosphate binders bind with phosphate in the digestive tract to form a compound that is not absorbed. It is therefore important that they are taken with meals and snacks which provide dietary phosphorus. There are three common types of phosphate binders: aluminium-based, calcium-based and aluminium-free/calcium-free phosphate binders.

Aluminium-based phosphate binders are very effective at controlling phosphorus. The most common binder of this type is aluminum hydroxide; however, aluminium is known to have toxic effects that can cause bone disease and damage the nervous system, so for this reason, aluminium-based phosphate binders are rarely used.

Calcium-based phosphate binders can be effective but do not bind phosphorus as well as aluminium. Common types of calcium-based binders used are calcium acetate and calcium carbonate. These binders can also serve as calcium supplements but taking too many will lead to an excess calcium load which can contribute to metastatic calcification in tissues and organs. Cardiac calcification can lead to heart damage and even death.

Aluminium-free/calcium-free phosphate binders, for example, sevelamar and lanthanum carbonate, are newer, more costly binders which have recently been introduced.

The appropriate prescription including the selection, dose and timing of phosphate binders is important for good phosphate control. The dietitian is the team member best suited to recommend when and how many phosphate binders patients should take. In some hospitals treatment protocols and patient group directions which allow the dietitian to both initiate and adjust phosphate binders independently of medical staff have been developed. These changes have been associated with improvements in patient care resulting in significantly better bone biochemistry.[71]

Sodium and fluid homeostasis

As kidney function deteriorates less sodium is excreted. The K/DOQI *Clinical Practice Guidelines on Hypertension and Antihypertensive Agents in Chronic Kidney Disease* recommend that most CKD patients should reduce sodium intake to 100 mmol/day to reduce extracellular fluid volume expansion and lower BP.[72] This is similar to the EDTNA/ERCA guidelines of 80–110 mmol/day, which is equivalent to a 'no added salt' diet.[62] A 'no added salt' diet is achieved by avoiding or minimising salt in cooking, not adding salt at the table and avoidance of too many processed foods. Salty foods, e.g. smoked or cured foods, should also be limited as much as possible. The use of herbs and spices are encouraged for flavouring. Patients are advised to avoid potassium-containing salt substitutes. Rarely some patients can be salt losers, identified by urinary sodium excretion, and may need sodium supplementation.

The recommended fluid intake for the majority of CKD patient's stage 1–4 is no different from the general population (30–35 mL/kg/IBW) as urine output is not reduced. However, a mild to moderate fluid restriction may be required for some patients especially if resistant oedema is present.

ERF (CKD stage 5)

Dialysis

Haemodialysis and peritoneal dialysis are only equivalent to approximately 10–15% of normal kidney function.

Peritoneal dialysis (PD)

In peritoneal dialysis (Figure 16.2) a Tenckhoff catheter is inserted into the peritoneal cavity and a 'glucose-based' dialysate is drained into the peritoneal cavity. The peritoneal membrane surrounding the intestine acts as a natural semi-permeable membrane. Uraemic toxins are removed from the blood into the dialysate by diffusion and fluid is removed by osmosis. In continuous ambulatory peritoneal dialysis (CAPD) the dialysate is drained into the peritoneum and after 4–6 hours drained out again. This process or exchange is repeated 4 or 5 times a day. Volumes of dialysate are 1–3 L and vary in concentration. Table 16.6 shows examples of different strengths of dialysate bags and the estimated energy absorbed from these bags. To optimise diabetic control and reduce peritoneal membrane exposure to glucose dialysis prescription regimens that

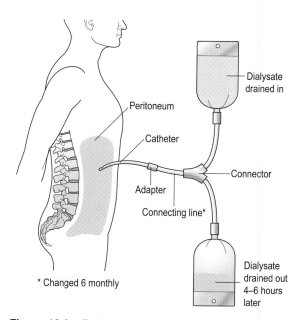

Figure 16.2 • Peritoneal dialysis.

Table 16.6 Examples of different strengths of 2-L PD bags and approximate energy absorbed from these

Strength of 2-L bag	Approximate energy absorbed
1.36% dextrose (light)	70 kcal
2.27% dextrose (medium)	120 kcal
3.86% dextrose (heavy)	200 kcal

incorporate less glucose and more glucose-free (amino acid, icodextrin) solutions are recommended.

In continuous cycler-assisted peritoneal dialysis (CCPD), also referred to as automated peritoneal dialysis (APD), a machine is programmed to carry out the exchanges usually overnight. The machine controls the fill volume, dwell time and length of treatment. This allows larger volumes of dialysate to be processed (up to 20 L). The patient usually has 2 L of dialysate fluid left in during the day and may need to carry out additional daytime manual exchanges.

Haemodialysis (HD)

In HD blood from the patient is pumped through a machine for the dialysis to take place. The dialysis machine contains a filtering unit called a dialyser or artificial kidney. This is a cylinder containing thousands of very small hollow tubes. Each of these hollow tubes is made of plastic and act as the dialysis membrane. Blood is pumped through the middle of these tubes and dialysis fluid is pumped around the outside, allowing dialysis to take place through the tiny holes of the tubes. HD is usually carried out three times a week, each session lasting between 3 and 5 hours. The length and frequency of dialysis sessions is adjusted individually to achieve optimal dialysis adequacy as measured by adequacy tests. Dialysis adequacy tests are performed in both PD and HD.

Protein and energy

Energy requirements are not influenced by dialysis and recommendations remain the same (30–35 kcal/kg IBW depending on age and activity). Energy requirements for PD patients also include the energy absorbed from the dialysate fluid (see Table 16.6). Interestingly, in CKD stage 5 a higher BMI or cholesterol level is not associated with an increased mortality rate.[73] Overnutrition is a well-known risk factor for CVD in the general population but in contrast seems to be protective and actually improves outcomes in dialysis patients. These paradoxical markers are referred to as *reverse epidemiology*. One explanation for this might be that overweight patients have more nutritionally complete diets and so meet their nutritional requirements.

A higher protein intake is recommended to compensate for the protein losses of dialysis (see Table 16.4). Studies have demonstrated that HD accelerates rates of whole body and muscle proteolysis, stimulating the release of amino acids from muscle breakdown.[74] The average loss of free amino acids in the dialysis fluid has been reported to be 5–8 g/dialysis during HD.[75] No difference in amino acid losses were reported between high and low flux membranes when dialysis dose and blood flow were adjusted.[76] It is estimated that protein lost across the peritoneum in PD can be 5–15 g/day and increase to 30 g/day during episodes of peritonitis.[77]

Malnutrition

Patients with CKD display a variety of metabolic and nutritional abnormalities and often show signs of protein–energy malnutrition. Studies estimate that 40–50% of HD and 18–50% of PD patients show some signs of malnutrition.[78–80] A strong relationship exists between the extent of malnutrition and mortality in CKD patients.[81,82] Reduced nutritional status prior to starting dialysis is a strong predictor of poor survival on dialysis.[83,84] In PD patients a poor outcome has been linked to a poor nutritional status.[85] In HD patients, a reduced appetite and anorexia have been associated with fourfold increase in mortality, greater hospitalisation rates and poor quality of life.[86]

Nutritional status should be assessed at the commencement of dialysis and at regular intervals thereafter to recognise the signs of malnutrition early so that the multidisciplinary team can work together to reduce the incidence of malnutrition. There is no single measurement which can be used to determine the presence of malnutrition. The renal association guidelines (RAG) 2007 recommend that nutritional screening should be carried out on all ERF patients and that a diagnosis of undernutrition should be considered with any of the following criteria:

* Unintentional fall in BMI or BMI < 18.5;
* Unintentional loss of oedema free weight > 10% in past 6 months;

- Subjective global assessment (SGA) score of B/C with 3-point scale or SGA score of 1–2 (severe undernutrition) or 3–5 (mild to moderate undernutrition) with 7-point scale.[87]

The use of the malnutrition universal screening (MUST) tool remains controversial in CKD patients. Although not ideal for use in CKD patients due to the significant changes in body fluid, a universal tool chosen for nutritional screening is more likely to be implemented. The SGA has been previously shown to be a valid and reliable tool to assess nutritional status among ERF patients.[78] Researchers do, however, caution the use of some of the modified SGA scores.[88] Handgrip strength, a simple, easily performed test, has been shown to be a marker of lean muscle mass and may be a useful part of the nutritional assessment procedure.[89]

It is important to remember that well-controlled biochemistry in CKD patients may reflect a poor dietary intake. Low creatinine and cholesterol levels have been found to be highly predictive of a poor outcome.[90] Hypoalbuminaemia, although not a good indicator of nutritional status in isolation, has been found to be a powerful predictor of both mortality and morbidity in EFR.[91]

Many of the causes of malnutrition are similar for both HD and PD as shown in Box 16.2. In addition, patients on PD can suffer from bloating and early satiety.[92] HD patients spend significantly more time at hospital than PD patients. An audit looking at eating patterns of HD patients found that 37% of the patients never or only sometimes ate at the meal time prior to HD and 21% of the patients never or only sometimes ate at the meal time after HD.[93]

Box 16.2

Causes of malnutrition in dialysis patients

Inadequate protein or calorie intake
Dietary restrictions
Anaemia
Metabolic acidosis
Inflammation/infection
Underlying illness
Gastroparesis
Depression
Time spent at hospital
Inadequate dialysis
Uraemic toxicity—nausea, vomiting, altered taste and
    anorexia
Catabolism secondary to the dialysis process
Protein losses from dialysis

Malnutrition is a significant problem in the elderly. It is not surprising then that nutritional problems are common in elderly patients with ERF and are a cause of morbidity in this group.[94] A poor dietary intake and diminished muscle mass can be a common occurrence in elderly patients, resulting in near normal levels of urea and creatinine. Caution is therefore needed when interpreting blood results.

It is believed that patients with CKD secondary to diabetes mellitus have a higher incidence of malnutrition as compared to nondiabetics. Reasons for this include poor glycaemic control, insulin resistance and gastroparesis.[95]

Researchers are questioning whether there are two types of malnutrition, one due to a poor intake and one due to an acute phase response releasing cytokines causing atherosclerosis and muscle wasting.[96] Research in the area of malnutrition suggests that malnutrition–inflammation complex syndrome (MICS), the combination of protein–energy malnutrition and chronic inflammation, is a common condition in dialysis patients.[97] MICS is suggested to be a significant contributor to reverse epidemiology and poor outcome.[98] A randomised clinical trial designed with an adequate sample size and optimal statistical power is required to evaluate the effect of nutritional or anti-inflammatory interventions in dialysis patients and whether these interventions can actually improve life expectancy in CKD patients.

Treatment for malnutrition

Once the patient has been identified as requiring nutritional support, this can be delivered in a number of ways. Firstly food as treatment is the priority and secondly it is important not to over-restrict CKD patients when their appetite is poor. Where oral intake is poor enteral nutrition is always the preferred method over parenteral nutrition. Gastrostomy feeding has been shown to be a successful way of improving nutritional status in HD patients.[99] It may be necessary to negotiate the dialysis regimen with the medical team to achieve the desired fluid allowance for nutritional support. Use of low volume, low electrolyte sip and enteral feeds may be more appropriate in some patients, depending on their clinical chemistry and fluid allowance. A high protein supplement may be particularly beneficial for dialysis patients who struggle to meet their protein requirements.

At the current time there is insufficient evidence to support the use of intradialytic parenteral nutrition (IDPN) as an effective therapy against malnutrition. IDPN is only given to the patient during HD sessions and does not meet full nutritional requirements. A number of studies have investigated this therapy but many of these studies have variations in research design and protocols, have small sample sizes or short follow-up periods and do not convincingly support the use of this expensive therapy which also carries risks of complications.[100] A study published in 2004 found that IDPN given to 31 patients for 6 months significantly improved nutritional status as measured by SGA, albumin and mid-arm circumference.[101] A prospective, randomised study where patients received oral nutritional supplements with or without IDPN for 1 year revealed no improvement in 2-year mortality, hospitalisation rate, BMI or laboratory markers of nutritional status.[102]

Short-term studies have suggested that amino acid-based peritoneal dialysate solutions, referred to as intraperitoneal amino acids (IPAA), can offer an alternative method of nutritional intervention in PD patients who cannot meet their protein requirements orally.[103,104] At present there is no convincing evidence for the use of IPAA for the treatment of PEM; however, it is used in diabetics as a non-glucose dialysate to reduce the exposure of glucose dialysate solutions.

Potassium

Hyperkalaemia is common in patients with a GFR < 10. Dialysis is successful in removing excess potassium so as PD is performed daily a potassium restriction is less likely. Conversely HD patients may require advice on potassium restrictions to prevent intradialytic hyperkalaemia. The RAG recommend maintaining a serum potassium of between 3.5 and 5.5 mmol/L in PD patients and between 3.5 and 6.5 mmol/L (pre-dialysis blood values) in HD patients.[105] Three to five percent of deaths in dialysis patients have been attributed to hyperkalaemia.[106] Non-compliance with the HD prescription and/or the dietary restrictions is the main cause of hyperkalaemia in dialysis patients.

Phosphorus

Dialysis alone does not remove sufficient phosphate, so good serum phosphate control depends on the combination of adequate dialysis, a careful diet and phosphate binders. Calcium levels are generally low in the earlier stages of CKD due to inadequate formation of 1,25-dihydroxycholecalciferol but may be elevated in CKD stage 5 secondary to the use of calcium-containing phosphate binders or vitamin D analogues. The RAG recommend in HD patients that serum phosphate should be between 1.1 and 1.8 mmol/L (pre-dialysis).[105] For patients with PEM the need to increase dietary protein takes precedence over the need to restrict dietary phosphorus.

Sodium and fluid homeostasis

A 'no added salt' restriction in CKD patients can help to prevent thirst and maintain an ideal fluid balance. As a guide the recommended fluid allowance for PD and HD patients is 800 mL plus previous day's urine output (PDUO) and 500 mL plus PDUO, respectively. It is important to keep intradialytic weight gain between HD sessions to 1.5–2.0 kg (i.e. 1.5–2 L fluid) or less than 4% actual body weight. In PD, patients should aim to keep their daily weight to within about 1 kg of their target weight. If patients gain too much fluid weight, this can cause swollen ankles, shortness of breath and hypertension. This often necessitates the need for longer dialysis sessions and stronger PD dialysate bags, and ultimately over time leads to a greater risk of CVD. Use of bags with high glucose concentrations is also associated with degradation of the peritoneal membrane and increased risk of PD failure.

Patients should be encouraged to use smaller cups, drink when thirsty rather than out of habit and use ice cubes to help moisten their mouths. Another practical and visual way to help with fluid restriction is for patients to mark an empty measuring jug with the amount of fluid allowed each day. Every time fluid is consumed the equivalent amount of water should be added to the jug to allow patients to visualise how much of their fluid allowance has been used. Foods with a high fluid content will also need to be counted, for example, soup, yoghurt, gravy, milk on cereal, and milk puddings.

Micronutrients and CKD

Renal failure alters the metabolism and nutritional requirements of micronutrients. Both deficiencies and abnormally high levels of vitamins occur in patients with CKD. Patients at stage 4 or 5 CKD are at high risk of vitamin deficiency for many reasons: impaired synthesis (e.g. 1,25-dihydroxycho-lecalciferol), anorexia causing a reduced food intake, dietary restrictions, altered metabolism of some vitamins and removal of water-soluble vitamins by dialysis. The most common deficiencies are 1,25-dihydroxycholecalciferol, folic acid, pyridoxine hydrochloride (vitamin B$_6$) and ascorbic acid (vitamin C).[107–109] Low levels of ascorbic acid have been reported in both HD and PD patients but care must be taken if supplementing with excess ascorbic acid as this can result in oxalate deposition.[110]

Plasma homocysteine levels are elevated in CKD patients and a folic acid supplementation of 5 mg/day has been shown to reduce these levels.[111] At the present time it is not known whether reducing homocysteine levels can subsequently reduce cardio-vascular risk and improve survival in CKD patients. A study called 'Folic Acid for Vascular Outcome Reduction in Transplantation' (FAVORIT) is currently examining whether lowering homocysteine levels with a multivitamin will reduce the occurrence of CVD outcomes in renal transplant patients. Routine supplementation of folic acid may be worthwhile when patients start erythropoietin therapy as folate is required for DNA synthesis during erythropoiesis.

There is currently insufficient evidence and no consensus on whether routine supplementation of CKD patients (particularly stage 4 and 5) with water-soluble vitamins is beneficial. Patients should be assessed on an individual basis.

Deficiency of fat-soluble vitamins (with the exception of vitamin D) is less common in CKD. Serum vitamin A levels are generally increased in HD patients and there appears to be a risk of vitamin A toxicity with supplementation.[112,113] Therefore CKD patients should aim to meet the reference nutrient intake (RNI) for vitamin A and avoid excessive supplementation. It therefore seems prudent to caution against supplements such as cod liver oil. CKD patients are known to be at risk of oxidative stress and CVD; however, conflicting results as to whether vitamin E supplementation is beneficial in CKD have been reported.[114,115] In contrast to vitamin A, vitamin E supplementation appears safe and may be beneficial in CKD.

Inadequate erythropoietin (EPO) production is the main cause of anaemia in CKD and recombinant human EPO (rhEPO) is used to treat this. In CKD patients iron requirements increase when EPO therapy is started. Treatment is most commonly with intravenous iron therapy, rather than oral supplements.

CKD patients should avoid taking alternative remedies unless these have been checked by a renal healthcare professional. All CKD patients should be advised to avoid star fruit as fatal side effects have been reported.

Exercise and CKD

The benefits of exercise are well known and CKD patients should be encouraged to exercise within their limitations. Studies investigating the effects of exercise during HD have found that as well as an improvement in a patient's physical function, stamina and QOL, a greater percentage of urea is removed, suggesting that exercise during dialysis enhances the treatment process.[116,117]

Acute kidney injury (acute renal failure)

Acute kidney injury (AKI) affects the body's homeostatic mechanisms in the same way as CKD; however, there are a number of differences between AKI and CKD as shown in Table 16.7.

The aims of dietary treatment for AKI are:

- To limit the build-up of waste products and help maintain fluid/electrolyte balance;
- To prevent metabolic complications (e.g. renal bone disease, acidosis, anorexia);
- To replace nutrient losses associated with the dialysis process/catabolic causes of AKI;
- To optimise/maintain nutritional status and minimise catabolism.

Table 16.7 Similarities and differences between CKD and AKI

Similarities	Differences
Biochemistry	AKI can be reversible and the patient may
Both may need	recover normal renal function
RRT	AKI has a rapid onset
Uraemic	AKI patient often has normal size kidneys
symptoms	AKI urine volume may be reduced, normal
Medications	or increased
High risk of	AKI mortality rate is high
malnutrition	

Table 16.8 Nutritional requirements of AKI patients are dependent on the underlying cause of renal failure

1	Normo-catabolic, e.g. dehydrated, drug overdose, obstruction
2	Moderately catabolic, e.g. infection, trauma
3	Hypercatabolic, e.g. burns, multiorgan failure

Table 16.9 A guide to protein requirements in AKI

	Protein requirements (g/kg)
Normo-catabolic	0.8–1 (not dialysed)
Moderately catabolic	1–1.2
Hypercatabolic	1.2–1.5

The nutritional requirements of patients with AKI depend very much on the cause of the injury/acute failure. AKI itself has little effect on energy requirements.[118] For example, a patient who has taken a drug overdose may go into AKI but still be classified as normo-catabolic as shown in Table 16.8. The aim of the medical management of AKI is to alleviate the cause of the underlying renal failure. Mortality rates are known to be high when AKI is severe enough to need dialysis, with overall mortality quoted at 40–60%. Mortality rates have been quoted to exceed 75% in AKI patients with sepsis or who are critically ill.[119]

If RRT is necessary this will either be as intermittent HD or continuous renal replacement therapy (CRRT). The dietetic management for intermittent HD will be similar for CKD patients. CRRT is delivered via haemofiltration or haemodiafiltration. The benefit of CRRT is the ability to remove fluid and waste products from very unstable patients and so allow an adequate volume for the nutritional support. A detailed description of the dietetic management of CRRT is beyond the scope of this chapter.

As a guide energy requirements will be approximately 30–35 kcal/kg body weight but these will need to be assessed individually using formulas and stress factors for catabolic patients. A reduction in mortality and morbidity of critically ill patients has been shown with strict control of blood glucose concentration and likewise hyperglycaemia adversely affects the prognosis for patients with AKI. Protein requirements will also be dependent on the cause of the AKI. Table 16.9 gives a guide to protein requirements in AKI.

Hyperkalaemia and hyperphosphataemia are common in AKI. Acute hyperkalaemia may need to be managed with intravenous calcium gluconate and dextrose/insulin infusions. Phosphate binders are often required for the management of hyperphosphataemia. The fluid and electrolyte requirements of AKI patients are known to change rapidly and so require daily monitoring.

Kidney transplantation

For many patients kidney transplantation can restore near normal function of the kidney and so present the best option. One study estimated that the long-term mortality rate was 48 to 82% lower among transplant recipients than patients on the transplant waiting list. The greatest benefits were found in younger patients.[120] Another study concluded that a successful transplant can triple the life expectancy of a patient.[121] Tables 16.10 and 16.11 show the percentage survival rates of a kidney transplant at 1, 2, 5 and 10 years.

One of the main benefits of a renal transplant is the end to the many dietary restrictions previously advised. However, the immunosuppressive drugs essential to prevent rejection of the transplanted kidney can cause side effects, for example, weight gain, dyslipidaemia, hypertension, diabetes and an increased risk of infection. For the majority of kidney transplant patients a low-fat healthy diet with an emphasis on food safety and adequate calcium intake, to compensate for the steroid therapy, should be advised. Although controversial in dialysis patients, statin therapy has been reported to be beneficial in transplant patients. In the ALERT study statin therapy reduced adverse cardiac events and the risk of cardiac death in transplant patients.[122,123]

Table 16.10 Long-term patient survival after deceased non-heart-beating donor kidney transplant

Year	% patient survival			
	1 year	2 years	5 years	10 years
1994–6	90	87	80	66
2000–2	92	89	80	
2003–6	96			

Data taken from the UK Blood and Transplant website.

Table 16.11 Long-term patient survival after living donor kidney transplant

Year	% patient survival			
	1 year	2 years	5 years	10 years
1994–6	98	97	94	89
2000–2	98	97	95	
2003–6	99			

Data taken from the UK Blood and Transplant website.

Components of grapefruit juice have been shown to inhibit an enzyme involved in the metabolism of the immunosuppressive drug cyclosporin. Some renal units recommend total avoidance of grapefruit juice whilst others recommend avoiding it 2 h either side of taking cylosporin. St John's Wort, a herbal supplement, is thought to have a similar effect so should also be discouraged. For further information please refer to the chapter on Drug–Nutrient Interactions.

Nephrotic syndrome

Nephrotic syndrome (NS) is a disorder which can develop gradually or suddenly at any age. In NS damaged glomeruli allow protein to leak into the urine. The features of NS include proteinuria, oedema, hypoalbuminaemia and hyperlipidaemia. Many diseases are known to cause NS including minimal change disease (a common cause in children), membranous nephropathy (sometimes called membranous glomerulonephritis, a common cause in adults), focal segmental glomerulosclerosis, diabetes nephropathy, amyloidosis and systemic lupus erythematosus. Sometimes the cause of NS is unknown.

Patients with NS may have periods of remission which require no dietetic input but others may present with progressive disease leading to CKD. The recommended dietetic management of NS is based on an energy intake of 30–35 kcal/kg IBW/day and approximately 1 g protein/kg IBW/day.[124,125]

Substituting saturated fat with poly- and monounsaturates should be encouraged but as lipid levels can be very high medication will often be required as treatment. When the protein losses are treated the lipid abnormalities will often resolve. A 'no added salt' diet is recommended and a fluid restriction may be beneficial in oedematous patients although diuretics will often allow the relaxation of fluid restrictions.

Key points

- CKD is classified into 5 stages based on GFR.
- CKD is now recognised as a global public health problem.
- Despite much research, the area of protein restriction and its possible effect of slowing the progression of CKD still remain controversial.
- Patients with CKD display a variety of metabolic and nutritional abnormalities and often show signs of protein–energy malnutrition. Reduced nutritional status prior to starting dialysis is a strong predictor of poor survival on dialysis.
- Nutritional status should be assessed at the commencement of dialysis and at regular intervals thereafter.
- Food as treatment is the priority for treating malnutrition and it is important not to over-restrict CKD patients when their appetite is poor.
- A poor dietary intake and diminished muscle mass can result in near normal levels of urea and creatinine. Caution is therefore needed when interpreting blood results.
- Factors other than diet can contribute to hyperkalaemia.
- The dietitian is the team member best qualified to recommend when and how many phosphate binders patients should take.
- A 'no added salt' restriction in CKD patients can help to prevent thirst and maintain an ideal fluid balance.

Case study

A 58-year-old lady who has been on HD for the past 6 months is referred to the dietitian as her appetite is reported to be poor and she has some unintentional weight loss. She was seen by the dietitian when she first started dialysis. At this time she was advised on a 1500-mL fluid restriction and to continue on a 'no added salt' diet. She was given some basic dietary advice on a potassium restriction but few dietary restrictions were really necessary and she was not prescribed phosphate binders. Her pre-dialysis blood results are shown in Table 16.12.

Intradialytic weight gain = 3 kg
PDUO = 500 mL
Weight = 62 kg
Height = 1.65 m

QUESTIONS

1. Review the clinical chemistry and comment on these results.
2. What are this patient's recommended calorie and protein requirements?
3. What are the fluid requirements for this patient?
4. Discuss why this patient is at high risk of malnutrition.

ANSWERS

1. Review the clinical chemistry and comment on these results.

   The patient is hyperkalaemic. The RAG recommends a pre-dialysis potassium level of 3.5–6.5 mmol/L. It is important to compare with previous clinical chemistry readings to see what the trend is and to check for causes of hyperkalaemia other than dietary, for example, medications, evidence of acidosis (her results reveal that this should be treated with bicarbonate), dialysis adequacy. The patient's diet history should be reviewed and her understanding/compliance with any previous advice checked. If she needs further potassium restrictions this must be tailored to her individual diet. Her appetite is poor so any restrictions should be kept to a minimum.

   Her phosphate levels are acceptable but these are likely to rise if an increase in dietary protein is recommended. The patient may then need a dietary phosphorus restriction and/or phosphate binders prescribed. Care must be taken with the patient's protein intake if restricting dietary phosphorus.

   It is important to look at the trends of her clinical chemistry results. Is her haemoglobin level dropping? Is this an acceptable level for her quality of life? What are the trends in her serum albumin levels? Are there signs of an inflammatory response? Are there any CRP results?

2. What are this patient's recommended calorie and protein requirements?

   This lady's BMI is approximately 23 and she has lost some weight unintentionally. It is important to prevent further weight loss. She may benefit from regaining any weight loss. Her recommended daily protein and energy intakes are 62–74 g protein, and 2170 kcal, respectively. Dietary advice should focus on food fortification, snacks and portions sizes to meet this. Dietary sip feeds may be necessary if this is not achievable by diet alone.

3. What are the fluid requirements for this patient?

   Her intradialytic weight gain is above the recommended level of 1.5–2 kg. Her urine output has reduced in volume, which makes her estimated fluid allowance now 1000 mL/day. It is important to check whether she has managed to achieve her previous 1500-mL fluid restriction. She may find a restriction of 1000 mL difficult if she is consuming a high salt intake and/or if she is advised to start on sip feeds. Consider the use of low volume, low electrolyte supplements.

4. Discuss why this patient is at high risk of malnutrition.

   CKD patients are known to be at high risk of malnutrition. This patient has a poor appetite and has unintentional weight loss. Multiple factors put her at risk of malnutrition, for example, inadequate protein or calorie intake, complex dietary restrictions and fear of eating the wrong foods, anaemia, metabolic acidosis, adjusting to dialysis and the time spent at hospital, catabolism secondary to the dialysis procedure, uraemic toxicity, tiredness and depression.

Table 16.12 Pre-dialysis blood results for case study

Pre-dialysis blood results		Reference range[a]
Potassium	6.5 mmol/L	3.5–5.2 mmol/L
Calcium (corrected)	2.25 mmol/L	2.2–2.6 mmol/L
Phosphate	1.40 mmol/L	0.8–1.4 mmol/L
Bicarbonate	18 mmol/L	22–32 mmol/L
Albumin	30 g/L	35–50 g/L
Haemoglobin	11 g/dL	11.5–16 g/Dl
Urea	23 mmol/L	2.5–6.5 mmol/L
Creatinine	695 µmol/L	40–130 µmol/L

[a]Values can vary depending on individual laboratory ranges.

Acknowledgements

Heather Sadler and Helena Jackson.

References

1. Klahr S, Levey AS, Beck GJ, et al. The effects of dietary protein restriction and blood-pressure control on the progression of chronic renal disease. Modification of Diet in Renal Disease Study Group. *N Engl J Med.* 1994;330:877–884.

2. Rigalleau V, Lasseur C, Perlemoine C, et al. Estimation of glomerular filtration rate in diabetic patients, Cockcroft or MDRD formula? *Diabetes Care.* 2005;28:838–843.

3. Levey AS, Bosch JP, Lewis JB, et al. A more accurate method to estimate glomerular filtration rate from serum creatinine: a new prediction equation. Modification of Diet in Renal Disease Study Group. *Ann Intern Med.* 1999;130:461–470.

4. Kidney Disease Outcomes Quality Initiative Guidelines (K/DOQI). Clinical practice guidelines for chronic kidney disease: evaluation, classification, and stratification. *Am J Kidney Dis.* 2002;39:S1–S266.

5. NICE clinical guideline 73. *Chronic Kidney Disease: Early Identification and Management of Chronic Kidney Disease in Adults in Primary and Secondary Care.* 2008.

6. Chan MR, Dall AT, Fletcher KE, et al. Outcomes in patients with chronic kidney disease referred late to nephrologists: a meta-analysis. *Am J Med.* 2007;120(12): 1063–1070.

7. Ansell D, Feehally J, Feest TG, et al. *UK Renal Registry Report.* Bristol, UK: UK Renal Registry; 2007. (The interpretation and reporting of these data are the responsibility of the authors and in no way should be seen as an official policy or interpretation of the UK Renal Registry of the Renal Association.)

8. Cirillo M, Lanti MP, Menotti A, et al. Definition of kidney dysfunction as a cardiovascular risk factor. *Arch Intern Med.* 2008;168(6):617–624.

9. Levey AS, Andreoli SP, DuBose T, et al. Chronic kidney disease: common, harmful and treatable— World Kidney Day 2007. *Am J Kidney Dis.* 2007;49:175–179.

10. Hsu C, McCulloch CE, Iribarren C, et al. Body mass index and risk for end-stage renal disease. *Ann Intern Med.* 2006;144:21–28.

11. Drey N, Roderick P, Mullee M, et al. A population-based study of the incidence and outcomes of diagnosed chronic kidney disease. *Am J Kidney Dis.* 2003;42:677–684.

12. Coresh J, Astor BC, Greene T, et al. Prevalence of chronic kidney disease and decreased kidney function in the adult US population: third National Health and Nutrition Examination Survey. *Am J Kidney Dis.* 2003; 41:1–12.

13. de Lusignan S. Identifying patients with chronic kidney disease from general practice computer records. *Fam Pract.* 2005;22:234–241.

14. Stevens PE, O'Donoghue DJ, de Lusignan S, et al. Chronic kidney disease management in the United Kingdom: NEOERICA project results. *Kidney Int.* 2007;72:92–99.

15. MacGregor MS. How common is early chronic kidney disease a background paper prepared for the UK Consensus Conference on Early Chronic Kidney Disease. *Nephrol Dialysis Transp.* 2007;22(suppl 9): ix8–ix18.

16. Ruggenenti P, Perna A, Loriga G, et al. Blood-pressure control for renoprotection in patients with non-diabetic chronic renal disease (REIN-2): multicentre, randomised controlled trial. *Lancet.* 2005;365: 939–946.

17. de Zeeuw D, Remuzzi G, Parving HH, et al. Proteinuria, a target for renoprotection in patients with type 2 diabetic nephropathy: lessons from RENAAL. *Kidney Int.* 2004;65:2309–2310.

18. Neter JE, Stam BE, Kok FJ, et al. Influence of weight reduction on blood pressure: a meta-analysis of randomized controlled trials. *Hypertension.* 2003;42:878–884.

19. Mulrow CD, Chiquette E, Angel L, et al. Dieting to reduce body weight for controlling hypertension in adults. *Cochrane Database Syst Rev.* 2000;(2):CD000484.

20. Franco V, Oparil S. Salt sensitivity, a determinant of blood pressure, cardiovascular disease and survival. *J Am Coll Nutr.* 2006;25(90003): 247S–255S.

21. Luft FC, Weinberger MH. Heterogeneous responses to changes in dietary salt intake: the salt-sensitivity paradigm. *Am J Clin Nutr.* 1997;65:612S–617S.

22. Peters RM, Flack JM. Salt Sensitivity and hypertension in African Americans: implications for cardiovascular nurses. *Prog Cardiovasc Nurs.* 2000;15(4): 138–144.

23. Johnson RJ, Herrera-Acosta J, Schreiner GF, et al. Subtle acquired renal injury as a mechanism of salt-sensitive hypertension. *N Eng J Med.* 2002;346:913–923.

24. He FJ, MacGregor GA. Effect of longer-term modest salt reduction on blood pressure. *Cochrane Database Syst Rev.* 2004;(3): CD004937.

25. Sacks FM, Svetkey LP, Vollmer WM, et al. DASH-Sodium Collaborative Research Group. Effects on blood pressure of reduced dietary sodium and the dietary approaches to stop hypertension (DASH) diet. *N Eng J Med.* 2001;344:3–10.

26. Scientific Advisory Committee on Nutrition (SACN). *Salt and Health.* London: Stationery Office; 2003.

27. Jones-Burton C, Mishra SI, Fink JC, et al. An indepth review of the evidence linking dietary salt intake and progression of chronic kidney disease. *Am J Nephrol.* 2006; 26(3):268–275.

28. Bazzano LA, He J, Ogden LG, et al. Dietary potassium intake and risk of stroke in US men and women: National Health and Nutrition Examination Survey I epidemiologic follow-up study. *Stroke.* 2001; 32(7):1473–1480.

29. Linas SL. The role of potassium in the pathogenesis and treatment of hypertension. *Kidney Int.* 1991;39(4):771–786.

30. Siani A, Strazzullo P, Giacco A, et al. Increasing the dietary potassium intake reduces the need for antihypertensive medication. *Ann Intern Med.* 1991;115: 753–759.

31. Nosadini R, Tonolo G. Blood glucose and lipid control as risk factors in the progression of renal damage in type 2 diabetes. *J Nephrol.* 2003;16(suppl 7): S42–S47.

32. Sustained effect of intensive treatment of type 1 diabetes mellitus on development and progression of diabetic nephropathy: the Epidemiology of Diabetes Interventions and Complications (EDIC) study. *JAMA.* 2003;290: 2159–2167.

33. The Diabetes Control and Complications Trial Research Group. The effect of intensive treatment of diabetes on the development and progression of long-term complications in insulin-dependent diabetes mellitus. *N Engl J Med.* 1993;329(14): 977–986.

34. Parikh NI, Hwang S-J, Larson MG, et al. Cardiovascular disease risk factors in chronic kidney disease overall burden and rates of treatment and control. *Arch Intern Med.* 2006;166:1884–1891.

35. Go AS, Chertow GM, Fan D, et al. Chronic kidney disease and the risks of death, cardiovascular events, and hospitaliztion. *N Engl J Med.* 2004;351:1296–1305.

36. Goodkin DA, Young EW, Kurokawa K, et al. Mortality among hemodialysis patients in Europe, Japan, and the United States: case-mix effects. *Am J Kidney Dis.* 2004;44(5 suppl 3): 16–21.

37. Harnett JD, Foley RN, Kent GM, et al. Congestive heart failure in dialysis patients: prevalence, incidence, prognosis and risk factors. *Kidney Int.* 1995;47(3):884–890.

38. Grutzmacher P, Marz W, Peschke B, et al. Lipoproteins and apolipoproteins during the progression of chronic renal disease. *Nephron.* 1988;50:103–111.

39. Krentz AJ. Lipoprotein abnormalities and their consequences for patients with type 2 diabetes. *Diabetes Obes Metab.* 2003;5(suppl 1):S19–S27.

40. Kronenberg F, Kuen E, Ritz E, et al. Lipoprotein(a) serum concentrations and apolipoprotein (a) phenotypes in mild and moderate renal failure. *J Am Soc Nephrol.* 2000;11:105–115.

41. Kronenberg F. Dyslipidemia and nephrotic syndrome: recent advances. *J Ren Nutr.* 2005;15: 195–203.

42. Kronenberg F, Lingenhel A, Lhotta K, et al. The apolipoprotein (a) size polymorphism is associated with nephrotic syndrome. *Kidney Int.* 2004;65:606–612.

43. Tonelli M, Isles C, Curhan GC, et al. Effect of pravastatin on cardiovascular events in people with chronic kidney disease. *Circulation.* 2004;110:1557–1563.

44. Athyros VG, Mikhailidis DP, Papageorgiou AA, et al. The effects of statins versus untreated dyslipidaemia on renal function in patients with coronary heart disease: a subgroup analysis of the Greek atorvastatin and coronary heart disease evaluation (GREACE) study. *J Clin Pathol.* 2004;57:728–734.

45. Fried LF, Orchard TJ, Kasiske BL. Effect of lipid reduction on the progression of renal disease: a meta-analysis. *Kidney Int.* 2001;59: 260–269.

46. Wanner C, Krane V, Marz W, et al. Atorvastatin in patients with type 2 diabetes mellitus undergoing hemodialysis. *N Engl J Med*. 2005;353:238–248.

47. Baigent C, Landray M. Study of heart and renal protection (SHARP). *Kidney Int*. 2003;84: S207–S210.

48. Rossert J, Fouqueray B, Boffa JJ. Anemia management and the delay of chronic renal failure progression. *J Am Soc Nephrol*. 2003;14(7 suppl 2): S173–S177.

49. Singh AK, Szczech L, Tang KL, et al. Correction of anemia with epoetin alfa in chronic kidney disease. *N Engl J Med*. 2006;355:2085–2098.

50. Hostetter TH. Chronic effects of dietary protein in the rat with intact and reduced renal mass. *Kidney Int*. 1986;30:509–517.

51. Mauer SM, Steffes MW, Azar S, et al. Effects of dietary protein content in streptozotocin-diabetic rats. *Kidney Int*. 1989;35:48–59.

52. Nath KA, Krens SM, Hostetter TH. Dietary protein restriction in established renal injury in the rat. *J Clin Invest*. 1986;1199–1205.

53. Fouque D, Laville M, Boissel JP, et al. Controlled low protein diets in chronic renal insufficiency: meta-analysis. *Br Med J*. 1992;304:2126.

54. Locatelli F, Alberti D, Graziani G, et al. Prospective, randomised, multicentre trial of effect of protein restriction on progression of chronic renal insufficiency. *Lancet*. 1991;337:1299–1304.

55. Levey AS, Adler S, Caggiula AW, et al. Effects of dietary protein restriction on the progression of moderate renal disease in the modification of diet in renal disease study. *J Am Soc Nephrol*. 1996;7:2616–2626.

56. Robertson L, Waugh N, Robertson A. Protein restriction for diabetic renal disease. *Cochrane Database Syst Rev*. 2007;(4): CD002181.

57. Kopple JD, Levey AS, Greene T, et al. Effect of dietary protein restriction on nutritional status in the modification of diet in renal disease study. *Kidney Int*. 1997;52:778–791.

58. Ikizler TA, Greene JH, Wingard RL, et al. Spontaneous dietary protein intake during progression of chronic renal failure. *J Am Soc Nephrol*. 1995;6:1386–1391.

59. National Kidney Foundation-K/DOQI. Clinical practice guidelines for nutrition in chronic renal failure. *Am J Kidney Dis*. 2000;35: S1–S140.

60. American Dietetic Association. *Medical Nutrition Therapy Evidence-Based Guides for Practice: Chronic Kidney Disease (Non-dialysis) Medical Nutrition Therapy Protocol*. Chicago: American Dietetic association; 2002.

61. Wiggins KL. Renal Dietitians Dietetic Practice Group, American Dietetic Association. *Guidelines for Nutritional Care of Renal Patients*. 3rd edn. Chicago: American Dietetic association; 2002.

62. EDTNA/ERCA. European guidelines for the nutritional care of adult renal patients. *Eur Dial Transplant Nurses Assoc/Eur Ren care Assoc J*. 2003;29:S1–S23.

63. Caring for Australians with Renal Impairment (CARI). *Nutrition and Growth in Kidney Disease Guidelines*. Australian Kidney Foundation and Australia New Zealand Society of Nephrology; 2005.

64. Cano N, Fiaccadori E, Tesinsky P, et al. ESPEN guidelines on enteral nutrition: adult renal failure. *Clin Nutr*. 2006;25:295–310.

65. Evidence Based Practice Guidelines for the Nutritional Management of Chronic Kidney Disease Nutrition and Dietetics. *J Dietitians Assoc Australia, including the J N Z Dietet Assoc*. 2006;63(2):S35–S45.

66. Martin KJ, Gonzalez EA. Metabolic bone disease in chronic kidney disease. *J Am Soc Nephrol*. 2007;18(3):875–885.

67. Llach F. Hyperphosphatemia in end-stage renal disease patients: pathophysiological consequences. *Kidney Int*. 1999;56:S31–S37.

68. Slatapolsky E, Brown A, Dusso A. Pathogenesis of secondary hyperparathyroidism. *Kidney Int*. 1999;73:S14–S19.

69. Block GA, Hulbert-Shearon TE, Levin NW, et al. Association of serum phosphorus and calcium × phosphate product with mortality risk in chronic hemodialysis patients: a national study. *Am J Kidney Dis*. 1998;31:607–617.

70. Eknoyan G, Levin A, Levin N. National Kidney Foundation. K/DOQI Clinical Practice Guidelines for Bone Metabolism and Disease in Chronic Kidney Disease. *Am J Kidney Dis*. 2003;42(suppl 3): S1–S201.

71. Hartley GH, Murray M, Rai EM, et al. Dietetic management of phosphate binder medication sustains improvement of bone biochemistry in hospital-based haemodialysis patients. In: *Book of Abstracts: British Renal Society Conference*. 2007.

72. National Kidney Foundation K/DOQI clinical practice guidelines on hypertension and antihypertensive agents in chronic kidney disease. *Am J Kidney Dis*. 2004;43(5 suppl 1): 1–290.

73. Lowrie EG, Lew NL. Death risk in hemodialysis patients: the predictive value of commonly measured variables and an evaluation of death rate differences between facilities. *Am J Kidney Dis*. 1990;15:458–482.

74. Ikizler TA, Pupim LB, Brouillette JR, et al. Hemodialysis stimulates muscle and whole body protein loss and alters substrate oxidation. *Am J Physiol Endocrinol Metab*. 2002;282:E107–E116.

75. Ikizler TA, Flakoll PJ, Parker RA, et al. Amino acid and albumin losses during hemodialysis. *Kidney Int*. 1994; 46:830–837.

76. Hyo-Wook G, Jong-Oh Y, Eun-Young L, et al. The effect of dialysis membrane flux on amino acid loss in hemodialysis patients. *J Korean Med Sci*. 2007;22:598–603.

77. Blumenkrantz MJ, Gahl GM, Kopple JD, et al. Protein losses during peritoneal dialysis. *Kidney Int*. 1981;19:593–602.

78. Enia G, Sicuso C, Alati G, et al. Subjective global assessment of nutrition in dialysis patients. *Nephrol Dial Transplant*. 1993;8:1094–1098.

79. Marckmann P. Nutritional status of patients on hemodialysis and peritoneal dialysis. *Clin Nephrol*. 1988;29(2):75–78.

80. Qureshi AR, Alvestrand A, Danielsson A, et al. Factors predicting malnutrition in hemodialysis patients: a cross-sectional study. *Kidney Int.* 1998;53:773–782.

81. Leavey SF, Strawderman RL, Jones CA, et al. Simple nutritional indicators as independent predictors of mortality in hemodialysis patients. *Am J Kidney Dis.* 1998;31(6):997–1006.

82. Lowrie EG, Huang WH, Lew NL. Death risk predictors among peritoneal dialysis and hemodialysis patients: a prelimary comparison. *Am J Kidney Dis.* 1995;26(11): 220–228.

83. Chung SH, Lindholm B, Lee HB. Influence of initial nutritional status on continuous ambulatory peritoneal dialysis patient survival. *Perit Dial Int.* 2000;20(1):19–26.

84. Kopple JD. Nutritional status as a predictor of morbidity and mortality in maintenance hemodialysis patients. *ASAIO J.* 1997;43(3):246–250.

85. Churchill DN, Taylor DW, Keshaviah PR. CANUSA Peritoneal Dialysis Study Group. Adequacy of dialysis and nutrition in continuous peritoneal dialysis: association with clinical outcomes. *J Am Soc Nephrol.* 1996;7(2):198–207.

86. Kalantar-Zadeh K, Block G, McAllister CJ, et al. Appetite and inflammation, nutrition, anemia, and clinical outcomes in hemodialysis patients. *Am J Clin Nutr.* 2004;80:299–307.

87. Renal Association. *Clinical Practice Guidelines. Module 2—Complications of CKD.* 4th edn. London: Royal College of Physicians of London and the Renal Association; 2007.

88. Campbell KL, Ash S, Bauer J, et al. Critical review of nutrition assessment tools to measure malnutrition in chronic kidney disease. *J Dietitians Assoc Australia, including the J N Z Dietet Assoc.* 2007;64(1):23–30.

89. Heimburger O, Qureshi AR, Blaner WS, et al. Hand-grip muscle strength, lean body mass, and plasma proteins as markers of nutritional status in patients with chronic renal failure close to start of

dialysis therapy. *Am J Kidney Dis.* 2000;36:1213–1225.

90. Lowrie EG, Lew NL. Commonly measured laboratory variables in hemodialysis patients: relationships among them and to death risk. *Semin Nephrol.* 1992;12:276–283.

91. Avram MM, Mittman N, Bonomini L, et al. Markers for survival in dialysis: a seven-year prospective study. *Am J Kidney Dis.* 1995;26:209–219.

92. Hylander B, Barkeling B, Rossner S. Changes in patients' eating behaviour: in the uremic state, on continuous ambulatory peritoneal dialysis treatment, and after transplantation. *Am J Kidney Dis.* 1997;29:691–698.

93. Collinson A, Stewart E, Leyland J. Haemodialysis: a contributing factor to malnutrition. In: *Book of Abstracts: Eleventh British Renal Symposium*; 2000.

94. Latos DL. Chronic dialysis in patients over age 65. *J Am Soc Nephrol.* 1996;7:637–646.

95. Park MI, Camilleri M. Gastroparesis: clinical update. *Am J Gastroenterol.* 2006;101: 1129–1139.

96. Stenvinkel P, Heimburger O, Lindholm B, et al. Are there two types of malnutrition in chronic renal failure? Evidence for relationships between malnutrition, inflammation and atherosclerosis (MIA syndrome). *Nephrol Dial Transplant.* 2000;15:953–960.

97. Kalantar-Zadeh K. The latest addition to the inflammatory homeboys in chronic kidney disease: interleukin-8. *Nephron Clin Pract.* 2006;102:c59–c60.

98. Kalantar-Zadeh K. Reverse epidemiology of conventional cardiovascular risk factors in patients with chronic heart failure. *J Am Coll Cardiol.* 2004;(8):1439–1444.

99. Sayce HA, Rowe PA, McGonigle RJS. Percutaneous endoscopic gastrostomy feeding in haemodialysis out-patients. *J Human Nutr Diet.* 2000;13(5): 333–341.

100. Foulkes CJ. An evidence-based evaluation of intradialytic parenteral nutrition. *Am J Kidney Dis.* 1999;33(1):186–192.

101. Czekalski S, Hozejowski R. Malnutrition Working Group. Intradialytic amino acids supplementation in hemodialysis patients with malnutrition: results of a multicenter cohort study. *J Ren Nutr.* 2004;14(2):82–88.

102. Cano NJM, Fouque D, Roth H, et al. Intradialytic parenteral nutrition does not improve survival in malnourished hemodialysis patients: a 2-year multicenter, prospective, randomized study. *J Am Soc Nephrol.* 2007;18: 2583–2591.

103. Jones M, Gehr T, Burkart J, et al. Replacement of amino acid and protein losses with 1.1% amino acid peritoneal dialysis solution. *Perit Dial Int.* 1998;18:210–216.

104. Kopple JD, Bernard D, Messana J, et al. Treatment of malnourished CAPD patients with an amino acid based dialysate. *Kidney Int.* 1995;47:1148–1157.

105. Renal Association. *Treatment of Adults and Children with Renal Failure: Standards and Audit Measures.* 4th edn. London: Royal College of Physicians of London and the Renal Association; 2007.

106. Morduchowicz G, Winkler J, Drazne E, et al. Causes of death in patients with end-stage renal disease treated by dialysis in a centre in Israel. *Isr J Med Sci.* 1992;28:776–779.

107. Kopple JD, Mercurio K, Blumenkrantz MJ, et al. Daily requirement for pyridoxine supplements in chronic renal failure. *Kidney Int.* 1981;19(5):694–704.

108. Milman N. Serum vitamin B12 and erythrocyte folate in chronic uraemia and after renal transplantation. *Scand J Haematol.* 1980;25(2):151–157.

109. Porrini M, Simonette P, Ciappellano S, et al. Thiamin, riboflavin and pyridoxine status in chronic renal insufficiency. *Int J Vitam Nutr Res.* 1989;59(3): 304–308.

110. Morgan SH, Maher ER, Purkiss P, et al. Oxalate metabolism in end-stage renal disease: the effect of ascorbic acid and pyridoxine. *Nephrol Dial Transplant.* 1988;3:28–32.

111. Arnadottir M, Brattstrom L, Simonsen O, et al. The effect of high-dose pyridoxine and folic acid supplementation on serum lipid and plasma homocysteine concentrations in dialysis patients. *Clin Nephrol.* 1993;40(4): 236–240.

112. Smith FR, Goodman DS. The effects of diseases of the liver, thyroid, and kidneys on the transport of vitamin A in human plasma. *J Clin Invest.* 1971;50: 2426–2436.

113. Yatzidis H, Digenis P, Fountas P. Hypervitaminosis A accompanying advanced chronic renal failure. *Br Med J.* 1975;3(5979):352–353.

114. Boaz M, Smetana S, Weinstein T, et al. Secondary prevention with antioxidants of cardiovascular disease in end stage renal disease (SPACE): randomised placebo-controlled trial. *Lancet.* 2000;356(9237):1213–1218.

115. Lonn E, Yusuf S, Hoogwerf B, et al. Effects of vitamin E on cardiovascular and microvascular outcomes in high-risk patients with diabetes: results of the HOPE and MICRO-HOPE substudy. *Diabetes Care.* 2002;25:1919–1927.

116. Cheema B, Abas H, Smith B, et al. Progressive exercise for anabolism in kidney disease (PEAK): a randomized, controlled trial of resistance training during hemodialysis. *J Am Soc Nephrol.* 2007;18:1594–1601.

117. Parsons TL, Toffelmire EB, King-VanVlack CE. Exercise training during hemodialysis improves dialysis efficacy and physical performance. *Arch Phys Med Rehabil.* 2006;87(5):680–687.

118. Schneeweiss B, Graninger W, Stockenhuber F, et al. Energy metabolism in acute and chronic renal failure. *Am J Clin Nutr.* 1990;52:596–601.

119. Hegarty J, Middleton RJ, Krebs M, et al. Severe acute renal failure in adults: place of care, incidence and outcomes. *QJM.* 2005;98: 661–666.

120. Wolfe RA, Ashby VB, Milford EL, et al. Comparison of mortality in all patients on dialysis, patients on dialysis awaiting transplantation, and recipients of a first cadaveric transplant. *N Engl J Med.* 1999;341:1725–1730.

121. Oniscu GC, Brown H, Forsythe JL. Impact of cadaveric renal transplantation on survival in patients listed for transplantation. *J Am Soc Nephrol.* 2005;16(6): 1859–1865.

122. Holdaas H, Fellstrom B, Jardine AG, et al. Effect of fluvastatin on cardiac outcomes in renal transplant recipients: a multicentre, randomised, placebo-controlled trial. *Lancet.* 2003;361:2024–2031.

123. Holdaas H, Fellstrom B, Jardine AG, et al. Beneficial effect of early initiation of lipid-lowering therapy following renal transplantation. *Nephrol Dial Transplant.* 2005;20:974–980.

124. Kaysen GA. Nutritional management of nephrotic syndrome. *J Ren Nutr.* 1992;2: 50–58.

125. Mansy H, Goodship THJ, Tapson JS, et al. Effect of a high protein diet in patients with the nephrotic syndrome. *Clin Sci.* 1989;77:445–451.

Useful websites

Kidney Patient Guide. http://www. kidneypatientguide.org.uk

National Kidney Federation. http:// www.kidney.org.uk

Renal Association. http://www.renal.org

K/DOQI guidelines. http://www.kidney. org/professionals/KDOQI

Nephrology at your fingertips. http:// www.nephronline.org

Renal registry. http://www.renalreg.com

Transplant data. http://www. uktransplant.org.uk

Recommended reading

Jackson H, James G, Cassidy A. *Eating Well with Kidney Failure: A Practical Guide and Cookbook*. London: Class; 2006.

Stein A, Wild J. *Kidney Failure Explained*. 3rd edn. London: Class; 2007.

Diabetes

Lindsay Oliver   Nick Lewis-Barned

LEARNING OBJECTIVES

By the end of this chapter the reader will be able to:

- Understand the nature, treatment and dietetic interventions appropriate in the management of diabetes;
- Be clear about the different types of diabetes and their unique management;
- Be aware of the long-term health implication and cost of diabetes and how risk factors can be managed;
- Be aware of the historical management of diabetes, and also of future developments; and
- Apply theoretical information to a case study.

Introduction

Food and lifestyle management is core to the prevention of type 2 diabetes and to the treatment of risk factors associated with the progression and development of long-term complications in all types of diabetes. However, agreement about what dietetic interventions are best is still debated, particularly in type 2 diabetes. Pragmatically it may be better to focus on the patient's own therapeutic goals and consider which dietetic intervention is evidence based in that instance.

Treatment goals could include any or all of the following:

- Blood glucose levels in the normal range, or as close to normal as safely possible (4.5–8 mmol/L pre-prandial) with an ideal HbA1c of 6–7% (DCCT) or 42–59 mmol/mol (IFCC);
- A lipid profile that reduces vascular disease (total cholesterol < 4 mmol/L, low density lipoprotein (LDL) < 2 mmol/L, triglyceride (TG) < 2 mmol/L);
- Blood pressure control (130/80 mmHg or 125/75 mmHg for those with renal impairment/microalbuminuria/proteinuria);
- Weight management (prevention of weight gain or weight loss);
- Maintenance of nutritional status particularly where other diagnosis are present; and
- Sustainability of dietary modifications by planning realistic, patient-centred changes.

When considering the options for individuals with diabetes, their current behaviour, barriers and goals need to be thought through, to develop concrete, individualised action plans.

In this section we will attempt to outline some of the differences in dietetic messages in relation to individual goals of treatment and the underpinning physiological problem.

Also refer to Chapter 18 on Obesity and Chapter 19 on Cardiovascular Disease.

Historical context

The first writings on diabetes were about diet and the earliest observers note that it was associated with dietary excess and advocated lifestyle change. Diet and lifestyle were the only options for managing diabetes until the discovery of insulin, in 1920, heralded the era of life-saving treatment for type 1 diabetes. From a dietary perspective this led to a focus mainly on carbohydrate. For almost five decades the importance of vascular risk management through food choice, weight management and physical activity, especially for those with type 2 diabetes, was largely overlooked. As technological advances in self glucose monitoring and insulin delivery have occurred, nutritional options have also developed.

Our method of measuring HbA1c is presently undergoing change. The Diabetes Control and Complications Trial (DCCT) values expressed as a % are being replaced with the International Federation of Clinical Chemistry and Laboratory Medicine (IFCC) values expressed as mmol/mol. At present both values are reported (www.diabetes.nhs.uk).

Pathophysiology and medical management of diabetes

Type 1 and type 2 diabetes are characterised by high levels of circulating glucose. Both arise from physiological problems with insulin whose main role is to transport glucose from the blood into cells either for use in metabolic processes or for storage as glycogen. However, in other respects the underlying causes of type 1 and type 2 diabetes are fundamentally different and this gives rise to different presentation and management (Table 17.1).

Despite this, type 1 and type 2 diabetes can sometimes be difficult to distinguish at presentation due to overlap in age, weight and symptoms. Initial

Table 17.1 Causes and characteristics of type 1 and type 2 diabetes

	Type 1 diabetes	Type 2 diabetes
Pathophysiology	Autoimmune destruction of β-cells in pancreatic islet tissue results in loss of insulin secretory capacity and *absolute* insulin deficiency	Insulin insensitivity (insulin resistance) gives rise to compensatory high insulin production. Secondary inability of insulin secretion to be maintained results in progressive hyperglycaemia due to *relative* insulin deficiency
Prevalence[1]	The prevalence for type 1 diabetes is estimated as 0.5% in the UK, with an annual incidence in of 14/100,000 in children. Risk is increased approximately 10-fold in first-degree relatives, but unexplained geographical variation and migrant studies suggests that environmental factors are also very important, but not well understood	The prevalence is 4–5% of the UK population. Risk factors include a family history of type 2 diabetes, age, increasing weight, physical inactivity. Type 2 diabetes is more common in ethnic minority groups in the UK. Between 25 and 30% of those with type 2 diabetes are undiagnosed
Typical features at presentation	Although β-cells failure may take place gradually over many years, onset is often abrupt with typical symptoms of hyperglycaemia occurring over a few weeks. About 10% present with severe insulin lack leading to marked hyperglycaemia, and fat breakdown. This results in formation of acidic ketone bodies (ketoacidosis), which is a medical emergency requiring intravenous fluid, insulin and electrolyte replacement	Glucose levels increase gradually over many years. It is possible to identify a 'latent' period of glucose abnormality before diabetes develops. Onset is therefore insidious and often asymptomatic. While typical symptoms of hyperglycaemia may occur, type 2 diabetes is often diagnosed as a result of active screening of high-risk groups
Management	Insulin replacement is always required. This must be given by subcutaneous injection. Peaks and troughs in the circulating insulin levels need to match the effects of timing and amounts of carbohydrate, and this forms the basis of dietary management	Initially this is directed at reducing insulin resistance through increased physical activity and weight management. Most patients will in time require tablet therapy either to reduce insulin resistance (metformin and thiazolidinediones) or to enhance insulin production (suplhonylureas). Thirty to 50% of patients will require supplementary insulin. Dietary management of cardiovascular risk and insulin resistance, however, remain key elements of management

management may be based on a clinical assessment of the likely type of diabetes, and careful observation of response to treatments. Where the type of diabetes is unclear, antibody tests for type 1 diabetes can be helpful.

Other forms of diabetes

While type 1 and type 2 diabetes account for the majority of those with diabetes, this can also arise from other causes.

Gestational diabetes

Gestational diabetes is defined as diabetes or impaired glucose tolerance that is identified for the first time during pregnancy and resolves following delivery. This is due to physiologically increased insulin resistance in pregnancy. Hyperglycaemia not only influences growth and development of the fetus, but also identifies affected women who are at increased risk of future type 2 diabetes. Management is dietary, although some women also require insulin treatment.

Pancreatic failure

Direct damage to the pancreas due to surgery or pancreatic inflammation (pancreatitis) may result in both insulin deficiency (partial or complete), and pancreatic enzyme deficiency causing malabsorption. This complex situation requires careful management of both aspects of pancreatic failure.

Monogenic diabetes

Formerly known as maturity onset diabetes in the young (MODY), this describes a rare group of inherited types of diabetes. All are characterised by non-insulin requiring diabetes with onset in childhood or young adulthood, and an autosomal dominant pattern of inheritance.

Long-term complications of diabetes

Glucose-related complications (microvascular complications)

High glucose levels over 4 or more years increase the risk of diabetes specific complications.[2,3] These result from structural and functional changes, including glycosylation of proteins and occlusion of small blood vessels. This most commonly affects light-sensitive retinal cells in the eye, renal glomeruli and peripheral nerves, resulting in visual impairment, kidney damage and pain or sensory loss especially in the feet. The degree of risk is directly related to the degree of glucose abnormality, with near normal glucose control minimising these risks. Systematic screening for microvascular complications and early treatment are part of routine care.

Vascular risk (macrovascular complications)

Both types of diabetes, but especially type 2 diabetes, are associated with a magnified risk of atherosclerosis resulting in heart disease, stroke and peripheral vascular disease.[4] While glucose control plays a part in this, the major contributors to risk are the same as for people without diabetes (blood pressure, lipid abnormalities, family history and age) except that the effects are magnified, and the relative protection experienced by pre-menopausal women is lost. Overall people with diabetes are at a two- to fourfold increased risk of macrovascular disease. Active management of these risk factors plays a key role in preventing macrovascular complications. Food choices, lifestyle and drug management are aimed at optimal control of risk factors.

Cost of diabetes care

Current estimates suggest that direct health cost of diabetes accounts for about 5% of the UK health budget, not including social costs related to sickness and disability and more than 10% of hospital bed days. These are largely the result of complications and their management. Government policy has increasingly focused on early identification, systematic care and self-management to reduce the personal and financial burden of this.[5]

Nutritional therapy in the management of diabetes

Prevention of diabetes

Preventative approaches to type 1 diabetes have so far all proved unsuccessful. Although environmental factors are thought to be important, type 1 diabetes is not directly caused by individual lifestyles and so there are no preventative lifestyle measures or strategies that can be implemented.[6]

However, the current epidemic of type 2 diabetes is likely to reflect lifestyle choices and increasing rates of overweight and obesity, with genetics playing a smaller but important role.

Some groups of the population have a higher risk of developing diabetes (see Table 17.2). Individuals in these categories should be screened for diabetes on a regular basis, although there is no evidence base to suggest how often. In practice it is suggested that fasting blood glucose should be checked annually. The risk of developing diabetes also increases with ages and is higher in some ethnic groups (Box 17.1).

People with impaired glucose tolerance (pre-diabetes) not only have a 10% annual risk of developing diabetes, but also have increased cardiovascular risk. This can be calculated using Joint British Societies risk tables.[7]

It is clear that lifestyle modification can prevent or delay type 2 diabetes. Both the Finnish Diabetes Prevention Study and the Diabetes Prevention Program in the USA strongly support this.[8,9] Lifestyle modification has been shown to be twice as

Box 17.1

Individual who are at increased risk of developing type 2 diabetes

Positive family history of type 2 diabetes
Personal history of:

- Gestational diabetes
- Impaired glucose tolerance
- Impaired fasting glucose
- Vascular disease (MI, PVD, angina, CVA, TIA)
- Central obesity (waist circumference: male > 100 cm, female > 90 cm)
- Increased blood pressure (pretreatment of > 130/85 mmHg)
- Increased lipid profile (HDL male < 1.0 mmol/L, female < 1.2 mmol/L fasting triglyceride > 2.0)

Iatrogenic factors: pancreatic surgery or steroid treatment

effective as metformin in the prevention of type 2 diabetes and the effects of lifestyle change were also shown to be additive, i.e. the more changes made, the more risk reduction.

Key recommendations from these programmes included:

- Moderate weight loss (5–7% of body weight);
- Regular physical activity (150 min/week); and
- Reduced fat intake (primary method of calorie reduction).

Of note, reduction of saturated fat has a strong, energy-independent impact on insulin resistance and so reduction of saturated fat should be the main focus of fat reduction. Whole grain foods have also been associated with improved insulin sensitivity, but studies looking at glycaemic index/load have been inconclusive in terms of preventing diabetes.[6]

Impaired glucose tolerance (IGT) and type 2 diabetes

IGT is not a disease in itself, but it is an indicator of risk for both cardiovascular disease (CVD) and type 2 diabetes. Individuals with IGT usually have features of the metabolic syndrome, including insulin resistance, and which is strongly associated with risk of developing diabetes and CVD (macrovascular risk). Once individuals progress to develop frank diabetes, they have blood glucose levels that, if not managed, can additionally lead to microvascular disease. (See Figure 17.1.)

Table 17.2 Dietary management of comorbid risk factors in diabetes

Risk factor	Evidence-based strategies
Weight management[10]	600-cal deficit approach Increased physical activity Reduced fat and alcohol Portion size Anti-obesity drugs Bariatric surgery
Lipid profile[11]	Reduced saturated fat (and trans fatty acids) Moderate monounsaturated fat Weight management
Cardio-protective messages	Eat fish containing omega-3 fatty acids (1–2 portions weekly, depending on presence of CVD)
Blood pressure[12,13]	Weight management Moderate alcohol Reduce salt DASH style pattern of eating (low saturated fat/7 portions of fruit and vegetables daily)

Figure 17.1 • Insulin resistance and type 2 diabetes.

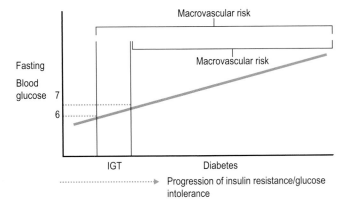

Management of impaired glucose tolerance

The goal of managing IGT is twofold and is aimed at:

1. Reducing the risk of progression to diabetes by reducing insulin resistance:

Insulin resistance has been shown to be made worse by increased weight, waist circumference and saturated fat intake. Physical activity improves insulin resistance.

2. Managing cardiovascular risk factors:

People with IGT should have their cardiovascular risk assessed using Joint British Society tables. Smoking cessation, aspirin, blood pressure management and the use of statins and cardio-protective dietary measures are all important aspects of risk reduction. They should be tailored to the risk profile of the individual. Weight management will have a global impact on all risk factors other than smoking.

There is a lack of dietary evidence specific to diabetes, IGT and cardiovascular risk, and so evidence is primarily extrapolated from more general studies (Table 17.2).

(See related chapter on cardiovascular disease.)

Management of type 2 diabetes

Individuals with type 2 diabetes usually have many of the features of metabolic syndrome and so will need monitoring, assessment and treatment of cardiovascular risk factors. In addition, they are now at risk of microvascular disease due to hyperglycaemia.

In dietary terms this means that all the messages related to insulin resistance will still be important, but in addition, for some people, the type and more specifically the amount of carbohydrate at any one time will also be important in determining day-to-day blood glucose excursions. This is represented diagrammatically in Figure 17.2.

Figure 17.2 • Nutritional messages and their impact on glucose control in type 2 diabetes.

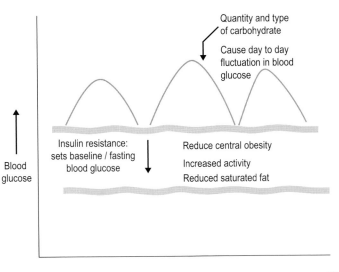

In reality what this means is that at different stages of the development of diabetes, individuals may need to focus on differing aspects of nutritional therapy.

Insulin resistance will determine fasting blood glucose levels and is nutritionally affected by central obesity, saturated fat intake and physical activity. Oral agents such as metformin will also improve insulin sensitivity. All of these therapies will improve fasting and thus to some extent preprandial blood glucose levels.

Day-to-day excursions in blood glucose will occur when the carbohydrate load exceeds the capacity of the pancreas to produce enough insulin to deal with both underlying insulin resistance and the carbohydrate load of any meal or snack. This is more likely to be a problem as diabetes progresses and pancreatic failure necessitates the use of sulphonyurea or/and insulin treatment. In practice type 2 diabetes requires a 'layering' or stepping up of all treatments as the condition progresses. For lifestyle advice this means:

Initial advice. *This is not necessarily provided by a dietitian*:

- Avoid food and drink with a very high glycaemic index/load, e.g. glucose-based drinks, boiled sweets, jelly;
- No need to buy diabetic products (usually high in fat).

Step one. *Dealing with insulin resistance*:

- Avoid foods high in fat, especially saturated fat (including for that reason 'diabetic' products);
- Promote monounsaturated fats as an alternative to saturated fats, but be cautious about amount in overweight clients;
- Manage weight through portion size and calorie sources, such as alcohol, especially if weight loss is not achieved though lower fat and lower sugar choices;
- Promote physical activity.

Step two. *Investigating day-to-day escalation in blood glucose levels*:

- Consider carbohydrate portion and 'glycaemic load' of carbohydrate foods;
- Carbohydrate 'awareness' may be useful for some people on insulin therapy, who demonstrate variability in day-to-day blood glucose level.

Weight management

In type 2 diabetes, weight loss has been directly linked to mortality and will influence most cardiovascular risk factors as well as glycaemic management via improved insulin resistance. In 1990 Mike Lean demonstrated that for people with type 2 diabetes, at 12 months from diagnosis, each 1 kg of weight loss was associated with 3–4 months increased survival.[14] In terms of interim measures of risk, a 10% reduction in weight can result in a:

- 30–40% reduction in diabetes-related deaths;
- 15% reduction in HbA1c;
- 30–50% reduction in fasting glucose; and
- 10% reduction in total cholesterol.

Without doubt weight loss should be a 'goal standard' outcome in type 2 diabetes.

However, weight loss can also be a sign of poorly controlled diabetes. Glycosuria can cause 'artificial' weight loss if blood glucose levels are persistently above the renal threshold, (usually blood glucose levels of 10 mmol/L or more). All medical therapies that correct hyperglycaemia will cause indirect weight gain, through reduced glycosuria and associated calorie loss. With insulin therapy this has been found to be a 5-kg weight gain for a fall in HbA1c of 2.5%.[15] This means as medical therapies are commenced, small deficits in calorie intake should be negotiated to limit weight gain. For some individuals, weight maintenance might be a more realistic option.

Carbohydrate and Type 2 diabetes

Amounts of carbohydrate

There is currently no evidence to support carbohydrate counting in type 2 diabetes, even if insulin treated. It is inappropriate to suggest a 'free' diet, with flexible insulin as for type 1 diabetes. Previous dietary guidelines have promoted high intakes of complex carbohydrates, but concerns about weight gain, worsening post prandial glucose and deterioration in lipid profile (triglyceride) have lead dietitians to look at more modest portion control of carbohydrate. Table 17.3 lists the diet's macronutrient components as suggested in the latest guidelines from the UK.[16] These recommendations allow for a higher proportion of monounsaturated fat to replace carbohydrate intake if clinically indicated.

There is no evidence to support the use of low carbohydrate diets (less than 130 g carbohydrate daily) as a management tool for blood glucose, and preliminary data from trials show no difference in outcome between low fat and low carbohydrate diets. The effect is mediated entirely by weight loss and indeed would indicate weight loss should be the primary nutrition therapy in type 2 diabetes.[16,17]

Table 17.3 Dietary guidelines for diabetes

Component	Proportion	
Protein	> 1 g per kg body weight	
Total fat	< 35% of energy intake	
Saturated and trans fat	< 10% of energy intake	
n-6 polyunsaturated fat } n-3 polyunsaturated fat	< 10% of energy intake To include some fish oils	
cis-monounsaturated fat	10–20% of energy intake	} 60–70%
Total carbohydrate of which sucrose	45–60% 10% of energy intake	

has no effect on glycaemic response. This means that modest amounts of sucrose-containing products can be consumed, without deterioration in glycaemic control.

The GI of individual foods is mediated by a number of factors, such as the type of starch, the pectin content, cooking processes and the disruption of grains and starch granules, as outlined in Table 17.4.[18] In addition, other macronutrients consumed at the mealtime will also impact on GI. Co-ingestion of fat and protein tends to reduce the glycaemic response to a meal.

However, the reproducibility of glycaemic response to individual foods can be quite varied, particularly once applied to the mixed meal scenario, which makes it difficult to use in practice.

Because of the number of variables, the GI can be difficult to teach and can lead to mixed messages for people with type 2 diabetes. For example, many high fat foods have a low GI, such as cake and chocolate. These foods are clearly not good choices for people with type 2 diabetes. Many people also believe that high fibre will equate to low GI. This is not the case for foods rich in insoluble fibre such as wholemeal bread.

Practically, it may be helpful to promote low fat, low GI foods *in place of* higher fat foods or other sources of carbohydrate, for example, the use of wholegrain bread and cereals, legumes, oats and lower GI fruits.

Types of carbohydrates: glycaemic index

The glycaemic index (GI) has been a topic of much debate in diabetes. A recent meta-analysis of low glycaemic index diet trials in people with diabetes showed such diets produce a 0.4% reduction in HbA1c, if applied to individuals who had an initial high GI diet.[18]

The GI has been useful for dispelling many misconceptions about carbohydrate foods. Research has shown that the 'chain length' of the carbohydrate

Table 17.4 Influences on the glycaemic index of food

Factor effecting GI	Mechanism	Example
Soluble fibre	Viscous fibres reduce rates of digestion by reducing enzyme action	Bean, oats, some fruit
Physical disruption of starch granules	Physical disruption of the starch granules provides greater surface area for digestion	Ground versus whole rice Whole fruit versus pureed fruit Puffed and extruded products
Gelatinisation of starches	Starch granules are heated using moist cooking methods, disrupting granules and increasing digestibility	Boiling potatoes
Resistant starch	Physically inaccessible starch, grain not physically disrupted, retrograded or ungelatinised starches	Wholegrains Cooled boiled potatoes Unripened bananas Partially cooked potato
Particle size of starch granules	Larger starch granules take longer to be digested	Pasta/rice slower than bread and potato
Amylose versus amylopectin	Amylopectin as a branch chain molecule has greater area for digestion	Some types of rice

All of this is unlikely to have an impact in itself and is simply fine tuning once other basic changes are in place, as outlined in the stepwise approach above. The exception to this is in pregnancy, where the post-prandial blood glucose is important to control and also in patients with type 1 diabetes using insulin pump therapy, where the infusion of mealtime insulin can be altered according to the glycaemic profile of the meal.

Fish oils and diabetes

The benefit of marine oils in diabetes has been a source of much debate. A particular source of confusion is the use of omega-3 fish oil supplements. Concern about the effect of fish oil supplements on deteriorating glycaemic control has not been confirmed by a recent meta-analysis.[19] Large therapeutic doses of 3–18 g/day, used to treat abnormal triglycerides, can increase LDL cholesterol, but this is not a problem with the 500 mg to 1 g dose.[20] Latterly DASH 2 has questioned the use of fish oil supplement in any clinical situation other than following myocardial infarction (MI; see the chapter on cardiovascular disease).[21] The forthcoming ASCEND trial will help answer this question. It will measure the cardiovascular events in people with diabetes who have no cardiovascular disease on entry to the study and are randomised to receive either 100 mg aspirin or 1 g omega-3 capsules.

Fish rich in omega-3 is of benefit to people who have had an MI, and who are advised to take 2–3 × 140 g portions each week. For people with diabetes who have not had an MI, then it is reasonable to have fish 1–2 times per week, one of which should be a source of omega-3.[22]

Alcohol

The main impact of alcohol in type 2 diabetes is in relation to its calorific value. In some overweight individuals alcohol alone will contribute to excess calorie intake and in theory alcohol reduction would be the primary weight management strategy.

In addition alcohol reduction should be considered for blood pressure management and severe hypertriglyceridaemia. Regular alcohol consumption may worsen painful peripheral neuropathy. Individuals with fatty liver and pancreatitis will need to consult their medical team for individualised advice about alcohol.

For those on sulphonylureas and on insulin, carbohydrate-free alcohol (wines and spirits) may cause delayed hypoglycaemia, and diabetes treatment may need to be manipulated to avoid such situations.

Insulin-treated Type 2 diabetes

Between 30 and 50% of people with type 2 diabetes are likely to require insulin. There is much debate about the best insulin regimes; however, a number of nutritional and educational messages are important for those on insulin:

- Insulin therapy in type 2 diabetes is a normal treatment, due to the progressive nature of diabetes;
- People who need insulin have not 'failed', nor does insulin therapy mean a more serious type of diabetes (there is no 'mild' diabetes);
- Insulin alone does not guarantee a good HbA1c;
- Insulin treatment does not replace the need for careful food choice and in fact to gain benefit from insulin therapy and to avoid weight gain, individuals need to be even more careful with lifestyle choices; and
- Ideally the trend in weight, prior to the commencement of insulin should be static/downward; otherwise, large weight gain should be anticipated.

Dietetic intervention is focused on minimising weight gain and ensuring lifestyle choices are as optimal as possible to gain benefits in glycaemic control.

Once insulin is established, blood glucose patterns should be examined, with a view to manipulating food portions to attain blood glucose targets without hypoglycemia.

In general people on insulin with type 2 diabetes do not need snacks. For some individuals who experience nocturnal hypoglycemia, there maybe a need for a small, low calorie carbohydrate-containing snack at supper time/before bed.

Management of type 1 diabetes

Managing blood glucose

In type 1 diabetes the main problem is a lack of insulin production. This leads to hyperglycaemia at diagnosis or if insulin is omitted. This requires insulin replacement. Nutrition education in this instance is therefore to help people with diabetes understand the impact of carbohydrate on their blood glucose levels and to balance this with insulin, so that the two are matched and create optimum blood glucose levels.

The choice of insulin therapy will depend on a number of factors, but key to the decision as to which regime to opt for will be the patient's desire for flexibility versus their preferences around the number of injections they wish to have. Pump therapy is an option for some (see later) but the core nutrition skills will be the same.

There are two core regimes:

A *twice daily premixed insulin* is suited to someone who tends to eat at similar times and with very little difference in the quantity of carbohydrate at specific mealtimes (Figure 17.3). It will be important to eat meals with consistent amounts of carbohydrate and to also include a mid-morning and bedtime snack.

A *multiple injection system* or basal bolus regimen is more flexible and can allow a much more varied approach to eating (Figure 17.4). On this system, short-acting insulin is taken to match the quantity of carbohydrate in the meal or snack (the bolus) and a long-acting insulin is used to provide the background insulin requirements (the basal). The more carbohydrate is eaten, the more short-acting insulin is needed to counteract it.

Neither insulin regime guarantees good diabetes control, and both require regular monitoring and adjustments to maintain glycaemic targets.

For both approaches it is invaluable to know the carbohydrate value of different types and amounts of food. This is normally calculated using a system of carbohydrate portions, where one carbohydrate portion (CP) is an amount of food containing 10 g of carbohydrate.

Carbohydrates

Virtually all carbohydrate-containing foods cause the blood glucose level to rise.

Figure 17.3 • The activity of twice-daily premixed insulin.

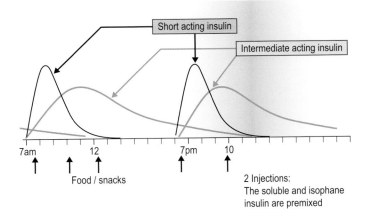

Figure 17.4 • The activity of multiple insulin injections.

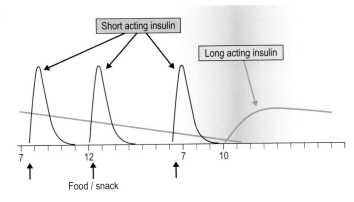

People with type 1 diabetes will benefit from being taught the following steps:

1. Identification of carbohydrate foods;
2. Types of carbohydrate: a simplified version of the glycaemic index; and
3. The quantity of carbohydrate in various types and amounts of food.

Identification of carbohydrate foods

It is an easy assumption to make that people will 'know' which food and drinks will affect blood glucose levels (Table 17.5). This is an important step in the teaching process; however, it needs to be emphasised that although some food and drink do not affect blood glucose, there may be other drawbacks to filling up on foods that do not directly cause the blood glucose levels to rise. For example, sorbitol and similar sweeteners have a laxative effect, and high fat foods will promote excess weight gain and may increase cardiovascular risk.

Types of carbohydrate

The glycaemic index can be a helpful tool for aiding dietetic understanding, but is complicated to understand, is frequently misinterpreted and is unhelpful in a mixed meal situation. In type 1 diabetes it is useful in dispelling myths about sweet foods and when discussing treatment of hypoglycaemia.

For the purposes of education of people with type 1 diabetes it may be best to consider carbohydrate in three discrete categories with associated key messages (Table 17.6).

The quantity of carbohydrate

This is the most important aspect of teaching about food and type 1 diabetes. The UK's most recent guidelines *The Implementation of Nutritional Advice for People with Diabetes* (2003) state that 'the amount of carbohydrate in meals or snacks has much greater influence than the source or type'.[16] This means that people with type 1 diabetes will need access to reliable carbohydrate portion guides, practical education encompassing estimation of commonly eaten foods, interpretation of carbohydrate values on food packets and strategies for eating out. Best practice for those who chose multiple injection therapy should be a self-management programme to teach accurate carbohydrate estimation and insulin adjustment.

Other factors affecting blood glucose control

Alcohol

In type 1 diabetes, alcohol, unless consumed in very small amounts, will have an impact on blood glucose levels. One to two units of alcohol will have very little effect on blood glucose levels. More than this will require some modification in food or insulin intake to prevent hypo- or hyperglycaemia. The impact will depend on the alcohol and carbohydrate content of the beverage.

Alcoholic drinks that have little or no carbohydrate make an individual prone to delayed hypoglycaemia, often hours after consumption. This is because alcohol prevents gluconeogenesis by the liver, once the individual is fasting. Typically this occurs through the night. To avoid hypoglycemia individuals should be encouraged to reduce their insulin dose or eat additional carbohydrate.

Alcoholic drinks that contain carbohydrate, such as beers, ciders, lagers and 'alcopops' will have the same impact on hypoglycemia, but will initially cause the blood glucose to rise, due to their carbohydrate content. In this instance, individuals should be given information according to their insulin regimen.

Ultimately the main concern in relation to alcohol and type 1 diabetes is the problem of hypoglycaemia, which can be severe due to the impact of alcohol on liver glucose release.

Physical activity

In type 2 diabetes, activity has a global benefit on most risk factors and on insulin resistance and thus blood glucose levels. This is not the case in type 1

Table 17.5 The effect of food and drink on blood glucose levels

Direct effect on blood glucose levels	No direct effect on blood glucose level
Cereals and grains	Protein foods: meat, fish,
Products made from flour	cheese, nuts, poultry and eggs
Most fruit and fruit juices	All vegetables except potatoes
Potatoes and potato products	Sour fruits, e.g. grapefruit, limes, lemon
Rice, pasta, couscous	Tea, coffee, sweeteners, herbs,
Milk, yoghurts	spices, sugar-free/diet drinks
Foods containing sugars: cola, ice cream, chocolate, biscuits, desserts, sweets	Vegetable oils, lard, butter, mayonnaise, salad cream dressings, cream
	Sorbitol-type sweeteners

Table 17.6 The impact of carbohydrate on blood glucose level

Category of carbohydrate	Key messages	Foods/drinks included:
Fast-acting carbohydrates	Fast-acting carbohydrates cause a rapid rise in the blood glucose level and injected insulin cannot match the speed at which the blood glucose level rises. If eaten ad lib will cause erratic blood glucose levels, and so are best avoided on a day-to-day basis. They do, however, have one important use, which is to treat hypoglycaemia (any blood glucose lower than 4 mmol/L). Their fast action is ideally suited to the swift treatment of a mild or moderate hypoglycaemia	Drinks and foods where glucose is the sole ingredient, such as ordinary soft drinks, glucose tablets, boiled sweets, jellies and mints
Medium-acting carbohydrates	Medium-acting carbohydrates have a broad glycaemic index, but are characterised by the fact they can be matched by injected insulin, if the quantity of carbohydrate is known	Starchy foods, e.g. bread, potato, cereals, rice, pasta, crisps Sugary foods where the sugar is mixed with other ingredients, e.g. biscuits, cakes, ice cream, yoghurts and chocolate Milk and fruit
Slow-acting carbohydrates	These types of carbohydrates have little or no impact on the blood glucose level and so they do not need insulin	Sorbitol, beans, peas and lentils (pulse vegetables), barley and sweetcorn

diabetes, where exercise and physical activity can cause blood glucose levels to vary, which necessitates insulin or carbohydrate manipulation to maintain levels.

In type 1 diabetes, hyperglycaemia can be caused if there is a lack of insulin circulating at the time of the exercise. This is due to the release of stored glucose, in a physiological response to exercise. If an individual has high blood glucose levels prior to exercise they should be encouraged to test for ketones, and if there are significant amount of ketones present, they should postpone exercise until high blood glucose levels are corrected.

In most instances, however, if significant activity occurs, the main risk is hypoglycaemia. To avoid hypoglycaemia during and potentially after prolonged exercise, individuals should reduce insulin or increase carbohydrate, depending on whether the activity is planned and whether they are attempting to lose weight. Alterations in therapy will depend on the intensity and duration of the activity and requires experienced specialist advice.

Illness

Illness can cause profound hyperglycaemia due to insulin resistance created by infection. There are a few key goals of managing illness:

- Avoidance of escalating blood glucose;
- Reduced production of ketones and thus susceptibility to diabetic ketoacidosis (DKA);
- Prevention of dehydration;
- Treatment of illness; and
- Prevention of unnecessary hospital admission.

People with diabetes should be given individualised advice. This will mean specific guidance about increasing insulin, even if not eating. There is usually no need to eat; however, fluids are very important and small amounts of carbohydrate, taken across the day, will help reduce ketone production. Occasionally an illness will cause hypoglycaemia, but this is less common. It is important that insulin is continued.

Sweeteners

Different types of sweetener have different properties, and varying effects on blood glucose and weight, depending on their calorific value.

Non-nutritive sweeteners

There are five non-nutritive sweeteners permitted for use in the UK: aspartame, saccharin, acesulfame potassium (acesulfame K), cyclamate and sucralose. Only very small amounts are needed because they are so intensely sweet. They are virtually free of calories and do not affect blood glucose levels.

Nutritive sweeteners

These include polyols such as sorbitol, maltitol, xylitol, isomalt and mannitol. Polyols have fewer calories and less effect on blood glucose levels than sucrose. Products containing polyols are safe to consume but should be eaten in moderation as excessive consumption can cause diarrhoea, flatulence and a laxative effect. In addition many products made with polyols are high in fat and so are unlikely to aid weight management. If polyols are consumed by people with type 1 diabetes, then they should be advised not to count the carbohydrate or take any insulin for the carbohydrate source in the product.

Fructose

Fruit sugar (fructose), when used as a sweetener, has no proven advantage over sucrose. It contains just as many calories as sucrose, still affects blood glucose levels and when eaten to excess can cause a laxative effect.

Life events

Young adults (16–25 years old)

Biologically this age group may still be growing. Insulin, appropriate nutrition and good glycaemic control all contribute to healthy growth and these should be reviewed closely. As growth levels off, calorie and insulin requirements will fall and this can lead to excess weight gain if individuals become over-insulinised and eat to prevent hypoglycemia. This can be extremely unhelpful in young people who are 'body conscious' and are likely to be comparing themselves with their peers/media images. It is well recognised that young people can underdose insulin to manipulate their weight and eating disorders are more prevalent in young people with diabetes than in the general population.[23]

The period of transition from paediatric to adult care can be extremely challenging. Transfer rates between paediatric and adult services vary from 29 to 71%, depending on how services are configured.[24] A key goal of transitional services should be to maintain engagement with young people and ensure they do not drop out of healthcare.

Young people find the added burden of living and coping with diabetes affects their management, especially if they are poorly supported or/and troubled by the stigma of diabetes. This occurs at a time of social upheaval for many young people, including leaving home or social care, starting work, learning to drive, exams, experimenting with relationships and peer groups and testing risky situations, e.g. drugs, alcohol.

One of the major challenges is the transition of care from the parent to the young person. It is common for young individuals to disengage from self-care and healthcare services at this time.[25] Healthcare providers need to work proactively to provide a service that people find useful and worthwhile attending, which includes smooth transitional care. Dietetics needs to be integrated into this process and should be always delivered on terms acceptable to the young person. Heavy-handed dietary advice rarely helps this group.

See Chapter 4, Transition to Adult Care.

Pregnancy and lactation

Pregnancy should be managed by a specialist multidisciplinary team.[26] Nutritional requirements and food safety measures are largely the same for people with and without diabetes. Prior to conception, all women with diabetes should be advised to take a supplement of folic acid, as a 5 mg/day dose. The goal of diabetes management prior to conception and during pregnancy is to obtain extremely tight diabetes control (HbA1c preferably less than 6.5% (DCCT) or 48 mmol/mol (IFCC)) and in type 1 diabetes, with the avoidance of severe hypoglycaemia and ketonaemia. In type 1 diabetes, this will mean closely matching insulin and carbohydrate, and increasing insulin in line with the requirements for pregnancy.

In gestational diabetes or for women with pre-existing type 2 diabetes, the goal of therapy is to avoid excess weight gain (and associated increases in insulin resistance) and to manage blood glucose levels, without the production of ketones due to excessive calorie restriction. This means choosing low fat, low glycaemic load foods spread evenly across the day to prevent pre- and postprandial hyperglycaemia, particularly for those on insulin therapy.

Women who develop gestational diabetes should be aware of their increased risk of developing type 2 diabetes in the future. They should receive individualised dietary advice to reduce the risk and should be screened a few months after delivery and annually after that.

Breastfeeding should be encouraged as it is associated with lower risk of diabetes in the child. Breastfeeding can cause hypoglycaemia for women with insulin-treated diabetes and it is usually suggested that women have a small carbohydrate-containing snack before or during breastfeeding.

Renal disease

Kidney disease is a common complication of poorly managed diabetes and the combination of a suitable dietary regime for both conditions can become quite restrictive, particularly as the kidney disease progresses.

The management of microalbuminuria or proteinuria should focus on treating an increased cardiovascular risk by the use of statins and asprin and on reducing the 'workload' of the kidneys by tight control of blood pressure, aiming for less than 125/75 mmHg. Other lifestyle measures such as smoking cessation are also important.

In terms of nutrition, this means a reiteration of 'usual' advice with a focus on salt reduction and if appropriate weight reduction. Good glycaemic management should also be encouraged, but is not as significant as blood pressure control in preventing further deterioration of the condition.

The avoidance of excessive protein intakes has been shown to reduce the rate of renal decline in type 1 diabetes. The UK dietary recommendations state that a 'pragmatic approach might be to reduce protein intake to 0.8–1 g/kg per day, which is little more than usual advice'.[16] In practice this often means keeping modest protein portions for meals and avoiding snacks/suppers with large quantities of protein, such as ad lib drinking of milk, or snacking on cheese or nuts.

Departure from 'usual dietary advice' will only be needed if the following occur:

- ACE inhibitors are commenced to treat blood pressure and cause blood potassium levels to rise. Individuals should be given basic potassium lowering information if this occurs.
- Kidney disease progresses, requiring specialist referral to the renal team.

Please refer to Chapter 16 on Renal Disease for further guidance on the management of renal disease in diabetes.

Older people

Older people who develop diabetes may be relatively healthy and so should receive the same information as younger people. However, the frail elderly need to have dietary advice that does not contribute to weight loss or malnutrition. It is recommended that for people in institutional care, they be served regular menus, with greater care over the portion size and regularity of carbohydrate. In such circumstances, liaison with catering service is vital for ensuring appropriate menu planning.[6]

Pancreatic disease

Conditions such as pancreatitis and pancreatic carcinoma can cause diabetes. The management of diabetes will depend on the extent of the pancreatic damage and its prognosis, but will often require use of sulphonylureas or insulin. In addition the other exocrine and endocrine functions of the pancreas need to be considered. This has implications particularly for insulin-managed patients. If glucagon production is altered or absent people are vulnerable to severe hypoglycaemia.

If the exocrine function is affected then enzyme replacement is needed for the digestion and absorption of foods. This means that if pancreatic enzymes are omitted, hypoglycaemia will be more likely to occur. In addition hypos will need to be treated exclusively with glucose and any backup (long-acting) carbohydrate should be administered with pancreatic enzymes.

In this instance patients need to match enzymes to fat intake and insulin to carbohydrate, and the failure to get this right might mean severe hypoglycaemia.

Even in those with a poor prognosis, it still may be important to manage the blood glucose levels adequately, since poor diabetes control will contribute to malnutrition and dehydration and osmotic symptoms can worsen quality of life.

Gastroparesis

This occurs when the autonomic nervous system is affected by diabetes, causing altered motility of the gut. It tends to occur more in type 1 diabetes where there has been a history of insulin omission and symptoms include nausea, vomiting, constipation, feeling of fullness and diarrhoea. People with gastroparesis will usually have other diabetes complications and some may have eating disorders. These patients are extremely complex and notoriously difficult to treat, but can be helped by lowering blood glucose levels, along with the use of specific drugs such as metoclopramide, erythromycin, domperidone or antiemetics/antibiotics.

In terms of nutrition the only effective strategy seems to be small, frequent amounts of food, using the patient's own preferences to guide this. In severe cases liquid or pureed food may be better tolerated. In addition any food that delays gastric emptying should be avoided, for example high fat foods. High fibre foods that are difficult to digest can cause the formation of bezoars. If a liquid or pureed diet is unsuccessful and nutritional status cannot be maintained, then jejunostomy feeding may be indicated.[6]

Nutrition support

If individuals with diabetes have concurrent medical conditions requiring nutrition support, then blood glucose levels should be managed using oral therapy or insulin. A core principle of treatment is that nutritional requirements should be met as the first priority and diabetes treatment should be individually tailored to feeding regimens. In theory all supplements are suitable for undernourished patients with diabetes and no restriction on high calorie foods should be in place.

Close working between the diabetes and nutrition support teams will be helpful to avoid 'mixed messages' to maintain good glycaemic control and to maximise the benefit of nutrition support, given that poor glycaemic control will contribute to dehydration and poor nutrition. For many cachexic individuals, insulin therapy may have anabolic benefits.

The aims of treatment are therefore:

- To meet the nutritional needs of the patient;
- To avoid clinically significant hypo- and hyperglycaemia, through adjustment of diabetes medication to match the glycaemic effect of the nutrition support; and
- To ensure nutritional support is not manipulated or withheld to improve glycaemic control.

There is very little quality research into the use of diabetes-specific formulas for people with diabetes who are enterally fed. A systematic review concluded that although these formulas demonstrated some benefit, methological limitations of the studies and limited evidence meant it was difficult to recommend specialist formulas.[26] None of the formulas produced a clinically beneficial reduction in HbA1c.

Any diagnosis of diabetes made during an acute hospital admission should be reviewed on resolution of the illness, as illness can precipitate temporary hyperglycemia.

How should interventions be delivered?

As the number of people with diabetes and other chronic diseases increases, self-management, structured education and group interventions have become more cost-effective methods of supporting lifestyle change and disease management. The evidence for isolated dietary counselling is poor and it is clear that good dietetic services should be holistic and integrated into the rest of diabetes care.[27]

Patient education programmes

Patient education programmes for type 1 and type 2 diabetes are in place across the UK. Several are under development and are being evaluated in line with NICE care criteria (www.diabetes.nhs.uk). The DAFNE (Dose Adjustment for Normal Eating) programme originates from a German Diabetes Teaching and Treatment Programme (DDP) in Intensive Insulin Therapy (IIT).[28] It has shown that people with type 1 diabetes can improve HbA1c by 1% without increased risk of hypoglycaemia or deterioration in cardiovascular risk with improvement in quality of life and psychological well-being. The programme has over 25 years of robust RCT evidence and has been adopted in many European countries.

An economic evaluation of DAFNE showed it to be cost effective based on the future saving in treating long-term complications.[29] Audit data from the DAFNE Collaborative also proves DAFNE has short-term economic benefits due to the reductions in severe hypoglycaemia and diabetic ketoacidosis (DKA), resulting in reduced paramedic attendance and hospital admissions.

Since the publication of DAFNE, education programmes have been seen as the 'way forward' in diabetes care, promoting self-management through structured education. These programmes should adhere to Department of Health (DH) guidance on structured education, which includes:

- A written, evidence-based curriculum;
- A clear philosophy;
- Delivery by trained educators; and
- Audits and quality assurance.[30]

Curriculums for people with type 2 diabetes will clearly be different from type 1 programmes. The focus will be on lifestyle modification and the management of glycaemic control and of other cardiovascular risk factors. An example of a successful type 2 diabetes education programme is the X-PERT Programme, developed by Dr Trudi Deakin in 2001 (www.xperthealth.org.uk).

Pump therapy

Pump therapy uses a continuous supply of short-acting insulin, delivered subcutaneously without the need to inject insulin. Users will, however, have to maintain their pump and site and be prepared to do a lot of blood glucose testing to calculate basal and bolus infusion rates. If the pump fails or is disconnected then this can lead to diabetic ketoacidosis due to the rapid clearance of insulin in the blood stream. Pumps require a motivated individual, training in the technical aspects of the pump and carbohydrate counting. Pumps still represent an expensive mode of insulin delivery. NICE has outlined criteria for pump therapy, most of which relate to the benefit of using an adaptable amount of basal insulin, which can help to avoid nocturnal hypoglycemia. Other benefits include the adaptability of basal insulin for physical activity and the ease of additional bolus use for snacks. What is unclear is the benefit of giving an individual this technology without DAFNE-style skills, or the added benefit of pump therapy (given the cost) over structured education programmes.

Consultation skills

Cognitive behavioural therapy, motivational interviewing and behaviour change skills are some of the techniques and models that have relevance in many dietetic consultations. At the heart of these is patient-centred care, moulding the dietetic intervention around the psychological factors that promote or inhibit an individual's ability to make lifestyle changes. Although the evidence for these interventions is difficult to interpret in a purely dietetic sense, it is likely that dietitians who master these skills have more tools at their disposal when working with clients.

Traditional dietary history taking and 'giving' of prescriptive information may be of limited value in diabetes care. This is in part because much of this will already have been experienced by the individual and so will have a repetitive feel to it and if used on a 'precontemplative' patient, will largely create resistance. In addition, people with weight problems and diabetes usually under-report their food intake, so any adaptations to reported food histories are likely to be flawed and unrealistic. The use of open questions, reflections and the exploration of patient perceptions of problems are likely to be more helpful as well as encouraging the person with diabetes to reflect on their previous attempts at change and their successes, and to set specific action plans based on the patient's own ideas.

Please refer to Chapter 3 on changing behaviour for further guidance on consultation skills in diabetes.

New and potential developments

In reality lots of developments are ongoing, but very few make their way into everyday practice or solve the current challenges of clinical care.

Genetic research

Research into the genetics of type 1, type 2 and monogenic diabetes is increasingly able to identify those at risk of developing diabetes. At present, however, the lack of interventions to prevent type 1 diabetes and the powerful influence of lifestyle factors in the development of type 2 diabetes mean that this is currently of limited practical use.

Insulin replacement technologies

These apply almost exclusively to patients with type 1 diabetes.

Closed loop insulin delivery

This refers to linking insulin pump delivery systems (see above) to subcutaneous glucose sensing technology to provide an 'artificial pancreas'. There is a delay between changes in blood glucose levels and glucose in interstitial fluid sensed by these systems and as yet the algorithms to overcome this have not been perfected.

Pancreas and islet cell transplant

This is at present limited to use in people having renal transplants. Pancreas transplants carry significant morbidity mostly associated with drainage of digestive enzymes from the donor pancreas. Islet cell transplants are less unpleasant but limited by the need for large numbers of donors and failure of full insulin replacement in the majority of patients within a few years.

Stem cell transplants

These may in future avoid the need for immunosuppressive therapy, produce large donor pools, and provide noninvasive islet cell replacement. They are not yet at the stage of clinical trials.

New drugs

New agents affecting gut motility and hormones involved in fuel metabolism (GLP-1 analogues and gliptins) offer potentially new approaches to managing glucose and perhaps weight. Their role and additional benefits over existing oral agents is as yet unclear.

Key points

- Food and lifestyle management is a core treatment for most risk factors associated with the development of long-term complications in all types of diabetes.

- High glucose levels over four or more years increase the risk of diabetes-specific complications due to structural and functional changes, including glycosylation of proteins and occlusion of blood vessels.
- The direct health cost of diabetes accounts for about 5% of the UK health budget and more than 10% of hospital bed days, making it one of the most costly chronic conditions.
- Lifestyle interventions have been shown to be highly effective in preventing type 2 diabetes, particularly if aimed at 'high risk groups', but there are currently no preventative strategies implementable for type 1 diabetes.
- Insulin resistance will determine fasting blood glucose levels in type 2 diabetes. It is nutritionally affected by central obesity, saturated fat intake and physical activity. Oral hypoglycaemic agents such as metformin will also improve insulin sensitivity.
- In type 2 diabetes weight loss should be an ideal treatment target. Due to the progressive nature of diabetes between 30 and 50% of people are likely to require insulin; however, insulin therapy does not replace the need for careful lifestyle choices.
- In type 1 diabetes the choice of insulin therapy is influenced by patient's eating patterns and by the desire for flexibility versus the frequency of injections they wish to have.
- The glycaemic index can be a helpful tool in dispelling myths about food and diabetes, but is complicated to understand, frequently misinterpreted and unhelpful in a mixed meal situation.
- In pregnancy, extremely tight diabetes control (HbA1c < 6.5%) is essential for good outcomes. Ideally in type 1 diabetes this should be achieved with the avoidance of severe hypoglycaemia and ketonaemia. In type 2 diabetes or gestational diabetes avoidance of excessive weight gain is also a desirable outcome.

Case studies

Mr Brown has just been diagnosed with impaired glucose tolerance. He is 55, weighs 108 kg and has a BMI of 35:

Waist measurement 102 cm
Blood pressure is 154/85 mmHg
Total cholesterol of 4.5, TG of 2.3, LDL of 3.5, HDL of 0.8
He has a family history of heart disease and is a nonsmoker.

FOOD DIARY

7.30am: Glass of fruit juice
2 slices of toast with marmalade and margarine
Cup of tea (1 teaspoon of sugar/semi-skimmed milk)
10.00am: Packet of crisps or 2 ginger nuts or handful of grapes
Cup of milky coffee (1 teaspoon of sugar)
12.30pm: Egg mayonnaise or beef or tuna mayonnaise or cheese savoury sandwich
2 ginger nuts or a banana or a mini roll
Can of diet cola
3.30pm: 2 ginger nuts
Milky coffee (no sugar)
5.30pm: Glass of fruit juice
Chicken Kiev or meat pie with potato or oven chips or spaghetti bolognese and garlic bread
Rice pudding or fruit and ice cream
Milky coffee (no sugar)
9.00pm: Cheese and crackers or bowl of crisps

Weekly: 2–3 chocolate biscuits
3 pints of real ale × 3 nights each week

QUESTIONS

1. Identify the main risks for this person's health and give ideal targets.
2. What key nutrients would help address these risks?
3. Suggest 3–4 changes to the food choices.
4. What other factors would influence these changes?
5. For each of these state how your food advice would alter and what other factors would you need to consider for each of the following:
   - A diagnosis of type 1 diabetes;
   - A newly diagnosed gestational diabetes;
   - A malnourished patient with pancreatitis;
   - An elderly lady in residential care with a BMI of 20 and an HbA1c of 9% on 'diet only'; and
   - Raised potassium levels on an ACE inhibitor.

ANSWERS

1. Identify the main risks for this person's health and give ideal targets.
   The key risks are an increased risk of developing diabetes and increased risk of a cardiovascular event (about 25% 10-year risk of cardiac event/cardiac death). Ideal targets are as listed in Table 17.7, but

Case studies (Continued)

these may not be realistic for the individual. Modifiable risk factors include weight and blood pressure and irrespective of the lipid profile, it recommended that those over 40 start a statin and aspirin regime regardless of cholesterol levels.

2. **What key nutrients would help address these risks?**

   Reducing calories aids weight management, particularly if combined with physical activity to create a 600Kcal deficit. Reduction of saturated fat also helps weight, insulin resistance and cardiovascular risk. Reducing salt, alcohol and weight will lower blood pressure. An intake of an omega-3 source will also be of benefit.

3. **Suggest 3–4 changes to the food choices.**

   Focusing on blood pressure and weight, there are many potential combinations of actions depending on the preference of the individual. For example:

   Omit supper of crisps/cheese and reduce to 2 pints of real ale twice weekly
   Or
   Cut out mayonnaise in sandwiches and avoid pastry and processed meats at main meal
   Or
   Cut out all biscuits.
   Also encourage 1–2 portions of fish weekly, including an omega-3-rich variety.

4. **What other factors would influence these changes?**

   Any number of factors could make a difference to the options chosen or indeed even if this advice is taken. For example:

   - Illness beliefs;
   - Concurrent life events;
   - Previous attempts at 'dieting';
   - Availability of alternative food choices;
   - Socialising;
   - Personal preferences;
   - Impact of other family members; and
   - Opportunities of exercise.

5. **For each of these state how your food advice would alter and what other factors would you need to consider for each of the following?**

Alternative scenarios

- **A diagnosis of type 1 diabetes**

  The role of the dietitian is to assess food intake, with a view to advising on a suitable insulin regimen and educating on carbohydrate and its impact on blood glucose levels. This eating pattern lends itself remarkably well to a twice-daily insulin regimen provided there aren't variable amounts of physical activity. The dietitian would need to educate the patient about types and amounts of carbohydrate and ensure that the carbohydrate content of each individual meal and snack was approximately the same. Mr Brown would need to make few changes to his food intake.

- **A newly diagnosed gestational diabetes**

  The key aims here would be to manage blood glucose levels on a day-to-day basis and prevent excessive weight gain, causing increased insulin resistance.

  In addition to the type of changes suggested for impaired glucose tolerance (i.e. reduced fat; such as crisps, mayonnaise, pastry, chicken Kiev and garlic bread), the glycaemic load at any one time should be reduced. This can be achieved by having modest main meal portions, for example, avoiding two carbohydrate sources at any one meal (i.e. having pasta or bread at the main meal, but not both), by having low GI desserts such as milk pudding, ice-cream and fruit several hours after the evening meal and by having small nutritious snacks (e.g. fruit, milk, yoghurt). In addition high GI goods such as fruit juice should be reduced to smaller portions or even omitted. All of this will be geared to blood glucose levels and other problems encountered throughout pregnancy (e.g. heartburn).

- **A malnourished patient with pancreatitis**

  The described food intake seems very good; therefore there are several possibilities. It could be that the actual portions eaten are minimal and so the calorific value is not that great. However, it is possible the patient has poor diabetes control and malabsorption. Tests should be performed to establish this and if so appropriate drugs to correct this instigated. People with pancreatitis should be treated as if they have type 1 diabetes, with minimal changes to their eating habits.

- **An elderly lady in residential care with a BMI of 20 and an HbA1c of 9% on 'diet only'**

  Although poor diabetes control is contributing to this lady's BMI, it is unlikely to be the sole factor. If dietetic advice is used to improve blood glucose levels, then weight loss may occur, so oral hypoglycaemic agents should be titrated up to achieve better control.

  Although this lady's diet is not ideal, it is likely that her portions aren't excessive as determined by her BMI.

- **Raised potassium levels on an ACE inhibitor**

  Milky coffee and crisps are likely to be the 'easy wins' here, in terms of correcting raised potassium. This may not be a popular decision with the person!

Table 17.7 Ideal targets

Measures	Ideal targets
Blood pressure	130/80 mmHg
Weight	A 5–7% weight loss
Waist	Less than 100 cm
Lipid profile	Total cholesterol < 4 mmol/L LDL < 2 mmol/L

References

1. Joint Health Surveys Unit. Health Survey for England 2006. *Cardiovascular Disease and Risk Factors*. Leeds: The Information Centre; 2008.

2. Gray A, Clarke P, Farmer A, Holman R. Implementing intensive control of blood glucose concentration and blood pressure in type 2 diabetes in England: cost analysis (UKPDS 63). *Br Med J*. 2002;325(7369):860.

3. Diabetes Control and Complications Research Group. The effect of intensive treatment of diabetes on the development and progressions of long-term complications in insulin-dependant diabetes mellitus. *N Engl J Med*. 1993;329:977–986.

4. Haffner S, Lehto S, Rönnemaa T, Pyörälä K, Laakso M. Mortality from coronary heart disease in subjects with type 2 diabetes and in nondiabetic subjects with and without prior myocardial infarction. *N Engl J Med*. 1998;339(4):229–234.

5. Department of Health. *National Service Framework for Diabetes*. London: Department of Health; 2001.

6. American Diabetes Association. Nutrition recommendations and interventions for diabetes. *Diabetes Care*. 2008;31(s):61–78.

7. FATS Steering Group. *FATS4 A District Wide Strategy for the Use of Cholesterol Lowering Drugs in Newcastle, North Tyneside and Northumberland*. The NHS in Newcastle, North Tyneside and Northumberland; 2006.

8. Lindstrom J, Louheranta A, Mannelin M, et al. The Finnish Diabetes Prevention Study (DPS) lifestyle intervention and 3-year results on diet and physical activity. *Diabetes Care*. 2003;26:3230–3236.

9. Knowler WC, Barrett-Connor E, Fowler SE, et al. Diabetes Prevention Program Research Group. Reduction in the incidence of type 2 diabetes with lifestyle intervention or metformin. *N Engl J Med*. 2002;346(6):393–403.

10. NICE Clinical Guideline 43. *Obesity: Guidance on the Prevention, Identification, Assessment and Management of Overweight and Obesity in Adults and Children*. 2008.

11. Mead A, Atkinson G, Albin D, et al., on behalf of the UK heart Health and Thoracic Dietitians Interest Group. Dietetic guidelines on food and nutrition in the secondary prevention of cardiovascular disease—evidence from systematic reviews of randomised controlled trials. *J Hum Nutr Diet*. 2006;19:401–419.

12. Williams B, Poulter N, Brown M, et al. British Hypertension Society. Guidelines for the management of hypertension. *J Hum Hypertens*. 2004;18:139–185.

13. Appel L, Moore T, Obarzanek E, et al. A clinical trial of the effects of dietary patterns on blood pressure. *N Engl J Med*. 1997;336(16):1117–1124.

14. Lean MEJ, Powrie JK, Anderson AS, Garthwaite PH. Obesity, weight loss and prognosis in type 2 diabetes. *Diabet Med*. 1990;7:228–233.

15. Davies M, Tringham J, Peach F, Daly H. Prediction of the weight gain associated with insulin treatment. *J Diabetes Nurs*. 2003;7:94–98.

16. Connor H, Annan F, Bunn E, et al. Nutrition Subcommittee of the Diabetes Care Advisory Committee of Diabetes UK. The implementation of nutritional advice for people with diabetes. *Diabet Med*. 2003;20:786–807.

17. Franz M, Bantle J, Beebe C, et al. Evidence-based nutrition principles and recommendations for the treatment and prevention of diabetes and related complications. *Diabetes Care*. 2002;25(1):148–198.

18. Brand Miller J, Hayne S, Petrocs P, Colagiuri S. Low-glycaemic index diets in the management of diabetes—a meta-analysis of randomised controlled trials. *Diabetes Care*. 2003;26:2261–2267.

19. Friedberg C, Janssen M, Heine R, Grobbee D. Fish oil and glycaemic controlin diabetes. A meta-analyis. *Diabetes Care*. 1998;21:494–500.

20. Montori V, Farmer A, Woolan P, Dinneen S. Fish oil supplementation in type 2 diabetes. A qualitative systematic review. *Diabetes Care*. 2000;23:1407–1415.

21. Burr MI, Ashfield-Watt PA, Dunstan FD, et al. Lack of benefit of dietary advice to men with angina: results of a controlled trial. *Eur J Clin Nutr*. 2003;57:193–200.

22. *Advice on Fish Consumption: Benefits and Risks*. London: HMSO; 2004.

23. Rodin G, Johnson L, Garfinkel P, Daneman D, Kenshole A. Eating disorders in female adolescents with insulin dependant diabetes mellitus. *Int J Psychiatry Med*. 1986;16(1):49–55.

24. Kipps S, Bahu T, Ong K, Ackland FM, Brown RS, Fox CT.

Current methods of transfer of young people with type one diabetes to adult services. *Diabet Med.* 2002;19:649–654.

25. Dovey-Pearce G, Doherty Y, May C. The influence of diabetes upon adolescent and young adult development: a qualitative study. *Br J Health Psychol.* 2007;12:75–91.

26. Elia M, Ceriello A, Laube H, Sinclaire AJ, Engfer M, Stratton RJ. Enteral nutritional support and use of diabetes-specific formulas for patients with diabetes: a systematic review and meta-analysis. *Diabetes Care.* 2005;28(9):2267–2279.

27. Nield L, Moore HJ, Hooper L, et al. Dietary advice for treatment of type 2 diabetes mellitus in adults. *Cochrane Database Syst Rev.* 2007;(3):CD004097.

28. DAFNE Study Group. Training in flexible, intensive management to enable dietary freedom in people with type 1 diabetes: dose adjustment for normal eating (DAFNE) randomised controlled trial. *Br Med J.* 2002;325:746.

29. Shearer A, Bagust A, Sanderson D, Heller S, Roberts S. Cost effectiveness of flexible intensive insulin management to enable dietary freedom in people with type 1 diabetes in the UK. *Diabet Med.* 2004;21(5):460–467.

30. Structured patient education working group. Report from the Patient Education Working Group. Department of Health; 2005.

Obesity

18

Linda Hindle   David Kendrick

LEARNING OBJECTIVES

Readers of this chapter will gain an appreciation of:

- The physical and psychological causes and consequences of obesity;
- The importance of assessment for weight management;
- Evidence-based approaches to the dietetic treatment of obesity;
- A psychological approach to weight management; and
- The use of drugs and surgery to manage obesity.

Background

The prevalence of obesity is increasing such that over half the population are now overweight or obese.[1,2] This has significant health consequences, causing an increase in the risk of diabetes, coronary heart disease and certain cancers.[3] In 2008 the UK Government's Foresight programme commissioned a report to project the future growth of obesity rates through to 2050 and to predict the consequences for health, health costs and life expectancy.[4] The worrying results estimate that by 2050, 60% of males and 50% of females and about 25% of all children under 16 will be obese. There is now considerable political, media and public focus on obesity and clear targets for the reduction of obesity. Governments across the world are setting targets and policies to stem the rising tide of obesity. Within this context, dietitians are in a key position to contribute to addressing the problem of obesity.

During the 1980s dietitians approached the treatment of obesity primarily from a technical perspective, taking the view that in order to lose weight people just needed information. In 1994 the Health Education Authority launched Helping People Change based on Prochaska and DiClemetes' Stages of Change Model.[5,6] This led dietitians to develop a patient-centred approach for the treatment of obesity as they began to understand the psychology of behaviour change and appreciate why changing lifestyles to lose weight is not as simple as following instructions in a diet sheet.

Nowadays obesity is seen as a specialist area. Many dietitians have developed skills in motivational interviewing, counselling and cognitive behavioural therapy (CBT) in order to support patients to lose weight. Medication is now available as an adjunct to dietetic advice and dietitians are working with patients who are undergoing surgery to manage their weight.[7] There has also been an expansion in the role of pubic health dietitians with the recognition of the importance of the prevention of obesity.[8,9]

Physiology

Obesity occurs when a person puts on weight to the point that it seriously endangers health. Obesity is defined in terms of body mass index (BMI), which is a measure of body fat based on height and weight (Table 18.1).

Obesity in children and adolescents is normally defined in clinical practice as a sex- and age-specific

Table 18.1 Classification of body mass index and risk of comorbidities[10]

Classification	BMI (kg/m^2)	BMI (kg/m^2) Asian origin[11]	Risk of comorbidities
Underweight	< 18.5	< 18.5	Low (but risk of other clinical problems increased)
Normal range	18.5–24.9	18.5–22.9	Average
Overweight	25.0–29.9	23–27.4	Increased risk
Obese class I	30.0–34.9	27.5–32.4	Moderate
Obese class II	35.0–39.9	32.5–37.4	Severe
Obese class III	> 40.0	> 37.5	Morbid obesity

BMI at or above the 98th percentile based on 1990 BMI percentile classification charts (91st percentile for overweight).[8] When population data are collected children are defined as obese if their BMI is > 95th percentile of the reference curve for age.

Although BMI is commonly used to assess the health risks associated with obesity, research suggests that measuring the waist circumference or waist-to-hip ratio is also a reliable method of estimating the health risks associated with an increase in weight (intra-abdominal fat mass).[10] This measure may also be more appropriate for Asian communities (Table 18.2).[8]

Some people are more genetically susceptible to obesity, but the basic cause of obesity is consuming more calories (units of energy) from food and drink than are expended in everyday activity. Most evidence suggests that the main reason for the rising levels of obesity is changing eating habits and less active lifestyles.

Psychological factors can play a significant part in the development and maintenance of obesity. These may include anxiety, depression, trauma and prolonged distress, low self-esteem and psychosocial problems.

Understanding the health consequences of obesity

Obesity is an important risk factor for many chronic diseases and the psychological and social burden of obesity can be significant. Social stigma, low self-esteem and a generally poorer quality of life are common experiences for many obese people.[12]

Estimates of relative risk give a broad indication of the strength of the association between obesity and the secondary disease types listed in Table 18.3, although the BMI range used to estimate risk varies between studies.

A weight loss of 10% will potentially bring significant health benefits for obese people with corresponding reductions in blood pressure, lipid profiles and blood sugars.

Table 18.2 Waist measurements as a predictor of health risk

	Men	Asian men	Women	Asian women
Waist circumference				
Increased risk	≥ 94 cm		≥ 80 cm	
Substantially increased risk	≥ 102 cm	≥ 90 cm	≥ 88 cm	≥ 80 cm
Waist-to-hip ratio				
Increased risk	≥ 1.0		≥ 0.87	

Adapted from WHO.[10]
Jung RT. Obesity as a disease. *Bri. Med. Bull.* 1997;53(2):307–321.

Table 18.3 Increased risk of developing associated disease for the obese[12]

Disease	Relative risk	
	Men	**Women**
Myocardial infarction	1.5	3.2
Type 2 diabetes	5.2	12.7
Hypertension	2.6	4.2
Stroke	1.3	1.3
Cancer of colon	3.0	2.7

Understanding the psychological and social consequences of obesity

Lack of understanding of the problems facing the obese is a serious problem. It is certainly fair to say that our society has a very negative view of people who are seen as being 'fat'. One of these problems is intense prejudice or discrimination which cuts across age, sex, religion, race and socioeconomic status, and can be experienced at school, in the workplace and in family and social situations.

Therefore, it is important for us to understand the social and psychological consequences of obesity if we are to successfully help treat the problem. Research evidence of stigma and discrimination agrees with the public values and attitudes commonly expressed by the media. They tell us that being fat is an extremely unattractive and undesirable way to be, indeed, that it is a state to be avoided at all costs. Obese women are less likely to find employment, more likely to have their performance rated negatively and less likely to be promoted.[13]

The perception of obesity

This derogatory view of obesity is not new. Some of the earliest research, published in the 1960s, examined children's attitudes, presumably because they tend to reflect prevailing adult opinion. In one of these studies 10- and 11-year-olds were presented with six line drawings of a child as physically normal and with each of five physical disabilities, one being overweight. Ranking the figures by asking which they liked best resulted in a robust order of preference, with the normal child at the top, and the overweight child at the bottom, below that of a child with facial disfigurement, in leg brace and crutches or in a wheelchair. In a second study children were asked to assign 39 adjectives to one of three silhouette drawings depicting a thin, a muscular and a fat body shape. The obese body shape was least frequently assigned as best friends, most frequently gets teased, and labelled as lazy, dirty, stupid, ugly, liars and cheats more often than the other body shapes.[14]

These two studies are important since they describe two principal features of the stigma of overweight. On one hand is the stigmatisation of bodily appearance; obesity is a highly visible but undesirable state. On the other is the stigmatisation of character; the moral view that holds the obese personally responsible for their own state and so blames them for their fatness.[15]

Cognitive behavioural features of obesity

One of the basic premises of cognitive behavioural psychology is that there is causal inter-relationship between the way a person thinks (cognition) and what they do (behaviour). Neither the cognition nor the behaviour has the dominant causal role; either can be responsible for eliciting the other at any time.[16] This relationship between thinking and doing can be very complex and difficult to understand, particularly by those who know they are engaging in maladaptive behaviour (e.g. overeating), leading to unwanted products of that behaviour (e.g. weight gain, diabetes), but can not seem to control the 'urge' or 'need' to do so.

The aim of a thorough cognitive behavioural assessment is to get as much information as possible about the behaviour under investigation and what the links are between the way the person thinks and behaves. The outcome of this assessment should lead the investigator to propose a functional analysis of the problem which focuses on explaining 'why' the person behaves the way they do. Once this is understood it is possible to give the client insight into the links between their own thinking and behaviour, which will hopefully better equip them to deal with the problems they are experiencing.

For instance, most people who are morbidly obese have tried to lose weight by a variety of dietary constraints and/or pharmacological methods. They have often been successful in losing weight, only then to regain it plus 'interest'! This subsequently leads to demoralisation over these 'failed' attempts to manage their obesity. It is important to understand how the individual handles this demoralisation in order to give them advice on how to plan their current/future attempt at weight loss by changing the 'rules' of their weight loss strategy.

It is similarly important to understand whether the person equates morbid obesity to a 'personal defect' or a 'behavioural problem'.

If it is seen as a personal defect, many compensate for this by overextending themselves at home, at work or with friends. They may have a tendency to take care of other people at the expense of their own health and well being, often assuming a 'caretaker' role, putting the needs of others above their needs, and being unable or unwilling to ask for help for themselves. Explaining and getting them to accept that obesity can be viewed as a behavioural problem rather than a character defect can increase the likelihood of successful weight loss and maintenance.

Finally, to what extent do they have control over their environment? Feeling helpless (or without control over one's environment) increases the risk for anxiety, depression and treatment non-adherence.[17]

Binge eating disorder

Binge-eating disorder (BED) is characterised by recurrent binge-eating episodes, without the compensatory weight control methods found in bulimia nervosa. Although obesity is not a criterion for BED, it is a condition frequently associated with this diagnosis. Compared to matched obese subjects who do not binge, obese binge-eaters experience higher levels of general and eating-related psychopathology. For example, they show more concerns with body shape, and some authors found that binge-eating is significantly correlated with the perception that body weight is above the ideal.[18]

Utilisation of social support

Research suggests that, for medical patients, social support is positively related to faster recovery and negatively related to premature mortality. Social support is also related to successful weight loss for people attending a general behavioural weight loss programme.[19]

It would appear that some patients are especially susceptible to weight regain when faced with adversity that distracts them from attending to self-management guidelines. Clinically, we see maladaptive eating behaviour (whether stress eating, emotional eating, binge eating or night eating) associated frequently with poor stress management and with an inability to effectively self-modulate intense emotions or internal sensations of arousal (whether positive or negative). A careful assessment of their ability to cope both with negative stressors (uncertainty, frustration, deadlines, depressed mood, anger, anxiety or boredom) and with positive stressors (a pay-rise, a promotion, a party or holiday) may indicate whether they need specific intervention to enable them to handle stress better and therefore increase the likelihood of successful weight control, and avoid simply substituting one maladaptive coping behaviour (eating) with another (e.g. alcohol or drug abuse).

Compliance with medical treatment and adherence to self-management regimens currently and in the past are indicators of the patient's potential attitude toward treatment.[20]

Nutritional therapy and dietetic application

Much about the management of obesity relates to the approach taken by the practitioner and the relationship established between the practitioner and client. Therefore the assessment, approach and interpersonal skills of the practitioner are key elements to successful weight management.

Assessment

It is well recognised that one size does not fit all when it comes to what will help someone to lose weight. The diet trials study followed participants on one of four commercially available weight management programmes (Weight Watchers, Slim Fast, Atkins Diet, Rosemary Conley).[21] The authors concluded that each approach could work effectively provided the client chose the approach most suited to their lifestyle and preferences. A thorough assessment is required to enable the therapist and client to identify the approach most likely to be effective. The assessment gives the client an opportunity to self-reflect and identify enablers and barriers and gives the therapist an understanding of the client's lifestyle, previous experiences of weight loss, history of weight gain, social circumstances and relationship with food.

The assessment is an opportunity to develop a rapport with the client and to demonstrate empathy in order that the client will have trust and confidence in the therapist's ability to support them to lose weight; therefore the assessment appointment must be relaxed and not feel like an interrogation.

Interviewer skills

The 'interviewer' must have a goal-directed, focused approach and needs to develop specific skills in order to overcome the patient's ambivalence or lack of resolve. This is one of the main obstacles that must be overcome if the person is to bring about the behavioural changes they need to ensure successful weight loss and maintenance.

Problem eating behaviour often takes the form of a conflict between the benefits and costs of both eating and restraint. It is important to attempt to get clients to identify, articulate and resolve this ambiguity, allowing them the opportunity to express (perhaps for the first time) the often confusing, contradictory and very personal feelings they have about themselves and their behaviour.

Direct persuasion is generally not an effective method of trying to resolve these issues. This may have been tried by family and friends attempting to be helpful, but tends to lead to the person becoming more resistant to change, resenting the help and the helpers, and increasing their belief in their own weakness. This in turn leads to more of the compensatory behaviour (i.e. eating).

The relationship between the client and the interviewer is very important and involves mutual respect. The person-centred approach allows the client to have their autonomy and freedom of choice. The client should respect the interviewer's expertise in the field but not feel as if they are in a purely recipient role. It is possible to develop this relationship in just one session provided the interviewer is well trained and experienced.

In summary, the primary intention of this type of motivational interviewing is to increase the client's readiness for change by allowing the client the opportunity to elaborate how they perceive the current situation. The skilled interviewer needs to be able to identify what the current conflicts are (discriminating between the critical and trivial issues), and then direct the person towards self-identification and subsequent problem solving. This gives the client 'ownership' of both the problem and its solution. They may need some form of intervention (e.g. skills training, cognitive restructuring, psycho-education) to enable them to satisfactorily resolve the problem but this is a secondary step to the initial phase of problem identification.

More directive or confrontational approaches should not be ruled out as motivational techniques. Some clients do respond well to having their beliefs confronted and deconstructed and alternatives proposed by the person carrying out the interview. They may not have had anyone able or willing to question their beliefs in a constructive way before. Use of logic, scientific facts and rationalising alternative thinking patterns can lead to the client being faced with information which is both novel and informative. This can be enlightening and give the client hope that there may be alternative strategies which they had not thought of and therefore may lead to an increased optimism of success.

The assessment interview will not necessarily follow any particular order; the flow will be determined by the client. However, the aim will be to cover the issues outlined below:

- History of weight gain;
- How the individual's weight or current eating habits are impacting on their life;
- Understanding of the client's social circumstances;
- What support the client has;
- Previous experiences of trying to lose weight;
- The client's realistic expectations, if any;
- Motivation and confidence to make lifestyle changes;
- Activity level;
- Comorbidities and medication;
- Measurements of weight, height, BMI and waist circumference; and
- Dietary assessment.

At the beginning as with all dietetic consultations, introduce yourself, set the scene by clarifying the purpose of the session with the client and explain how long the appointment will take. The room setup is important: clients should feel comfortable and care should be taken that seating is appropriate for obese clients by avoiding chairs with arms or chairs that are too low.

A traditional diet history or 24-hour recall may not provide the most useful information about a client's eating habits. Overweight and obese clients are known to under-report their intake by as much as 30–50%.[22] Overweight people may feel that they will be judged and therefore may not divulge the amount they eat. Equally they may not be fully aware of what they regularly consume. Overeating is usually associated with feelings of guilt which makes sharing this difficult. Asking about patterns rather than specifics can result in a more enlightening response. Questions that may be useful include:

- Are there any foods that are a problem for you?/If you were to overeat, what foods would you generally choose?
- Are there any times of the day when it is more difficult for you to control your eating?
- Do you eat regularly?/Do you ever miss meals?
- Do you tend to eat in response to emotions such as anger, being upset or because you are bored?
- Do you ever feel that your eating is out of control/feel that you can't stop eating?
- Do you ever get up in the middle of the night to eat?
- Do you ever use laxatives or vomiting in an attempt to control your weight?
- How would you describe your portion sizes?
- How frequently do you eat out or have takeaways?
- What do you usually drink (including alcohol)?
- What do you think is the reason you are gaining weight?

The information obtained from this method of questioning will enable the therapist and client to identify key problems to be addressed such as irregular meals, snacking, types of food consumed and binge eating. The use of a food diary may give more detail if the client is able to complete it in adequate detail. This can be useful for refining advice at a later date but is not generally required initially.

A thorough assessment will require at least 45 minutes to do well.

Dietetic therapy

The dietetic approach chosen will be driven by the outcomes of the assessment.

There is no one size fits all with respect to choosing a weight loss approach; however, there are a number of principles supported by the evidence that are most likely to result in a successful outcome. These are described below.

Combination of diet, activity and behaviour modification

Weight management programmes that combine diet and physical activity treatments with behaviour modification support are most effective at supporting people to lose weight.[7] Approaches that focus on only one lifestyle element are less likely to support long-term weight loss.

Importance of regular meals

Many people struggling to control their weight follow an erratic meal pattern, frequently missing meals. This may be as a conscious effort to diet or restrain eating or as a lifestyle choice or habit. Ignoring internal hunger cues in order to stick to a diet may disrupt normal caloric regulation as demonstrated in Keys' starvation studies.[23] These studies of conscientious objectors during World War II highlighted the impact of prolonged calorie restriction. The participants underwent experimental starvation to reduce their weight by 25% followed by a refeeding programme. As a result of the starvation phase, they became more obsessed by food (hording food, eating very slowly and taking interest in cookery books) and during the period of refeeding, many became disinhibited and 'lost control' of their eating, consuming large quantities without feeling satiated. It has been suggested that habitual dieters display marked overcompensation in eating behaviour similar to binge eating observed in eating disorders.[24] By the same mechanisms, dieters who frequently miss meals are more likely to overeat at other points in the day; therefore one of the key aspects of supporting weight management is to help the client to develop a structured eating pattern including regular meals.[25] The basis for these effects of starvation is both physical and psychological. Prolonged periods between meals result in depleted glycogen and blood glucose stores which may lead to cravings for food, particularly that which is energy dense.

Low calorie diets

Reducing calorie intake to lower than energy expenditure will inevitably result in weight loss. Emphasis has been placed on a 600-calorie deficit diet as an effective low calorie diet. This involves estimating an individual's energy requirements and then subtracting 600-kcal. Formulas to estimate this have been published based on modified Schofield

Table 18.4 Formula to calculate energy requirements

Age range	Male	Female
BMR equals		
10–17 years	17.7 × weight (kg) + 657	13.4 × weight (kg) + 692
18–29 years	15.1 × weight (kg) + 692	14.8 × weight (kg) + 487
31–59 years	11.5 × weight (kg) + 873	8.3 × weight (kg) + 846
60+ years	11.7 × weight (kg) + 587	9.1 × weight (kg) + 658
Account for activity factor		
Inactive	BMR × 1.4	BMR × 1.4
Light	BMR × 1.5	BMR × 1.5
Moderate	BMR × 1.78	BMR × 1.64
Heavy	BMR × 2.1	BMR × 1.82

Adapted from Schofield.[26]

equations (Table 18.4).[26] And on a simplified predictive equation for resting energy expenditure proposed by Mifflin and St Jeor[27]:

Females
$$REE = 9.99 \times weight\ (kg) + 6.25 \times height\ (cm) - 4.92 \times age - 161$$
Males
$$REE = 9.99 \times weight\ (kg) + 6.25 \times height\ (cm) - 4.92 \times age + 5$$

A review of 13 randomised controlled trials (RCTs) using 600-calorie deficit diets have demonstrated that this is an effective method of weight loss for some, resulting in an average weight loss of 5.32 kg after 12 months, compared to usual care.[28] This is the energy deficit that clients are most likely to be able to adhere to over the time required to achieve weight loss; greater deficits increase the risk of non-compliance.[29,30] This approach, however, will not suit everyone as it does require clients to plan meals and measure their intake.

The dietary assessment will support the dietitian to determine which clients are likely to benefit from this approach. These diets are generally based on the healthy eating principles. The use of low energy density foods, i.e. those with a high volume to calorie ratio, may support clients to follow an energy-deficit diet. This is based on the principle that the volume of food consumed rather than the calorie content influences satiety.[31,32]

Low fat diets

Low fat diets have been encouraged both to support weight loss and to improve cardiovascular risk. Fat is more energy dense than other macronutrients and therefore reducing the proportion of fat in the diet can be a successful way of reducing the total calorie content. A meta-analysis of 16 trials has reviewed the effectiveness of low fat diets eaten ad libitum to achieve weight loss.[33] This analysis found that low fat diets resulted in an average weight loss of 3.2 kg lower than that of controls. There is, however, a paucity of research examining the efficacy of low fat diets on weight loss as many studies have not investigated weight change as a primary outcome.

Meal replacements

Meal replacements are generally considered to be 'portion controlled products that are vitamin and mineral fortified and replace one or two meals in the day allowing one low calorie meal using standard foods (and snack/s)'.[34] A meal replacement approach will usually provide in the region of 1200–1600 kcal per day and should not be confused with very low calorie diets that provide less than 800 kcal/day. Meal replacement products are not designed to be a complete source of nutrition and therefore are not usually recommended for use without the inclusion of foods in the diet, although they do provide protein, fibre, vitamins and minerals.

This approach is popular among consumers and recent research has indicated that it is an effective and safe method of weight loss.[34,35] Part of the efficacy of the meal replacement approach may relate to the structured nature of the plan and the emphasis on regular eating. Meal replacements can simplify food choices by lessening the 'pressure' of food selection, providing confidence in the number of calories consumed and reducing the variety of foods to choose from while maintaining an element of food choice. Meal replacements can be used to train clients in the skills of stimulus control and relapse prevention by using the meal replacements in situations where binging behaviour would be likely.[36]

Very low calorie diets (VLCDs)

VLCDs are defined according to the international CODEX standardisation and legislation by the US Food and Drugs Administration and European Union as total diet replacements with an energy content < 800 kcal and > 450 kcal/day. VLCDs are designed to produce the most rapid weight loss possible while preserving muscle mass. This is done by providing a high proportion of dietary protein (70–100 g/day). They are also required to contain (or be supplemented with) 100% of the recommended daily amount of vitamins and minerals. Typically no other foods are allowed and individuals are expected to consume at least 2 L of water.

These diets should not be used continuously for more than 12 weeks at a time and must be under medical supervision.[7] A typical course includes the very low calorie diet for 12 weeks followed by a refeeding phase lasting approximately 6 weeks during which foods are gradually reintroduced and then a weight stabilisation phase. For patients who need to lose large amounts of weight the VLCD phase may be repeated several times with refeeding periods between each 12-week phase. VLCD programmes are generally run by commercial companies offering varying degrees of support from lay counsellors to specialist weight management clinics. Medical supervision is required for individuals undergoing a VLCD; this ideally involves a physician visit and blood test every two weeks of the diet phase, although this level of support is not always available. Medical examination is to rule out contraindications.

In the short term VLCDs are very successful, producing weight losses in the region of 9–26 kg.[37,38]

There is less good evidence that these diets are any more effective that low calorie diets in the longer term. In the NIH clinical guidelines four RCTs were identified comparing VLCD of 400–500 kcal/day with low calorie diets of 1000–1500 kcal/day for a period of 6 months to 5 years. Although the VLCD produced greater initial weight loss, after 1 year VLCDs were no more effective than the more conventional dietary treatment. This finding was supported by a Cochrane review which explored long-term non-pharmacological weight loss interventions in type 2 diabetes and found VLCDs were no more effective over the longer term than low calorie diets.[39]

VLCDs do have a role in weight management but will not be appropriate for the majority of overweight and obese patients.

Low carbohydrate diets

Low carbohydrate diets include 20–40 g carbohydrate per day during the weight loss phase, with a gradual increase in carbohydrate for weight maintenance. The diet relies on foods high in protein and does not limit fat intake. The weight loss mechanism is promoted to be a switch from a carbohydrate-burning metabolism to a fat-burning metabolism, resulting in the loss of body fat.[40] The benefits promoted are rapid initial weight loss without feeling hungry. The initial 1- to 2-kg weight loss achieved with a low carbohydrate diet is mostly due to glycogen and associated fluid losses.[41] The satiating effects of protein seem to help control appetite and have been shown to enhance weight loss over 6 months.[42]

Low glycaemic index diets

In theory choosing foods with a low glycaemic index (GI) can keep the glycaemic impact of the diet constant, i.e. avoid fluctuations in blood sugar. The theory follows that this would improve satiety and thereby facilitate regular meals and minimise overeating.[43] Currently there is inconsistent evidence as to whether this effect is seen in practice. A review by Raben found no difference in weight loss or satiety on low versus high GI diets.[44] A study by Ebbeling also found little effect of a low GI diet over their whole sample; however, it was effective for those who had high insulin secretions, suggesting that a low GI diet may be of benefit to support weight loss in those with hyperinsulinaemia.[45] Further studies are ongoing to determine the impact of low GI diets for weight management.

Cognitive–behavioural approach to managing obesity

Cognitive–behavioural therapy is a scientifically based programme developed after years of research on the most effective approaches to weight loss. Cognitive–behavioural treatment for weight loss/maintenance consists of three basic stages:

Changing eating behaviours

- Learning to recognise and adjust destructive eating patterns;
- Gaining control over binges;
- Learning about nutritional needs and hunger;
- Identifying alternatives to social and emotional eating;
- Starting a manageable exercise programme;
- Restricting calories for steady and healthy weight loss; and
- Self-monitoring (this is an extremely effective behavioural change technique when applied correctly, and warrants further explanation).

Self-monitoring is a very important component of behaviour therapy for obesity and involves keeping daily records of food intake and physical activity, and checking weight regularly. Self-monitoring records can provide information needed to identify links in the behaviour chain that can be targeted for intervention. In addition, record keeping can enhance compliance with dietary and physical activity interventions. Some people, however, find self-monitoring aversive, leading to increased feelings of inadequacy or loss of control. Should this be the case, self-monitoring should be discontinued either permanently or until they are able to recognise the benefits that can be gained from use of this powerful monitoring device.[46]

The most common time for self-monitoring to take place is post-behaviour, i.e. recording food eaten after it has been consumed. This can give a precise measure of the amount of food consumed, and other information about time, location, etc, and therefore should be used during the assessment phase of any behaviour change programme to give the most reliable data about these aspects of the client's eating behaviour. Post-behaviour recording can also lead to change in eating behaviour by the reactive effect of having to record it, and this in itself can be a very effective change technique. However, to gain maximum reactive effect from self-monitoring, clients should be asked to record the food they are going to eat before they eat it (pre-behaviour monitoring). The effect of this is to make the client think about the food they are going to eat and have to justify to themselves actually eating it.

Challenging cognitions, or the psychological patterns and dysfunctional thinking that gets in the way of healthy eating

- Identifying cognitive distortions;
- Adjusting thinking to promote success rather than shame and hopelessness;
- Reducing depression and anxiety;
- Increasing social support and improving existing relationships;
- Learning stress management skills; and
- Improving body image and self-confidence.

Long-term maintenance of weight loss

- Development of individualised weight management plans;
- Prevention of weight regain;
- Maintaining motivation for a healthy lifestyle; and
- Strengthening coping skills for challenging situations and future setbacks.

Cognitive restructuring teaches patients to think in a positive manner and to correct thoughts that undermine weight management efforts. Cognitive techniques also help patients accept realistic, but less-than-desired, weight losses. Inappropriate feelings of failure after achieving modest but clinically important weight loss can lead to relapse and weight regain.

Pharmacology

Lifestyle modification is the cornerstone of obesity management; however, many patients require additional therapy with drugs. At the time of writing there is only one drug licensed to treat obesity in the UK; this acts by

> decreasing absorption of fat from the gastrointestinal tract (Orlistat)

Royal College of Physicians and NICE have given guidance on the use of anti-obesity medications.[7]

Surgery

Surgery is now an option for weight management in those with a BMI over 40 and significant health risks related to their weight or with a BMI over 50.[7] Essentially restrictive surgical procedures are vertical banded gastroplasty (VBG) and adjustable gastric banding (AGB) which involve a band being positioned around the stomach to create a small stomach pouch. This pouch effectively becomes the stomach and thereby restricts the intake and will hopefully cause the individual to feel full after a small amount of food. A sleeve gastrectomy (SG) is similar to a VBG but relies purely on the surgical formation of a small stomach pouch or sleeve without any additional restrictive banding.

Other procedures used include duodenal switch and gastric bypass which redirects the gut from the upper part of the stomach to a lower part of the small intestine, thereby both reducing the size of the stomach and the absorptive capacity of the gut. Some surgeons will perform a two-stage procedure on super-obese patients for whom surgery is a major risk. They will initially complete a SG, which should reduce the patient's weight to a more acceptable (less risk) level, and then a bypass to help with continued and satisfactory weight loss. All bariatric surgery has medical, dietary and psychological implications and therefore multiprofessional assessment and management is essential.

Psychological assessment presurgery

Bariatric surgery is a procedure that can not only reconfigure a patient's eating behaviour (and therefore body shape), but also significantly affect their psychological well being (either positively or negatively). It is therefore of paramount importance to carry out an assessment of the psychological status of the patient prior to surgery.[7]

The presurgical assessment attempts to ascertain whether the candidate is adequately prepared, from a psychosocial perspective, to go forward with bariatric surgery and whether there is evidence of any issues that may compromise patient safety and/or with the patient's adjustment to the surgical procedure.

Some clinicians may elect to incorporate some level of intervention into the assessment process. Intervention may include education about the surgery and the requirements of success, skill-building, reframing faulty cognitions or psycho-education.

In the same way that a surgeon assesses patients for bariatric surgery in an attempt to ascertain features of their general health, establishing those for whom surgery is too risky and/or those who have conditions that preoperative intervention is indicated, psychological health specialists need to make an assessment on similar lines. Whilst no prediction of outcome can be definite, a psychological assessment can identify psychosocial risk factors and make recommendations to both the client and the other members of the team that are aimed at facilitating the best possible outcome for the patient.

When problematic presurgery psychosocial factors are identified, the clinician is able to inform and alert both the treatment team and the patient, and make appropriate recommendations, which may include pharmacological interventions, psycho-education or specific psychotherapy to address potential post-surgery stumbling blocks. It may also be in the patient's best interest if the clinician can identify, recommend and perhaps initiate preoperative psychological intervention should the client's problems be assessed to require more long-term therapy.

Postoperatively, patients must make some major behavioural and cognitive adjustments. There are no rules as to how difficult or easy the individual will find making these changes, but the clinician needs to assess numerous aspects of the patient's current psychological functioning in order to make a judgement about the prognosis of a successful long-term outcome. Part of this assessment must involve ascertaining the degree of understanding the individual has about their own eating behaviour and changes they will need to make postoperatively, together with a judgement about whether making such changes will be possible.

Whilst there are no definitive rules on what must be included in a pre-bariatric surgery psychological assessment, common categories of assessment include the following.

Behavioural

Previous attempts at weight management and patterns of weight loss and regain can provide valuable information regarding the psychological (behavioural and cognitive) factors associated with the patient's success/failure to control weight gain.

Included in this part of the assessment would be a review of the candidate's past and current eating and dietary styles which can also provide the clinician with vital information on both the client's readiness for surgery and factors that will either support or interfere with post-surgical compliance and adherence.

Tracking eating behaviours over time and across situations (e.g. work, home or holidays) can offer information regarding how environmental factors affect cognition and therefore behaviour, helping the client predict and prepare for these situations and make appropriate changes.

Behavioural information of this sort can be indicative of post-surgical prognosis and therefore that pre-surgery intervention and post-surgery monitoring and/or intervention are required.

Maladaptive eating behaviour

This term covers a number of different eating patterns including binge eating, bulimia nervosa, overeating, grazing and night eating disorder.

All maladaptive eating behaviours are not functionally similar. It can be useful initially to delineate maladaptive patterns of eating that are subsequent to dieting and restriction versus those styles of eating that are clearly emotionally driven.

Substance use

While the assessment of substance use is standard practice for nearly all healthcare practitioners, when assessing obese people it is useful to examine any links between the person's use of a substance and his/her judgment of the benefits and dangers of the substance and how well the individual can control its usage. To this end, some indication of the individual's coping strategies under different situations, proneness to addictive behaviours, compulsive tendencies and real/perceived need to self-medicate can be useful indicators of their ability to control their behaviour post-surgery.

Health-related risk-taking behaviour

These include behaviours likely to be impulsive, compulsive or habitual in nature.

Impulsive behaviour is one which is preceded by little if any consequential thinking. Bariatric surgery candidates with impulse control problems raise concerns because postoperative safety and success relies on a high degree of compliance, which in turn relies on a high degree of cognitive control. Patients with impulsive tendencies may be at higher risk for the resumption of disordered eating, including the consumption of less healthy foods with high caloric

value and ignoring initial post-surgery dietary restrictions (liquid and pureed food intake) and turn to eating solids too soon, thus risking pouch-related problems.

Compulsive behaviour serves to distract an individual from unpleasant or unwanted thoughts or feelings. In obese patients typical compulsive behaviours include emotional eating, stress eating and cigarette smoking. Obese patients who are known to exhibit compulsive behaviour are at high risk post-surgery for substituting other behaviours when food is no longer readily available or a usable option.

Habitual behaviour is an action executed automatically. However, new habit acquisition often requires deliberate thinking. In order to change a habit, the individual must be able to respond repeatedly in a deliberate way to specific cues in his/her external environment or to thoughts/feeling they may experience. Evaluation of the role that food has played across the patient's life and the extent to which their eating behaviour is based on habitual thinking is very important because it may indicate specific psychological input is necessary to enable the patient to make changes to their established pattern of habitual behaviour.

Cognitive and emotional

Cognitive functioning and ability

It is important that candidates for bariatric surgery ideally should have the cognitive functioning and ability to be able to fully understand the surgical procedure, the associated risks and the behavioural changes required following surgery. It is of prime importance to establish preoperatively whether the patient is capable of understanding the profound changes that he/she needs to put in place postoperatively in order to ensure the greatest chance of a successful outcome in the long term.

Knowledge of morbid obesity, surgical interventions and outcome

It is not uncommon to find that patients have little or confused information about their condition, bariatric surgery and the problems they may have to face and overcome. It goes without saying that all patients need to be fully aware of all the facts before they can make an informed decision.

Many do not understand the dietary restrictions they must endure and the permanent change in eating and dietary habits that they must live with for the rest of their lives. Many are expecting a 'quick fix' which will relieve them of all the problems they experience around food. They also believe that being thinner is going to be the thing that will totally transform their lives; all will be well when they are thin.

Motivation and expectations

It is essential to assess patient motivation and reasons for pursuing surgery. What is motivating the candidate to pursue a bariatric surgical procedure at this time?

What expectations does the patient have concerning psychosocial, emotional and lifestyle challenges and adjustments post-surgery, both short and long-term? Unrealistic expectations may lead to the perception of failure when those expectations cannot be met. This failure may then become linked to 'throwing in the towel' and to giving in to old habits and unhealthy choices. Abstract expectations like 'to be happy' need to be seen in more concrete terms to ensure the patient isn't setting themselves up to fail.

Psychopathology

Psychopathology need not preclude a candidate from having a bariatric surgical procedure.[47] Before surgery, however, as with the assessment of cognitive functioning, it is necessary to determine and document that the candidate is emotionally stable, adequately informed and understanding of the risks both of surgery and of a psychiatric episode or an emotional crisis after surgery. There should also be a precautionary mental health action plan in place which has been agreed and accepted by all involved in the patient's care.

Current life situation

Any psychological assessment in this field needs to evaluate whether the candidate is suffering any current life stressors that may be seen to be contributory or causal to their weight control problems; any historical major stressors still affecting them; or any major stressors expected in the next year. A decision needs to be taken as to whether the client will be able to cope with the additional stress related to rapid, extensive post-surgery changes.

Dietetic management of patients undergoing bariatric surgery

Adjustable gastric banding

A gastric band produces a smaller stomach pouch which helps the individual to adhere to a weight-reducing diet by facilitating smaller meals and improving satiety between meals. The band restricts the passage of food ingested from the stomach pouch. The band can be inflated or deflated to achieve optimal restriction. For the first month after surgery patients are generally encouraged to follow a liquid diet or small amounts of blended food. After 4 weeks patients gradually progress to a soft diet and then to a normal diet. Typically weight is lost at a rate of 0.5–1 kg per week.

In the longer term patients should be encouraged to eat normal texture foods and avoid drinking with food. Liquid and soft textures can easily pass through the band and therefore do not effectively restrict intake. There is no reduced absorption; therefore supplementation should not be required, although most centres do recommend precautionary multivitamins and minerals.

Gastric bypass

This involves the creation of a smaller stomach pouch and a bypass of part of the intestine. Therefore weight loss effects are caused by restricted intake as with gastric banding and by slightly reducing the absorption of nutrients from the food ingested. Bypass operations are more complex and are usually reserved for those with the most weight to lose and who have serious comorbidities. Initial advice after surgery is not dissimilar to that used after a gastric banding as patients are getting used to a smaller stomach pouch.

Longer term, dietitians need to be aware of the risk of malnutrition caused by a combination of restricted intake and malabsorption. The nutrients most commonly affected are protein, iron, calcium and vitamin B_{12}. Most centres recommend routine use of a multivitamin and mineral preparation and some give B_{12} injections. A full blood count should be carried out on a regular basis. Dietitians need to support patients to consume a balanced diet. Patients often suffer from dumping syndrome when they eat foods high in refined carbohydrate.

Websites providing further information about the surgical management of obesity are included at the end of the chapter.

Special considerations

This chapter has primarily focused on obesity in adults although many of the issues discussed are equally relevant to subgroups of the population. This section briefly discusses the specific considerations of particular subgroups.

Obesity in children

It is generally agreed that children should be the target for reducing the obesity epidemic from both the perspective of preventing the development of obesity and management in children who are already obese. Factors that have been linked to the development of obesity in children include:[48–50]

- Sedentary lifestyles;
- Lack of physical activity;
- High intakes of energy-dense foods;
- Advertising of energy-dense foods;
- Lack of breastfeeding;
- High intakes of sugar-rich drinks;
- Poor sleep patterns;
- TV viewing;
- Parental obesity (one or both parents); and
- Early adiposity rebound.

Parents recognise that they have the greatest role to play in preventing obesity in their children but there are significant barriers to improving diets and lifestyles in children including a lack of recognition by parents of their child's weight status or associated risks; parental beliefs that healthy lifestyles are too challenging; pressure on parents that undermines healthy food choices such as advertising or peer pressure; and pressure on parents that reduces opportunities for active lifestyles such as work and financial pressures.[51]

There is limited evidence-based models for the effective treatment of obesity in children; however, research suggests that successful interventions will use a multifaceted approach incorporating increased lifestyle activity, reduced sedentary activity, emotional support, nutrition and exercise advice and social support. They will involve parents and have frequent appointments with prolonged duration.[52]

Obesity in older adults

The ageing process results in a loss of lean body mass. This can be masked in obese older adults by excess fat. The combination of reduced lean body mass and obesity can result in obese older adults becoming increasingly frail and immobile. As activity levels decrease weight gain may exacerbate. Obesity can also mask malnutrition if the quality of the diet is poor. Supporting older people to lose weight requires particular attention to the energy density of the diet.

Obesity in people with learning disabilities

People with learning disabilities are at an increased risk of obesity; it has been suggested that over 60% of people with learning disabilities are classified as overweight or obese.[53] Reasons for this can relate to specific syndromes such as Down's syndrome or Prader Willi or relate to the lifestyle circumstances of the individual. People with learning disabilities are more likely to have a sedentary lifestyle and have a lower knowledge of healthy eating or skills to put this into practice; they are likely to be reliant on others for food provision and frequently food will be inappropriately used as a reward by carers.[54]

Work to support people with learning disabilities to manage their weight will need to focus on environmental change and work with carers as well as equipping individuals with skills and knowledge to make healthy lifestyle decisions.

Obesity in South Asians

People in lower socio-economic groups, especially women, and some ethnic groups, e.g. black Caribbean and Pakistani women, are more at risk of becoming obese than the rest of the population.

Surveys of BMI have generally found that South Asian and European men have similar BMIs, although in South Asian women BMIs are higher than in European women.[55] Reliance on BMI as a measure of obesity has limitations when comparing ethnic groups because:

- There is uncertainty about whether the relationship between weight for height and percentage of body fat is the same in all ethnic groups;
- Ideal weight criteria are based on European data and may be inappropriate for South Asians because of differences in body frame size; and
- The metabolic consequences of obesity are related to the distribution of fat on the body as well as the quantity of fat in proportion to lean body mass.

At a given level of BMI, South Asian men and women have thicker trunk skin folds and higher mean waist-to-hip ratios than Europeans. About one-third of South Asian men and women aged over 40 years have waist-to-hip ratios above those considered to increase health risk (Table 18.2).

South Asians are also characterised by having higher blood pressure, greater insulin resistance, higher triglyceride and lower HDL levels. Thus rates of CHD are 40% higher than in Europeans and the prevalence of type 2 diabetes is five times higher.

Key points

- The prevalence of obesity is increasing and requires significant investment and focus to change the current trajectory.
- Dietitians can play a key role in the prevention and management of obesity through involvement in strategy and policy development, training, public health and clinical services.
- Treatment and prevention of obesity requires an understanding of the psychological as well as the physiological mechanisms involved in eating and activity.
- The assessment stage is critical to the treatment of obesity in the individual, just as an understanding of the target population is key to the prevention of obesity.
- Effective interventions are those where the individual can achieve and maintain an energy deficit. Different approaches will work for different individuals; the key is to match the intervention to the individual.
- Weight maintenance support is needed to ensure that the focus on the treatment of obesity is not wasted.

Case study

Jane is a 39-year-old single mother of two. She has always struggled with her weight but gained 7 kg as a result of each of her pregnancies and has gradually increased weight since then. She now weighs 96 kg; she is 155 cm tall. She has a part-time job in a local supermarket. Her social life is limited, because of her childcare responsibilities and financial circumstances. Jane used to enjoy going out but now she prefers to stay in because her self-confidence has decreased. Her children are aged 7 and 11; one is starting to become overweight. She is conscious of this and has attempted to alter the family meals; however, the children are reluctant to try new foods and she likes to treat them. Jane tries to avoid sweet foods and snacks but she does buy them for the children. Mornings are very busy and therefore she frequently misses breakfast. She always has lunch in the canteen at work and usually nibbles at what the children are having when she makes their dinner. Evenings are the most difficult time for Jane; she has a tendency to snack once she has put the children to bed and she relaxes with a glass or two of wine. Jane has tried numerous diets in the past; she is usually able to stick to them for about 2 weeks but then gets bored and frustrated with slow weight loss. She is busy at work but otherwise does not participate in any form of exercise. Jane is approaching 40 and wants to reinvent herself.

QUESTIONS

1. What else would you want to find out?
2. What are her motivations to change?
3. What might she find difficult?
4. What goals would you plan to discuss with her?
5. What other issues may need to be addressed?

ANSWERS

1. What else would you want to find out?
   - How does she feel her weight is impacting on her life?
   - How important is it for her to make changes now?
   - How confident is she that she can do this?
   - What does she feel will get in the way?
   - What are her expectations?
   - What access to support does she have?
2. What are her motivations to change?
   - Her age—she is reaching a milestone, which is causing her to focus on her future.
   - Her children—she is concerned about her children's weight.
   - She may hope to improve her appearance and self-confidence as this has decreased.
3. What might she find difficult?
   - It is likely that she has previously tried strict diet approaches to lose weight, which may be why she has tired of them so quickly; this may be linked to unrealistic expectations of weight loss.
   - She has a limited budget to buy food.
   - She is buying foods to suit her children which may be high fat/sugar foods.
   - She does not exercise regularly; this may be due to a variety of reasons such as time, cost, enjoyment, perception of ability.
   - She has a tendency to eat in the evenings; she may fear that this will be difficult to break.

Case study (Continued)

- She may have an 'all or nothing approach' to weight loss, which may cause her to feel that she has failed if she lapses.

4. What goals would you plan to discuss with her? These will be led by the client but may include:

    - Regular meals, especially eating breakfast and dinner;
    - Increasing activity, by building more activity into daily life, possibly undertaking activities with her children or making time to join an exercise class/go swimming where she may also meet new friends;
    - Reduce availability of high fat and high sugar snack foods in the house; and

- Reduce alcohol intake, which may be affecting her tendency to pick by disinhibiting her food choice, in addition to the direct source of calories.

5. What other issues would you want to address?

    - Access to support/social network—where could she get this from?
    - Realistic expectations;
    - Aiming for a lifestyle change rather than a diet and focusing on making changes for the whole family rather than just herself; and
    - Reasons for picking in the evening—is this just related to irregular meals or is she also eating for psychological reasons?

References

1. *Health Survey for England 2006, vol. 1: Cardiovascular Disease and Risk Factors in Adults*. The Information Centre; 2008. Available at: http://www.ic.nhs.uk/pubs/HSE06CVDandriskfactors.

2. Ogden CL, Caroll MD, Flegan KM. High body mass index for age among US children and adolescents 2003–6. *JAMA*. 2008;299(20):2401–2405.

3. Health Development Agency. *Evidence for the Effective Prevention and Treatment of Obesity*. London: HDA; 2004.

4. Foresight. *Trends and Drivers of Obesity: A Literature Review for the Foresight Project on Obesity*. 2007. Available at: http://www.foresight.gov.uk/obesity/Literature_Review.pdf.

5. Health Education Authority. *Helping People Change*. HEA; 1994, rev. 1997.

6. Prochaska JO, DiClemente CC. Towards a comprehensive model of change. In: Miller WR, Heather N, eds. *Treating Addictive Disorders: Process of Change*. New York: Plenum; 1986:3–27.

7. National Institute for Health and Clinical Excellence (NICE) (2006). *Obesity: The Prevention, Identification, Assessment and Management of Overweight and Obesity in Adults and Children*.

Available at: http://www.nice.gov.uk.

8. National Heart Forum. *Healthy weight; healthy lives: A toolkit for developing local strategies*; 2008.

9. Department of Health. *Healthy Weight, Healthy Lives: A Cross Government Strategy for England*. London: Department of Health; 2008.*http://www.dh.gov.uk/en/publichealth/healthimprovement/obesity/DH082383*.

10. World Health Organization (WHO). *Obesity: Preventing and Managing the Global Epidemic*. Report of a WHO Consultation on Obesity, Geneva, 3–5 June 1997, Geneva: WHO; 1998.

11. WHO Expert Consultation. Appropriate body mass index for Asian populations and its implications for policy and intervention strategies. *Lancet*. 2004;363:157–164.

12. National Audit Office. *Tackling Obesity in England*. London: HMSO; 2001.

13. Goldstein DJ. *The Management of Eating Disorders and Obesity*. 2nd edn. Clifton, NJ: Humana Press; 2005.

14. Hill AJ. Self-image and the stigma of obesity. In: Voss L, Wilkin T, eds. *Adult Obesity: A Paediatric Challenge*. London: Taylor and Francis; 2003:61–72.

15. Eisenberg ME, Neumark-Sztainer D, Story M. Associations of weight-based teasing and emotional well-being among adolescents. *Arch Pediatr Adolesc Med*. 2003;157:733–738.

16. Bandura A. *Social Learning Theory*. Prentice Hall: Englewood Cliffs, NJ; 1977.

17. Faith MS, Matz PE, Jorge MA. Obesity-depression co variations in the population. *J Psychosom Res*. 2002;5:935–942.

18. Dingemans AE, Bruna MJ, van Furth EF. Binge eating disorder: a review. *Int J Obes*. 2002;26: 299–307.

19. Cooper Z, Fairburn CG, Hawker DM. *Cognitive-Behavioural Treatment of Obesity*. New York: Guilford Press; 2003.

20. Meichenbaum D, Turk DC. *Facilitating Treatment Adherence: A Practitioner's Handbook*. New York: Plenum; 1987.

21. Truby H, Baic S, deLooy A, et al. A randomised controlled trial of four commercial weight loss programmes in the UK: initial findings form the BBC Diet Trials. *Br Med J*. 2006; 332(7553):1309–1314.

22. Lichtman SW, Pisarska K, Berman ER, et al. Discrepancy between self reported and actual caloric intake and exercise in obese subjects. *N Engl J Med*. 1992;327: 1893–1898.

23. Keys A, Brozek J, et al. *The Biology of Human Starvation*. Vol 2. Minneapolis: University of Minnesota Press; 1950.

24. Polivy J, Heman CP. Dieting and binging: a causal analysis. *Am Psychol*. 1985;40:193–201.

25. Haus G, Hoerr SL, Mavis B, Robison J. Key modifiable factors in weight maintenance: fat intake, exercise and weight cycling. *J Am Diet Assoc*. 1994;94(4):409–413.

26. Schofield WN. Predicting basal metabolic rate: new standards and review of previous work. *Hum Nutr Clin Nutr*. 1985;39C(suppl 1.5):41.

27. Mifflin MD, St Jeor ST, et al. A new predictive equation for resting energy expenditure in healthy individuals. *Am J Clin Nutr*. 1990;51:241–247.

28. Avenell A, Broom J, Brown J, et al. *Systematic Review of the Long-term Effects and Economic Consequences of Treatments for Obesity and Implications for Health Improvements*. Winchester, UK: Health Technology Assessment; 2004.

29. Lean MEJ, James WPT. Prescription of diabetic diets in the 1980. *Lancet*. 1986;1:723–725.

30. Frost G, Masters K, King C, et al. A new method of energy prescription to improve weight loss. *J Hum Nutr Diet*. 1991;15:287–295.

31. Bell EA, Rolls BJ. Energy density of foods affects energy intake across multiple levels of fat content in lean and obese women. *Am J Clin Nutr*. 2001;73:1010–1018.

32. Lowe M, Annunziato R, Riddell L, et al. Reduced energy density eating and weight loss maintenance: 18 month follow up results from a randoimised controled trial. *Obes Rev*. 2003;11s:A22.

33. Astrup A, Ryan L, Grunwalk GK, et al. The role of dietary fat in body fatness: evidence from a preliminary meta-analysis of ad libitum dietary intervention studies. *Br J Nutr*. 2000;83(suppl 1):s25–s32.

34. Heymsfield SB, van Mierlo CAJ, van der Knaap HCM, Heo M, Frier HI.

Weight management using a meal replacement strategy: meta and pooling analysis from six studies. *Int J Obes*. 2003;27(5):537–549.

35. Ashley JM, St Jeor ST, Perumean-Chaney S, Schrage J, Bovee V. Meal replacements in weight intervention. *Obes Res*. 2001;9(suppl 4): 312S–320S.

36. Heber D. Meal replacements in the treatment of obesity. In: Fairburn CG, Brownell KD, eds. *Eating Disorders and Obesity: A Comprehensive Handbook*. 2nd edn. New York: Guildford Press; 2002.

37. Anderson JW, Konz EC, Frederich RC, Wood CL. Long term weight loss maintenance: a meta-analysis of US studies. *Am J Clin Nutr*. 2001;74(5):579–584.

38. Saris WHM. Very low calorie diets and sustained weight loss. *Obes Res*. 2001;9(suppl 4):295–301.

39. Norris SL, Zhang X, Avenell A, et al. Long term non-pharmacological weight loss interventions for adults with type 2 diabetes mellitus. *Cochrane Database Syst Rev*. 2005;(2):CD004095.

40. Atkins RC. *Dr Atkins' New Diet Revolution*. New York: Avon Books; 1998.

41. Kreitzman SN, Coxon AY, Szaz KF. Glycogen storage: illusions of easy weight loss excessive weight regain, and distortions in estimates of body composition. *Am J Clin Nutr*. 1992;56(1 suppl):292s–293s.

42. Skov AR, Touboro S, Ronn B, Holm L, Astrup A. Randomised trial on protein versus carbohydrate in *ad libitum* fat reduced diet for the treatment of obesity. *Int J Obes*. 1999;23:528–536.

43. Brand-Miller JC, Holt SHA, et al. Glycaemic index and obesity. *Am J Clin Nutr*. 2002;76(suppl): 281S–285S.

44. Raben A. Should obese patients be counselled to follow a low glycaemic index diet? No. *Obes Rev*. 2002; 3:245–256.

45. Ebbeling CB, Leidig MM, Feldman HA, Lovesky MM,

Ludwig DS. Effects of a low-glycemic load vs low-fat diet in obese young adults: a randomized trial. *JAMA*. 2007; 297:2092–2102.

46. Haynes SN, Wilson CG. *Recent Advances in Behavioural Assessment*. San Francisco: Jossey-Bass; 1979.

47. Kinzl JF, Schrattenecker M, Traweger C, Mattesich M, Fiala M, Biebl W. Psychosocial predictors of weight loss after bariatric surgery. *Obes Surg*. 2007;16(12):1609–1614.

48. Campbell K, Waters E, O'Meara S, et al. Interventions for preventing obesity in children. *Cochrane Database Syst Rev*. 2002;(2):CD001871.

49. World Health Organization. *Diet, Nutrition and the Prevention of Chronic Diseases*. Geneva: WHO; 2003.

50. Reilly JJ, Armstrong J, Dorosty AR, et al. Early life risk factors for obesity in childhood: cohort study. *Br Med J*. 2005;330:1357.

51. Jebb S, Steer T, Holmes C. *The 'Healthy Living' Social Marketing Initiative: A Review of the Evidence*. Cambridge: Medical Research Council Human Nutrition Research; 2007.

52. Summerbell CD, Ashton V, Campbell KJ, Edmunds L, Kelly S, Waters E. Interventions for treating obesity in children. *Cochrane Database Syst Rev*. 2003;(3): CD111872.

53. Marshall D, McConkey R, Moore G. Obesity in people with intellectual disabilities: the impact of nurse-led screenings and health promotion activities. *J Adv Nurs*. 2003;41(2): 147–153.

54. Jefferys K. Managing and treating obesity in people with learning disabilities. *Learning Disability Practice*. 2000;2(4):30–34.

55. CRV Report 5: Reviews of literature and guidance for purchasers in the area of cardiovascular disease, mental health and haemoglobinopathies (ethnicity and health). NHS Centre for Reviews and Dissemination, Social Policy Research Unit; 1996.

Useful web sites

Dietitians in Obesity Management UK. http://www.domuk.org

British Obesity Surgery Patient Association. http://www.bospa.org

http://www.WLSinfo.co.uk

Cardiovascular disease

Katherine E. Paterson   Kenneth C-W. Wong
Hari K. Parthasarathy   Isma Rafiq

LEARNING OBJECTIVES

By the end of this chapter the reader will be able to:

- Understand the pathophysiology of cardiovascular disease (CVD) and the causal role of modifiable risk factors;
- Describe how nutritional interventions may complement medical management of CVD or risk factors;
- Evaluate the effectiveness of nutritional interventions in preventing and managing CVD;
- Implement practical dietetic strategies; and
- Critically appraise the role of omega-3 fatty acids in reducing cardiovascular mortality/morbidity.

Pathophysiology and risk factors

Introduction

Cardiovascular diseases encompass three main conditions: peripheral vascular disease, coronary heart disease and stroke. Whilst cardiovascular disease (CVD) has been the major cause of death and disability in developed countries for many years, its emergence as the major cause of death worldwide is a relatively recent statistic. It is estimated that 3.8 million men and 3.4 million women, worldwide, die each year from coronary heart disease (CHD) together with over five million total deaths from stroke.[1] Regional differences still occur with the highest incidence in countries where the main risk factors of hypertension, high plasma cholesterol, smoking, lack of physical activity and poor diet are prevalent. Whilst the incidence of CHD has declined in many developed countries, where various forms of intervention have been developed, the incidence in many emerging nations has increased dramatically during the past 30 years. For example, in the age range 35 to 75 the incidence has declined by over 40% in men and women in Sweden and the UK and by about 30% in the USA, whilst the incidence in Croatia has increased by over 60% in men and women and by about 40% overall in the Ukraine.[1]

CVD remains the major cause of death in the United Kingdom, accounting for about 198,000 deaths a year, with nearly half attributed to CHD and about a quarter from stroke. CVD remains one of the major causes of premature death in both men and women.[2] Like many other developed nations, where various strategies have increased public awareness of the major risk factors, such as smoking, lack of exercise and poor diet, the UK has seen a significant decline in the incidence of CHD in the last ten years. For people under the age of 75, the incidence has declined by 40%. Whilst medical and surgical treatment has made a significant contribution to the improved statistics, it is estimated that some 58% of the mortality decline during the past 30 years is attributable to a reduction in major risk factors.[2] Encouraging though these global figures are, they mask a number of trends related to factors such as age, regional, socioeconomic and ethnic differences.[2]

- The decline in the incidence of CHD is less marked in the younger age groups.
- The incidence of CHD remains higher and is declining less rapidly in the UK than in several other developed nations.

- Death rates from CHD are higher in Scotland and Northern England than in the rest of the UK. Premature death rates for men are 65% higher in Scotland than in south-west England and 112% higher for women.
- Premature deaths remain significantly higher in manual than in non-manual workers in both men (50%) and women (73%).
- Ethnic differences show a higher incidence of premature death in men (112%) and women (146%), living in the UK but born in South Asia, whilst for men born in the Caribbean and West Africa, but living in the UK, the incidence is lower than the national average.[3] Government and voluntary agencies have targeted all of the major risk factors for CVD, with particular emphasis on smoking, exercise and diet, with the aim of reducing the incidence of CVD.

The National Service Framework for Coronary Heart Disease set a series of standards to reduce the overall incidence of CHD in the population with a particular emphasis on addressing the regional, socioeconomic and ethnic inequalities outlined above.[4] Table 19.1, collated by the British Heart Foundation, summarises the major targets that have been set in England, Scotland and Wales.[2] Despite the unequal decline in the incidence of CHD in the population, the rate of decline in recent years shows that the UK has already achieved many of its 2010 targets.

The emphasis of this chapter is clearly focused on diet as improvement in cardiovascular health in recent years has involved a series of initiatives to improve nutritional standards in the general population.

Pathogenesis of cardiovascular disease

CVD encompasses a group of diseases affecting the heart and cerebral and peripheral vasculature. The term can refer to any disease affecting these structures but is usually used to refer to those conditions that result from the development of atherosclerosis in the heart, resulting in CHD or ischaemic heart disease (IHD); in the brain, causing a cerebrovascular accident (CVA); or in peripheral blood vessels causing peripheral vascular disease (PVD). The leading cause of death involves the coronary blood vessels, resulting in the development of ischaemic conditions in the heart, which may cause a heart attack or myocardial infarction (MI).

It is widely accepted that atherosclerosis develops as a result of mild endothelial damage, causing an inflammatory response with recruitment of circulating monocytes. Atherogenic lipoproteins such as low density lipoproteins (LDL) then enter the subendothelial space, where they become oxidised. Together with subendothelial monocyte-derived macrophages and T lymphocytes, fatty streaks develop, one of the earliest pathological lesions in atherosclerosis. Oxidised lipids can be taken up by macrophages to form lipid-laden macrophages called 'foam cells'. These foam cells in turn produce growth factors that promote cell proliferation, especially that of smooth muscle cells. Smooth muscle cells can also migrate from the muscular layers of the vessels (tunica media), ingest lipids and become foam cells themselves. Atherosclerosis occurs when these substances including the collagen secreted by smooth muscle cells, build up in the walls of arteries and form hard lesions called plaques. Besides lipid-laden cells, advanced plaques also contain extracellular cholesterol deposits released from dead cells. Calcified deposits can also develop between the muscular layers and the outer portion of the plaque, a result of intracellular microcalcification of smooth muscle cells and smooth muscle cell death. In addition, a fibrous cap usually forms between the endothelium and this lipid plaque. The overall result of all these processes is an atheromatous fibrolipid plaque, leading to narrowing and stiffening of arteries (though initially coronary arteries will enlarge in response to plaque formation in order to compensate). Note that arterial-associated macrophages can interact with high density lipoprotein (HDL) particles with transfer of cholesterol to the latter; this cholesterol will eventually be taken up by the liver. This is thought to be an important process limiting the progression of atheromatous plaques in peripheral arteries.

Figure 19.1 shows the mechanism for the development of thrombosis on plaques in two stages.

Atheromatous plaques are prone to rupture, leading to exposure of the prothrombotic contents (e.g. subendothelial collagen) of the plaque to circulating blood. Platelets start to aggregate and a thrombus develops, with subsequent partial or complete occlusion of the vessel. Some platelet-derived factors such as thromboxane A_2 can lead to localised vasospasm, which further limits blood flow. Severe limitation of blood flow can lead to an infarction in which the ischaemic conditions can lead to tissue damage and cellular death in the area(s) affected. When this happens in coronary arteries it results in a myocardial

Table 19.1 CVD mortality targets for the United Kingdom

England[a,b]

CVD—target	To reduce the death rate from CHD, stroke and related diseases in people under 75 years by at least two-fifths by 2010—saving up to 200,000 lives in total
CVD—milestone	To reduce the death rate from CHD, stroke and related diseases in people under 75 years by at least one-quarter by 2005
CVD—inequalities target	To reduce the inequalities gap in death rates from CHD, stroke and related diseases between the fifth of areas with the worst health and deprivation indicators and the population as a whole in people under 75 years by 40% by 2010

Wales[c,d]

CHD—health outcome target	To reduce CHD mortality in 65–74-year-olds from 600 per 100,000 in 2002 to 400 per 100,000 in 2012
CHD—health inequality target	To improve CHD mortality in all groups and at the same time aim for a more rapid improvement in the most deprived groups
Stroke	To reduce stroke mortality in 65–74-year-olds by 20% by 2012

Scotland[e]

CHD—target	To reduce mortality rates from CHD among people under 75 years by 60% between 1995 and 2010, from the 1995 baseline of 124.6 to 49.8 per 100,000 population (standardised to the European Standard Population)
CHD—inequalities target	To reduce the death rate from coronary heart disease (CHD) of those aged under 75 years living in the most deprived 15% of areas in Scotland. Reduce mortality from CHD among the under 75s in deprived areas
Stroke—target	To reduce mortality rates from stroke among people under 75 years by 50% between 1995 and 2010, from the 1995 baseline of 37.5 to 18.8 per 100,000 population (standardised to the European Standard Population)

Northern Ireland[f]

No target set

Reprinted from Allender S, Peto V, Scarborough P, Kaur A, Rayner M. *Coronary Heart Statistics 2008*. London: British Heart Foundation, 2008, with kind permission. Available at: http://www.heartstats.org

[a]Department of Health. *Our Healthier Nation*. London: Department of Health, 1999.

[b]Department of Health. *National Standards, Local Action: Health and Social Care Standards and Planning Framework 2005/06 and 2007/08*. London: Department of Health, 2004.

[c]Welsh Assembly Government (2005). See Chief Medical Officer Wales website http://www.cmo.wales.gov.uk/content/work/health-gain-targets/the-targets-e.htm#chd

[d]Welsh Assembly Government (2005). See Chief Medical Officer Wales website http://www.cmo.wales.gov.uk/content/work/health-gain-targets/the-targets-e.htm#olderpeople

[e]Scottish Executive (2008). Spending Review 2007, Scottish Government. The Scottish Executive: http://www.scotland.gov.uk/Publications/2007/11/30090722/34 and http://www.scotland.gov.uk/Publications/2007/12/11103453/6

[f]New strategies for CVD in Northern Ireland are currently being developed by the Department of Health, Social Services and Public Safety.

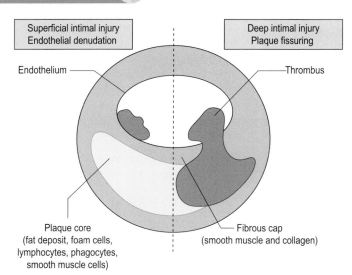

| Superficial intimal injury Endothelial denudation | | Deep intimal injury Plaque fissuring |

Endothelium ——
———Thrombus

Plaque core
(fat deposit, foam cells,
lymphocytes, phagocytes,
smooth muscle cells)

—— Fibrous cap
(smooth muscle and collagen)

Figure 19.1 • The mechanism for the development of thrombosis on plaques. Reproduced from Kumar P and Clark M (eds), *Clinical Medicine*, 5e, 2002, with permission from Elsevier Ltd.

infarction or heart attack. Figure 19.2 shows an acute coronary thrombus.

Whilst IHD may result from a number of causes, such as coronary artery spasm, vasculitis affecting coronary arteries, severe anaemia or severe trauma, atherosclerosis remains the commonest cause and provides the focus for many of the nutritional targets and interventions detailed in this chapter.

Definitions and symptoms

Stroke may result from haemorrhage, due to the rupture of weakened blood vessels, but is commonly associated with ischaemic conditions resulting directly or indirectly from abnormal thrombotic states, in particular arteriosclerosis.

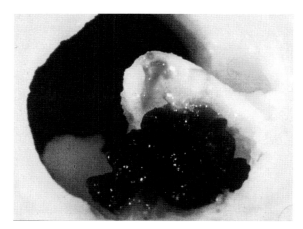

Figure 19.2 • Acute coronary thrombus. Reproduced from Kumar P and Clark M (eds), *Clinical Medicine*, 5e, 2002, with permission from Elsevier Ltd.

Stroke is defined by the World Health Organization as a clinical syndrome consisting of rapidly developing clinical signs of focal (or global in case of coma) disturbance of cerebral function lasting more than 24 hours. A transient ischaemic attack (TIA), often referred to as mini stroke, is caused by a temporary disturbance of blood supply to a restricted area of the brain, resulting in brief neurologic dysfunction that persists, by definition, for less than 24 hours. The form taken by a stroke and the symptoms displayed will depend on the blood vessels affected by the underlying event. The sudden onset of face weakness, arm drift and abnormal speech are the most common symptoms displayed. Since the vascular event will usually affect one side of the brain, the symptoms commonly affect one side of the body (please refer to Chapter 20 on Management of Stroke, for further information).

PVD refers to atherosclerosis of arteries supplying the limbs, usually affecting the lower limbs. It is characterised by the development of pain in the muscles of the leg on exertion due to intermittent claudication and in severe cases by pain even at rest. Whilst severe ischaemic conditions can result in gangrene and the need to amputate, there is a far greater risk of the individual developing atheromatous complications resulting in ischaemic heart disease or a stroke if the underlying causes are not addressed.

IHD is a continuum of disorders, from asymptomatic plaques in coronary arteries to full-blown heart attacks or MI.

Stable angina is exertional chest pain that settles readily with rest and/or glyceryl trinitrate spray.

Unstable angina is brought on much more easily and sometimes happens at rest. It also tends to last longer than a typical episode of stable angina attack.

Decubitus angina means angina precipitated by lying flat.

Prinzmetal's angina is rare and caused by coronary artery spasm; although it is not caused by atherosclerosis, it can certainly coexist with the latter.

Myocardial infarction is a major ischaemic event leading to myocardial damage, and can be subdivided into ST elevation MI and non-ST elevation MI, abbreviated as STEMI and NSTEMI, respectively. ST elevation is where the vessel is blocked completely by a fibrin-rich thrombus (traditional heart attack). A non-ST elevated MI is where the vessel is severely narrowed by a platelet-rich thrombus.

The term *acute coronary syndrome* (ACS) is an umbrella term that includes unstable angina, NSTEMI and STEMI.

Figure 19.3. shows the different states of the coronary artery vessel wall and the corresponding clinical syndromes. Figure 19.4 shows an angiogram of a STEMI.

Chronic heart failure (CHF) is a complex syndrome that can result from any structural or functional cardiac disorder that impairs the ability of the heart to function as a pump to support the circulatory system.[5] The incidence has doubled during the past 20 years. One in 6 adults over the age of 85 has CHF and it accounts for over 5% of hospital admissions. IHD is the leading cause of heart failure in the UK, accounting for more than 70% of the incidence. Whilst excessive alcohol intake, hypertension and obesity are significant risk factors and may also contribute to the development of atherosclerosis, strategies to reduce heart failure are aimed predominantly at reducing the risk factors associated with atherosclerosis and IHD.[6]

Investigations and diagnosis of CVD

PVD is usually diagnosed on the basis of symptoms displayed. Blood pressure measurements taken in the ankle may provide evidence of vascular occlusion. Imaging techniques are useful if the diagnosis is uncertain or if surgery is required.

The investigation and diagnosis of stroke following the recognition of the signs and symptoms relies on patient history, neurological examination and various imaging techniques. There is no blood test specific to stroke, although blood tests may be useful in establishing the underlying cause (please refer to the chapter on Management of Stroke, for further information).

The diagnosis of an MI usually requires at least two of the three of the following criteria:

- A typical history;
- The establishment of electrocardiogram (ECG) changes; and
- Cardiac enzyme elevation.

An ECG is the first investigation to be done if a chest pain is suspected to be cardiac in origin. The 12 leads on an ECG can indicate which area(s) of the heart, and which coronary artery, is involved in an MI.

Figure 19.3 • Relationship between the state of coronary artery vessel wall and clinical syndromes. Reproduced from Kumar P and Clark M (eds), *Clinical Medicine*, 5e, 2002, with permission from Elsevier Ltd.

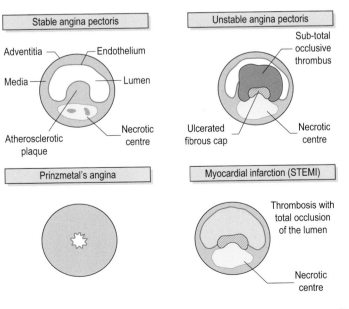

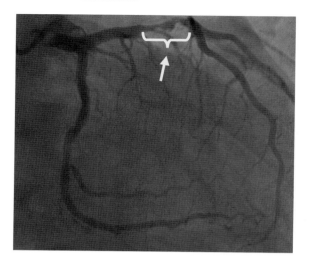

Figure 19.4 • Coronary Angiogram. The arrow shows the plaque and thrombus in the left anterior descending artery leading on to Anterior ST segment Elevation Myocardial Infarction (STEMI). Reproduced with permission from Papworth Hospital NHS Foundation Trust.

There are ECG criteria to differentiate between a STEMI and an NSTEMI, for which there are different management strategies.

Troponin T and troponin I are very sensitive and specific markers for myocardial damage. The cardiac troponins T and I are released from damaged cardiac cells within 4–6 hours of an MI and remain elevated for up to 2 weeks. They have nearly complete tissue specificity and are now the preferred markers for assessing myocardial damage. Creatine kinase is also released from heart muscle when it is damaged and may also be used as a marker.

Careful analysis of the changing pattern of released cardiac markers and ECG recordings can provide an accurate assessment of the timing and extent of cardiac damage. Whilst the troponins are also elevated in other conditions, notably pulmonary embolism and renal failure, the pattern of elevation seen following an MI compared to other conditions allows differentiation of the conditions. Figure 19.5 shows the damage to the heart after an MI.

Risk factors for atherosclerosis and cardiovascular disease

As indicated above, atherosclerosis and the development of ischaemic conditions in the circulation and heart remain the overwhelming major cause of CVD and risk factor analysis is focused in this area.

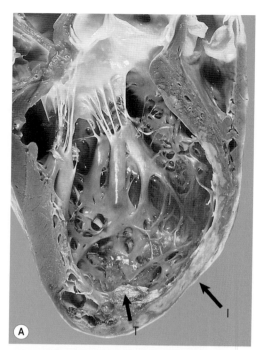

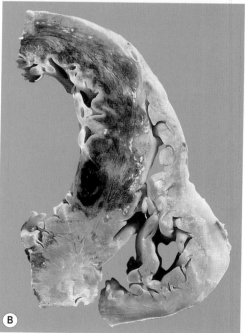

Figure 19.5 • Pathology specimen photo of an infarcted heart. A-Longitudinal section of an infarcted heart. I-Infarcted and thinned out myocardium. T-Organized Thrombus. B Cross section of an infarcted heart showing areas of necrosis. Reproduced with kind permission of Elsevier Ltd.

Framingham and risk factors

The Framingham heart study is a longitudinal prospective cohort study originally directed by the National Heart Institute (now the National Heart, Lung and Blood Institute), which started in 1948.[7] Its goal has been to identify risk factors or characteristics which contribute to the development of CVD in a cohort free from CVD at the start of the study. Over 5000 adults between the ages of 30 and 62 from Framingham, Massachusetts, have been reviewed comprehensively and periodically since 1948. Through this surveillance, major CVD risk factors, such as high blood pressure, serum cholesterol levels, smoking, obesity, diabetes and physical inactivity, along with others such as triglyceride level, age, gender and psychosocial factors, have been identified. In 1971 a second generation group was enrolled and in 2002 a third generation.

The epidemiology of CVD is still not fully understood and assessment of risk is inexact, hence the need for ongoing surveillance. An increasing proportion of CVD morbidity in individuals formerly without disease occurs in people over the age of 60. In this case, it is less predictable when new patients will present with CVD. Furthermore, patterns of disease incidence are changing. Alterations in health behaviours relating to nutrition, cigarette smoking and exercise, for example, along with improvements in medical treatment may affect future CVD death and illness rates.[7]

Risk factors can be divided into two groups—those that cannot be modified or influenced by or for the individual and those that can.

Non-modifiable risk factors

- Gender: affects males more than females up to the age of 70, as females are thought to be protected by oestrogens until menopause. After the age of 70, males and females have similar incidences;
- Age: the risk increases with age;
- Family history: ACS in a first-degree relative at less than 55 years of age;
- Ethnicity; and
- Previous medical history.

Modifiable risk factors

- Hypertension;
- Dyslipidaemia;
- Smoking;
- Obesity;
- Diabetes and glucose intolerance;
- Fibrinogen;
- Drug abuse;
- Behavioural factors/stress; and
- Physical inactivity.

Hypertension

Blood pressure (BP) has a skewed normal distribution in a population and there is no fixed dividing line between normal blood pressure and blood pressure that is slightly raised. In the population as a whole, the target is to have a blood pressure of 140/85 mmHg (140 systolic and 85 diastolic). In those with diabetes, or disease of the heart and circulation the target is below 130/80 mmHg.[8] The British Hypertension Society suggests that the ideal blood pressure is 120/80 mmHg and normal is less than 130/80 mmHg.[8]

Hypertension can occur in the systemic, pulmonary or even portal circulations, although as a term it is usually used to describe high blood pressure in the systemic arteries. Using a threshold of 140/90, about 40% of the UK population have hypertension and the prevalence increases with age. In fact, isolated systolic hypertension affects more than 50% of the over-60 population.

Most cases (around 95%) of hypertension have no known medical cause and are termed essential or primary hypertension and the minority of cases are secondary hypertension.

Secondary hypertension can be due to:

1. Renal disease including intrinsic renal disease (e.g. glomerulonephritis) or renovascular diseases (e.g. secondary to atherosclerosis in renal arteries);
2. Endocrine disorders (e.g. Cushing's syndrome, Conn's syndrome);
3. Drugs (e.g. steroids, oral contraceptive pills);
4. Pregnancy; and
5. Rarer causes such as coarctation of aorta.

Hypertension is usually asymptomatic; hence screening is essential. Occasionally symptoms such as headache and blurred vision can occur, especially with malignant hypertension (i.e. a hypertensive emergency with papilloedema and other evidence of target organ damage). BP fluctuates significantly and can even go up only when measured by a healthcare professional, giving rise to the so-called 'white coat hypertension'. It is crucial to repeat BP measurements and to consider ambulatory BP monitoring, also known as 24-hour BP monitoring, in some cases.

For adults aged between 40 and 69 years, every 20 mmHg rise in typical systolic blood pressure or 10 mmHg rise in diastolic blood pressure doubles the risk of death from IHD. Within the INTERHEART case control study those with hypertension had nearly double the risk of MI. In Western Europe it was estimated that 22% of MIs were due to a history of hypertension.[9] Hypertension is the largest risk factor for stroke. Reducing blood pressure significantly reduces the risk of CVD. In people with diabetes reducing blood pressure in addition reduces the risk of microvascular complications.[10]

The classification of blood pressure levels developed by the British Hypertension Society is shown in Table 19.2 and the threshold blood pressures for treatment are shown in Table 19.3.[11]

Table 19.2 Classification of blood pressure

	Systolic BP (mmHg)	Diastolic BP (mmHg)
Optimal	< 120	< 180
Normal	< 130	< 85
High-normal	139	85–89
Hypertension		
Grade 1: Mild	140–159	90–99
Grade 2: Moderate	160–179	100–109
Grade 3: Severe	≥ 180	≥ 110
Isolated systolic hypertension (Grade 1)	140–159	< 90
Isolated systolic hypertension (Grade 2)	≥ 160	< 90

After British Hypertension Society by permission from Macmillan Publishers Ltd. *Journal of Human Hypertension* © (2004).[11]
BP, blood pressure.

Dyslipidaemia

Dyslipidaemia refers to an abnormal pattern of lipid levels. A population is thought to be unhealthy when its average plasma cholesterol is greater than 5 mmol/L (LDL > 3 mmol/L).[12] In the UK the average cholesterol level is 5.9 mmol/L.[12] A 1% decrease in total cholesterol is associated with a 3% reduction in IHD risk at a population level. On the other hand, for every 1% decrease in HDL cholesterol there is thought to be a 2–3% increase in the risk of IHD.[13] Some believe that the total cholesterol: HDL cholesterol ratio is a more optimal predictor for CVD risk than LDL cholesterol alone. Experts vary in their opinion as to what constitutes an ideal, desirable or abnormal lipid level. Reference ranges based on the distribution of blood cholesterol levels in a normal population do not reflect ideal levels. It is important to consider the levels in the context of existing CVD or other CVD risk factors (see the section Calculation of Cardiovascular Risk).

The commonly measured lipids in clinical practice include:

- Total cholesterol;
- LDL cholesterol;
- Total cholesterol:HDL ratio;
- HDL cholesterol; and
- Total triglyceride.

Table 19.3 shows target or 'optimal' levels for total and LDL cholesterol and desirable values for other lipid fractions recommended by the Joint British Societies.[8] The National Institute of Health and Clinical Excellence (NICE) does not make any targets in primary prevention for total or LDL cholesterol.[14] For secondary prevention the targets are < 4 and < 2 mmol/L for total and LDL cholesterol, respectively.[14] There is evidence that reducing absolute cholesterol from baseline level may help to achieve greater risk reduction than through meeting specific targets alone. For this reason, NICE set no target for total or LDL cholesterol levels post MI.[15] It should be noted that at the time of an ACS, total, LDL cholesterol and HDL cholesterol levels diminish. These decreases generally do not last longer than 6–8 weeks unless there are complications.[8] A lipid profile within 1 day of symptoms presenting can give an acceptable approximation.

There are many different types of primary hyperlipidaemia with different underlying biomolecular defects and different lipid profiles. It is helpful, clinically, to consider this wide spectrum of disorders in terms of whether cholesterol or triglyceride or both are elevated. They are summarised in Table 19.4.

Elevated lipid levels could also be secondary to or associated with other conditions or factors, which must be excluded before starting patients

Table 19.3 Cardiovascular disease prevention: lifestyle, risk factors and therapeutic targets for all people at high risk and their families

	Asymptomatic people at high risk (CVD risk $\geq$ 20% over 10 years)	People with atherosclerotic cardiovascular disease
Blood pressure[a]		
	$\leq$ 140/85 mmHg	$\leq$ 130/80 mmHg (includes people with diabetes)
Lipids[a,b]		
	TC < 4 mmol/L (or a 25% reduction) LDL-C < 2 mmol/L (or a 30% reduction)	TC < 4 mmol/L (or a 25% reduction) LDL-C < 2 mmol/L (or a 30% reduction)
Fasting plasma glucose		
	$\leq$ 6 mmol/L	$\leq$ 6 mmol/L
Pharmacotherapy[c]		
Antiplatelet drugs	Aspirin 75 mg/day (once BP controlled to audit standard)[a]	Aspirin 75 mg/day
Statins[d]	For all persons to meet cholesterol targets	For all persons to meet cholesterol targets
ACE inhibitors/all receptor blockers		For persons with heart failure or left ventricular dysfunction. Consider in others with heart disease and normal LV function if BP is not at target
Beta blockers		For all persons post-myocardial infarction
Calcium channel blockers		Consider in persons with heart disease when goal BP is not achieved
Anticoagulants		Consider in persons at high risk of systemic vessel occlusion
Lifestyle		
Smoking habit	Stop smoking	Stop smoking
Diet[e,f]	Cardioprotective diet: five portions of fresh fruit and vegetables per day at least Regular consumption of fish and other sources of omega-3 polyunsaturates Total fat intake $\leq$ 30% total energy • Saturated fat $\leq$ 10% total energy • Replace saturates with monounsaturates • Dietary cholesterol < 300 mg/day Alcohol: $\leq$ 14 units per week for women; $\leq$ 21 units per week for men Salt: $\leq$ 6 g/day ($\leq$ 100 mmol/2.4 g sodium/day)	
Adiposity	Waist circumference Asians: men < 90 cm, women < 80 cm. White Caucasians: men < 102 cm, women < 88 cm; BMI 20–25.	
Physical activity		
	Regular aerobic physical activity for a minimum of ½ hour per day nearly every day e.g. swimming/fast walking.	

Modified from British Cardiac Society et al[8]

TC, total cholesterol; LDL-C, low density lipoprotein cholesterol; HDL-C, high density lipoprotein cholesterol; BP, blood pressure.

[a]Audit standards for blood pressure and lipids are different: BP < 150/90 mmHg; < 145/80 mmHg for diabetes; TC < 5 mmol/L, LDL < 3 mmol/L, i.e. minimum standard of care.

[b]Desirable lipid levels: triglycerides < 1.7 mmol/L; HDL-C > 1 mmol/L (men), > 1.2 mmol/L (women); non-HDL-C < 3 mmol/L (non-HDL-C is total minus HDL-C).

[c]Indications for medications and doses of medications for individuals with diabetes mellitus may differ.

[d]Simvastatin is the first choice of statin preparation; lower dose or alternative preparation may be indicated if clinical contraindication.

[e]NICE recommends replacing saturates with unsaturates.[14]

[f]NICE does not routinely recommend plant sterols/stanols or omega 3 supplementation for primary prevention.[14]

Table 19.4 Summary of the subtypes of hyperlipidaemia

Disorder with lipid levels where appropriate	Fredrickson classification	Estimated prevalence in European adults (%)	Molecular defect	Elevated lipoprotein	Total cholesterol	Total triglyceride	Clinical features/comorbidities
Familial hyper-cholesterolaemia	IIa	0.2 (heterozygous)	AD, absent or malfunctioning LDL receptors	LDL	↑	Normal	Tendon xanthoma (specific), corneal arcus, xanthelasma
Polygenic hyper-cholesterolaemia	IIa	20–80	Mechanism unclear	LDL	↑	Normal	As above but no tendon xanthoma
Familial combined hyperlipidaemia/ combined Hyperlipidaemia: TG 2–10 mmol/L	IIb	10+	AD, mechanism unclear	LDL, VLDL	↑	↑	Corneal arcus, xanthelasma (Often DM, obesity or hypertension present)
Familial or sporadic hypertriglyceridaemia TG 2–10 mmol/L	IV	1	AD, mechanism unclear	VLDL	Normal	↑	Recurrent pancreatitis, eruptive xanthoma, lipaemia retinalis, hepatosplenomegaly (Often secondary to DM, obesity, pancreatitis, alcoholism and/or hypothyroidism)
Familial hyper-chylomicronaemia TG > 10 mmol/L	I	0.1	Deficient lipoprotein lipase or apo C-II	Chylomicrons	Normal	↑	Recurrent pancreatitis, eruptive xanthoma, lipaemia retinalis, hepatosplenomegaly
Remnant particle disease TG 5–20 mmol/L cholesterol typically 7–12 mmol/L	III	0.02	AR, defective clearance of remnants at hepatic remnant receptor	Chylomicron remnant, IDL	↑	↑	Palmar xanthoma, tubero-eruptive xanthoma (Often associated with obesity, hyperuricaemia and DM)
Type V hyper-lipoproteinaemia TG > 10 mmol/L	V	Rare	Similar mechanism to type I	Chylomicrons, VLDL	↑	↑	Eruptive xanthoma, lipaemia retinalis, hepatosplenomegaly (may be associated with DM or excessive alcohol intake)

Adapted from Durrington.[99]

AD, autosomal dominant; AR, autosomal recessive; DM, diabetes mellitus; TG, triglyceride; LDL, low density lipoprotein; VLDL, very low density lipoprotein; IDL, intermediate density lipoprotein.

on lipid-lowering agents. Examples of secondary hyperlipidaemia include:

- Endocrine disorders—hypothyroidism, diabetes mellitus;
- Renal disorders—nephrotic syndrome, renal failure;
- Drugs—e.g. thiazide diuretics, isotretinoin;
- Gastrointestinal disorders—biliary obstruction; and
- Dietary factors—high intakes of saturates are associated with raised total and LDL cholesterol and triglycerides; obesity and diets high in refined carbohydrates, excessive alcohol or energy intake are associated with raised triglycerides.

Figure 19.6 shows the endogenous and exogenous pathways in lipid metabolism. The endogenous pathway handles synthesised lipids, while its counterpart deals with dietary fat.

Traditionally it was thought that LDL cholesterol was the main culprit in CVD and it is well established that high total cholesterol and/or LDL cholesterol is a risk factor. However, several other lipoproteins are also atherogenic, namely chylomicron remnants, very low density lipoprotein (VLDL), intermediate density lipoprotein (IDL) and small, dense LDL. VLDL and IDL are rich in triglycerides, and this is in keeping with hypertriglyceridaemia being an independent risk factor for IHD. Hypertriglyceridaemia is associated with an elevated VLDL level. In the presence of high VLDL levels, cholesterylester transfer protein (CETP) can facilitate exchange of triglycerides on VLDLs for cholesterol esters on either HDL or LDL. The result is twofold:

1. HDL becomes more readily excreted by the kidneys, resulting in a reduction in HDL cholesterol levels. This explains why there is a strong inverse relationship between triglyceride levels and HDL levels. Note that low HDL levels are associated with an increased risk of IHD.

2. The now triglyceride-rich LDL can undergo further hydrolysis catalysed by various lipases, and the result is a small, dense LDL particle which is highly atherogenic due to its susceptibility to oxidation and its high penetration through endothelial layers. It tends to bypass the usual route of LDL receptor mediated uptake which is an important regulatory mechanism.

This is the biochemical picture seen in the metabolic syndrome X, which is also a risk factor for IHD. Individual risk approaches that of full diabetes and if it is uncontrolled it results in type 2 diabetes and should be managed accordingly. Box 19.1 shows the features of the metabolic syndrome.

Smoking

Cigarette smoking is a major factor in the development of coronary heart disease, stroke and PVD.

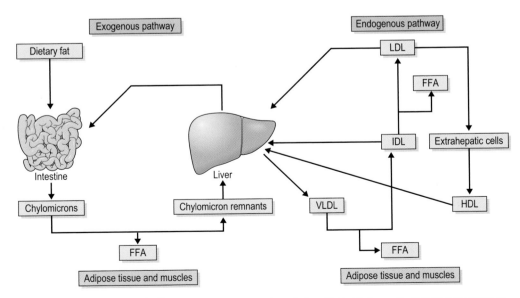

Figure 19.6 • Lipid metabolism. Reproduced with kind permission of Dr Hari Parthasarathy. FFA, free fatty acids; LDL, low density lipoprotein; VLDL, very low density lipoprotein; IDL, intermediate density lipoprotein; HDL, high density lipoprotein.

Box 19.1

Metabolic syndrome[a]

Diagnosed if three or more of the features below are present:

- Hypertension ($\geq$ 130/85 mmHg or active treatment for hypertension)
- Central obesity: increased waist circumference $\geq$ 102 cm in men and $\geq$ 88 cm in women; $\geq$ 90 cm for Asian men, $\geq$ 80 cm Asian women
- Insulin resistance
- Hypertriglyceridaemia ($\geq$ 1.7 mmol/L)
- Low HDL cholesterol ($<$ 1.03 mmol/L for men; $<$ 1.29 mmol/L for women)
- Fasting blood glucose ($>$ 5.6 mmol/L or active treatment for hyperglycaemia)

[a]Definition from the American Heart Association and the National Heart, Lung, and Blood Institute.[16]

Smoking is one of the major causes of CVD and smokers are almost twice as likely to have a heart attack as people who have never smoked. It can increase the risk of developing several different types of cancer and is the main cause of some lung diseases. Smoking increases the risk of elevation in fibrinogen and increased blood viscosity. The British doctors cohort study found that mortality from CHD was 50% higher in smokers and over 75% higher in heavy smokers, than in non-smokers. It is estimated that in 2000 around 30,600 deaths or 27% of all smoking attributable deaths were due to CVD.[17]

Obesity

Overweight and obesity increase the risk of CHD. As well as being an independent risk factor, obesity is also a major risk factor for high blood pressure, raised blood cholesterol, diabetes and impaired glucose tolerance.[18]

The distribution of excess weight is an important factor and the impact is greatest when the fat is concentrated in the abdomen, assessed by the waist-to-hip ratio or waist circumference.

The World Health Organization's World Health Report 2002 estimated that over 7% of all disease burden in developed countries was caused by raised body mass index (BMI), and that around a third of CHD and ischaemic stroke and almost 60% of hypertensive disease in developed countries were due to being overweight.[19]

More recently the INTERHEART case-control study estimated that 63% of heart attacks in Western Europe and 28% of heart attacks in Central and Eastern Europe were due to abdominal obesity, as assessed by a high waist-to-hip ratio and those with abdominal obesity were at over twice the risk of a heart attack compared to those without.[9] This study also found that abdominal obesity was a much more significant risk factor for heart attack than BMI.

Diabetes mellitus and insulin resistance

Diabetes substantially increases the risk of CHD. There are two main types of diabetes: type 1 and type 2 diabetes. Men with non-insulin-dependent diabetes (type 2) have a two- to fourfold greater annual risk of CHD than normal and in women with type 2 diabetes they are at an even higher, three- to fivefold, increased risk.[20] Diabetes not only increases the risk of CHD but also magnifies the effect of other risk factors for CHD such as raised cholesterol levels, raised blood pressure, smoking and obesity.

The recent INTERHEART case-control study estimated that 15% of heart attacks in Western Europe and 9% of heart attacks in Central and Eastern Europe are due to diagnosed diabetes, and that people with diagnosed diabetes are at three times the risk of a heart attack compared to those without.[9]

Fibrinogen

Fibrinogen is a strong predictor of CHD, fatal or non-fatal, new or recurrent and of death from an unspecified cause, for both men and women. Its effect is only partially attributable to other coronary risk factors, the most important of which is smoking.[21] Whilst the assessment of cardiovascular risk is usually made on the basis of a number of established risk factors, the suggestion that fibrinogen, C-reactive protein (CRP) and homocysteine should be included in such assessments does not have universal support. For example, a factfile from the British Heart Foundation developed for GPs in February 2007 concludes that there is no clear indication that measuring novel potential risk factors, such as CRP, fibrinogen and homocysteine, is of any value in predicting risk of CHD. Similar conclusions apply to the prediction of CVD risk. However, measurement of homocysteine may be indicated in patients with a demonstrated, strong predisposition to venous and arterial thromboses.[22]

Behavioural factors/stress

Inadequate social support, depression (including anxiety), personality (chiefly hostility) and work stress are the four psychosocial factors most often correlated with a raised risk of CHD.[2] More men than women appear to lack social support. The Health Survey for England data, in 2005, show that 18% of men compared with 11% of women reported a severe lack of social support.[23] In the same survey over one-third of men from Pakistan and Bangladesh described a severe lack of social support compared with 18% in the general population.

Women report higher levels of psychological distress than men. For example, in the 2005 Health Survey for England, 15% of women compared with 11% of men had high 'GHQ12' scores (General Health Questionnaire score assessing degree of psychological distress).[23] In the same survey, the GHQ12 score is negatively associated with income. Geographically, men residing in the south-east of England were 50% less likely to have a high GHQ12 score than their counterparts in the north-east of England. Amongst men in the UK, the highest levels of psychological distress were seen in men from Bangladeshi communities and secondly in men from Indian communities. For women, the highest scores were seen in those from the Pakistani and Black African communities.

Psychosocial factors may modify risk of CHD in a number of ways. They may have an effect on habits such as diet, smoking or alcohol which then affect CHD risk. They also may be the basis for pathophysiological changes. Lastly, psychosocial factors may influence access to and availability of healthcare.[24]

The Department of Health recognises that 'working in jobs which make very high demands, or in which people have little or no control, increases the risk of CHD and premature death. Inadequate social support or lack of social networks can also have a harmful effect on health and on the chances of recovering from disease'.[25] To date there are no estimates of CHD mortality due to adverse psychosocial health. We also do not know whether the CHD mortality rate would improve if psychosocial health was improved.[2]

Drug abuse

Recreational drug misuse is an increasingly important, yet often overlooked, risk factor for CVD. Around 3 million people use at least one illicit drug each year in the UK.[26] In 2007–2008 730,000 people are reported to have used cocaine in the year prior to the aforementioned survey. Many recreational drugs, such as cocaine, amphetamine and 'ecstasy' (a derivative of amphetamine), activate the sympathetic nervous system, thereby leading to hypertension. These drugs could also directly lead to myocardial ischaemia via various mechanisms, such as coronary artery spasm and increase in myocardial oxygen demand. Individuals between 18 and 25 years of age have the highest rate of cocaine use, and hence cocaine is an important contributor to MI among the young.[27] Other recreational drugs that have been reported to cause myocardial ischaemia include psilocybin ('magic mushrooms') and inhaled volatile substances.

Physical inactivity

Recent research from the World Health Organization highlighted the importance of physical inactivity as a major risk factor for CHD. The 2002 World Health Report estimated that around 3% of all disease burden in developed countries was caused by physical inactivity, and that over 20% of CHD and 10% of stroke in developed countries were due to physical inactivity, i.e. less than 2.5 hours per week moderate intensity activity or 1 hour per week vigorous activity.[19] People who are regularly active have a lower risk of heart disease. The activity needs to be regular and aerobic and to use the major muscle groups of the body. Since the mid-1990s Government initiatives have attempted to increase the level of activity in all sections of the community.[28,29] However, physical activity levels are low in the UK. Health Survey for England data show that, in 2006, only 40% of men and 28% of women met the current physical activity guidelines suggested by the Government. In 2006 around one-third of English adults were inactive, that is, participated in less than one occasion of 30 minutes activity a week.[30]

Calculation of cardiovascular risk

The new NHS Health Check programme aims to prevent heart disease, stroke, diabetes and kidney disease in adults aged 40–74 without existing CVD. All Primary Care Trusts in England have been asked to employ a standardised vascular risk assessment and management plan for people in this age group who have not already been diagnosed with one of these conditions. Individuals will be invited (once every 5 years) to have a vascular check to assess their risk of developing these diseases. They will then be provided with the appropriate help to manage that risk as appropriate.[31]

For the primary prevention of CVD, NICE recommends employing the Framingham 1991 10-year risk equations to measure CVD risk in this age group.

$$\text{CVD risk}$$
$$=$$
$$\text{10-year risk of fatal and non-}$$
$$\text{fatal stroke including TIA}$$
$$+$$
$$\text{10-year risk of CHD.}$$

The Joint British Societies risk charts are based on these equations and electronic calculators based on this algorithm are available.[8,32]

The data required to estimate risk include:

- Age;
- Gender;
- Mean systolic blood pressure;
- Total and HDL cholesterol;
- Presence of left ventricular hypertrophy; and
- Smoking status.

Various adjustments can be made for factors affecting risk such as family history of premature CHD, ethnicity, obesity, serum triglyceride ≥ 1.7 mmol/L; HDL levels < 1 mmol/L for men or < 1.2 for women.[8,14]

It is inappropriate to use the calculator for persons with established CVD, diabetes, familial dyslipidaemia, TC:HDL-C ratio ≥ 6, renal dysfunction or persistently high blood pressure.

If the 10-year CVD risk $\geq 20\%$, NICE recommends that lifestyle changes be reviewed and optimised before offering lipid lowering treatment.

Table 19.3 shows interventions and targets recommended for adults who have a $\geq 20\%$ 10-year risk of developing CVD and for those with established CVD.

Nutritional therapy and dietetic application

Table 19.3 summarises the components of diet recommended for people at high risk of developing CVD or those with established disease. It includes recommendations for other lifestyle measures integral to reducing risk. Our discussion will focus on the dietary recommendations. Most dietary research relating to those with established CVD has been carried out in patients post MI.

The Mediterranean diet

Population studies show a reduced risk of CVD in those consuming a traditional 'Mediterranean' diet.[33] A traditional Mediterranean diet, which has an emphasis on fresh foods, is recommended by NICE for survivors of MI, to include more bread, fruit, vegetables and fish and less meat; and to replace butter and cheese with products based on vegetable and plant oils.[15] Evidence for this comes from the Lyon Heart Study in which survivors of an MI in the experimental group who were advised to follow a traditional Mediterranean diet experienced a significant reduction in all cause and cardiovascular mortality along with a reduction in cardiac events compared with the control group.[34] After 27 months the trial was stopped early because of improved outcomes in the intervention group: mortality was 2.6% for the intervention group compared with 6% for the control group. Improvements were also seen at an extended follow up more than 1 year later. The experimental group ate significantly less saturated fat, cholesterol and omega-6 polyunsaturates (PUFA), but more monounsaturates (MUFA) and alpha linolenic acid (ALA) and significantly more fruit and vegetables. The advantages of the Mediterranean diet here did not appear to be due to changes in established risk factors such as raised cholesterol and blood pressure as at the end of the investigation when the intervention group and control group were compared, there were few distinctions between them. In light of such evidence, the American Heart Association acknowledged in its revised dietary guidelines in 2000 that an approach wider than conventional cholesterol lowering by diet to help prevent CHD was appropriate.[35]

The recent INTERHEART case control study suggests that 'Western' style diets that are high in meat, fat and salt are associated with higher risk of MI when compared to 'prudent' diets rich in fruit and vegetables.[36]

Other evidence to support dietary modification to reduce CVD risk or risk factors is outlined below.

Salt (sodium) and other electrolytes

There has been a 10% decrease in the salt intake of the adult population, from 9.5 g in 2001 to 8.6 g per day in 2008.[37,38] In the UK about three-quarters of salt intake comes from processed foods. On average between 10–15% is added at the table. If the population target of $\leq$6 g/day is achieved, it is estimated that this will correspond to a 13% reduction in stroke and 10% reduction in IHD.[13,39,40]

Sodium acts with other minerals in the regulation of blood pressure. Habitual consumption of sodium during early life is thought to be linked to hypertension in later life.[39] Observational data show a strong positive association between sodium intake and blood pressure within and between countries.

Reducing salt from 10 to 5 g per day lowers BP by about 5/2 mmHg, with greater reductions seen in older people and those with higher initial BP levels.[11,41,42] Although dietary advice to restrict salt has proved beneficial, the effect appears to decrease with time.[41,43,44] Effective lifestyle interventions can reduce the need for antihypertensive medication, augment pharmacological effect and reduce the need for multiple drug therapies.[11,45] The greatest reductions in blood pressure appear to be when a diet rich in fruits, vegetables and low fat dairy products and reduced in saturates is combined with a reduced salt diet.[39]

The Dietary Approaches to Stop Hypertension (DASH) study compared a typical high fat American diet with the efficacy of a diet rich in wholegrains, fruit and vegetables and low fat dairy products, reduced in both saturated fat and total fat intake, as outlined in the DASH eating plan below. It demonstrated that blood pressure can be reduced even without changes in weight or sodium intake in the short term.[46]

The DASH sodium study gives strong evidence of additional benefit from further restriction in salt intake on blood pressure (3 g versus 6 g versus 9 g salt/day).[47] Recommendations in primary and secondary prevention remain at $\leq$ 6 g salt per day, despite evidence that reducing sodium further

would reduce blood pressure further.[18,39,44] This perhaps relates to what is realistically achievable with minimum reductions in sodium in our food supply.

The DASH diet is recommended in the USA for patients with hypertension in the national guidelines of the American Heart Association.[45] It should be noted that in the DASH study participants were provided with their meals to ensure that their dietary intake met the required nutrient profiles and appropriate energy levels. This included 8–10 servings of fruit and vegetables per day. Had it examined the effect of such a diet in the form of 'dietary advice', the results may have been different. A follow-up of a subsample from the DASH sodium 1 year after discontinuation concluded that DASH diet participants continued to eat more fruits and vegetables than at baseline and had sustained reductions in BP despite increased sodium intake.[43]

The 6 g Salt DASH eating plan/day

- Total fat   27% energy
- Saturated fat   6% energy
- Carbohydrate   55% energy
- Protein   18% energy
- Potassium   4.7 g
- Calcium   1.25 g
- Sodium   2.3 g
- Magnesium   0.5 mg
- Cholesterol   1.5 mg
- Fibre   30 g

Salt restriction appears to have effects on cardiovascular health besides reducing blood pressure which merit further investigation. In 2007, Cook et al. examined the effect of reduction in dietary sodium intake on cardiovascular events using data from two completed randomised controlled trials 10–15 years earlier.[48] Participants between the ages of 30 and 54 with blood pressure between 120/80 and 139/89 mmHg received intensive dietary counselling to restrict sodium over 18 months in the first trial and over a time period of 36–48 months in the second. The target individual sodium intake to be achieved at 6 months and maintained during follow-up was < 1.8 g per day. Only 21% of individuals achieved this at 6 months.[49] The net decrease in sodium excretion from baseline in the intervention groups was 44 and 33 mmol/24 h, respectively, at the end of the two periods. Net changes in blood pressure were small at this time: −1.7/−0.8 mmHg. Ten to 15 years after the original trials, there was a 30% lower incidence in CVD events compared with the control group, irrespective of gender, age or BMI. There was no reduction in total mortality, however.

There is increasing evidence that high sodium intakes increase extracellular sodium concentrations and may affect vascular reactivity and growth and promote myocardial fibrosis.[39,48]

A 24-year follow-up of the Nurses Prospective Cohort Study has reported that a 'DASH' type diet is associated with a lower risk of stroke and IHD among middle-aged women.[50]

Potassium, calcium and magnesium

Although calcium, potassium and magnesium are all inversely associated with hypertension in population studies, results from supplementation studies have been inconsistent and their use is not supported. Further research is required.[11,44] Inverse associations have been shown with blood pressure for diets rich in fruits and vegetables. The mechanism by which increasing fruit and vegetable intake may lower blood pressure is unclear, though it may relate to increasing potassium intake (Figure 19.7).[11]

Nitrates

A recent preliminary study employing 500 ml daily beetroot juice in healthy volunteers suggests that the nitrate content of vegetables may be the factor in vegetables which reduces blood pressure.[51] Further research is required.

Fruit and vegetables: antioxidants

The average intake of fruit and vegetables in adults in the UK population is 2.8 portions per day.[37] For primary and secondary prevention CVD, people are advised to consume 400 g fruit and vegetables per day, i.e. 5×80 g portions.

This recommendation is based on observational evidence. Meta-analyses of cohort studies have shown negative correlations between consumption of fruit and vegetables and the occurrence of stroke and IHD, suggesting a protective effect of fruit and vegetables.[52]

Antioxidant supplementation is not recommended for the treatment or prevention of CVD. Many prospective cohort studies have shown an inverse

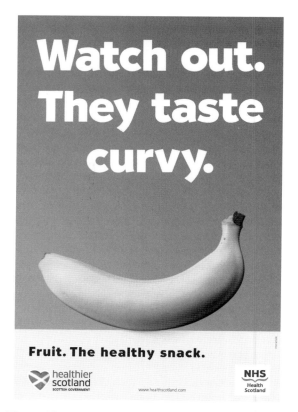

Figure 19.7 • An example of a government incentive to encourage healthy eating. Reproduced from NHS Health Scotland with permission.

association between vitamin E and cardiac morbidity and mortality. However, systematic reviews show no benefit on CVD risk factors either alone or in combination with other antioxidants in primary or secondary prevention.[53,54] The same appears to be true for other antioxidant vitamins alone or in combination.[55] Doses of vitamin E ≥ 400 IU appear to increase risk of all cause mortality in secondary prevention.[56] This negative effect has also been seen with beta carotene supplementation.[55,57] Fruit and vegetables contain vitamins and minerals and fibres. They are also important sources of potassium. Antioxidant vitamins in experimental studies appear to reduce lipoprotein oxidation.

High plasma homocysteine concentrations are associated with increased risk for CVD. Although intervention studies with B vitamins in individuals with established CVD have shown reductions in homocysteine levels, none have shown any clear benefit in CVD risk reduction.[58–60] However, a 25% reduction in stroke risk was seen in one trial.[61]

Further trials are underway but with the exception of rare genetic disorders, to date there appears to be no place for B vitamin supplementation in individuals with pre-existing CVD.

Intake of fat and type of fat

The average intake of total fat and saturated fat in UK adults is 35.5% and 13.3% of food energy, respectively.[37]

Table 19.3 shows target cardioprotective fat recommendations suitable for managing dyslipidaemia.[8] The population average recommendation for total fat is 33% of total energy.[13] Replacing saturates (SFA) with unsaturates is recommended by some for primary and secondary prevention of CVD, whereas others recommend MUFA alone for replacement, in keeping with the Mediterranean-style diet.[8,14,62,63]

A small significant reduction in cardiovascular events is found in trials that assess the effect of advice to modify fat intake, over a period of at least 2 years, in high-risk individuals.[62] We are unclear whether a low fat or modified fat diet or both together is most protective in preventing CVD morbidity. Ongoing clinical trials may help to clarify this.

A meta-analysis of short-term metabolic studies shows that a lipid-lowering diet that replaces 60% of SFA with unsaturated fats and reduces dietary cholesterol can lower total cholesterol by about 10–15% (about 0.8 mmol/L), with four-fifths of this reduction being in LDL cholesterol.[64]

In clinical trials assessing effectiveness of dietary counselling interventions in free living individuals lasting at least 6 months, total blood cholesterol level reductions on average of 5% can be achieved.[65] Higher reductions can be seen in the short term. More intensive recommendations to reduce saturated fat and cholesterol than are generally recommended in the UK do not always yield larger reductions in blood cholesterol. Lack of adherence to dietary advice seems to be the main reason for no further cholesterol reductions in trials. There is some suggestion, though, that individuals at high risk are perhaps more motivated to change their diet and may achieve greater reductions in blood cholesterol in some studies but not in others.[62,64]

In clinical practice there is a wide degree of responsiveness to diet and studies suggest LDL reduction ranges from 5–40%.[66] Statin therapy reduces serum cholesterol by 18–28% and is indicated along with lifestyle advice for people at high risk or with existing CVD.[8,67] We should remember that in most pharmacological lipid-lowering trials, dietary treatment had been commenced before starting the drug. One short-term trial employing cholesterol lowering dietary advice with simvastatin showed LDL cholesterol reductions of 10.8% with the diet, 29.7% with simvastatin and 40.5% in combination.[68]

In population studies partial replacement of SFAs and *trans* fatty acids (TFAs) with unsaturated fat appears to be more protective than decreasing total fat alone.[69]

The influence of dietary fat on blood lipids

Increasing saturates as a proportion of dietary energy significantly increases total cholesterol and LDL cholesterol and therefore CVD risk. Current thinking is that MUFA have cholesterol-lowering properties similar to those of omega-6 PUFA[70]. However, replacing SFA with MUFA can increase the HDL:LDL ratio and provide a better lipid profile as omega-6 PUFA decreases both LDL and HDL. There is also concern that LDL is more prone to oxidation with high intakes of omega-6 PUFA and the Department of Health recommended that individual intakes of omega-6 PUFA should not exceed 10% of dietary energy.[13] This limit has since been questioned in the USA.[71] Current adult intakes of *cis*-omega-6 PUFA are 5.4% of food energy in the UK.[37]

Trans fatty acid (TFA)

Prospective and experimental studies show that even small amounts of TFA have a deleterious effect on CVD risk, similar to that of saturated fat. They have been widely used in margarines, commercial cooking and manufactured foods. However, in Europe hydrogenated vegetable oils used in margarines and cooking fat have largely been replaced with ingredients that have low levels of TFA and this probably accounts for both the UK adult population average and the low income adult average intake now being below the dietary reference value of $\leq$ 2% food energy.[72]

Dietary cholesterol

Most individuals consume 300–500 mg per day of dietary cholesterol. Intakes over 500 mg/day are seen in individuals whose saturated fat intake is high. The influence of dietary cholesterol on blood cholesterol is thought to be small and individuals vary in their response to dietary cholesterol. However, the most significant contribution to raising LDL cholesterol level is saturated fat. Reducing SFA also reduces dietary cholesterol.

Eggs

A 50-g egg contains 213 mg cholesterol, 5 g fat, of which about 3.5 g is SFA. Eggs are also a significant source of B vitamins, such as biotin.

Omega-3 PUFA

The recommendation for long chain omega-3 PUFA for primary prevention of CVD is 450 mg per day.[73] In primary prevention two portions of fish a week are recommended, one of which is oily. A standard portion size is regarded as 140 g. As much as 83% of people in the UK do not eat any oily fish.

High intakes of omega-3 PUFA > 3 g/day may lower blood pressure, especially in older people and those with hypertension. The antihypertensive effect of lower doses of fish oil, however, remains to be established.[45]

A recent large study showed a protective effect of 1800 mg eicosapentaenoic acid (EPA) daily when added to statin treatment on reducing major coronary events in hypercholesterolaemic Japanese patients over a period of almost 5 years.[74] The result was significant for the group with existing coronary artery disease but not for those without. There is a low rate of IHD mortality in Japan and a high consumption of fish. Further trials are required to see the effect of this dose in different populations.

The influence of omega-3 PUFA on risk of CVD

EPA displaces arachidonic acid (AA) in platelets, reducing thromboxane synthesis, resulting in reduced platelet aggregation. Platelet count and fibrinogen are also reduced. Also omega-3 PUFA lowers monocyte adhesion and migration, reduces the expression of endothelial cytokines, improves endothelial function and has anti-arrhythmatic properties which are all thought to contribute to the cardioprotective effect in the above trials.[75]

NICE recommends that survivors of MI consume at least 7g omega-3 PUFA per week, from two to four portions of oily fish per week.[15]

- For patients who have had an MI and are not achieving the oily fish target amount of consider providing 1 g daily of omega 3-acid ethyl

esters (460 mg EPA and 380 mg DHA (docosahexaenoic acid) treatment licensed for up to 4 years).

- Initiation of omega-3-acid ethyl esters supplements is not routinely recommended for patients who have had an MI more than 3 months earlier.

This evidence comes from two large randomised control trials with post-MI patients which both showed a significant decrease in all cause mortality in the omega-3 PUFA intervention groups. The first showed a 29% reduction in all cause mortality in patients randomised to oily fish advice compared to those not advised at 2 years.[76] In the second, the GISSI-P trial, those randomised to receive 1 g omega-3-acid ethyl esters (Omacor®, Figure 19.8) daily experienced a 20% risk reduction in mortality at 3.5 years compared with the control group.[77] Further analysis revealed that those individuals whose diet was most similar to the traditional Mediterranean diet suffered fewer events than those whose diet was least similar.[78]

In the Diet and Reinfarction trial (DART) compliance to dietary advice to eat 200–400 g oil-rich fish per week over two or more occasions, equivalent to 3.5–5.6 g omega 3 PUFA/week, was high in the intervention group and they received periodic dietetic follow-up over the 2 years. Fourteen percent of patients at 6 months and 22% at 2 years received total or partial omega-3 PUFA replacement as they did not like or tolerate the fish. The authors concluded that any benefit from fish consumption was likely to be independent of any changes in saturated fat and cholesterol intake as serum cholesterol levels tended to rise in the fish advice group compared with those not so advised.

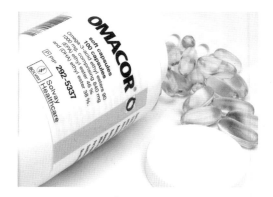

Figure 19.8 • Omacor®. The only omega-3-acid ethyl esters currently licensed in the UK for prescribing post MI. Image from Solvay Healthcare Ltd, used with their permission.

It has been customary to apply the same omega-3 PUFA advice to people with all forms of CVD.[79] However, the outcome of a trial cast doubt onto the potential benefits of omega-3 PUFA supplements in stable angina patients.[80] A recent meta-analysis that examines the influence of omega-3 PUFA in CVD found no benefit in terms of cardiovascular endpoints.[81] However, this analysis was criticised for including the above trial on stable angina and thus including trials with different endpoints. Clearly further trials are required in stable angina patients.

Further trials are required to assess the outcome of supplementation with omega-3 PUFA post-MI with patients receiving the latest medical treatments. At the time of writing we await publication in a peer reviewed journal of the OMEGA trial which looked at the effects of 1 g omega-3-acid ethyl esters daily on reduction in sudden cardiac death after MI at 1 year. It should be noted that in both the DART trial and GISSI-P trial, like the Lyon Heart Study, improved survival was apparent very early on in the treatment group.[34,76,77] This compares with statin medication where improved survival is not seen until after 2 years.[82]

A recent study lasting nearly 4 years by the same investigators showed a small but significant effect in reduced mortality and hospital admissions in patients with heart failure taking the same dose of omega 3-acid ethyl esters.[83] The patients were already prescribed standard medications for heart failure so the effect was additive. It is unclear whether the treatment effect would have been larger if patients were not already on standard drugs. The mechanism and optimal dose remain to be elucidated.

Safe intakes of omega-3 PUFA and oily fish

The Food Standards Agency recommends an upper limit of oily fish of four portions per week for adults except in pregnancy and breastfeeding where the limit is two.[73] Safe upper limits have been advised due to high levels of polychlorinated biphenyl and dioxin build-up in oily fish, causing increased risk of cancer. Their levels are decreasing and levels in the environment are now lower than when the DART trial was conducted in the 1980s. As stated earlier, 83% of UK adults do not consume any oily fish.

There are concerns that pharmacological doses of 'fish oil' above 3 g/day may adversely affect glycaemic control and LDL cholesterol levels in individuals with type 2 diabetes.[84] A recent systematic review of short-term trials concluded that omega-3 PUFA supplementation (mean daily dosage of 3.5 g/day) in people with type 2 diabetes may raise LDL cholesterol and has no statistically significant effect on glycemic control or fasting insulin.[85] Longer term trials are required. Nearly a quarter of patients admitted into hospital with an MI have diabetes and the cardioprotective daily dose of 1 g omega-3-acid ethyl esters daily is not contraindicated.[15,84]

Species of oily fish include herring, hilsa, mackerel, sardines, pilchards, sild, skippers, kippers, trout, salmon, sprats, fresh tuna and whitebait.

Plant sources of omega-3 PUFA

Plant-based sources of omega-3 PUFA are important for non-fish eaters. Most research has employed long chain omega-3 PUFAs and the cardioprotective role of the shorter chain omega-3 PUFA, such as α-linolenic acid is less well established. The recent substantial decline in IHD in Eastern Europe may be due to increased consumption of high ALA plant oils.[86] There is no established cardioprotective dose of ALA, but non-fish eaters should be encouraged to consume foods rich in ALA, such as rapeseed oil, walnuts, soy oil and linseed oil, as outlined in Box 19.2.

Novel sources of omega-3

The number of omega-3-enriched foods is increasing. These include eggs, milk, yoghurt drinks and margarines. Some contain long chain omega-3 PUFA, whereas others contain ALA. It is important to advise patients to look at labels to calculate the amounts of EPA and DHA.

Sterols/stanols

NICE does not routinely recommend products with these added in primary prevention. Intake of dietary plant sterols is inversely related to serum total and

---

Box 19.2

Plant sources of ALA

Oils/seeds—rapeseed, walnut, soya, flax, linseed, pumpkin
Nuts—walnuts, pecan, peanuts, almonds
Soya—beans, tofu
Vegetables—dark green leafy, sweet potato, sprouted pulses and grains

LDL cholesterol.[87] Short-term clinical trials assessing efficacy of plant sterols show that consumptions of around 2g per day of plant sterols (or stanols) have been shown to reduce total and LDL cholesterol in a variety of populations with no impact on triglycerides or HDL cholesterol. Their hypocholesterolaemic effect appears additive to statin therapy.[88]

Average reductions of LDL cholesterol of 10% can be achieved, though there is considerable variation between individuals. Generally speaking the cholesterol-lowering effect is proportionally higher in diets with higher amounts of fat and cholesterol. Intakes above 3 g appear to show no further benefit. There have been no randomised controlled trials identified which examine the effectiveness of plant stanols/sterols in primary or secondary prevention relating to cardiovascular outcomes. Indeed NICE has recommended that research over 2 years should be undertaken to find this out.[14]

Stanols and sterols may be suitable for patients resistant to statins or as an adjunct to medication if target cholesterol is not reached. They can reduce cholesterol absorption by up to 50%. It is thought that they compete with cholesterol for absorption into the mixed micelle. Amounts larger than would occur naturally are added to products such as margarine, yoghurts and milk as a vehicle for consumption. It is important for patients to follow consumer advice on the packaging. Usage of such products could cost patients up to £70 per year.

Familial phytosterolaemia is a very rare autosomal recessive disorder where increased absorption of sitosterol and campesterol leads to premature atherosclerosis. In the heterozygous condition, although sitosterol absorption is increased, the ability to excrete the excess remains.

Soya and legumes

The average daily intake of soya in the UK is about 2–3 g. The Joint Health Claims initiative agreed the claim that 'the inclusion of at least 25 g soya protein per day as part of a diet low in saturated fat can help reduce blood cholesterol'.[89] To carry this claim a product must include a minimum of 5 g of soya protein and intact isoflavone in each serving of food.

A recent meta-analysis of clinical trials in adults with normal or mild hypercholesterolaemia lasting 4 weeks–1year including modest amounts of soya protein (average 26.9 g) resulted in small, significant reductions in total and LDL cholesterol, with a 6% LDL reduction.[90]

A previous meta-analysis of studies employing larger amounts of soya showed a greater average reduction in cholesterol. The hypolipidaemic effect appears stronger when baseline cholesterol is greater. There are several possible cardioprotective effects of soya: it is high in omega-6 PUFA, it has an antioxidant effect due to the presence of isoflavones and it is also a substitute for animal protein. There is debate whether it is soya protein alone or a combination of the protein and isoflavones that reduce cholesterol. Using soya and other legumes may also help people reduce overall saturated fat in the diet. A wide range of soya products is now available.

Nuts

According to epidemiological studies, nuts in general are associated with a decrease risk of CVD. Nuts are high in unsaturated fat and fibre and low in saturates so influence the lipid profile. Nuts contain fibre and also antioxidants. Advice to eat them should consider their energy content. Clinical studies are short term and consumption of 50–100 g nuts on five or more occasions per week as part of a healthy heart diet may significantly lower LDL and total cholesterol in the short term.

Soluble fibre

Short-term intervention studies suggest that soluble fibre from plant foods such as oats, psyllium and guar gum may be effective in lowering total cholesterol and LDL when taken in an appropriate form and quantity.[91] The mechanism by which fibre lowers cholesterol is not yet clear. Beta glucan found in oats forms a viscous non-starch polysaccharide in the gut which delays bile absorption. It is possible that some of the effect is due to substitution for dietary fat. More recently there have been short-term trials with functional foods containing barley beta glucans showing significant decreases in total and LDL cholesterol.[92]

Low glycaemic index (GI) diets

The glycaemic index is a measure of how rapidly carbohydrate is absorbed from the gastrointestinal tract. The carbohydrate in foods with a high GI is absorbed rapidly but is absorbed slowly from those with a low GI. Diets with a low GI have been associated with low IHD risk in prospective cohort studies. Foods such as beans, peas, spaghetti and barley and some fruits have a low GI. Some low GI foods are high in soluble fibre, such as oats, peas and beans. There is some evidence that they increase HDL cholesterol and lower LDL and thus may be cardioprotective. However, there appears to be insufficient evidence to recommend these diets to reduce lipids or CVD mortality/morbidity.[93] Please refer to Chapter 17 on diabetes for further information on the glycaemic index.

Obesity

Although abdominal adiposity is more predictive of cardiovascular risk than BMI alone, BMI may be less prone to measurement error in clinical practice than waist circumference and therefore a more reliable measure.[94] Weight loss is known to reduce risk factors, such as hypertension and dyslipidaemia. Please refer to Chapter 18 on obesity for guidance on the management of obesity.

Alcohol

An excess alcohol intake, greater than 21 units weekly for men and 14 units weekly for women, is a risk factor for high blood pressure and poor cardiovascular health. Excessive intake can also cause resistance to antihypertensive therapy. Alcohol is a major risk factor for hypertriglyceridaemia. Drinking 1 to 2 units per day may provide some protection against heart disease, particularly in those over 40 years of age.

Under the age of 40 any alcohol consumption is linked with an increased mortality because IHD rates are low and deaths due to injury are high. The cardioprotective effect starts to increase in men at the age of 40 and women at 50. An intake of 1–2 units of alcohol per day increases HDL cholesterol by 12%, on average. Alcohol also has significant antithrombotic actions, which have been compared to aspirin. There is no evidence to show that any particular type of wine confers any additional benefit.[95]

Know your units?

In the UK 1 unit = 8 g or 10 mL pure alcohol.

1 unit = volume of drink (mL) × % alcohol/10.

So 125 mL glass wine at 13% = 1.6 units.

Garlic supplements

There is insufficient evidence to recommend garlic or garlic supplements to reduce serum lipids.[96]

Dietary management of chronic heart failure (CHF)

More research is recommended into effective dietary treatments for this group of patients.[5,97]

Dietary recommendations for CHF include:[5]

- Restrict salt intake to ≤ 6 g/day to improve blood pressure. Avoid low salt substitutes because of risk of hyperkalaemia.
- In hyponatraemia, assessment of fluid intake and personal advice to restrict fluid intake is required.
- Weigh daily at a set time and follow-up by GP, or specialist, of any weight gain of more than 1.5 to 2 kg in 2 days.
- Limit alcohol intake or avoid it, particularly if it has caused CHF.

The relation between obesity and CHF is complex. Although obesity causes abnormalities in diastolic and systolic function and predisposes to CHF, obese patients with CHF appear to have a better clinical prognosis, including survival and event-free survival. In one 2-year study, a higher percentage of body fat appeared to be the strongest predictor of event-free survival. It is unclear whether the link is causal or merely an association. It could be related to increased nutritional and metabolic reserve. Further studies are required to elucidate the mechanism of this reverse epidemiology.[98]

Dietary management of familial hypercholesterolaemia and other hyperlipidaemias

Familial hypercholesterolaemia (FH) is the main clinical syndrome that leads to premature IHD that is possible to identify and treat at present. Manifestation of IHD may begin after the teenage years in heterozygotes and in childhood for homozygotes. FH accounts for 5% premature mortality from IHD in Europe and although it is common, only 20% of cases are identified.

Diagnosis of FH

Criteria for the diagnosis of FH are outlined below.[63] A definite diagnosis of FH can be concluded in the presence of criteria 1 + 2 or 1 + 3. A probable diagnosis requires 1 + 4 or 1 + 5 below:

1. Total cholesterol > 7.5 mmol/L or LDL-C > 4.9 mmol/L in an adult (levels either pretreatment or highest on treatment);
2. Tendon xanthomas in patient, or in first-degree relative or in second-degree relative;
3. DNA-based evidence of an LDL receptor mutation of defective apolipoprotein B;
4. Family history of myocardial infarction: < 50 years of age in second-degree relative or < 60 years of age in first-degree relative; and
5. Family history of raised total cholesterol: > 7.5 mmol/L in adult first- or second-degree relative or > 6.7 mmol/L in child or sibling aged younger than 16 years.

NICE recommends that individuals with FH are offered individualised nutritional advice from a healthcare professional with specific expertise in nutrition.[63] This general lifestyle advice, including a cardioprotective diet, as shown in Table 19.3, applies to individuals with FH. There is insufficient evidence of dietary interventions in this group from which to make separate recommendations to diet distinct from that in Table 19.3, though NICE recommends replacement of saturates by either PUFA or MUFA.[63]

It would be unusual for dietary measures alone to lower serum cholesterol to an ideal level. So it is recommended that lipid-lowering medication is started without delay. Where individuals choose to take stanol/sterol-containing products, they are advised to take them consistently and in sufficient quantities to confer benefit. This may be important for individuals who do not tolerate medication.

The advice for individuals with serum triglycerides (TG) between 2 and 10 mmol/L (phenotype type IV) is similar to that of all patients with hyperlipidaemia.

As the TG level increases, further overall fat restriction is required. When TG level is > 11 mmol/L, most patients have chylomicronaemia (usually type V or more rarely type I hyperlipoproteinaemia). These patients are at increased risk of acute pancreatitis particularly when TG levels > 20–30 mmol/L. This condition is often associated with excess alcohol intake and obesity. Advice to limit or avoid alcohol intake is essential.

In chylomicronaemia, the diet must be low in fat of all types. A decrease to a total fat intake of 10–25% of dietary energy per day is necessary.

This is because the triglyceride-rich chylomicrons are made in the gut in response to all long chain fatty acids in the diet. The only realistic energy alternative is carbohydrate. Glucose polymers or Medium chain triglyceride (MCT) oil may be indicated. This substitution may itself cause an endogenous hypertriglyceridaemia. So creating a balance between exogenous and endogenous hypertriglyceridaemia must be considered when devising a suitable diet.

Supplements of essential fatty acids such as linoleic (omega-6 PUFA) acid and ALA are likely to be required along with fat soluble vitamins. Skimmed milk may be a useful source of protein.

Key points

- Diet and lifestyle changes are an integral part of disease prevention and management whether drug therapy is employed or not.
- Dietary advice known to reduce morbidity and mortality should be prioritised in patients with CVD over reducing individual risk factors;
- Two to four portions per week of oily fish or 1 g omega-3-acid ethyl esters daily after an MI improves survival.
- Adopting a Mediterranean dietary pattern improves survival and reduces cardiac events in post-MI patients.
- Dietary advice to modify fat intake in high-risk CVD patients appears to have a modest effect in reducing CVD morbidity if followed for at least 2 years.
- Although compliance with dietary advice to reduce salt intake decreases with time, reductions in long-term cardiovascular morbidity have been observed in individuals without CVD and high normal blood pressure at the outset, despite modest reductions in blood pressure.
- Hypertension and dyslipidaemia are treated in the overall context of cardiovascular risk in primary prevention of CVD.
- It is important to take a considered approach to interpreting guidelines and translating them into advice for patients.

Case study

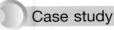

Mary is a 56-year-old lady who works in an office. She is overweight with a BMI of 31 and does not smoke.

Doctors diagnosed her as having a myocardial infarction (a STEMI as seen in Figure 19.4). Her total cholesterol was measured on admission as 6 mmol/L. She was normotensive.

Since leaving hospital she has chosen to stop taking the simvastatin because of cramps in her legs. She is struggling to achieve the two portions of oily fish a week target recommended to her in hospital. Her GP, reluctant to prescribe omega-3-acid ethyl esters because of local prescribing restrictions, asked her whether she would like to see the local dietitian at the surgery the following week for dietary counselling.

QUESTIONS

1. Based on current evidence from randomised controlled trials, which dietary interventions are most likely to improve Mary's chances of survival?

2. What considerations would you make about including stanol/sterol products in her diet? Justify your reasoning.

3. She informs you that she dislikes sardines and tuna and that is why she is struggling to take two portions of oily fish per week. List the strategies you might employ to help her include two portions of oily fish in her diet per week.

4. If she was to manage one portion of oily fish per week and you were to advise her to purchase an omega-3 supplement, how much omega-3 PUFA would you ask her to find in a daily supplement?

5. Mary tells you that her husband has stable angina and asks how much oily fish he should eat per week or whether he should take a fish oil supplement. What are your considerations before advising Mary?

ANSWERS

1. Based on current evidence from randomised controlled trials, which dietary interventions are most likely to improve Mary's chances of survival?

To improve her omega-3 PUFA intake to target amounts, i.e. 2–4 portions of oily fish per week or 1 g per day as omega-3 PUFA supplements, and to follow a Mediterranean type diet.

2. What considerations would you make about including stanol/sterol products in her diet? Justify your reasoning.

It may be worth considering. First of all, assess her overall diet for other changes she can make first such as modifying fat intake and reducing energy intake to lose weight. Other considerations include cost of stanol/sterol products to patient and ensuring she takes the stanol/sterol products in optimal amounts.

3. She informs you that she dislikes sardines and tuna and that is why she is struggling to take two portions of oily fish per week. List the strategies you might employ to help her include two portions of oily fish in her diet per week.

Present her with other examples of oily fish to ensure she knows what is considered oily fish. Suggest she try those she has never tried before. Suggest practical ways she can include these in her diet.

4. If she was to manage one portion of oily fish per week and you were to advise her to purchase an omega-3 supplement, how much omega-3 PUFA would you ask her to find in a daily supplement?

About 0.5 g omega-3 PUFA/day as EPA/DHA.

5. Mary tells you that her husband has stable angina and asks how much oily fish he should eat per week and whether he should take a fish oil supplement. What are your considerations before advising Mary?

The population recommendation is two portions of fish a week, one of which should be oily. The Food Standards Agency recommends a maximum of four oily fish portions a week. The evidence as it stands appears to be that people post-MI will benefit from two to four portions of oily fish per week. We are less clear about the benefit of this amount in other forms of heart disease. One trial which has been criticised for poor design showed an increase in mortality in stable angina patients taking omega-3 PUFA supplements, as outlined in the text.

Acknowledgements

We thank C. Eddy, C. Hames and A. Mead for their comments on an earlier draft of this chapter.

References

1. World Health Organization. *The Atlas of Heart Disease and Stroke*. Geneva: World Health Organization; 2009. Online. Available at: http://www.who.int/cardiovascular_diseases/en/cvd_atlas_14_deathHD.pdf.

2. Allender S, Kaur A, Peto V, et al. *Coronary Heart Disease Statistics*. London: British Heart Foundation; 2008. Online. Available at: http://www.heartstats.org/datapage.asp?id=7998.

3. Harding S, Rosata M, Teyhan A. *Trends for CHD and Stroke Mortality among Migrants in England and Wales 1979–2003*. Cited in Allender et al.[2]

4. Department of Health. *National Service Framework for Coronary Heart Disease*. London: Department of Health; 2000.

5. National Institute of Clinical Excellence. *Chronic Heart Failure: National Clinical Guideline for Diagnosis and Management in Primary and Secondary Care*. 2003. Online. Available at: http://guidance.nice.org.uk/CG5.

6. Schocken DD, Benjamin EJ, Fonarow GC, et al. Prevention of heart failure: a scientific statement from the American Heart Association Councils on Epidemiology and Prevention, Clinical Cardiology, Cardiovascular Nursing, and High Blood Pressure Research; Quality of Care and Outcomes Research Interdisciplinary Working Group; and Functional Genomics and Translational Biology Interdisciplinary Working Group. *Circulation*. 2008;117:2544–2565.

7. National Heart, Lung and Blood Institute and Boston University. *Epidemiological Background and Design: The Framingham Study*. 2009. Online. Available at: http://www.framinghamheartstudy.org/about/background.html. Accessed July 2009.

8. British Cardiac Society, British Hypertension Society, Diabetes UK, et al. JBS 2: Joint British Societies' guidelines on prevention of cardiovascular disease in clinical practice. *Heart*. 2005;91(suppl V):v1–v52.

9. Yusuf S, Hawken S, Ounpuu S, et al. Effect of potentially modifiable risk factors associated with myocardial infarction in 52 countries (the INTERHEART study): case-control study. *Lancet*. 2004;364:937–952.

10. Adler AI, Stratton IM, Neil HA. Association of systolic blood pressue with macrovascular and microvascular complications of type 2 diabetes: prospective observational study. *Br Med J*. 2000;321:412–419.

11. Williams B, Poulter NR, Brown MJ, et al. The BHS guidelines working party guidelines: report of the fourth working party of the British Hypertension Society, 2004-BHS IV. *J Hum Hypertens*. 2004;18:139–185.

12. Bhatnagar D, Soran H, Durrington PN. Hypercholesterolaemia and its management. *Br Med J*. 2008;337:503–508.

13. Department of Health. *Nutritional Aspects of Cardiovascular Disease. Report of the Cardiovascular Review Group Committee on Medical Aspects of Food Policy*. Report on Health and Social Subjects 46, London: HMSO; 1994.

14. National Institute for Health and Clinical Excellence. *Lipid Modification: Cardiovascular Risk Assessment and the Modification of Blood Lipids for the Primary and Secondary Prevention of Cardiovascular Disease*. London: NICE; 2008. Online. Available at: http://www.nice.org.uk/CG67.

15. National Institute of Clinical and Health Excellence. *MI: Secondary Prevention in Primary and Secondary Care for Patients Following a Myocardial Infarction*. London: NICE; 2007. Online. Available: http://www.nice.org.uk/CG48.

16. American Heart Association/National Heart Lung and Blood Institute Scientific Statement. Diagnosois and management of the metabolic syndrome. *Circulation*. 2005;112:2735–2752.

17. Petersen S, Peto V. *Smoking Statistics*. London: British Heart Foundation; 2004. Online. Available at: http://www.heartstats.org/datapage.asp?id=3916.

18. World Health Organization. *Obesity—Preventing and Managing the Global Epidemic. Report of a WHO consultation on obesity*. Geneva: World Health Organization; 2000.

19. World Health Organization. *The World Health Report 2002. Reducing Risks, Promoting Healthy Life*. Geneva: World Health Organization; 2002.

20. Garcia MJ, McNamara PM, Gordon T, et al. Morbidity and mortality in the Framingham population: sixteen year follow-up. *Diabetes*. 1974;23:105–111.

21. Woodward M, Lowe GD, Rumley A, et al. Fibrinogen as a risk factor for coronary heart disease and mortality in middle-aged men and women: the Scottish Heart Health Study. *Eur Heart J*. 1998;19(1):55–62.

22. British Heart Foundation. *Novel Risk Factors and the Prediction of Coronary Heart Disease Risk*. British Heart Foundation Fact file 2. London: British Heart Foundation; 2007.

23. Joint Health Surveys Unit. *Health Survey for England, 2005*. London: TSO; 2005. Cited in Allender et al.[2] 2008.

24. Hemingway H, Marmot M. Psychosocial factors in the aetiology and prognosis of coronary heart disease: systematic review of prospective cohort studies. *Br Med J*. 1999;318:1460–1467.

25. Department of Health. *Saving Lives: Our Healthier Nation*. London: Department of Health; 1999.

26 Hoare J, Flatley J. Home Office Statistical Bulletin. *Drug Misuse Declared: Findings from the 2007/08 British Crime Survey England and Wales*. London: Home Office.

27. McCord J, Jneid H, Hollander JE. Management of cocaine-associated chest pain and myocardial infarction. A scientific statement from the American Heart Association acute cardiac care committee of the council on clinical cardiology. *Circulation*. 2008;117:1897–1907.

28. Department of Health. *At Least Five a Week: Evidence on the Impact of Physical Activity and Its Relationship*

to Health. London: Department of Health; 2004.

29. Department of Health. Choosing Activity: A Physical Activity Action Plan. London: Department of Health; 2005.

30. Department of Health. Health Survey for England 2006. London: TSO. Cited in Allender et al. 2008.[2]

31. Department of Health. NHS Health Check: Vascular Risk Assessment and Management Best Practice Guidance. London: Department of Health; 2009.

32. Patient UK: Primary Cardiovascular Risk Calculator. 2008. Online. Available at: http://www.patient.co.uk/doctor/Primary-Cardiovascular-Risk-Calculator.htmx.

33. Sofi F, Francesca C, Abbate R, et al. Adherence to Mediterranean diet and health status: meta-analysis. Br Med J. 2008;337:a1344.

34. de Lorgeril M, Salen P, Martin JL, et al. Mediterranean diet, traditional risk factors, and the rate of cardiovascular complications after myocardial infarction: final report of the Lyon Diet Heart Study. Circulation. 1999;99:779–785.

35. Krauss RM, Eckel RH, Howard B, et al. American Heart Association Dietary Guidelines: revision 2000: a statement for healthcare professionals from the Nutrition Committee of the American Heart Association. Stroke. 2000;(11):2751–2766.

36. Iqbal R, Anand S, Ounpuu S, et al. on behalf of the INTERHEART Study Investigators. Dietary patterns and the risk of acute myocardial infarction in 52 countries: results of the INTERHEART study. Circulation. 2008;118(19):1929–1937.

37. Office for National Statistics. National Diet and Nutrition Survey: Adults Aged 19–64 Years. Vol 5. London: TSO; 2003.

38. National Centre for Social Research. An assessment of dietary sodium levels among adults (aged 19–64) in the UK general population in 2008, based on analysis of dietary sodium in 24 hour urine samples. Online. Available at: http://www.food.gov.uk/multimedia/pdfs/sodiumreport08.pdf.

39. Scientific Advisory Committee on Nutrition and Health. Salt and Health. London: TSO; 2003.

40. He FJ, Macgregor GA. How far should salt intakes be reduced? Hypertension. 2009;42:1093–1099.

41. Hooper L, Bartlett C, Davey Smith G, et al. Advice to reduce dietary salt for prevention of cardiovascular disease. Cochrane Database Syst Rev. 2004;(1):CD003656.

42. Whelton PK, Appel LJ, Espeland MA, et al. for the TONE Collaborative Research Group. Sodium reduction and weight loss in the treatment of hypertension in older persons: a randomized controlled trial of nonpharmacologic interventions in the elderly (TONE). JAMA. 1998;279:839–846.

43. Ard JD, Coffmann CJ, Lin PH, et al. One year follow up study of blood pressure and dietary patterns in dietary approaches to stop hypertension (DASH)-sodium participants. Am J Hypertens. 2004;17:1156–1162.

44. NICE. Hypertension: Management of Hypertension in Adults in Primary Care. Online. Available at: http://www.nice.org.uk/CG34.

45. American Heart Association scientific statement. Dietary approaches to prevent and treat hypertension. Hypertension. 2006;47:296–308.

46. Appel LJ, Moore TJ, Obarzanek E, et al. A clinical trial of the effects of dietary patterns on blood pressure. N Engl J Med. 1997;336:1117–1124.

47. Sacks FM, Svetkey LP, Vollmer WM, et al. Effects on blood pressure of reduced dietary sodium and the dietary approaches to stop hypertension (DASH) diet. DASH-Sodium Collaborative Research Group. N Engl J Med. 2001;344:3–10.

48. Cook NR, Cutler JA, Obarzanek E, et al. Long term effects of dietary sodium reduction on cardiovascular disease outcomes: observational follow-up of the trials of hypertension prevention (TOHP). Br Med J. 2007;334(7599):885–888.

49. Kumanyika SK, Cook NA, Cutler JA. Sodium reduction for hypertension prevention in overweight adults: further results from the Trials of

Hypertension Prevention Phase II. J Hum Hypertens. 2005;19:33–45.

50. Fung TT, Chiuve SE, McCullough ML, et al. Adherence to a DASH-style diet and risk of coronary heart disease and stroke in women. Arch Intern Med. 2008;168:713–720.

51. Webb AJ, Patel N, Loukogeorgakis S, et al. Acute blood pressure lowering, vasoprotective, and antiplatelet properties of dietary nitrate via bioconversion to nitrite. Hypertension. 2008;51:784–790.

52. He FJ, Nowson CA, Lucas M, MacGregor GA. Increased consumption of fruit and vegetables is related to a reduced risk of coronary heart disease: meta-analysis of cohort studies. J Hum Hypertens. 2007;21:717–728.

53. Shekelle PG, Morton SC, Jungvig LK, et al. Effect of supplemental vitamin E for the prevention and treatment of cardiovascular disease. J Gen Intern Med. 2004;19:380–389.

54. Eidelman RS, Hollar D, Hebert PR, et al. Randomized trials of vitamin E in the treatment and prevention of cardiovascular disease. Arch Intern Med. 2004;1552–1556.

55. Morris CD, Carson S. Routine vitamin supplementation to prevent cardiovascular disease: a summary of the evidence for the U.S. preventive services task force. Ann Intern Med. 2003;139:56–70.

56. Miller ER, Pastor-Barriuso R, Dalal D, et al. Meta-analysis: high-dosage vitamin E supplementation may increase all-cause mortality. Ann Intern Med. 2005;142(1):37–46.

57. Vivekananthan DP, Penn MS, Sapp SK, et al. Use of antioxidant vitamins for the prevention of cardiovascular disease: meta-analysis of randomised trials. Lancet. 2003;361:2017–2023.

58. Albert CM, Cook NR, Gaziano JM, et al. Effect of folic acid and B vitamins on risk of cardiovascular events and total mortality among women at high risk for cardiovascular disease: a randomized trial. JAMA. 2008;299:2027–2036.

59. Homocysteine lowering with folic acid and B vitamins in vascular disease—the Heart Outcomes Prevention Evaluation (HOPE)

2 results. *N Engl J Med.* 2006;354:1567–1577.

60. Homocysteine lowering and cardiovascular events after acute myocardial infarction—results of the NORVIT study. *N Engl J Med.* 2006;354:1578–1588.

61. Lonn E, Yusuf S, Arnold MJ, et al. Heart Outcomes Prevention Evaluation (HOPE) 2 Investigators. Homocysteine lowering with folic acid and B vitamins in vascular disease. *N Engl J Med.* 2006;354(15):1567–1577.

62. Hooper L, Summerbell C, Higgins JPT, et al. Dietary fat intake and prevention of cardiovascular disease: systematic review. *Br Med J.* 2001;322:757–763.

63. National Institute of Health and Clinical Excellence. *Familial Hypercholesterolaemia: Identification and Management of Familial Hypercholesterolaemia.* London: NICE; 2008.

64. Clarke R, Frost C, Collins R, et al. Dietary lipids and blood cholesterol: quantitative meta-analysis of metabolic ward studies. *Br Med J.* 1997;314:112–117.

65. Tang JL, Armitage JM, Lancaster T, Silagy CA, Fowler GH, Neil HAW. Systematic review of dietary intervention trials to lower blood total cholesterol in free-living subjects. *Br Med J.* 1998;316: 1213–1220.

66. Reckless J, Morrell J. *Lipid Disorders: Your Questions Answered.* Edinburgh: Churchill Livingstone; 2005.

67. Scottish Intercollegiate Guidelines Network. Secondary prevention of coronary heart disease following myocardial infarction. In: Mead A, Atkinson G, Albin D, et al., eds. Dietetic guidelines on food and nutrition in the secondary prevention of cardiovascular disease—evidence from systematic reviews of randomized controlled trials (*second update, January 2006*). *J Hum Nutr Diet.* 2000;19:401–419.

68. Jula A, Marniemi J, Huupponen R, et al. Effects of diet and simvastatin on serum lipids, insulin, and antioxidants in hypercholesterolemic men: a randomized controlled trial. *JAMA.* 2002;287: 598–605.

69. Oh K, Hu FB, Manson JE, et al. Dietary fat intake and risk of coronary heart disease in women: 20 years of follow-up of the nurses' health study. *Am J Epidemiol.* 2005;161:672–679.

70. Durrington PN. *Hyperlipidaemia Diagnosis and Management.* 3rd edn. London: Hodder Arnold; 2007.

71. Harris WS, Mozaffarian D, Rimm E, et al. Omega-6 fatty acids and risk for cardiovascular disease: a science advisory from the American Heart Association Nutrition Subcommittee of the Council on Nutrition, Physical Activity, and Metabolism; Council on Cardiovascular Nursing; and Council on Epidemiology and Prevention. *Circulation.* 2009;119(6):902–907.

72. Nelson B, Erens B, Bates B, et al. *Low Income Diet and Nutrition Survey, vol. 2. Food Consumption Nutrient Intake.* London: TSO; 2007.

73. Scientific Advisory Committee on Nutrition and Health, Committee on Toxicity. *Advice on Fish Consumption Benefits and Risks.* London: TSO; 2004.

74. Saito Y, Yokoyama M, Origasa H, et al. Effects of eicosapentaenoic acid on major coronary events in hypercholesterolaemic patients (JELIS): a randomised open-label, blinded endpoint analysis. *Lancet.* 2007;369:190–198.

75. Kris-Etherton PM, Harris WS, Appel LJ, et al. Fish consumption, fish oil, omega-3 fatty acids, and cardiovascular disease. *Circulation.* 2002;106:2747–2757.

76. Burr ML, Fehily AM, Gilbert JF, et al. Effects of changes in fat, fish, and fibre intakes on death and myocardial reinfarction: diet and reinfarction trial (DART). *Lancet.* 1989;2:757–761.

77. GISSI-P Investigators. Dietary supplementation with n-3 polyunsaturated fatty acids and vitamin E after myocardial infarction: results of the GISSI-Prevenzione trial. Gruppo Italiano per lo Studio della Sopravvivenza nell'Infarto miocardico. *Lancet.* 1999;354:447–455.

78. Barzi F, Woodward M, Marfisi RM. Mediterranean diet and all-causes mortality after myocardial infarction: results from the GISSI-

Prevenzione trial. *Eur J Clin Nutr.* 2003;10:604–611.

79. Hooper L. Dietetic guidelines: diet in secondary prevention of cardiovascular disease. *J Hum Nutr Diet.* 2001;14:297–305.

80. Burr ML, Ashfield-Watt PA, Dunstan FD, et al. Lack of benefit of dietary advice to men with angina: results of a controlled trial. *Eur J Clin Nutr.* 2003;57:193–200.

81. Hooper L, Thompson RL, Harrison RA, et al. Risks and benefits of omega 3 fats for mortality, cardiovascular disease, and cancer: systematic review. *Br Med J.* 2006;332:752–760.

82. Scandinavian Simvastatin Survival Study Group. Randomised trial of cholesterol lowering in 4444 patients with coronary heart disease: the Scandinavian Simvastatin Survival Study (4S). *Lancet.* 1994;344: 1383–1389.

83. Gissi-HF Investigators. Effect of n-3 polyunsaturated fatty acids in patients with chronic heart failure (the GISSI-HF trial): a randomised, double-blind, placebo-controlled trial. *Lancet.* 2008;372:1223–1230.

84. Diabetes UK. *Position Statement on Fish and Fish Oil.* London: Diabetes UK; 2009.

85. Hartweg J, Perera R, Montori V, et al. Omega-3 polyunsaturated fatty acids (PUFA) for type 2 diabetes mellitus. *Cochrane Database Syst Rev.* 2008;(1) CD003205.

86. Zatonski W, Campos H, Willet W. Rapid declines in coronary heart disease mortality in eastern Europe are associated with increased consumption of oils rich in alpha linolenic acid. *Eur J Epidemiol.* 2008;23:3–10.

87. Andersson SW, Skinner J, Ellegård L. Intake of dietary plant sterols is inversely related to serum cholesterol concentration in men and women in the EPIC Norfolk population: a cross-sectional study. *Eur J Clin Nutr.* 2004;58: 1378–1385.

88. Katan MB, Grundy SM, Jones P, et al. Efficacy and safety of plant stanols and sterols in the management of blood cholesterol levels. *Mayo Clin Proc.* 2003;78: 965–978.

89. Joint Health Claims Iniative. *Generic Claim Soya Protein and Blood Cholesterol*. London: JHCI; 2002.

90. Harland A, Haffner T. Systematic review, meta-analysis and regression of randomised controlled trials reporting an association between an intake of circa 25 g soya protein per day and blood cholesterol. *Atherosclerosis*. 2008;200(1): 13–27.

91. Brown L, Rosner B, Willett W, Sacks FM. Cholesterol-lowering effects of dietary fiber: a meta-analysis. *Am J Clin Nutr*. 1999;69:30–42.

92. Keenan JM, Goulson M, Shamliyan T, et al. The effects of concentrated barley beta-glucan on blood lipids in a population of hypercholesterolaemic men and women. *Br J Nutr*. 2007;97: 1162–1168.

93. Kelly S, Frost G, Whittaker V, Summerbell C. Low glycaemic index diets for coronary heart disease. *Cochrane Database Syst Rev*. 2004;(4):CD004467.

94. Graham I, Atar D, Borch-Johnsen K, et al. European guidelines on cardiovascular disease prevention in clinical practice: full text. Fourth Joint Task Force of the European Society of Cardiology and other societies on cardiovascular disease prevention in clinical practice (constituted by representatives of nine societies and by invited experts). *Eur J Cardiovasc Prev Rehabil*. 2007;(suppl 2):S1–S113.

95. Rimm EB, Williams P, Fosher K. Moderate alcohol intake and lower risk of coronary heart disease: meta-analysis of effects on lipids and haemostatic factors. *Br Med J*. 1999;319(7224):1523–1528.

96. Ackermann RT, Mulrow CD, Ramirez G, et al. Garlic shows promise for improving some cardiovascular risk factors. *Arch Intern Med*. 2001;16:813–824.

97. Scottish Intercollegiate Guidelines Network. *Guideline 95: Management of Chronic Heart Failure*. Edinburgh: SIGN; 2007. Online. Available at: http://www. sign.ac.uk/pdf/sign95.pdf.

98. Lavie CJ, Mehra MR, Milani RV. Obesity and heart failure prognosis: paradox or reverse epidemiology? *Eur Heart J*. 2005;26:5–7.

99. Durrington PN. Dyslipidaemia. *Lancet*. 2003;362(9385):717–731.

Bibliography

Betteridge DJ, Morrell JM. *Clinicians Guide to Lipids and Coronary Heart Disease*. 2nd edn. London: Arnold; 2003.

British National Formulary 56. London: BMJ Group and RPS Publishing; 2008. Online. Available at: http:// bnf.org/bnf/.

Camm AJ, Bunce NH. Cardiovascular disease. In: Kumar P, Clark M, eds. *Kumar and Clark Clinical Medicine*. 6th edn. Edinburgh: Elsevier Saunders; 2005:725–871.

Lipids Online. *Educational Resources in Atherosclerosis and Coronary Heart Disease*. Houston: Baylor College of Medicine. Online. Available at: http://www.lipidsonline.org. Accessed 24 June 2008.

Longmore M, Wilkinson I, Turmezei T, et al. *Oxford Handbook of Clinical Medicine*. 7th edn. Oxford: Oxford University Press; 2007.

Mead A, Atkinson G, Albin D, et al. Dietetic guidelines on food and nutrition in the secondary prevention of cardiovascular disease—evidence from systematic reviews of randomized controlled trials (second update, January 2006). *J Hum Nutr Diet*. 2006;19:401–419.

National Institute of Clinical Excellence. *Diagnosis and Initial Management of Acute Stroke and Transient Ischaemic Attack (TIA)*. London: NICE; 2008. Online. Available at: http://guidance. nice.org.uk/CG68.

Reckless J, Morrell J. *Lipid Disorders: Your Questions Answered*. Edinburgh: Churchill Livingstone; 2005.

Stanner S. *Cardiovascular Disease: Diet, Nutrition and Emerging Risk Factors. A Report of the British Nutrition Foundation Task Force*. Oxford: Blackwell; 2005.

Thomas B, Bishop J. *Manual of Dietetic Practice*. 4th edn. Oxford: Blackwell; 2007.

Patient information resources

British Dietetic Association. *Heart Disease and Omega 3 Fats Information Leaflet*. 2nd edn. 2007. Online. Available at: http://www. bda.uk.com.

British Heart Foundation. *Food Should Be Fun …. And Healthy!*. London: BHF; 2005. Online. Available at: www.bhf.org.uk. (healthy eating plan and some delicious, mouth-watering recipes from around the world).

Heart UK. *Dietary Advice to Help Lower Your Cholesterol and Keep Your Heart Healthy*. Available at: http://www. heartuk.org.uk/ Suitable for individuals with FH from a variety of cultures.

National Institutes of Health. *Your Guide to Lowering Your Blood Pressure with DASH. DASH Eating Plan. Lower Your Blood Pressure*. Online. Available at: http://www. nhlbi.nih.gov/health/public/heart/ hbp/dash/new_dash.pdf.

Food Standards Agency. For advice on alcohol units; food labelling and salt. Available at: http://www.eatwell.gov. uk.

Povey R, Morrell J, Povey R. *Eating for a Healthy Heart*. London: Sheldon Press; 2005.

Management of stroke

20

Marion Ireland

LEARNING OBJECTIVES

By the end of this chapter, the reader will be able to:

- Gain knowledge of the background to and pathophysiology of stroke, and identify the relevance of nutritional screening and assessment in stroke management;
- Demonstrate a critical understanding of the effective management of dysphagia in stroke patients, including the roles of enteral nutrition, texture modified diets, oral nutritional support and the key importance of hydration;
- Understand some of the complexities of the ethical considerations relating to enterally fed stroke patients; and
- Gain insight into the dynamic process of neurorehabilitation, and of the approach required to secondary prevention and discharge planning in stroke patients.

Introduction

Stroke is a major cause of morbidity and mortality in the UK, and the third major cause of death, accounting for 11% of all deaths.[1] Most people survive a first stroke, but are often left with significant morbidity.

Stroke is defined as a sudden interruption in the blood supply to an area of the brain, depriving the affected point of oxygen and causing death of brain tissue, the neurological consequences of which can be profound, resulting in long-term disability, especially in the elderly.[2] In addition, the World Health Organization definition includes that the focal or global signs of disturbance of cerebral function will last more than 24 hours or leading to death with no apparent cause other than that of vascular origin.[3]

A transient ischaemic attack (TIA) is defined as stroke symptoms and signs that resolve within 24 hours, which can in fact resolve within minutes or a few hours of onset.[4]

In recent years, there is a growing body of evidence for more effective primary and secondary prevention of stroke, recognising that it is a preventable and treatable disease, rather than a consequence of ageing that inevitably results in death or severe disability.[4]

Epidemiology of stroke

Stroke is the third most common cause of death in the Western populations, following ischaemic heart disease (IHD) and cancer, and remains a major health problem in the UK. The incidence of stroke is strongly age-related, with more than 75% of strokes occurring in people aged above 65 years. Approximately 125,000 new or recurrent strokes occur each year in the UK, but up to 350,000 people are affected at any one time, of which ~50% will make a full recovery with no obvious residual disability.[5]

Between 20 and 30% of people die within the first month of a stroke occurring and it remains the largest cause of adult disability. Approximately one-third of people who have a stroke are left with a long-term disability. Stroke also has a causative role in further morbidities such as depression, dementia and epilepsy.

Types of stroke

There are two main types of stroke which occur:

- Ischaemic or cerebral infarction—this accounts for ~80% of strokes; caused by a clot narrowing or blocking cerebral blood vessels, which results in brain cell death due to oxygen deprivation.
- Haemorrhagic stroke: intracranial haemorrhage ~10%, subarachnoid haemorrhage ~5%, ~5% unknown origin. This is a bursting of weakened or damaged blood vessels, resulting in bleeding within the brain, or on the brain's surface, both of which cause damage.[5]

Risk factors

As with any vascular disease process, there are several factors involved that can increase risk of stroke, many of which are modifiable. Risk factors which contribute to the development of atherosclerosis include hypertension, smoking, diabetes mellitus, excessive alcohol consumption and raised lipids.

Additionally, the presence of other cardiovascular conditions such as ischaemic heart disease, peripheral vascular disease, coronary artery stenosis, atrial fibrillation, prosthetic valves and cardiomegaly are directly associated with increasing the risk of ischaemic stroke.[5]

There are some obvious nutrition-related risk factors, such as hypertension, raised lipids, obesity, impaired glucose tolerance, all of which can be affected and improved by modification of dietary intake. There is also a growing evidence base for factors such as raised homocysteine levels, which are associated with poor dietary intake of folate and vitamins B_6 and B_{12}, and this is associated with increased cardiovascular risk, further emphasising that nutrition has a part to play in both primary and secondary prevention of stroke.

Pathophysiology of stroke

Residual deficits can depend on the location and extent of a stroke. Some deficits are permanent in some patients, but can resolve in others, depending on the damage the brain has incurred.

The pathophysiology of stroke can include:

- Aphasia—a loss of language, affecting speech, reading and interpretation;

- Apraxia—disordered skilled purposeful movement, e.g. affecting ability to feed self;
- Ataxia—tremor or poor motor control;
- Altered appetite control;
- Behavioural difficulties, e.g. inappropriate social behaviours;
- Changes in mobility, balance;
- Cognitive impairment;
- Continence problems;
- Depression;
- Dysphagia—difficulties in swallowing;
- Dysphasia—impairment of speech and verbal comprehension;
- Emotional lability;
- Fatigue;
- Hemianopia—visual problems;
- Hemiplegia—paralysis affecting one side of the body;
- Impaired memory and perception;
- Neglect; and
- Sensory loss—altered taste or smell.

Although dysphagia is closely associated with undernutrition in stroke patients, many of these features of stroke have a significant impact on nutritional intake and require appropriate management of these deficits to ensure that nutritional status does not suffer as a result. The practicalities of mealtimes in patients with significant residual disabilites can make the process of 'plate to mouth' a complex one. For example, a patient with apraxia or ataxia may be unable to feed themselves; a patient with neglect or hemianopia may only be able to see or access half of their plate of food; or a patient with impaired memory may forget to eat, or have forgotten that they have already eaten.

Nutritional screening

Nutritional screening should be a simple procedure that can be carried out by any member of the multidisciplinary team, to detect each patient's risk of nutritional problems, and a plan of action for the management of them. Screening of all patients should ideally be carried out within 48 hours of admission to hospital and repeated regularly throughout the episode of care.[6] Baseline information required should include height, weight, body mass index and percentage weight change.[7] Malnutrition occurs in approximately 15% of all patients admitted to hospital, increasing to approximately 30% within the first week. It carries with it a strong association with poorer functional outcome and slower rate of recovery.[8]

In addition, SIGN 78 recommends that a nutritional screening tool for use in stroke patients should focus on the effects of stroke on nutritional status, e.g. presence of dysphagia, ability to eat, rather than solely focusing on pre-existing nutritional status.[9]

Nutritional screening helps to identify any immediate or pre-existing nutritional problems, and helps direct appropriate action required to manage this in the short term. It should also direct referral to a dietitian for assessment and management of nutritional risk. However, as with all screening tools, it is important that all staff carrying out screening still use clinical judgement to avoid inappropriate referrals, or more importantly, if there is cause for concern when a patient is *not* identified as high risk by a nutritional screening tool.

Nutritional therapy and dietetic intervention

Nutritional assessment

Nutritional assessment of patients is a more detailed evaluation of each patient's nutritional requirements and current nutritional status. It should involve an in-depth assessment of a patient's clinical condition, and any physiological changes therein affecting nutritional status, biochemical and anthropometric measurements, prescribed medications and any dietary factors which will influence current intake.

The prevalence of malnutrition, and the impact that this has on the patient's condition, is well documented, including increased frequency of infection, increased rate of pressure sores, increased morbidity and mortality, increased length of hospital stay, increased levels of apathy and depression and poorer functional outcomes.[10]

The risk of malnutrition in stroke patients varies, but it is recognised that nutritional status can worsen during admission, and that undernutrition following admission is associated with increased case fatality and poor functional status at 6 months.[11] It is important to assess beyond merely swallowing problems and poor intake, and look thoroughly at the mechanics of plate to mouth and the entire meal process, to ensure that the impact of any residual disabilities is minimised.

Nutritional assessment and estimation of requirements are based on predictive equations such as Schofield, which allow estimation of basic requirements of energy and protein and fluid, along with micronutrients, e.g. trace elements.[12] The outcome of a patient's swallow assessment is integral to ensure that nutritional intervention is delivered appropriately in patients with identified dysphagia.

It is unclear to what extent hypermetabolism and hypercatabolism occur post-stroke, with estimations for the increase in metabolic rate following stroke ranging from 10 up to 50%, depending on the severity and clinical consequences of the stroke, and clinical judgement is required when estimating the increase in resting energy expenditure.[13] Catabolic effects vary according to the individual, but usually persist for the first few weeks, then begin to resolve in the following weeks and months.

Hyperglycaemia following stroke occurs as part of the metabolic response to injury, related to the stress hormone levels. Optimisation of blood glucose control is essential in order to minimise the risk of worsening the effects of stroke, and some studies have shown that even in the absence of diabetes, an initially high blood glucose following stroke is a predictor of poor outcome.[14] Insulin therapy is recommended in all patients with diabetes to ensure that blood glucose is controlled within the recommended levels.[4]

Undernutrition, in stroke patients in particular, is associated with a higher stress response, increased frequency of infections, poor functional status and reduced survival.[5] Risk of undernutrition and dehydration are significant in stroke patients, and their causes are complex and often multifactorial. This emphasises the importance of good management of undernutrition at each stage of the patient's journey, to ensure the minimum impact on nutritional status is made. The management of dysphagia in stroke patients is of the utmost importance, due to the risk of undernutrition that accompanies it. However, even in patients without dysphagia, risk of undernutrition is significant in stroke, ensuring that robust measures for nutritional support should be in place in all stroke units, and for all stroke patients.

Swallow screening

Dysphagia, which is a difficulty in swallowing, is a common and clinically significant complication following stroke which can result in aspiration.[8] Aspiration can be defined as when solids or liquids that should be swallowed into the stomach are instead breathed into the respiratory system, and the presence of aspiration is associated with an increased risk of developing an aspiration pneumonia, and other bronchopulmonary infections.[9]

Both NICE 2004 and SIGN 78 recommend that, following acute stroke, all patients should be screened for dysphagia by an appropriately trained healthcare professional before being given food, drink or medication.

A water swallow test is often used to help identify a patient's risk of aspiration (Figure 20.1). This involves giving the patient teaspoons of water, and then observing for any signs such as delayed initiation of swallowing, coughing or altered voice quality. This type of test has good reported clinical sensitivity of > 70%, and between 22 and 66% sensitivity for prediction of aspiration.[15]

As with all screening tools, clinical judgement is essential for ensuring appropriate referral to a speech and language therapist, for full assessment of swallow, and appropriate management of dysphagia, and to prevent patients from being put at risk if aspiration is not clearly identified on screening.

NICE 2008 recommends that if the admission screen indicates a swallowing problem, that a specialist assessment should take place within 72 hours of admission.[4]

Dysphagia defined

Dysphagia, which is a difficulty in swallowing either food or fluids or both, is a significant complication in patients following stroke. In stroke patients, it presents as difficulty in safely moving food or fluid from the mouth to the stomach without aspiration often due to difficulties at the oral preparation stage with chewing and tongue control.[9] Incidence varies greatly, ranging from 64 to 90% in patients conscious during the acute phase, with aspiration rates, including silent aspiration, ranging from 22 to 42% on videofluoroscopy.[8]

Dysphagia has serious implications for patients following stroke, such as increased potential for undernutrition and dehydration, if it is not managed effectively. With increased risk of aspiration, there is a higher risk of respiratory infection, which may develop into aspiration pneumonia. Nutritional problems tend to be exacerbated by the presence of dysphagia, and patients with pre-existing malnutrition are at even greater risk.

Management of dysphagia

Effective management of dysphagia is of key importance following stroke, in order to prevent undernutrition and dehydration from occurring as far as possible. This must involve multidisciplinary working and good communication between involved practitioners. Once a full assessment of dysphagia by a speech and language therapist has taken place, the appropriate route of feeding can be identified, making it more attainable to meet nutrition and hydration requirements.

The route of feeding initially is often a combination of oral and enteral feeding, and the management of each transition through the different stages of this spectrum is a crucial part of effective dysphagia management.

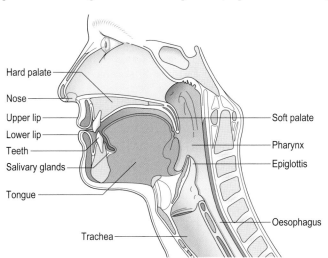

Figure 20.1 • Swallowing mechanism.

Hard palate

Nose

Upper lip

Lower lip

Teeth

Salivary glands

Tongue

Trachea

Soft palate

Pharynx

Epiglottis

Oesophagus

Enteral nutrition

Nutritional intervention following stroke can often involve enteral feeding in patients who are unable to meet their requirements safely or consistently via oral diet and fluids, and for some patients, oral intake is contraindicated completely.

Enteral feeding is the introduction and delivery of nutrients via the gastrointestinal tract, by means other than eating.[16] Contraindications to enteral nutrition are patient refusal, patients with a non-functioning gastrointestinal (GI) tract, and where it is inappropriate to feed for ethical reasons.[17] Enteral feeding in stroke tends to focus on nasogastric and gastrostomy feeding, both of which are used in patients unable to meet their requirements or who are at risk of disease-related malnutrition.

Nasogastric feeding

Tube placement involves a fine-bore nasogastric tube being inserted transnasally into the stomach. The tubes are usually between 6 and 9 mm French gauge, made from polyurethane, PVC or silicone. Nasogastric feeding is ideal in the acute setting, for patients who require short-term feeding, identified as less than 4 weeks.[2] It can be used longer term if other options such as gastrostomy feeding are contraindicated or not appropriate.[19]

Care is needed in the insertion of nasogastric tubes, which should be carried out by suitably trained personnel, particularly in stroke patients where there is impaired or absent swallow, as getting patients to swallow during tube placement can help with insertion. The position of the tube should be confirmed by aspiration of stomach contents and checking that the pH of aspirate is < 5.5, indicating gastric contents, as per the National Patient Safety Agency Guidelines from 2005.[20] The position of a nasogastric tube should be confirmed before *each* use by aspiration of stomach contents, and radiological confirmation should only be used when there is ongoing difficulty in obtaining aspirate, or concern regarding the tube position that cannot be otherwise resolved.

Consent should be obtained for placement of all feeding tubes, and this can prove difficult in stroke patients, as there may be cognitive impairment, and significant communication difficulties, along with confusion and poor understanding, particularly immediately post stroke. Medical staff usually take responsibility for obtaining consent for procedures considered invasive, or identifying when patients do not have the capacity to consent, and putting alternative arrangements for procedures to take place, such as per the guidance for consent and capacity from the British Medical Association in England and Wales, or the Adults with Incapacity Act in Scotland.

Results from the FOOD Trial indicated that early enteral feeding, clarified as within 7 days, may reduce mortality, and that dysphagic stroke patients should be offered enteral feeding via nasogastric tube within the first few days of admission. However, it also identified worse quality of life in patients allocated early tube feeding, concluding that early feeding may keep patients alive, but in a severely disabled state when they would otherwise have died.[21] The RCP Stroke Guidelines go a step further, indicating that patients should be fed within the first 24 hours, based on the recommendations of the FOOD Trial and the observed reduction in mortality, with further consultation with patient representatives regarding the timing of initiation of feeding for maximum benefit.

Refeeding syndrome

Early enteral feeding is recommended in stroke patients, but in circumstances where a patient has received little or no nutritional intake for more than 5 days, risk of refeeding should be identified and managed appropriately.[21] Refeeding is defined as 'severe fluid and electrolyte shifts and related metabolic implications in malnourished patients undergoing refeeding',[16,18] and there are established guidelines regarding the replacement of electrolytes and the reintroduction of fluids and nutrients in at risk patients, such as those developed by Oxford Radcliffe Hospitals in 2003.

Nasal bridle tubes

Nasal bridle tubes are enteral feeding tube retaining devices that are increasing in use in patients who repeatedly displace nasogastric tubes, e.g. in patients who are confused following stroke. The use of nasal bridle loops has been shown to have few complications and minimal discomfort for the patients, and in one prospective study showed a reduction in 30-day gastrostomy mortality, in part due to better selection of patients for gastrostomy, and also that bridle loops allowed patients an average 10 days' nutrition prior to either recovery or gastrostomy placement.[22] The NICE Guideline for management of acute stroke endorses the consideration of using nasal bridle tubes in stroke patients who are unable to tolerate a nasogastric tube.[4]

Gastrostomy feeding

Gastrostomy feeding is generally used for patients requiring longer term nutritional support, usually identified as more than 4 weeks.[4] Gastrostomy tubes are placed directly into the stomach, endoscopically, surgically or radiologically, and each patient should be fully assessed prior to placement, to ensure that there are no contraindications to placement, e.g. previous abdominal surgery.

Previously, a number of studies comparing nasogastric to gastrostomy feeding showed that there was better success in the administration of feed, less interruption to feeding regimen and lower risk of aspiration with gastrostomy feeding. As a result, patients were more consistently hydrated and fed, and nutritional status improved, and with it many of the functional measures associated with poor nutrition, such as increased frequency of infection, increased risk of pressure areas, depression and loss of muscle mass.

However, the FOOD Trial found that there were no clinically significant benefits of gastrostomy feeding compared to nasogastric feeding, and also found a reduction in poor outcomes with nasogastric feeding.[21] The recommendation from this was to use nasogastric feeding initially for the first 2–3 weeks post stroke, unless there was a clear practical reason to use gastrostomy. An additional finding of interest was that the gastrostomy group had a higher rate of pressure sores, which raised the possibility that these patients may move less or be nursed differently.

Poor outcome following gastrostomy insertion, as concluded by the FOOD Trial, must consider that patient selection is a factor, as those requiring gastrostomy are patients with poor nutritional intake and status, and the poorest prognosis. This links in with the finding that, although early enteral feeding is recommended, and does not cause any harm, this can keep patients alive but in a severely disabled state where they would otherwise have died; that is, survival itself does not equate to survival with good outcome.

Please refer to the chapter on enteral nutrition for further guidance on this aspect of patient care.

Texture modified diets

For patients not identified as 'nil by mouth' by bedside or instrumental assessment, the speech therapist will provide clear guidance regarding the appropriate consistency of diet and fluids.

Dietary modification involves the altering of the texture and viscosity of food and fluids to allow safe bolus transport, to maximise the control of the rate that food or fluid passes through the pharynx and to minimise risk of aspiration in patients with dysphagia. Thickening agents, derived from food starch, can be added to both food and fluids to achieve the correct consistency, and these are prescribable products for dysphagia.[23]

The National Descriptors for Texture Modification in Adults gives a comprehensive classification of the different consistencies of food and fluids used in dysphagia management, although many places may have local guidelines based on the National Descriptors successfully implemented (Tables 20.1 and 20.2, Box 20.1).[24]

Patient medications also need careful review in patients with identified dysphagia, and alternative presentations may be required. It is not always appropriate to crush tablets and administer via the enteral route, as this may affect the efficacy of the medication, and advice from pharmacists should be sought on the most appropriate method and formulation of administering medication.

Similarly, particular attention should be given to oral hygiene in dysphagic patients, not just those on enteral feeding, due to the difficulties that may occur by the nature of dysphagia. Many problems such as pocketing of food or inability to mouth clear may occur which can impact on oral hygiene if not closely monitored.

For stroke patients who have experienced a significant impairment of swallow, a common starting point would be a trial diet of pureed consistency, usually teaspoonfuls only at each meal, designed to reintroduce swallowing to the patient. If this is successful, the patient would progress on to a full pureed diet and thickened fluids. Of course, neither of these options would meet nutrition or hydration requirements, due to the constraints of texture modification, and the quantity of diet and fluids required to be consumed in order to meet these requirements. Hopefully, patients then continue to progress through the different consistencies on to a normal diet and fluids, but of course each patient has a

Table 20.1 Texture modification—fluid

Texture	Description of fluid texture	Fluid example
Thin fluid	Still water	Water, tea, coffee without milk, diluted squash, spirits, wine
Naturally thick fluid	Product leaves a coating on an empty glass	Full cream milk, cream liquers, Complan, build-up (made to instructions), nutriment, commercial sip feeds
Thickened fluid	Fluid to which commercial thickener has been added to thicken consistency	
Stage 1	<ul><li>Can be drunk through a straw</li><li>Can be drunk from a cup if advised or preferred</li><li>Leaves a thin coat on the back of a spoon</li></ul>	
Stage 2	<ul><li>Cannot be drunk through a straw</li><li>Can be drunk from a cup</li><li>Leaves a thick coat on the back of a spoon</li></ul>	
Stage 3	<ul><li>Cannot be drunk through a straw</li><li>Cannot be drunk from a cup</li><li>Needs to be taken with a spoon</li></ul>	

From *National Descriptors for Texture Modification*, 2009, published by the British Dietetic Association, reproduced with permission.

Table 20.2 Modification texture—food

Texture	Description of food texture	Food examples
A	<ul><li>A smooth, pouring, uniform consistency</li><li>A food that has been pureed and sieved to remove particles</li><li>A thickener may be added to maintain stability</li><li>Cannot be eaten with a fork</li></ul>	<ul><li>Tinned tomato soup</li><li>Thin custard</li></ul>
B	<ul><li>A smooth, uniform consistency</li><li>A food that has been pureed and sieved to remove particles</li><li>A thickener may be added to maintain stability</li><li>Cannot be eaten with a fork</li><li>Drops rather than pours from a spoon but cannot be piped or layered</li><li>Thicker than A</li></ul>	<ul><li>Soft whipped cream</li><li>Thick custard</li></ul>
C	<ul><li>A thick, smooth, uniform consistency</li><li>A food that has been pureed or sieved to remove particles</li><li>A thickener may be added to maintain stability</li><li>Can be eaten with a fork or spoon</li><li>Will hold its own shape on a plate, and can be moulded, layered and piped</li><li>No chewing required</li></ul>	<ul><li>Mousse</li><li>Smooth fromage frais</li></ul>
D	<ul><li>Food that is moist, with some variation in texture</li><li>Has not been pureed or sieved</li><li>These foods may be served or coated with a thick gravy or sauce</li><li>Foods easily mashed with a fork</li><li>Meat should be prepared as C</li><li>Requires very little chewing</li></ul>	<ul><li>Flaked fish in thick sauce</li><li>Stewed apple and thick custard</li></ul>

Continued

Table 20.2 Modification texture—food—Cont'd

Texture	Description of food texture	Food examples
E	• Dishes consisting of soft, moist food • Foods can be broken into pieces with a fork • Dishes can be made up of solids and thick sauces or gravies • Avoid foods which cause a choking hazard (see list of high-risk foods in Box 20.1)	• Tender meat casseroles (approx. 1.5 diced pieces) • Sponge and custard
Normal	Any foods	Include all foods from 'High Risk Foods' list

From *National Descriptors for Texture Modification*, 2009, published by the British Dietetic Association, reproduced with kind permission of the British Dietetic Association.

Box 20.1

High risk foods

- Stringy, fibrous texture, e.g. pineapple, runner beans, celery lettuce
- Vegetable and fruit skins including beans, e.g. broad, baked, soya, black-eye peas, grapes
- Mixed consistency foods, e.g. cereals which do not blend with milk, such as muesli; mince with thin gravy, soup with lumps.
- Crumbly items, e.g. bread crusts, pie crusts, crumble, dry biscuits
- Hard foods, e.g. boiled and chewy sweets and toffees, nuts and seeds
- Husks, e.g. sweetcorn and granary bread

From *National Descriptors for Texture Modification*, 2009, published by the British Dietetic Association, reproduced with kind permission of the British Dietetic Association.

---

different rate and degree of progression, so there are many variables within this spectrum.

Patients remaining on texture modified diets for longer periods of time can easily become disillusioned or bored with their diet, due to the limited food choices available, or poor presentation or texture of the food provided. Efforts should be made to try and provide aesthetically pleasing diets of uniform consistency, such as pre-moulded meals, and choice offered at each meal where possible.

Oral nutritional supplements

Routine nutritional supplementation is not recommended in patients with acute stroke who are adequately nourished on admission.[4] However, nutritional support should be initiated in stroke patients at risk of undernutrition.

When a patient commences on a texture modified diet, nutritional requirements should be reassessed, as they are unlikely to be met by diet alone. In the case of low intake that requires supplementation, this may be met either by enteral nutrition (as previously discussed) or by oral nutritional supplements (ONS), if able to be taken. This should also involve a food fortification approach, from within the constraints of hospital catering, to increase nutrient density, i.e. to maximise the calories and protein provided by the texture modified diet consumed.

ONS are a useful addition to a patient's diet when it is nutritionally incomplete. ONS are nutrient dense, providing energy, protein and micronutrients. There are now a large variety of types and flavours available as prescribable products, so it should be possible to find a product to suit each patient. Some ONS may require thickening, depending on the prescribed fluid consistency for that particular patient, and may be required on an ongoing basis. The use of ONS in stroke patients should be regularly reviewed alongside oral intake and nutritional status, to ensure that prescription is current and appropriate over time.

Hydration

Fluid intake in stroke patients is of key importance, and may need to be supplemented if unable to be met orally, most commonly by subcutaneous or intravenous fluids in the acute phase of treatment. Once an alternative feeding route is established, most likely nasogastric tube in the acute phase, this can serve a dual purpose of providing nutrition and hydration, and should be the route of choice for meeting an individual's requirements until oral intake of food and fluids improves.

Many factors can make risk of dehydration in stroke patients more likely, such as decreased sense of thirst, fear of incontinence, inadequate intake of thickened fluids required to meet requirements, inability to self-feed and communication difficulties, e.g. difficulties in expressing thirst or need for a drink to carers. Again, with good observation of patients at ward level, coupled with robust assessment measures, these risks can be managed, thus decreasing the likelihood of dehydration occurring.

Dysphagia is a dynamic process, and many patients experience great improvements in their swallow ability, with dysphagia resolving completely in some patients. However, progress varies greatly between individuals, and some patients can remain static at a certain level of dysphagia for a considerable time. In these patients in particular, close monitoring is essential to ensure that their nutritional needs are being met consistently over time.

After a period of time, a patient may reach the point where oral nutrient intake is adequate and weight is stable. At this point, it may be appropriate to phase out nutritional support, and replace with appropriate advice on a balanced diet, based on the five main food groups, adapted within the constraints of the texture modified diet advised.

It is important to have dietetic involvement throughout these different stages in the process of dysphagia, to ensure adequate management of each transitional stage, and overall adequacy of nutritional intake over time, but all members of the multidisciplinary team are involved in the monitoring and effective treatment of dysphagia; from observation of mealtimes to provision and use of adapted cutlery, each member has an important role to play.

Ethical considerations in enteral nutrition

The complexities of enteral feeding, and insertion of enteral feeding tubes should lead us to concentrate more closely on the decision to feed in the first instance, and the ethical considerations surrounding the initiation of feeding in stroke patients as an intervention. However, particularly in this patient group, this is a complex and multifactorial decision, as many of the functional measures initially impaired can improve, but at very different rates in each individual, thus making it hard to predict how each patient will progress. For example, one study recorded that

dysphagia had a mean duration of 8 days, and 86% who survived regained the ability to swallow within 14 days.[25] Each patient's capacity to contribute to this decision needs to be assessed, and if not deemed able to consent, then additional measures should be put in place regarding consent and capacity to do so.

Enteral nutrition is regarded as an aspect of medical treatment and it is recommended that in cases where the benefits of nutrition support are uncertain, a 'time-limited' trial should be undertaken.[4] Whilst it is important to avoid nutritional status deteriorating in the acute phase of stroke, the decision to feed severely disabled patients with little prospect of neurological recovery is difficult, and all aspects of survival need to be taken into account. This needs to be a medical decision, and any previously expressed wishes, e.g. living will or advanced directive, should be adhered to.

Once the decision to feed is taken, a nasogastric tube remains the most appropriate measure in the short term. The decision to place a gastrostomy should be addressed at around the 4-week mark, as this is the point where feeding moves into being considered longer term, but each individual's circumstances and progress needs to be evaluated as part of this process. The decision to place a gastrostomy in patients following stroke should not solely focus on a patient's swallow and ability to eat, but also the stage of illness that the individual is at. Quality of life must be considered, along with the longer term implications of feeding, particularly following discharge, along with social circumstances and prognosis.[17] Once again, this is a decision that can only be dealt with on an individual basis, and all aspects of treatment and prognosis need to be considered by experienced practitioners before being made.

With all this considered, sometimes the practicalities of trying to manage confused patients repeatedly removing nasogastric tubes, and thus compromising their already fragile nutritional state, can prove difficult at ward level, and if life expectancy is reasonable, gastrostomy tubes or nasal bridles must be considered as more practical and successful means of feeding and hydrating stroke patients moving towards rehabilitation.

Withdrawal of feeding

There are no real ethical dilemmas in withdrawing enteral feeding when it is successful; i.e. a patient is now able to maintain nutrition and/or hydration via the oral route.[17] In practice, stroke patients can often require hydration beyond the point where they are meeting nutritional requirements, and feeding is discontinued. This is often due to the constraints of remaining on thickened fluids, and consuming adequate volumes of these to achieve adequate hydration; patients may need to receive additional hydration via the established enteral route until hydration needs are being consistently met orally.

Difficulties can arise when nutrition is established, and nutritional status is maintained or improved following stroke, but neurological function does not improve, or perhaps even deteriorates, e.g. if a patient suffers another stroke. A decision to withdraw enteral feeding must be handled similarly to a decision to initiate feeding when it is unclear which course of action is right. The views of the patient, family and carers, along with all members of the multidisciplinary team, should be sought and taken into consideration, to enable a holistic decision that encompasses all aspects of patient care, including quality of life issues, to be made.

Management of transition from acute care to rehabilitation

Most acute hospitals should now have dedicated Stroke Units based on multidisciplinary models as recommended by bodies such as NICE and SIGN.

The National Clinical Guidelines for Stroke (second edition) recommend that a specialist stroke team should ideally consist of consultant physician specialising in stroke medicine; nurses; a physiotherapist; an occupational therapist; a speech and language therapist; a neuroradiologist; a dietitian; a clinical psychologist; a pharmacist; and a social worker.

All staff should have a specialised knowledge of stroke and adequate support in training.

Ideally, if a stroke patient is unable to be discharged home from acute care; hospital-based rehabilitation should be provided for patients who remain dependent for their activities of daily living. Stroke-specific rehabilitation has the best outcomes for stroke patients particularly if an individual goal-centred model is used.[8,26,27]

Neurorehabilitation

Neurorehabilitation is a dynamic process, commencing at the point of acute admission, and continuing on beyond discharge back into the community. Thus, when a patient moves from acute care to rehabilitation, ongoing assessment and monitoring of nutritional goals should occur and be adapted to the patient's changing requirements.

Patients moving into the rehabilitation phase should be medically stable, and thus the effects of the initial increased metabolism and catabolism should have stabilised. Undernutrition or malnutrition should be expected in some patients, usually related to the severity of stroke, or if there is pre-existing malnutrition, often seen in elderly stroke patients. Thorough handover from acute care ensures good continuity of care for all patients entering a rehabilitation unit.

A reassessment of nutritional requirements should take place after the first few days, to ensure that nutritional goals remain current. Goals at this stage should be directed towards improving compromised nutritional status and aiming to replace some of the losses incurred during the acute phase. In addition, they should aim to enable the patient to resume as near normal eating habits as possible within the constraints of any persisting neurological deficits.[4]

Cognitive impairments can adversely affect a patient's ability to participate in therapy to varying degrees, and it is recommended that all patients are screened when entering the rehabilitation phase, so that the impact on activity and participation can be assessed.[8] In a rehabilitation unit, there are different drivers that need to be taken into account, in particular a full therapy programme for each individual, usually involving increased time with each member of the multidisciplinary team, often scheduled as daily sessions. This can be problematic when inheriting patients on enteral feeding regimens, which often do not lend themselves to the change of routine. For example, it may not be ideal to feed overnight patients who are nasogastrically fed but with significant dysphagia, due to positioning in bed and increased risk of aspiration. Therefore, it can be a challenge to match a daytime feeding regimen with an intensive therapy programme, and often use of bolus regimens or time-limited feeding periods become essential to allow the patient the maximum benefit from their therapy programmes, and from time spent in neurorehabilitation.

Nutritional assessment in the rehabilitation phase needs to take into account all the differing factors that can impact on nutritional status, such as dysphagia, ability to self-feed, weight loss incurred in the acute phase of illness and effective management of all residual deficits, to ensure that nutritional intake is adequate. Verbal assessment can be problematic in patients with cognitive impairment, memory or concentration problems or communication difficulties such as expressive or receptive dysphasia. Alternative methods of obtaining useful information, for example using pictorial examples, closed questioning, or involving family and carers can be useful. Similarly, robust assessment tools, such as food record and fluid balance charts, along with observation of patient mealtimes, should be utilised as part of establishing an accurate record of a patient's current intake.

Effective management of stroke patients through each of the transitional stages, from enteral feeding and trial diet and fluids, through each of the stages of consistency modification, with or without the adjunct of nutritional support, requires regular review to ensure nutritional adequacy. Progression through the differing transitional stages varies greatly with each individual, as does the timescale involved. Some patients can progress very rapidly through the different stages once oral intake is reintroduced, whilst in others it can be a much more static process, with progression from stage to stage taking weeks or months rather than days. Ensuring nutritional adequacy of whichever combination of oral intake with enteral feeding or oral nutritional support is a dynamic and often rapidly progressing process, so regular monitoring of progress and review of dietary intervention is essential.

When enteral nutrition is in the process of being reduced or discontinued, dietary intake often requires supplementation, via either food fortification or oral nutritional supplements, or a combination of both. Texture modified diets are in the main nutritionally incomplete, and require supplementation to ensure that nutritional requirements are being met, and should be regularly re-evaluated to ensure that estimated intake remains current.

Hydration is important throughout the patient's journey in stroke, but of particular importance during the transitions through the different consistencies of diet and fluids. Robust monitoring of fluid balance needs to occur regularly, in particular for dysphagic patients who remain on thickened fluids. Many patients do not enjoy thickened fluids, and most find it difficult to drink the amount required for adequate hydration, usually 1500–2000 mL/day. This can result in enteral routes being utilised for hydration to ensure fluid needs are met, even after enteral nutrition has been discontinued. In addition, if patients are experiencing continence and toileting difficulties, they may self-limit oral fluids, to avoid the inconvenience, either to themselves or to others, of going to the toilet, or to prevent bladder accidents, which may be embarrassing to the patient. This aspect should be of particular concern, and requires careful management, as urinary continence is a recognised predictor of stroke morbidity and mortality, but has also been linked to the deterioration of nutritional status in stroke patients.[5] In all stroke patients, adequate fluids should be encouraged consistently by all staff, as the consequences of dehydration are both unpleasant and avoidable.

Stroke patients are also at high risk of constipation, due to a variety of factors including decreased fluid intake, decreased fibre intake, decreased mobility, decreased gut motility and perhaps some medications. Management consists of increasing fluid intake by whichever means is suitable, and increasing the consumption of more fibre-rich foods, matched with whichever dietary constraints the patient may have, e.g. texture-modified diet. The use of fibre feeds in long-term enterally fed patients is recommended for general bowel health, but is essential if the patient is prone to constipation.

The nutritional needs of stroke patients change as their functional status changes throughout the patient's journey, and all members of the multidisciplinary team have a role to play in the monitoring of all aspects of care, from weighing patients to observing mealtimes, from adapted cutlery, beakers and utensils to facilitate self-feeding, through to assessing progress of muscle strength in exercise sessions.

Secondary prevention of stroke

Patients who have suffered a stroke are at high risk of a subsequent stroke, of between 30 and 43% within the first 5 years, and also carry increased risk of other vascular events such as myocardial infarction.[4]

Lifestyle advice regarding modifiable risk factors, such as smoking, weight and activity levels, should be given to patients in an appropriate format, depending on the nature of their residual deficit. The dietary objectives for secondary prevention are the same as for primary prevention, but the nature and delivery may differ due to residual disabilities, cognitive impairment or communication difficulties. This should be tailored to the individual's needs, and may take the form of pictures to illustrate advice, large print versions of information, recorded information for visually impaired patients or converting dietary advice into easy prompts for patients with memory problems. Additionally, the patient may remain on a texture modified diet, and the limitations of this must be incorporated into secondary prevention advice.

Physical disabilities may also affect the practicalities of healthy eating advice, such as food shopping, meal preparation and the consumption of foods. Liaison with occupational therapists and carers is essential to ensure that this aspect of care is addressed.

The secondary prevention advice itself consists of the same messages as that of a cardioprotective diet, with slightly more focus on antihypertensive measures and anticoagulation control:

- Increase of omega-3 fats and oils;
- Increase of fruit and vegetable consumption;
- Avoidance of excess sodium consumption;
- Decrease of saturated fat intake;
- Weight management;
- Alcohol consumption within safe limits; and
- Optimal management of diabetes.

Although research has failed to categorically show that reduced dietary sodium can affect future cardiovascular events, it is a generally agreed point of good practice that reducing salt intake can lower blood pressure, which is likely to be of benefit.

Optimum control of diabetes is also desirable, as the presence of diabetes usually carries with it hypertension and altered lipid metabolism, along with accelerated degeneration of blood vessels. Again, although there is no clear trial evidence to support that tight glucose control reduces the risk of stroke, it does reduce the risk of microvascular complications, so it seems reasonable to extrapolate that good glucose control is a sensible preventative measure in stroke.

Discharge planning

Prior to discharge, most patients will have an environmental visit, in order to identify and address any issues in terms of the practicalities of returning to their residence. This usually involves joint working with local authorities to ensure that the correct package of care for that patient on discharge, and usually includes adaptations required such as doors widened to accommodate wheelchair width, handrails in bathrooms, etc. as a result of the occupational therapy assessments.

Communication of all appropriate food and fluid advice should be conveyed to both the patient (in appropriate format) and carers. Provision of nutritional products on discharge, e.g. nutritional supplements, thickening agents, will vary from region to region, but a reasonable discharge supply should always be given.

For the ongoing management of the patient's dysphagia, hydration and bladder and bowel function, good communication with the patient's GP is essential, along with the relevant community dietitian or enteral feeding team, depending on the needs of the patient.

Support for carers varies throughout the country, but organisations such as Headway provide support via groups and practical advice and it is part duty of care of a rehabilitation team to ensure that carers have access to such support to ensure that they have their own needs met, which in turn has an impact of the care that they can provide.

Key points

- Between 20 and 30% of people die within the first month of a stroke occurring and it remains the largest cause of adult disability. Approximately one-third of people who have a stroke are left with a long-term disability.
- The prevalence of malnutrition is high in stroke. Its impact includes increased frequency of infection, increased rate of pressure sores, increased morbidity and mortality, increased length of hospital stay, increased levels of apathy and depression and poorer functional outcomes.
- The extent of hypermetabolism and hypercatabolism following stroke ranges from 10 up to 50%, depending on the severity and clinical consequences of the stroke.
- Hyperglycaemia following stroke occurs as part of the metabolic response to injury and incurs risk of worsening the effects of stroke. An initially high blood glucose level following stroke is a predictor of poor outcome.
- Risk of undernutrition and dehydration are significant in stroke patients, and their causes are complex and often multifactorial. The management of dysphagia in stroke patients is of the utmost importance, due to the risk of undernutrition that accompanies it.
- The incidence of dysphagia in stroke varies greatly, ranging from 64 to 90% in patients conscious during the acute phase, with aspiration rates, including silent aspiration, ranging from 22 to 42% on videofluoroscopy.

- In all stroke patients, adequate fluids should be encouraged consistently by all staff, as the consequences of dehydration are both unpleasant and avoidable.
- The FOOD Trial found that early nasogastric enteral feeding, within 7 days, may reduce mortality. It found no clinically significant benefits of gastrostomy feeding compared to nasogastric feeding, in the early stage, with a reduction in poor outcomes with nasogastric feeding.

- Stroke-specific rehabilitation has the best outcomes for stroke patients particularly if an individual goal-centred model is used.
- Patients who have suffered a stroke are at high risk of a subsequent stroke, of between 30 and 43% within the first 5 years, and also carry increased risk of other vascular events such as myocardial infarction.

Case study

A 68-year-old male presents with an ischaemic stroke, which results in significant neurological deficits. Water swallow test indicates high risk of aspiration and following assessment by a speech and language therapist, the patient is identified as 'Nil by Mouth' awaiting videofluoroscopy. The patient is hydrated initially by IV fluids and after 48 hours the decision to pass a nasogastric tube is taken. The patient remains confused and agitated and removes four nasogastric tubes within a 24-hour period. His pre-morbid weight is 55 kg, height 1.7 m.

QUESTIONS: ACUTE PHASE

1. What would be your suggested immediate management of this patient's nutritional needs?
2. What additional considerations do you need to take into account?

Three weeks later, this patient is transferred to a neurorehabilitation unit. He now has a gastrostomy tube in situ, but often disconnects his feed from the pump. Videofluoroscopy recommendations have allowed him to commence a pureed diet and thickened fluids, but he still needs feeding and remains very distracted at meal times. He has now developed antibiotic associated diarrhoea, following a course of antibiotics for a urinary tract infection. His weight is now 52 kg, height 1.7 m.

QUESTIONS: NEUROREHABILITATION

1. What would be your ongoing management of this patient's nutritional needs?
2. Which members of the multidisciplinary team should be involved, and what would their role be?
3. What measures can be put in place to improve the patient's nutritional status?

ANSWERS: ACUTE PHASE:

1. What would be your suggested immediate management of this patient's nutritional needs?

- Medical review for agitation, patient needs to be more settled to allow basic care needs to be met, e.g. hydration, nutrition, toileting;
- Ensure patient is not at risk of refeeding;
- Repass nasogastric tube, but continue meeting hydration needs via IV until ascertained whether tube will remain in situ; and
- Consider use of nasal-bridle tube, preferably using an experienced practitioner to place.

2. What additional considerations do you need to take into account?

- When appropriate, meet hydration needs enterally once route is secure;
- Patient is underweight, so further increase in requirement will be needed once feeding is established; and
- Oral hygiene needs.

ANSWERS: NEUROREHABILITATION

1. What would be your ongoing management of this patient's nutritional needs?

- Change patient onto bolus regimen, to manage feed disconnecting;
- Ensure fibre-containing feed is used. Anecdotally lower density feeds have fewer problems in patients with AAD; and
- Increase protein, calories and fluid as able within the bolus regimen.

2. Which members of the multidisciplinary team should be involved, and what would their role be?

- Nursing staff, to manage behaviour—may need to be isolated initially at mealtimes, to allow less distraction;
- SLT—under constant review from speech therapy re dysphagia and communication, plus supervision and management of behaviour at mealtimes
- OT and physio—ongoing work on ADLS especially around mealtimes and feeding, etc.; and
- Medical/psychology—if agitation does not improve.

Continued

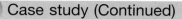

Case study (Continued)

3. What measures can be put in place to improve the patient's nutritional status?
   - Bolus regimens have good success in agitated patients;
   - Fortification of texture modified diet and fluids as able;
   - Weekly weights; and
   - Monitor +++.

References

1. British Heart Foundation. *Coronary Heart Disease Statistics*. London: BHF; 2004.

2. Thomas B, Bishop J. *Manual of Dietetic Practice*. 4th edn. Oxford: Blackwell; 2007.

3. World Health Organization. *Cerebrovascular Disease Prevention, Treatment and Rehabilitation*. Geneva: WHO; 1971.

4. National Institute for Health and Clinical Excellence. *Stroke—Diagnosis and Initial Management of Acute Stroke and Transient Ischaemic Attack*. Clinical Guideline 68. 2008.

5. Gariballa S. *Nutrition and Stroke: Prevention and Treatment*. Oxford: Blackwell; 2004.

6. Nursing and Midwifery Practice Development Unit. *Nutrition: Assessment and Referral in the Care of Adults in Hospital—Best Practice Statement*. Edinburgh: NMPDU; 2002.

7. Malnutrition Advisory Group of British Association for Parenteral and Enteral Nutrition. Nutritional Screening of adults: a multidisciplinary responsibility; 2003.

8. Royal College of Physicians. *National Clinical Guidelines for Stroke*. London: RCP; 2004.

9. Scottish Intercollegiate Guidelines Network. *Management of Patients with Stroke: Identification and Management of Dysphagia*. Clinical Guideline 78. Edinburgh: SIGN; 2004.

10. McWhirter JP, Pennington CR. Incidence and recognition of malnutrition in hospital. *Br Med J*. 1994;308:945–958.

11. Dennis MS, Lewis SC, Warlow C, FOOD Trial Collaboration. Routine oral nutritional supplementation for stroke patients in hospital: a multicentre randomised controlled trial. *Lancet*. 2005;365:755–763.

12. Schofield WN. Predicting basal metabolic rate, new standards and review of previous work. *Hum Nutr Clin Nutr*. 1985;39(C suppl 1): 5–96.

13. Finestone HM, Greene-Finestone LS, Foley NC, Woodbury MG. Measuring longitudinally the metabolic demands of stroke patients: resting energy expenditure is not elevated. *Stroke*. 2003;34:2502–2507.

14. O'Neill PA, Davies I, Fullerton KJ, Bennett D. Stress hormone and blood glucose response following acute stroke in the elderly. *Stroke*. 1991;22:842–847.

15. Perry L, Love CP. Screening for dysphagia and aspiration in acute stroke: a systematic review. *Dysphagia*. 2001;16(1):7–18.

16. National Institute for Health and Clinical Excellence. *Nutrition Support in Adults*. Clinical Guideline 32. London: NICE; 2006.

17. Lennard-Jones JE. *Ethical and Legal Aspects of Clinical Hydration and Nutritional Support. A report for the British Association for Parenteral and Enteral Nutrition*, Redditch, Worcs: BAPEN; 2000.

18. Parenteral and Enteral Nutrition Group of the British Dietetic Association. *A Pocket Guide to Clinical Nutrition*. 3rd ed. Birmingham: BDA; 2004.

19. McAtear CA, ed. *Current Perspectives on Enteral Nutrition in Adults*. BAPEN Working party report. Redditch, Worcs: BAPEN; 1999.

20. National Patient Safety Agency. *Patient Safety Alert: Reducing the Harm Caused by Misplaced Nasogastric Feeding Tubes*. London: NPSA; 2005.

21. Dennis MS, Lewis SC, Warlow C. FOOD Trial Collaboration. Effect of timing and method of enteral tube feeding for dysphagic stroke patients: a multicentre randomised controlled trial. *Lancet*. 2005;365: 764–772.

22. Johnston RD, O'Dell L, Patrick M, Cole AT, Cunliffe RN. Outcome of patients fed via a nasogastric tube retained with a bridle loop: do bridle loops reduce the requirement for percutaneous endoscopic gastrostomy insertion and 30-day mortality? *Proc Nutr Soc*. 2008; 67(OCE):E116.

23. British National Formulary published jointly by the British Medical Journal Group and the Royal Pharmaceutical Society – updated 6 monthly, version used was March 2009. Information found in Appendix 7: Borderline Substances, under Feed Thickeners and pre-thickened foods.

24. British Dietetic Association. *National Descriptors for Texture Modification in Adults*, Birmingham: BDA; 2009.

25. Gordon C, Hewer RL, Wade DT. Dysphagia in acute stroke. *Br Med J*. 1987;295:411–414.

26. Stroke Unit Trialists' Collaboration. Organised inpatient care for stroke. *Cochrane Database Syst Rev*. 2001;(1):CD000197.

27. Scottish Intercollegiate Guidelines Network. *Management of Patients with Stroke: Rehabilitation, Prevention and Management of Complications, and Discharge Planning*. Clinical Guideline 64. Edinburgh: SIGN; 2002.

Neurological conditions

Karen Green

21

LEARNING OBJECTIVES

By the end of this chapter the reader will be able to:

- Appreciate the impact of Parkinson's disease (PD) or a head injury (HI) on nutritional status and nutritional requirements;
- Understand the role of the dietitian in the management of people living with PD or HI;
- Assess the nutritional status of people living with PD or HI; and
- Advise on the suitability of different types of nutrition support and provide appropriate dietary counseling.

Brief scene setting/historical context

The UK Department of Health launched the National Service Framework for Long-Term Conditions in March 2005 and it has a particular focus on the needs of people with neurological conditions and brain or spinal injuries.[1] The role of the dietitian in the management of these patients is highlighted in this key policy. It is now recognised that the dietitian is as an important team member of any neurological multidisciplinary team (MDT) responsible for the care of the neurological patient.

The incidence and prevalence of head injury (HI), and Parkinson's disease (PD) in the UK is considerable.

The incidence of new HI cases in the UK is 175 per 100,000 of the population per year; all require hospital admission and lead to long-term problems.[1]

In the case of PD, there are approximately 120,000 people living with this condition in the UK.[1]

Appropriate and timely nutrition support for the management of HI and PD has been well documented.[2,3]

Head injury

Physiology

There are two general categories of HI: closed and penetrating. A closed head injury is one in which the skull is not broken open, which can be caused by a direct blow to the head. In a penetrating injury, the skull is broken open, and damage occurs to the brain as well. This can occur when an object, e.g. a bullet, passes through the skull into the brain. Both closed and penetrating HI can cause damage that ranges from mild to very serious. In the most severe cases, HI can result in death.[4]

Pathophysiology

HI can take many forms. These include skull fractures (broken bones in the skull), blood clots between the brain and the skull and damage to the brain itself. Brain damage can occur even if the skull itself is undamaged. The brain may move around inside the skull with enough force to cause bruising and bleeding.

Bleeding such as an intracranial haemorrhage inside the skull may accompany a HI and may cause additional damage to the brain. A blood clot (haematoma) may also form between the brain and the skull. The clot can press against the brain and interrupt the flow of blood and oxygen through the brain. A reduced flow of oxygen prevents the brain from functioning normally.

Several types of intracranial haemorrhage can occur, including the following:

- Extradural haematoma (EDH) occurs inside the head. It results in a collection of blood in between the skull and dura matter (the outer protective lining that covers the brain). EDH is usually caused by fractured bones of the skull.
- Subdural haematoma (SDH) is a collection of clotting blood that forms in the subdural space (the area between two of the meninges that form the dura matter). The associated mortality rate is high, approximately 60–80%.
- Intracerebral haemorrhages (ICH) occur when a diseased blood vessel within the brain bursts, allowing blood to leak inside the brain. The most common cause of ICH is hypertension.
- Intraventricular haemorrhage (IVH) tends to occur due to a rupture of aneurysm accounting for ~25% of IVH in adults; or brain tumour; or arterio-ventricular malformation (AVM).
- Subarachnoid haemorrhage (SAH) can occur spontaneously or be due to trauma, resulting in ruptured aneurysms. About 10–15% die before medical care can be administered, and ~50% die within two weeks. It may lead to a communicating hydrocephalus if blood products obstruct the arachnoid villi or in the event of a non-communicating hydrocephalus secondary to a blood clot obstructing the third or fourth ventricle.[5]

Severity of HI can be determined using the Glasgow Coma Scale (GCS) within 48 hours of injury.[6] This scale is based on a patient's ability to open his or her eyes, give answers to questions and respond to physical stimuli, such as a doctor's touch. A person can score anywhere from 3 to 15 points on this scale. A score of less than 8 points on the scale suggests the presence of serious brain damage.[7]

The lowest possible GCS (the sum) is 3 (deep coma or death), whilst the highest is 15 (fully awake). Generally comas are classified as:

- Severe, with GCS < 8;
- Moderate, GCS 9–12; and
- Minor, GCS > 13.

Common symptoms of HI include loss of consciousness, confusion, drowsiness, cognitive decline, personality change, swallowing difficulties, headache, nausea and vomiting or in some cases speech and language difficulties. HI accounts for about 30% of traumatic deaths and long-term disability.[8]

The immediate objective in severe HI is to prevent secondary damage from hypoxia or raised intracranial pressure (ICP); therefore the initial priorities are to maintain (a) oxygenation and (b) adequate cerebral circulation.

Intubation and ventilation may also be necessary to help in the control of cerebral vasodilation and prevent a rise in ICP.[9] Special attention should be given to the following to prevent secondary complications, thus ensuring a smooth progression to rehabilitation:

- Timely and appropriate nutrition and fluid balance to meet the increased metabolic demands;
- Prevention of contractures;
- Maintenance of postural reflexes;
- Bladder and bowel management;
- Skin care to avoid pressure sores; and
- Management of agitation/confusion.

Attention to these details is all too easily forgotten in the process of saving a patient's life. However, the development of limb contractures or pressure sores at this stage can take months to heal later. Ideally the rehabilitation team should be involved in the patient's care as early as possible to ensure that these aspects are addressed.[9]

Once the patient is stable enough to leave intensive care, they should be transferred to an acute specialist brain injury rehabilitation unit. These patients frequently have continuing medical and surgical requirements, so immediate post-acute rehabilitation often needs to be provided in an acute hospital setting. As the patient's condition continues to improve, continuation of the rehabilitation programme on a day-patient or outpatient basis may be appropriate. These programmes and needs will vary from patient to patient as they move from the differing stages of rehabilitation. Therefore a network of integrated

MDT services must be provided, with excellent communication systems, so that the patient can pass from one level to another in a seamless continuum of care.[9]

Nutritional therapy and dietetic application

Severe undernutrition can exacerbate complications caused by a HI, and can continue throughout the course of rehabilitation.[10] Undernutrition has been shown to increase length of stay (LOS) by up to 28 days on rehabilitation units compared with patients who were well nourished also having sustained a HI. Therefore this highlights the importance of providing continuous monitoring and review of the patient's nutritional status and nutrition provision throughout their admission.[10]

Underfeeding should be avoided at all costs.[11] At least 60% of patients who are admitted to rehabilitation units were found to exhibit severe undernutrition.[12] Feeding difficulties in these patients can be attributed to unconsciousness, drowsiness, being in a vegetative state, bulbar paralysis/palsy, dysphagia, agitation and facial trauma.[10]

Nutritional requirements

Energy

The severe hypermetabolic (HM) response to traumatic HI has been well documented since the 1980s.[13–16] The brain normally regulates metabolism through the sympathetic nervous system. In HI the normal regulatory mechanisms of the brain are disrupted and a disordered HM state develops.[17]

It has been found that an acute severe HI, even in a patient that is sedated and paralysed, is accompanied by energy expenditure values 130–135% above the predicted basal metabolic rate (BMR).[10,18,19] BMR will further escalate due to agitation, spasticity, autonomic storming and vegetative dysfunction and also when both the sedation and paralysing agents are discontinued.[10,20] Agitation is common in these patients and can be associated with fever, posturing, tachycardia, hypertension and diaphoresis. This stress response is known as autonomic storming. It is also thought to be a stage of recovery from severe HI. Other well-documented, associated complications such as infections, fever, septicaemia and pressure sores can affect the patient's energy requirements.[10]

An increased metabolic rate, with rapid protein breakdown in patients with moderate and severe HI during the early, post-injury phase and the related depletion of muscle mass and depressed immuno-function, are reported to increase complication rates and worsen long-term outcome.[21–23]

One suggested preventative approach has been to provide nutrition in accordance with the accelerated metabolism;[24] unfortunately, evidence-based guidelines in this area are lacking.

It has been found that only 27% of patients are able to spontaneously eat post-HI.[25] They often require artificial nutritional support because of their accelerated metabolism and a prolonged inability to eat.[25] The duration of the HM state is variable, lasting from 1 week to 1 year post-HI.[26] Because of this duration, even patients who have recovered and are in rehabilitation facilities may be HM and at risk of developing malnutrition.

The aim of nutritional therapy during this highly variable HM phase is to supply adequate caloric intake to meet the increased metabolic demand.[27] It is important to note that when providing and maintaining optimal nutritional status in the acutely ill HI patient that the dietitian has realistic expectations of what artificial nutrition support can accomplish. It is unlikely that a positive nitrogen (N) balance and significant weight gain can be achieved by meeting or exceeding energy expenditure at the hypermetabolic/catabolic state.[3]

At this stage overfeeding does not prevent muscle wasting and may exacerbate hyperglycaemia, which can induce anaerobic metabolism in the brain, increasing lactate levels, which in turn may contribute to secondary neuronal damage.[18,28–30] In addition to this, overfeeding with high carbohydrate/glucose-based formulas in particular can increase oxygen consumption and therefore yield excess carbon dioxide (CO_2) production. Hypercapnia increases a patient's requirement for artificial ventilatory support, and can cause dilation of cerebral vessels, thereby increasing ICP and the risk of further brain injury.[30]

Protein

Unfortunately very few studies have looked at the protein requirements of critically ill patients. However, early nutrition support in the HI patient has been shown to improve the profound negative N balance caused by excessive protein catabolism.[27,31] Optimal protein use has been found to be heavily dependent on the adequacy of caloric intake.

As already discussed, energy requirements increase in severe HI and N excretion also increases.[32]

In a normal fasting human, the N catabolism is in the region of 3–5 g N/day. In severely head injured patients, N catabolism has been found to be 14–25 g N/day.[33,34] This can be equated to a 10% decrease in lean muscle mass in 7 days.[35] Underfeeding for 2–3 weeks could result in a weight loss of 30%, which is potentially detrimental and has been observed in clinical practice.[35]

Excessive protein intakes, like excessive energy intakes, are unlikely to correct negative N balance in critically hypermetabolic/catabolic patients.[3] This is particularly true during the first 2 weeks following HI. Achieving the lowest possible level of negative N balance should be the goal during this early catabolic period.[27]

Some research has demonstrated that N excretion sharply increases throughout the weeks post-HI, peaking in the second week, and remaining increased well above normal throughout hospital admission.[25,36] Young et al. studied the protein losses of head injured patients and concluded that negative N balance persisted even when protein intake exceeded 1.5 g/kg/day.[25,37]

Studies providing high intakes of N (>17 g/day) via artificial nutrition support have found that less than 50% of N is retained by the body. Therefore, the level of N intake that generally results in less than 10 g of N loss per day is 15–17 g N/day, or 0.3–0.5 g N/kg. This equates to about 2 g protein/kg/day (20% of the caloric composition of a 50 kcal/kg/day feeding protocol). Twenty percent is the maximal protein content and amino acid content of most enteral nutrition support (ENS) and parenteral nutrition support (PNS) formulations.[38]

In a HM patient, N equilibrium is rarely achievable, although it has been shown that increasing the N content of enteral feeding from 14 to 20% does result in improved N retention.[39] The survival rate is better when an increased protein diet is commenced within 1–10 days post-injury versus the same diet administered more gradually or after a long period.[25,40] Ishibashi and colleagues measured protein balance in a critically ill population; each group was randomised to receive intakes of protein ranging from 0.9 to 1.5 g/kg/day.[41] Although the patients in all groups were reported to be in a negative protein balance, protein intake of 1.2 g/kg/day was found to be associated with a 50% improvement in the protein balance. Intakes >1.2 g/kg/day conferred no further benefit.

Some studies have noted that exact values for individual therapy cannot be reliably calculated using clinical predictive formulas and are further distorted in individual patients because of treatment with barbiturates, paralytics and sedatives, and the presence or absence of infection, fever and the severity of injury/depth of coma.[25] For these reasons, routine repeated monitoring of a patient's energy and protein needs should ideally be carried out using indirect calorimetry and urinary urea or total N measurements. Energy expenditure is quantified under specific conditions (usually resting) by measuring respiratory gases (oxygen consumed and carbon dioxide produced) usually undergoing mechanical ventilation on ICU. *The measurement of energy expenditure is the most accurate method for assessing energy needs, especially in acutely ill patients.* Although accurate, this method is expensive, is not readily accessible and requires technical expertise.

Which method of artificial nutrition support is best used in HI?

Infections are a frequent complication in patients with traumatic HI. Early nutritional intervention can clearly combat the development of severe malnutrition, although its effect on improving outcome is not clear. Studies have demonstrated that early ENS is the preferred route of nutritional support in ventilated patients with a functioning gastrointestinal (GI) tract.[24,42,43] The advantage of ENS is less risk of hyperglycaemia, low risk of infection and reduced cost.[38]

In the vast majority of ventilated HI patients, the general trend is to maintain nutrition via the enteral route. In many cases although provision of ENS is adequate, its absorption in the GI tract may be impaired.[44,45] Early intolerance to ENS can be attributed to gastric dysmotility during periods of raised intracranial pressure,[44] prolonged paralytic ileus, abdominal distension, aspiration pneumonitis and diarrhoea.[46,47] Drugs such as anaesthetics and sedatives, opioids and catecholamines can also cause or augment GI dysmotility.[48]

The use of prokinetic agents, such as metaclopramide and erythromycin, during delayed gastric dysmotility can be beneficial when administered intravenously.[49] The effects of erythromycin to improve gastric emptying and to improve tolerance to ENS have been confirmed by studies of critically ill and mechanically ventilated patients.[50,51] However, some intensive care units do not use erythromycin as first-line treatment due to the rising incidence of microbial resistance and the association between erythromycin and ventricular dysrhythmias.[52,53] Metoclopramide on the other hand has been used for the past 35 years for treating gastric dysmotility and is commonly used as a first-line treatment.[48] The only adverse effect of its use is the development of extrapyramidal motor reactions and symptoms of drowsiness, agitation, fatigue and dystonic reactions in long-term usage.[54] Metoclopramide, however, is usually discontinued once normal gastric motility returns. If, however, a post-pyloric feeding tube can be safely inserted, then nasojejunal feeding may be another useful alternative method for providing optimal nutrition.

Attempts at achieving nutrient goals in this case presents a great challenge to the dietitian to maintain optimal energy requirements. Despite this many researchers have demonstrated that the development of enteral feeding protocols and continuous education of critical care staff may improve delivery of ENS.[55,56] Patients should be monitored carefully for signs of gastric dysmotility and subsequent feed intolerance during enteral feeding, so that appropriate treatment can be instigated early to prevent complications such as reflux and aspiration; and optimise nutrition provision.[57]

Enteral nutrition support (ENS) versus parenteral nutrition support (PNS)

Studies have demonstrated that more energy in the form of calories and protein are provided by the PNS route than ENS when administered to patients with severe HI.[44,58] It has been recommended that PNS should be considered as an adjunct therapy, while other researchers believe that early PNS improves the outcome after severe HI.[10,31,47] Many studies have demonstrated that, with nearly equivalent quantities of feeding, the mode of administration has no effect on neurologic outcome and either PNS or ENS is equally effective when prescribed according to individually measured energy expenditure (EE) and N excretion.[25,32,46] Agreement concerning the feeding technique of patients with severe HI should be established within the ICU team, to ensure the appropriate nutritional therapy is followed.[10]

Fluid and sodium

Appropriate fluid management of patients with HI can be challenging for many clinicians as it plays an important role in the maintenance of cerebral perfusion pressure (CPP) and ICP.[30,59] A negative fluid balance (approx <600 mL/day) has been associated with a significant negative effect on outcome, whereas previously it was believed that a negative fluid balance reduced cerebral oedema.[30,60]

It is fairly common for patients following HI to experience difficulties with sodium and water regulation. Both hyper- and hyponatraemia can lead to detrimental consequences, such as altered mental status, for these patients, and can prolong or exacerbate the underlying condition.[30,61]

Syndrome of inappropriate antidiuretic hormone (SIADH) and cerebral salt wasting (CSW)

Hyponatraemia is a common neuromedical problem seen in survivors of central nervous system injury. The aetiology of this hyponatraemia is often diagnosed as 'syndrome of inappropriate diuretic hormone' (SIADH) or cerebral salt wasting (CSW). SIADH is a disorder of sodium and water balance characterised by hypotonic hyponatraemia and impaired water excretion in the absence of renal insufficiency, adrenal insufficiency or any recognised stimulus for the antidiuretic hormone (ADH).[62] Fluid restriction is usually the first line of treatment. However, this can exacerbate vasospasm and produce resultant ischaemia. CSW is a syndrome of renal sodium loss that may occur commonly after central nervous system injury, yet remains unrecognised. Treatment of CSW consists of hydration and salt replacement. Typically, urinary sodium levels are found to be elevated with a low serum osmolality and a serum sodium (Na) level of < 134 mmol/L.[30]

Without adequate evaluation of volume status, patients with CSW may be mistaken for those with SIADH.[63] This is concerning because inappropriate fluid restriction may result in volume depletion and potential cerebral ischaemia in the HI population.[62] The primary mechanism of CSW is still not understood but likely reflects a role for the disturbance of atrial naturetic peptide.[60] Table 21.1 specifies the differential diagnosis of both types of hyponatraemic conditions.

Maintaining electrolyte balance in patients with HI

Patients with severe HI are at risk of developing hypomagnesaemia, hypophosphataemia and hypokalaemia.[63] HI may precipitate polyuresis through a

Table 21.1 Criteria for diagnosis of SIADH and CSW

Parameters	SIADH	CSW
Weight	Increased	Decreased
Dehydration	Absent	Present
Urine Na	Increased	Increased
Serum Potassium (K)	Decrease or no change	Increase or no change
Osmolality	Decreased	Increased or normal
Serum Na	Decreased	Decreased
Blood urea Nitrogen (N)	Normal	Increased
Uric acid	Decreased	Normal

Adapted from Clifton et al.[60]

variety of mechanisms or can be induced through medication, e.g. mannitol. Mannitol is used clinically to reduce acutely raised ICP.

These electrolytes must be monitored daily especially during the acute phase of injury and supplemented accordingly via the enteral or intravenous route.[30]

Key points

- HI has the potential to promote visceral protein depletion and wasting of skeletal musculature through being bed-bound, inadequate nutrition or hypercatabolism and hypermetabolism caused by the insult.[64,65]
- The generally accepted goals of nutrient delivery in patients with HI are to:
  - Provide early nutritional intervention consistent with the patient condition;[27,64,66] and
  - Prevent nutrient deficiencies, which can be achieved by avoiding overfeeding and underfeeding during the hypermetabolic/catabolic state.[66] Overfeeding at this stage may lead to metabolic complications.[25] Underfeeding particularly at the rehabilitation stage causes patients to exhibit severe malnutrition.[12]

- ENS is the preferred route of feeding in ventilated patients with a functioning GI tract.[45–47]
- The dietitian plays a very important role in the continuous and timely monitoring of the patient's nutritional status and provision of adequate nutrition support. This is imperative with respect to gut motility disturbances, whereby an individually tailored treatment is used to prevent further exacerbation of existing motility disturbances.[67]

Developing issues

- Use of indirect calorimetry to determine patient's energy and protein needs. Increased utilisation of indirect calorimetry would facilitate individualised patient care and should lead to improved treatment outcomes;
- Glutamine supplementation may also be beneficial to decrease incidence of infection rate, but it has yet to be adequately studied in HI; and
- Use of and requirements for vitamin, mineral and trace element in patients with post-HI.

Parkinson's disease (PD)

Pathophysiology

PD is a progressive neurodegenerative disorder. It is characterised by tremor, rigidity, akinesia and postural instability, resulting from dopamine depletion in the substantia nigra area of the brain.

Dopamine is a neurotransmitter that allows messages to be sent from the brain to the muscles to activate voluntary movements.[68] This helps us to perform smooth, coordinated movements. The symptoms of PD usually appear when at least 80% of the dopamine is lost. The level of dopamine will continue to decline over many years.

Most cases of PD are of unknown cause. PD is not one disease but the most common form of Parkinsonism.[68] This is the name for a group of disorders, e.g. progressive supranuclear palsy (PSP) or multiple-systems atrophy (MSA), with similar symptoms and all resulting from the loss of dopamine-producing nerve cells.

Onset of PD is usually between the ages of 55 and 65, known as 'late-onset' PD, but between 5 and 10% of patients are under the age of 40, known as 'young-onset' or 'early-onset' PD.[69] It can significantly impair the quality of life, especially physical and social functioning.[70] The impact of having young-onset PD is often most profound in terms of the psychological, emotional and social effects on a person's life.[71] It is worth noting that patients may live with this illness for up to 30 years.[72]

There is no cure at present for PD, although the treatments available are directed at minimising the symptoms and disabilities of the patient.[72–74] The type of medication used varies between individuals according to the nature and severity of symptoms. Since many of the available drugs have significant side effects, the aim of drug therapy is to find a balance between effective symptom control and avoidance of side effects.

Some of the drugs used in the management of PD are levodopa, dopamine agonists, anticholinergics, amantadine and catechol-O-methyl transferase (COMT) inhibitors. Levodopa is used to replace or mimic dopamine in the brain and is used alongside COMT inhibitors to limit the conversion of levodopa to dopamine in the peripheral tissues, therefore enabling a greater proportion of levodopa to cross the blood–brain barrier. Dopamine agonists (mimics dopamine) are usually the first drugs prescribed for those diagnosed with young-onset PD, such as apomorphine hydrochloride and cabergoline.[75] It is also used in conjunction with levodopa.

The effectiveness of drug therapy in PD tends to decrease with time and the duration of benefit after each dose becomes progressively shorter; this is known as 'end-dose failure'. Side effects of levodopa such as dyskinesia may also begin to appear.

Patients on long-term therapy may also suffer from 'on/off syndrome', causing sudden changes in or loss of functional ability. These 'off' periods are unpredictable and may last for only a few minutes or many hours. The main feature of the "off" period is increased muscle tone, and increased involuntary movements during the on period. Drug adjustment is often titrated in an attempt to overcome this problem.

Nutritional therapy and dietetic application

The nutritional issues faced by people living with PD are complex and diverse, in particular weight loss. Weight loss is often accompanied by malnutrition and is a very common observation among healthcare professionals. Weight loss in this particular group of patients had not received much attention until recently.[76–78]

Weight loss is reported frequently by patients living with PD.[79] They exhibit lower body weight and weight loss can occur during the early stages of the disease.[80–83] This can be associated with increased risk of fall and fractures due to low bone mineral density, and is multifactorial.[77,84,85] The symptoms of PD are outlined in Table 21.2.

People living with PD are therefore at considerable risk of malnutrition as a result of these symptoms and the side effects of its treatment.[76] Good nutrition is important at all stages of PD and attention to the dietary elements of treatment can lessen the symptoms of the condition by improving nutritional status, and the efficiency of drug therapy.[86]

Nutritional assessment

Early nutrition support could potentially avert problems associated with weight loss and reduce the burden of healthcare costs.[87] Table 21.3 outlines the dietary management of those at high risk of malnutrition, as identified by a validated nutrition screening tool (e.g. the Malnutrition Universal Screening Tool, MUST), who require nutritional support.[88]

Nutritional requirements

The daily energy requirements of PD are unclear. Recent data suggest that some individuals with chronic diseases such as PD have energy requirements at or below current recommendations, while others have elevated energy needs.[89]

Energy

Energy requirements can vary between the stages of the disease and the severity of the patient's symptoms.[86] Clinical experience has shown that some people living with PD can consume more than 3000 kcal per day; yet, they continue to lose weight. This has also been found in other studies.[82,85] This may be caused by rigidity, tremor and levodopa-induced dyskinesia.[77,78,90] It has been suggested that levodopa may enhance glucose metabolism, resulting in enhanced energy expenditure.[78,90] Therefore energy intake should be estimated accordingly.[86]

Table 21.2 The symptoms of PD and how they can contribute to unintentional weight loss

Symptom	Action	Result
Tremor in hands	Increase in spillages	Embarrassment and reluctance to eat in front of others—resulting in social isolation
Rigidity and stiffness in muscles	Inability to prepare food and manually feed themselves	Difficulties with chewing and swallowing food may develop, requiring assistance, which can demoralise the patient
Bradykinesia	Slow movements can prolong the time taken to eat a meal	Food may be abandoned either because it has become cold and unappetising or because of fatigue arising from the sheer effort involved in eating
Motor fluctuations	Unpredictable 'off' periods around mealtimes and for extended periods during the day	Can affect ability to eat and drink enough, thus having a direct impact on nutritional intake and weight
Dyskinesia	Uncontrolled 'jerky' movements	This uses up more energy than the patient consumes, thought to be due to increased energy consumption by skeletal muscle[80]
Mood changes	Anxiety, depression, irritability, restlessness and cognitive decline	This may impair appetite. Side effects of some anti-Parkinsonian drugs may also exacerbate these problems
Drug side effects	Some neuropsychiatric side effects such as confusion, insomnia, hallucinations or psychosis OR gastrointestinal side effects may include nausea, vomiting, dry mouth or constipation	Many of the side effects of anti-Parkinsonian drugs have nutritional implications such as reduced appetite, forgetting to eat, or early satiety
Dysphagia	Inability to control/tolerate certain textures and consistencies increasing the risk of aspiration	Certain textures such as puree can be nutritionally dilute and therefore not adequately energy dense to prevent weight loss

Table 21.3 Nutritional assessment for nutrition support

Aims	Action
1. Identify and avoid nutritional inadequacies as early as possible	Thorough in-depth, individualised diet history
2. Instigate measures to correct deficiencies or nutrition-related problems	Dietary counselling, use of oral sip feeds, nutritional supplementation, e.g. calcium and vitamin D, supplementary and/or ENS
3. Identify ways to minimise any practical difficulties associated with eating/swallowing	Close liaison with the speech and language therapist, occupational therapist, physiotherapist combined with dietary counseling
4. Prevent undesirable weight gain or weight loss	Agree a goal weight with the patient/carer, especially if being fed by ENS
5. Preserve lean muscle mass	Provide tailored, individual guidance on ways to provide optimal nutrition and energy balance
6. Monitor nutritional status	Regular review of weight and BMI, tolerance to nutrition support prescription as the disease progresses; rescreen using MUST
7. Encourage high intake of fibre and fluid to prevent or manage constipation	All oral sip feeds and/or enteral preparations should be high in fibre. Advice on ways to increase fluid intake should be given to the patient/carer

The dietitian ideally needs to work in collaboration with other healthcare professionals, e.g. the MDT, to ensure that these aims are achieved.

Calculating estimated energy requirements is based on the Schofield equation. Clinical judgment is required to determine how much of a weight gain factor your patient requires, e.g. adding 600–1000 kcal to the basal metabolic rate or 25–35 kcal/kg ideal body weight initially and review regularly.[91]

Protein

Levodopa is a large neutral amino acid (LNAA). For levodopa to be absorbed, it must attach itself to carrier molecules in the wall of the intestine, which then carry it across the intestinal wall to the blood. Anything (e.g. protein) that also uses this carrier system can compete with levodopa.[86]

Levodopa disappears from the blood very quickly, usually within 60–90 minutes after administering the drug. It is absorbed from the small intestine into the bloodstream, crosses the blood–brain barrier and then is enzymatically converted to dopamine in the brain. Meals high in fat or protein and also constipation can delay emptying of the stomach's content into the small bowel, preventing adequate absorption of levodopa. The blood–brain barrier is the major site of interference between levodopa and protein, in particular, of the large neutral amino acids, e.g. phenylalanine, tyrosine and tryptophan.[92]

Throughout the late 1980s and more recently, it has been advocated that reduction, manipulation or redistribution of dietary protein intake may help counteract the decrease in the long-term effectiveness of the drug and so help provide symptom relief.[93–99] Patients with PD may also be advised to take their medication 45 minutes before a meal. However, it should be borne in mind that these are experimental techniques, and that the benefits have not been sufficiently established for them to be regarded as standard practice. They may be a viable option in some instances when symptom control on medication is failing or inadequate but, in any patient where nutritional intake is already inadequate (especially in patients with advanced disease), there is a considerable risk that such dietary manipulations could seriously compromise nutritional status.

In light of the risk of exacerbating malnutrition and recent advances in treatment, such as controlled release levodopa and new surgical techniques, including deep brain stimulation (DBS), this type of dietary manipulation has declined.[100]

In practice, these patients often enforce very strict and drastic dietary changes and some will devise their own experimental modification of their diet. It is the dietitian's responsibility to make them aware that adequate dietary protein is recommended to maintain optimal health and if following this diet, it should not be followed for more than two weeks if it does not confer any benefit.[98] Patients should be closely monitored by their PD team, i.e. neurologist, clinical nurse specialist and dietitian while following this dietary change. The diet could affect the patient's response to levodopa, and could increase risk of nausea, dyskinesias and episodes of hallucinations. Those restricting daytime protein intake for two months reduce their intake of protein, calcium, phosphorous, iron, riboflavin and niacin.[98] Careful monitoring of nutritional intake is needed while following this diet. This is important especially if the normal intake for these patients is only marginally nutritionally adequate or when patients are at risk of bone disease, e.g. osteoporosis.

Calculating protein requirements is based on using 1 g protein/kg ideal body weight or using the dietary reference values (DRVs) for men and women. Intakes of greater than 1.2 g/kg body weight were found to correlate with poor levodopa absorption.[101]

Fibre and fluid

Approximately 60–80% of patients with PD complain of constipation, which usually appears about 10–20 years before motor symptoms become evident.[102] It is thought to be caused by damage to the peripheral or central nervous system.[103–105]

Fluid requirements should be assessed according to age and weight (kg), i.e. < 60 years, 35 mL/kg, or if > 60 years, 30 mL/kg. Fibre requirements do not differ from the DRVs.

Micronutrients

Calcium and vitamin D

Osteoporosis is often diagnosed in patients with PD and correlation between disease severity and bone density has been found. Patients with PD have been found to have a defect in the renal synthesis of 1,25-dihydroxy–vitamin D (1, 25-[OH]$_2$D).[106] It has been suggested that PD patients should be supplemented with 1-alpha-hydroxyvitamin D3—the more active form of vitamin D, which can help increase bone density and dramatically lower the risk of fracture in these patients.[106] This is essential for patients who are bed bound or immobile. Calcium

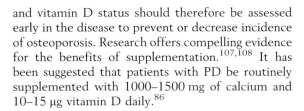

and vitamin D status should therefore be assessed early in the disease to prevent or decrease incidence of osteoporosis. Research offers compelling evidence for the benefits of supplementation.[107,108] It has been suggested that patients with PD be routinely supplemented with 1000–1500 mg of calcium and 10–15 µg vitamin D daily.[86]

Enteral nutrition support (ENS)

The importance of interventions to maintain nutrition and fluid intake in neurogenic dysphagia via ENS should not be delayed unless declined by the patient (assuming they are cognitively intact) or clinically inappropriate.[109] In chronic neurodegenerative conditions it often helps to anticipate artificial feeding at an early stage by discussing it with the patient and/or carer supported by the MDT.[110]

Dysphagia needs to be addressed promptly to prevent weight loss and malnutrition. Approximately 95% of PD patients experience swallowing difficulties.[111] It occurs in the later stages of the disease compared to atypical Parkinsonian syndromes, e.g. PSP or MSA.[112] Significant problems with swallowing require expert assessment from a speech and language therapist (SALT) and guidance regarding appropriate food texture modification. Since texture modified diets, e.g. puree, may be nutritionally dilute and not energy dense enough to prevent weight loss, additional use of supplementary enteral nutrition support may be indicated.

Confusion is common and may be accompanied by delusions and hallucinations. Drug dosage to control motor dysfunction may have to be reduced in order to produce a more settled psychological state. The consequent worsening of motor symptoms is likely to increase the risk of eating and swallowing difficulties requiring dietetic involvement. Active nutritional support via the enteral route, e.g. nasogastric tube for short-term feeding or if indicated a percutaneous endoscopic gastrostomy (PEG) could be considered for long-term feeding. PEG is being used increasingly in the treatment of patients with neurogenic dysphagia to prevent or reverse nutritional deficits,[113] and thus improve fitness and quality of life for those patients unable to take sufficient oral nutrients. Through appropriate and timely intervention, it may also prevent the problem of aspiration in patients with swallowing disorders.[114,115]

Special considerations for the needs of the ageing population

- Malnutrition risk and body weight in those living with PD must be routinely monitored as the disease progresses;
- Worsening motor symptoms, e.g. dyskinesias should also be monitored to prevent or reverse weight loss in people living with PD; and
- Dietitians have the skills to help people living with PD to optimise their nutritional status and manage nutrition-related symptoms at all stages of the disease.

Conclusion

All patients newly diagnosed with PD should be advised to follow the 'Balance of Good Health' guidelines. In the later stages of the disease there is an increased risk of poor oral intake, dysphagia, dyskinesia, medication side effects, drug–nutrient interactions, constipation, weight gain and cognitive decline. Good nutrition is essential to the well being of the PD patient and this is why it is important to establish and maintain good eating habits throughout the course of the disease.

Key points

- Approximately 95% of people living with PD will develop swallowing difficulties at some stage of the disease.
- Dietetic intervention is essential for preventing or correcting nutritional inadequacies at an early stage.
- Dietetic intervention is essential for preventing undesirable weight gain or loss.
- The patient's nutritional status should be closely monitored as the disease progresses.
- A focused multidisciplinary team approach is the key to successful treatment outcomes for this group of patients.

Case study

BACKGROUND

Mrs Y, who is 74 years old, was diagnosed with Parkinson's in 1984. She has been under the care of the MDT PD clinic at the local community hospital since 2005. Her first nutritional, speech and swallowing assessments were conducted and appropriate advice was given.

PAST MEDICAL HISTORY

Oct 2006—UTI
Dec 2007—Fractured (L) hip post-fall on icy footpath
May 2008 ongoing—Recurrent chest infections
Currently admitted to hospital.

CLINICAL SYMPTOMS

- Excessive drooling;
- Dysphagia to solids and thin fluids;
- 25% weight loss over past 3–6 months;
- Decreased mobility (sits in chair most of day) and poor gait;
- Quiet speech;
- Moderate dyskinesia;
- Unable to communicate fully;
- Constipation; and
- Poor response to current medication regime.

REASON FOR LATEST HOSPITAL ADMISSION

- Review medication/simplify medication regime;
- Assess state of disease progression;
- PT assessment to review mobility;
- SALT assessment to review swallow and speech impairments;
- Treat constipation—BNO × 10 days;
- Dietetic assessment to review nutritional status and explore appropriateness for artifical nutrition support; and
- OT assessment to review ADLs.

ASSESSMENT

- Anthropometry;
- Weight on admission: 57 kg;
- Height: 1.74 m;
- BMI: 18.8 k g/m^2;
- Estimated oral intake: 850 kcal, 28 g protein, 1200 mL over a 24-hour period; and
- Diet as per SALT recommendations: puree diet and syrup thick fluids.

QUESTIONS

1. A dietary care plan was developed between the patient, nursing staff and dietitian.
   a) What are the goals of dietary intervention at this stage of the patient's admission?
   b) How would you estimate the patient's nutritional requirements?
   c) What intervention would you advise?
2. What should be considered to provide appropriate and effective dietary management of this patient?
3. What would be the desired outcome of evaluation following this admission?

ANSWERS

1. A dietary care plan was developed between the patient, nursing staff and dietitian.
   a) What are the goals of dietary intervention at this stage of the patients admission?
   Goals that should be considered are:
   - Prevent/minimise further weight loss;
   - Aim for weight gain to ideal body weight;
   - Provide suitable puree meal choices;
   - Provide sufficient fluids throughout the day, e.g. 30 mL/kg; and
   - Prescribe use of oral sip feeds/desserts suitably pre-thickened.

   b) How would you estimate the patient's nutritional requirements?
   Estimated nutritional requirements:
   Energy—BMR + 0% stress + 30% mobility plus dyskinesia + 600–1000 kcal weight gain factor)
   Protein—1 g/kg or DRV
   Fluids—30 mL/kg
   c) What intervention would you advise?
   Strict food and fluid balance charts for 3 days
   Puree menu and suitable puree snacks
   Puree fruit to help ease discomfort of constipation
   Prescribe suitable oral sip feeds × 1–2 per day initially and then review
   Weekly weight

2. What should be considered to provide appropriate and effective dietary management of this patient?
   - Patient's agreement to treatment;
   - Patient's wishes and goals for weight gain;
   - Detailed dietary intake to establish eating patterns and habits;
   - Swallowing and chewing difficulties;
   - Dental and oral health;

Continued

Case study (Continued)

- Medications including vitamin and mineral preparations;
- Investigation of any self-imposed dietary restrictions or unconventional diets;
- Determination of level of physical activity and mobility;
- Establishment of level of disabilities, if any, that may impact on dietary intake;
- Activity (dyskinesia/akinesia) and rest patterns;
- Medical and physical condition; and
- Other risk factors/socio-economic circumstances.

3. What would be the desired outcome of evaluation following this admission?
- Improved eating and drinking due to prescribed oral sip feeds and pre-thickened drinks and decreased nausea caused by medication;
- Weight stabilised;
- Revised SLT/PT and OT regimens;
- Simplified medication regimen; and
- Carer support via local carers' group.

References

1. Department of Health. *The National Service Framework for Long-Term Conditions*. London: The Stationery Office; 2005.

2. Cushing ML, Traviss KA, Calne SM. Parkinson's disease: implications for nutritional care. *Can J Diet Pract Res*. 2002;63(2):81–87.

3. Reid C. Nutritional requirements of surgical and critically-ill patients: do we really know what they need? *Proc Nutr Soc*. 2004;63:467–472.

4. NICE. *Head Injury: Triage, Assessment, Investigation and Early Management of Head Injury in Infants, Children and Adults*. Clinical Guideline 4. 2007.

5. McCaffrey P. *The Neuroscience on the Web series. CMSD 636. Neuropathologies of Language and Cognition. Traumatic Brain Injury: Effects of Closed Head Injury 1998–2008*. Available at: http://www.csuchico.edu/~pmccaffrey//syllabi/SPPA336/336unit11.html.

6. Jennett B. The Glasgow Coma Scale: history and current practice. *Trauma*. 2002;4(2):91–103.

7. Teasdale G, Jennett B. Assessment of coma and impaired conciousness: a practical scale. *Lancet*. 1974;2:81–84.

8. Greenwood R. Head injury for neurologists. *J Neurol Neurosurg Psychiatry*. 2002;73(2):8–16.

9. Das-Gipta R, Turner-Stokes L. Traumatic brain injury. *Disabil Rehabil*. 2002;24(13):654–665.

10. Denes Z. The influence of severe malnutrition on rehabilitation in patients with severe head injury. *Disabil Rehabil*. 2004;26(19):1163–1165.

11. Annoni JM, Vuagnat H, Frischknecht R, Uebelhart D. Percutaneous endoscopic gastrostomy in neurological rehabilitation: a report of six cases. *Disabil Rehabil*. 1998;8:308–314.

12. Brook MM, Barbour PG, et al. Nutritional status during rehabilitation after head injury. *J Neurol Rehabil*. 1989;3:27–33.

13. Clifton GL, Robertson CS, Choi SC. Assessment of nutritional requirements of head injured patients. *J Neurosurg*. 1986;64:895–901.

14. Bivins BA, Twyman DL, Young AB. Failure of non-protein calories to mediate protein conservation in brain-injured patients. *J Trauma*. 1986;26:980–986.

15. Ott L, McClain C, Young B. Nutrition and severe brain injury. *Nutrition*. 1989;5:75–79.

16. Sunderland PM, Heilbrun MP. Estimating energy expenditure in traumatic brain injury: comparison of indirect calorimetry with predictive formulas. *Neurosurgery*. 1992;31:246–253.

17. Chiolero R, Schutz Y, Lemarchand T, et al. Hormonal and metabolic changes following severe head injury or non-cranial injury. *JPEN J Parenter Enteral Nutr*. 1989;13:5–12.

18. Weekes E, Elia M. Observations on the patterns of 24-hour energy expenditure changes in body composition and gastric emptying in head-injured patients receiving nasogastric tube feeding. *JPEN J Parenter Enteral Nutr*. 1996;20:31–37.

19. Bruder N, Raynal M, Pellissier D, Courtinat C, François G. Influence of body temperature, with or without sedation, on energy expenditure in severe head-injured patients. *Crit Care Med*. 1998;26:568–572.

20. McCall M, Jeejeebhoy K, Pencharz P, Moulton R. Effect of neuromuscular blockade on energy expenditure in patients with severe head injury. *JPEN J Parenter Enteral Nutr*. 2003;27:27–35.

21. Dickerson RN, Guenter PA, Gennarelli TA, Dempsey DT, Mullen JL. Increased contribution of protein oxidation to energy expenditure in head-injured patients. *J Am Coll Nutr*. 1990;9:86–88.

22. Quattrocchi KB, Issel BW, Miller CH, Frank EH, Wagner Jr FC. Impairment of T-cell function following severe head injury. *J Neurotrauma*. 1992;9:1–9.

23. Peterson SR, Jeevanandam M, Harrington T. Is the metabolic response to injury different with or without severe head injury? Significance of plasma glutamine levels. *J Trauma*. 1993;34: 653–660.

24. Suchner U, Senftleben U, Eckart T, et al. Enteral versus parenteral nutrition: effects on gastrointestinal function and metabolism. *Nutrition*. 1996;12:13–22.

25. Borzotta AP, Pennings J, Papasadero B. Enteral versus parenteral nutrition after severe closed head-injury. *J Trauma Injury Infect Crit Care*. 1994;37:459–468.

26. Deutschman CS, Konstaninides FN, Raup S, Thienprasit P, Cerra FB. Physiological and metabolic response to isolated closed-head injury. *J Neurosurg*. 1986;64: 89–98.

27. Pepe LJ, Carlos AB. The metabolic response to acute traumatic brain injury and implications for nutritional support. *J Head Trauma Rehabil*. 1999;14:462–474.

28. Streat SJ, Beddoe AH, Hill GL. Aggressive nutritional support does not prevent protein loss despite fat gain in septic intensive care patients. *J Trauma*. 1987;27: 262–266.

29. Hart DW, Wolf SE, Herndon DN, et al. Energy expenditure and caloric balance after burn. Increased feeding leads to fat rather than lean mass accretion. *Ann Surg*. 2002; 235:152–161.

30. Reid C. Optimising nutritional care of head injury patients. *Clin Nutr Update*. 2002;7:8–10.

31. Rapp RP, Young B, Twyman D, et al. The favourable effect of early parenteral feeding on survival in head injury. *J Neurosurg*. 1983;58: 906–912.

32. Hadley MN, Graham TW, Harrington T, et al. Nutritional support and neurotrauma: a critical review of early nutrition in forty-five acute head injury patients. *Neurosurgery*. 1986;19:367.

33. Akkersdijk WL, Roukema JA, van der Werken C. Percutaneous endoscopic gastrostomy for

patients with several cerebral injury. *Injury*. 1998;29:4–11.

34. Gadisseux P, Ward JD, Young HF, Becker DP. Nutrition and the neurosurgical patient. *J Neurosurg*. 1984;60:219.

35. Duke JH, Jorgensen SD, Broell JR, Long CL, Kinney JM. Contribution of protein to caloric expenditure following injury. *Surgery*. 1970; 68:168.

36. Clifton GL, Robertson CS, Choi SC. Assessment of nutritional requirements of head-injured patients. *J Neurosurg*. 1986;64: 895–901.

37. Young B, Ott L, Norton J, et al. The metabolic and nutritional sequela of the nonsteroid treated injury patient. *Neurosurgery*. 1985;17:784.

38. Darba A. Nutritional requirements in severe head injury. *Nutrition*. 2001;17:71–72.

39. Clifton GL, Robertson CS, Contant CF. Enteral hyperalimentation in head injury. *J Neurosurg*. 1985;62:186–193.

40. Young B, Ott L, Twyman D, et al. The effect of nutritional support on outcome from severe head injury. *J Neurosurg*. 1987;67:668–676.

41. Ishibashi N, Plank LD, Sando K, Hill GL. Optimal protein requirements during the first 2 weeks after the onset of critical illness. *Crit Care Med*. 1998; 26:1529–1535.

42. Moore FA, Feliciano DV, Andrassy RJ, et al. Early enteral feeding, compared with parenteral, reduces septic complications. The result of a meta-analysis. *Ann Surg*. 1992;216:172–183.

43. Jeejeebhoy KN. Enteral and parenteral nutrition: evidence based approach. *Proc Nutr Soc*. 2001;60: 399–402.

44. Norton JA, Ott LG, McClain C, et al. Intolerance to enteral feeding in the brain-injured patient. *J Neurosurg*. 1988;68:62–66.

45. Margarson MP, Soni N. Serum albumin: touchstone or totem? *Anaesthesia*. 1998;53:789–803.

46. Young B, Ott L, Phillips R, McCain C. Metabolic management of the patients with head injury. *Neurosurg Clin N Am*. 1991;2:301.

47. Ott L, Young B, Phillips R, et al. Altered gastric emptying in the

head injured patients: relationship to feeding intolerance. *J Neurosurg*. 1991;74:738–742.

48. Herbert MK, Holzer P. Standardized concept for the treatment of gastrointestinal dysmotility in critically ill patients—current status and future options. *Clin Nutr*. 2008;27:25–41.

49. Bradley C. Erythromycin as a gastrointestinal prokinetic agent. *Intensive Crit Care Nurs*. 2001;14:117–119.

50. Dive A, Miesse C, Galanti L, et al. Effects of erythromycin on gastric motility in mechanically ventilated critically ill patients: a double-blind, randomised, placebo-controlled study. *Crit Care Med*. 1995;23: 1356–1362.

51. Chapman MJ, Fraser RJ, Kluger MT, Buist MD, De Nichilo DJ. Erythromycin improves gastric emptying in critically ill patients intolerant of nasogastric feeding. *Crit Care Med*. 2000;28: 2334–2337.

52. Seppälä H, Klaukka T, Vuopio-Varkila J, et al. The effect of changes in the consumption of macrolide antibiotics on erythromycin resistance in group A streptococci in Finland. Finnish Study Group for Antimicrobial Resistance. *N Engl J Med*. 1997;337:441–446.

53. Katapadi K, Kostandy G, Katapadi M, Hussain KM, Schifter D. A review of erythromycin-induced malignant tachyarrhythmia-torsade de pointes. A case report. *Angiology*. 1997;48:821–826.

54. Tonini M, Cipollina L, Polluzi E, et al. Review article: clinical implications of enteric and central D2 receptor blockade by antidopaminergic gastrointestinal prokinetics. *Aliment Pharmacol Ther*. 2004;19:379–390.

55. Petros S, Engelmann L. Enteral nutrition delivery and energy expenditure in medical intensive care patients. *Clin Nutr*. 2006;25:51–59.

56. Woien H, Bjork IT. Nutrition of the critically ill patient and effects of implementing a nutritional support algorithm in ICU. *J Clin Nurs*. 2006;15(2):168–177.

57. Corke C. Gastric emptying in the critically ill patient. *Crit Care Resusc.* 1999;1:39–44.

58. Datta G, Gnanalingham KK, van Dellen J, O'Neill K. The role of parenteral nutrition as a supplement to enteral nutrition in patients with severe brain injury. *Br J Neurosurg.* 2003;17:432–436.

59. Rhoney DH, Parker D. Considerations in fluids and electrolytes after traumatic brain injury. *Nutr Clin Pract.* 2006; 21(5):462–478.

60. Clifton GL, Miller ER, Choi SC, Levin HS. Fluid thresholds and outcome from severe brain injury. *Crit Care Med.* 2002;30:739–745.

61. Parobek V, Alaimo I. Fluid and electrolyte management in the neurologically-impaired patient. *J Neurosci.* 1996;23:322–328.

62. Zafonte RD, Mann RD. Cerebral salt wasting syndrome in brain injury patients: a potential cause of hyponatraemia. *Arch Phys Med Rehabil.* 1997;78(5):540–542.

63. Polderman KH, Bloemers FW, Peerdeman SM, Girbes AR. Hypomagnesemia and hypophosphatemia at admission in patients with severe head injury. *Crit Care Med.* 2000;28: 2022–2025.

64. Ghanbari C. Protocols for nutrition support of neuro intensive care unit patients: a guide for residents. *Internet J Emergency Intensive Care Med.* 1999;3(1).

65. Brain Trauma Foundation. Nutrition. *J Neurotrauma.* 2007;24(suppl 1):S77–S82.

66. Stapleton RD, Jones N, Heyland DK. Feeding critically ill patients: what is the optimal amount of energy? *Crit Care Med.* 2007;35(suppl 9):S535–S540.

67. Fruhwald S, Holzer P, Metzler H. Intestinal motility disturbances in intensive care patients pathogenesis and clinical impact. *Intensive Care Med.* 2007;33(1):36–45.

68. Lang AE, Lozano AM. Parkinson's disease:second of two parts. *N Engl J Med.* 1998;339(16):1130–1143.

69. Calne DB. Parkinson's disease is not one disease. *Parkinsonism Relat Disord.* 2001;7(1):3–7.

70. Schrag A, Ben-Schlomo Y, Brown R, Marsden CD, Quinn N. Young-onset Parkinson's disease revisited—clinical features, natural history and mortality. *Mov Disord.* 1998;13(6):885–894.

71. Schrag A, Jahanshahi M, Quinn N. How does Parkinson's disease affect quality of life? A comparison with quality of life in the general population. *Mov Disord.* 2000; 15(6):1112–1118.

72. McCall B. Young-onset Parkinson's disease: a guide to care and support. *Nurs Times.* 2003;99(30):28–31.

73. Calne DB, Calne S. Treatment of Parkinson's disease. In: Ancil RJ, Holliday SG, Mithani AH, eds. *Therapeutics in Geriatric Neuropsychiatry*. Chichester: Wiley; 1997:1–12.

74. Calne DB. Treatment of Parkinson's disease. *N Engl J Med.* 1993;329:1021–1027.

75. Uitti R, Ottman R, Goldman SM, et al. Parkinson's disease. *Neurosci News.* 1999;2:36–43.

76. Rascol OFJJ, Thalamas CGM, Montastruc JL. Dopamine agonists: their role in the management of Parkinson's disease. In: Calne DB, Calne SM, eds. *Parkinson's Disease, Advances in Neurology*. Philadelphia: Lippincott, Williams and Wilkins; 2001:301–309.

77. Beyer P, Palarimo M, Michalek D, et al. Weight change and body composition in patients with Parkinson's disease. *J Am Diet Assoc.* 1995;95(9):979–983.

78. Bachmann CG, Trenkwalder C. Body weight in patients with Parkinson's disease. *Mov Disord.* 2006;21(11):1824–1830.

79. Kashihara K. Weight loss in Parkinson's disease. *J Neurol.* 2006;253(suppl 7):VII/38–VII/41.

80. Lorefält B, Ganowiak W, Pålhagen S, et al. Factors of importance for weight loss in elderly patients with Parkinson's disease. *Acta Neurol Scand.* 2004;110(3):180–187.

81. Levi S, Cox M, Lugon M, Hodkinson M, Tomkins A. Increased energy expenditure in Parkinson's disease. *Br Med J.* 1990;301:1256–1257.

82. Davies KN, King D, Davies H. A study of the nutritional status of elderly patients with Parkinson's disease. *Age Ageing.* 1994;23: 142–145.

83. Markus HS, Cox M, Tomkins AM. Raised resting energy expenditure in Parkinson's disease and its relationship to muscle rigidity. *Clin Sci.* 1992;83:199–204.

84. Chen H, Zhang S, Hernán M, Willett WC, Ascherio A. Weight loss in Parkinson's disease. *Ann Neurol.* 2003;53:676–679.

85. Sato Y, Kaji M, Tsuru T, Oizumi K. Risk factors for hip fracture among elderly patients with Parkinson's disease. *J Neurol Sci.* 2001;182(2): 89–93.

86. Lorefalt B, Ganowiak K, Wissing U, Granérus AK, Unosson M. Food habits and intake of nutrients in elderly patients with Parkinson's disease. *Gerontology.* 2006;52(3): 160–168.

87. Carter J, Nutt J. Dietary issues in Parkinson's disease. In: Koller W, Paulson G, eds. *Therapy of Parkinson's Disease*. New York: Marcel Dekker; 1995:443–461.

88. Holden K. Unintentional weight loss and its management in patients with Parkinson's disease. *Nutr Clin Care.* 2001;4(3):131–139.

89. BAPEN. *Malnutrition Universal Screening Tool*. Available at: http:// www.bapen.org.uk/must_tool.html.

90. Starling RD, Poehlman ET. Assessment of energy requirements in elderly populations. *Eur J Clin Nutr.* 2000;54(suppl 3): S104–S111.

91. NICE. *Nutrition Support in Adults*. Clinical Guidance 32. 2006.

92. Pålhagen S, Lorefalt B, Carlsson M, et al. Does L-dopa treatment contribute to reduction in body weight in elderly patients with Parkinson's disease? *Acta Neurol Scand.* 2005;111(1):12–20.

93. Karstaedt PJ, Pincus JH. Protein redistribution diet remains effective in patients with fluctuating Parkinsonism. *Arch Neurol.* 1992;49:149–151.

94. Frankel JP, Kempster PA, Bovingdon M, et al. The effects of oral protein on the absorption of intraduodenal levodopa and motor performance. *J Neurol Neurosurg Psychiatry.* 1989;52:1063–1067.

95. Tsui JK, Ross S, Poulin K, et al. The effect of dietary protein on the efficacy of L-dopa: a double blind study. *Neurology.* 1989;39: 549–552.

96. Carter JH, Nutt JG, Woodward WR, Hatcher LF, Trotman TL. Amount and distribution of dietary protein affects clinical response to levodopa in Parkinson's disease. *Neurology.* 1989;39:552–556.

97. Pincus JH, Barry KM. Plasma levels of amino acids correlate with motor fluctuations in Parkinsonism. *Arch Neurol.* 1987;44:1006–1009.

98. Riley D, Lang AE. Practical application of low protein diet for Parkinson's disease. *Neurology.* 1998;38:1026–1031.

99. Pare S, Barr SI, Ross SE. Effect of daytime protein restriction on nutrient intakes of free-living Parkinson's disease patients. *Am J Clin Nutr.* 1992;55:701–707.

100. Berry EM, Growdon JH, Wurtman JJ, Caballero B, Wurtman RJ. A balanced carbohydrate: protein diet in the management of Parkinson's disease. *Neurology.* 1991;41:1295–1297.

101. Novakova L, Ruzicka E, Jech R, et al. Increase in body weight is a non-motor side effect of deep brain stimulation of the subthalamic nucleus in Parkinson's disease. *Neuro Endocrinol Lett.* 2007; 28(1):21–25.

102. Marczewska A, De Notaris R, Sieri S, et al. Protein intake in Parkinsonian patients using the EPIC Food Frequency Questionnaire. *Mov Disord.* 2006;21(8):1229–1231.

103. Ueki A, Otsuka M. Life style risks of Parkinson's disease: association between decreased water intake and constipation. *J Neurol.* 2004;251(suppl 7):VII/18–VII/23.

104. Pfeiffer RF, Quigley EMM. Gastrointestinal motility problems in patients with Parkinson's disease—epidemiology, pathophysiology and guidelines for management. *CNS Drugs.* 1999;11(6):435–448.

105. Stocchi F. Disorders of bowel function in parkinsonism. In: Fowler CJ, ed. *Neurology of Bladder, Bowel and Sexual Dysfunction.* London: Butterworth, Heinemann; 1999:255–264.

106. Edwards LL, Quigley EM, Harned RK, Hofman R, Pfeiffer RF. Characterisation of swallowing and defecation in Parkinson's disease. *Am J Gastroenterol.* 1994;89: 15–25.

107. Sato Y, Kikuyama M, Oizumi K. High prevalence of vitamin D deficiency and reduced bone mass in Parkinson's disease. *Neurology.* 1997;49:1273–1278.

108. Jackson C, Gaugris S, Sen SS, Hosking D. The effect of cholecalciferol (vitamin D_3) on the risk of fall and fracture: a meta-anaylsis. *QJM.* 2007;100:185–192.

109. Boonen S, Lips P, Bouillon R, et al. Need for additional calcium to reduce the risk of hip fracture with vitamin D supplementation: evidence from a comparative meta analysis of randomized controlled trials. *J Clin Endocrinol Metab.* 2007;92(4):1415–1423.

110. Park RH, Allison MC, Lang J, et al. Randomised comparison of percutaneous endoscopic gastrostomy and nasogastric tube feeding in patients with persisting neurological dysphagia. *Br Med J.* 1992;304:1406–1409.

111. Rehman HU. Progressive supranuclear palsy. *Postgrad Med J.* 2000;76:333–336.

112. Logemann JA, Boshes B, et al. Speech and swallowing evaluation in the differential diagnosis of neurological disease. *Neurol Neurocir Psichustr.* 1997;18: 71–78.

113. Müller J, Wenning GK, Verny M, et al. Progression of dysarthria and dysphagia in post-mortem-confirmed Parkinsonian disorders. *Arch Neurol.* 2001;58:259–264.

114. Britton JER, Sipscomb PD, Mohr PD, Rees WD, Young AC. The use of percutaneous endoscopic gastrostomy (PEG) feeding tubes in patients with neurological disease. *J Neurol.* 1997;244(7):1432–1459.

115. Pennington C. To PEG or not to PEG. *Clin Med.* 2002;2(3): 250–255.

Mental health

Ursula Philpot

LEARNING OBJECTIVES

By the end of this chapter the reader will be able to:

- Give an overview of the key drivers, stakeholders and changes to mental health services;
- Critically discuss the changing role of the dietitian within mental health services;
- Critically evaluate the key issues in assessment, communication and treatments in serious mental illness and eating disorders; and
- Critically discuss some of the ethical and legal issues involved in treating mental illness.

OUTLINES

The area of mental health (MH) and nutrition is vast, and cannot be covered within the remit of this chapter. Instead this chapter aims to give a critical overview of recent changes to MH services, the key drivers for change and the advanced practice role of the MH dietitian within mental illness and eating disorders. There is a strong focus on the areas of eating disorders, practical assessment approaches and new ways of working. The more complex and challenging aspects of dietetic practice within each area is critically discussed. Emerging new developments are also examined.

Introduction

MH dietetics covers three large areas: learning disabilities, eating disorders and more general mental health. A high percentage of MH dietitians sit within services for eating disorders, chronic fatigue, learning disabilities and serious mental illness. Dietitians in MH work with individuals from all age groups and within a wide range of clinical specialties. They work across many sectors and settings including health, education, social services, primary care, secondary care, and the independent and voluntary sectors. These are clinically very different, but share commonality in complexity, policy, treatment approaches and ways of working.

The white paper 'Choosing Health: Supporting the Physical Health Needs of People with Severe Mental Illness' states:

> People with diagnoses of severe and enduring mental illness (SMI) such as schizophrenia and bipolar disorder are at increased risk for a range of physical illnesses and conditions, including coronary heart disease, diabetes, infections, respiratory disease and greater levels of obesity. They are almost twice as likely to die from coronary heart disease as the general population and four times more likely to die from respiratory disease.[1]

Medication used to treat mental illness can have marked side effects including hyperglycaemia, hyperlipidaemia, diabetes, obesity and gastrointestinal disorders, which need long-term dietary management. Self-neglect, cognitive impairment and disorganised lifestyles may also result in malnutrition or overnutrition. In addition the above disorders may be exacerbated by food refusal and other disordered eating patterns such as high caffeine intakes, polydypsia and food phobias. The most common types of mental illness that dietitians are likely to encounter are:

- Mood affective disorders (depression, bipolar disorder, anxiety and mania);
- Schizophrenia;

- Dementia;
- Anxiety;
- Personality disorders (PD); and
- Borderline personality disorders (BPD).

PD and BDP, although not categories of mental illness but disorders of personality and behaviour, are also likely to be met and require an understanding of the diagnosis and management issues. The impact of some of the above conditions on nutritional status is outlined in Table 22.1.

The impact of drug treatments on physical health is enormous. Drug-induced weight gain, leading to an increased risk of metabolic syndrome and type 2 diabetes, is one of the most common problems. Examples of these are outlined in Appendix 22.1. Also refer to Chapter 6 on Drug Nutrient Interactions.

The evidence base for many MH interventions is very limited. With a paucity of high quality evidence on which to base decisions, clinical consensus, clinical reasoning and critical thinking are essential skills. Evaluation of emerging evidence, its quality and its implementation are key skills for the advanced level practitioner in the field of mental health.

Background

There is a changing paradigm within mental health services in the UK that has seen an overhaul of psychiatric services and the physical health needs of service users put high on the agenda for many MH trusts. This has led to a number of sweeping changes in the way that services are delivered and a significant increase in the number of Allied Health Professionals (AHP) employed in MH services. This is creating an exciting and dynamic time for dietitians working in this area.

The initiative 'New Ways of Working' (NWW), from the Department of Health, was established in 2005 as part of the National Institute for Mental Health for England's workforce programme.[2] It aims to change workforce practice and is a current key driver for change in the mental health sector. NWW, together with a growing evidence base linking physical and mental health, is driving a shift towards a broader, holistic, and more multidisciplinary team (MDT) approach to MH services as discussed below.

Table 22.1 Impact of mental health on nutritional status

Mood disorder	Possible influences on food intake	Possible nutritional consequences
Depression	Apathy and disinterest in food	Undernutrition, weight loss
	Anorexia	
	Feeling not worthy of food	
	Food refusal	
	Loss of thirst sensation	Dehydration
	Fluid refusal	Constipation; impacted faeces
	Distorted food intake	Unbalanced diet, weight gain
	Carbohydrate craving	Obesity
Anxiety	Frequent loose stools	Selective food avoidance
	Abdominal pain or discomfort	Food refusal
Mania	Drug side effects causing dry mouth or altered taste	Difficulties in chewing or swallowing Altered taste sensation
	Increased appetite	Weight gain
	Hyperactivity	Increased energy requirements
	Erratic eating habits	Unbalanced diet; weight gain

MGH advanced practice MH training 2008 (Helen Webb).

Significantly there has been a move away from the traditional medical modes of working and the emergence of models for new ways of working. An example of this changing philosophy is the use of the 'recovery model'. This model challenges conventional thinking around recovery and cure, providing a holistic view of mental illness that focuses on the person and not just their symptoms, believing recovery from severe mental illness is possible. It aims to help people with MH problems, not to become symptom free, but rather despite symptoms, to move forward and carry out activities and develop relationships that give their lives meaning.

Reflecting the principle that physical and mental health is intrinsically linked, the previously overlooked physical heath agenda has now been given a very high priority within MH settings. New policies and key documents such as 'Choosing Health: Supporting the Physical Needs of People with Severe Mental Illness' from the Department of Health in 2006 highlight the need for change and for physical health needs of service users to be addressed in order to support their mental health.[1] This has led to an increase in physical monitoring and new developments such as healthy living groups.

Following on from this is a fast-growing interest in the link between nutrition and MH. Increasing numbers of high quality trials are providing evidence to support the link, and large stakeholders such as 'Food and Behaviour Research' and 'Sustain' are beginning to influence policy at a parliamentary level.[3]

In summary there is a cultural change in the delivery of MH services which includes the development of new, enhanced and changed roles for staff and the redesigning of systems and processes to support staff to deliver effective, person-centred care. Rather than looking at traditional services, teams and roles, new approaches place the service user at the centre and redesign around the holistic needs of the service user. It is a person-centred values-based approach where services and roles are responsive and flexible and provides the most benefit to service users and carers. In practice this means that AHPs, such as dietitians, will take on extended or non-traditional roles, for example, dietitians as the clinical lead for an eating disorders or learning disabilities service, passing and changing feeding tubes, taking service users out to eat/shop/cook, running group therapy sessions and undertaking home visit assessments. This has also led to a blurring of traditional professional roles and management structures. For example, a dietitian may be professionally led by an occupational therapist, operationally managed by a nurse and supervised by a psychologist. This situation may bring with it both opportunities and threats. It can both enhance and broaden MDT working, offering a greater understanding of close MDT working and enhanced service user care. Or it may increase difficulties where clashes in working style or work priorities, or misunderstanding regarding roles leads to tensions between professional groups.

Ways of working

Strategic working

Despite a significant increase in the number of dietitians in MH services, there is a chronic shortage in certain specialist and geographic areas.[3] Dietitians may need to shift focus from traditional ways of working and instead work very strategically in their role. In some cases doing no service user work at all, but instead focusing on the creation of a trust-wide food and nutrition policy. Such efforts include influencing trust processes and infrastructure, and implementing National Institute for Health and Clinical Excellence (NICE) guidance, screening tools, and training and education programmes through trust steering groups and clinical governance at board level.

Embedding nutrition into essential physical monitoring and assessment at ward level may involve the development of complex care pathways and adaptations of tools such as the Malnutrition Universal Screening Tool (MUST) for use in particular patient groups.[4] This also includes designing, implementing and evaluating training for staff based upon Skills for Health competence-based approaches (see http://www.Skillsforhealth.org.uk).

Ethical considerations

One of the most contentious barriers to change that dietitians must manage comes from the tension between 'human right' and 'duty of care' in MH services. Is it a service user's human right to eat only takeaways that are impacting on his/her health, or is it our 'duty of care' to support them to follow a diet that improves mental well being? Working through policy and clinical governance is essential to resolving such difficult conflicts within MH settings.

Assessment

Like complex physical conditions, assessments are largely multidisciplinary in approach, with much greater emphasis on holistic assessment and integrated treatments. Assessment in MH is similar in approach to assessing physical health for long-term lifestyle conditions, with service users managing an array of symptoms that fluctuate, with the emphasis on self-management. The dietitian uses enhanced communications skills to assess the impact of disease on the life of the service user and explore the underpinning psychopathology, with a focus on establishing the background to the condition, current scenario and support and to eliciting thoughts and feelings that relate to food behaviours, to aid insight into what is important to the service user.

Training and education for fellow healthcare professionals (HCPs) is vital and screening tools are often an invaluable first-line assessment tool. To meet NICE and Quality Improvement Scotland (QIS) Standards for Food, Fluid and Nutritional Care in Hospitals the use of MUST or a similar tool is recommended[5]:

> The initial assessment includes screening for risk of undernutrition. This screening is carried out using a validated tool appropriate to the patient population, and which includes criteria and scores that indicate action to be taken. (QIS Standard 2.2)[4]

However, such tools are not validated for MH settings. They often fail to capture service users who are obese and thus need dietetic and physical activity support, as well as those who were undernourished. Consequently, screening tools have been adapted by many services in MH and learning disabilities in partnership with clinical effectiveness departments. The QIS and NICE specify the use of a 'validated' screening tool. The validity of any assessment tool can be described in a number of ways. In some cases, validity can be assessed qualitatively, but for others quantitative analysis is required. Table 22.2 shows an example of the process of validating a new screening tool.

Table 22.2 Process for validating a new screening tool in mental health

'Qualitative' validity

Face validity	Does it seem like a realistic assessment of nutritional needs?
Content validity	Is it based on a checklist of things that should be included in a tool like this? The screening tool should be based on current best practice, outlined in: NICE, *Nutrition Support in Adults* (Clinical Guideline 32[5])
External validity	Would this tool work for other people, in other places, and at other times? Does it pick up obesity? It would seem reasonable to assume that this tool could be used by other organisations
Convergent validity	Is it similar to comparable projects? The screening tool shares certain characteristics of the MUST tool, e.g. both attempt to identify malnourished and obese patients; both use BMI as part of the assessment; both check for any unplanned weight loss; both consider ability to consume food and fluid, and the patient's general physical health

'Quantitative' validity

Predictive validity	Is it able to predict who will have additional nutritional requirements in the future? This tool does not require predictive validity, as it is an assessment of current, rather than future, needs
Construct validity	Does it measure what it claims to measure? Identification of the number of patients who are referred, and the reasons for referral Analysis of dietetic input for referred patients Dietetic opinion on the appropriateness of referral Further audit work could also include reviewing the patients identified above after one year. This could consider whether any referrals were made to dietetics after the initial assessment. This would help to identify any additional factors to include when the tool is reviewed

An example of a validated screening tool can be found in Appendix 22.2

Single assessment

With a move towards single assessment within MH services, dietitians may find that they form part of a wider holistic assessment of the service user, where health professionals cross-populate areas of the assessment tool. Many HCPs working in the field of MH are dual trained (OT, medical and nursing), which allows them to take on the role of care coordinator and to undertake risk assessments. Very few dietitians are dual trained and so cannot be legally responsible for certain areas of assessment such as risk to self. An example of a MDT single assessment tool is provided in Table 22.3.

Nutrition and aetiology of mood disorders

There is growing interest in the hypothesis that nutritional deprivation may contribute significantly to psychiatric disorders, with the implication that enhanced nutrition may exert a positive influence on mental health.

Converging lines of evidence from epidemiologic studies, clinical samples and treatment outcome studies suggest that nutrition may play a role in mental health. They may also offer new hypotheses about the aetiology and treatment of certain psychiatric conditions, particularly those that involve deregulated affect, for example: bipolar disorder, depression and borderline personality disorder.

Epidemiological evidence suggests that sugar intake is positively correlated with the incidence of depression and other recent dietary changes may be partly responsible for an increase in mood disorders due to increased consumption of processed foods.[6,7] For example, there has been an increased intake of sugar, *trans* fats, saturated fats and omega-6 fatty acids and a reduction in the intake of fibre, folate and omega-3 fatty acids.[8]

Emerging data regarding the role of omega-3 fatty acids suggest effects of nutrition on mood.[9–13] Rates of both unipolar and bipolar depression have been correlated inversely with seafood consumption and it is proposed that omega-3 fatty acid deficiencies may result in changes in membrane structure that could impair serotonin release and uptake.[14–17]

Brain serotonin affects mood and low levels contribute to the aetiology of depression in some people.[18]

Table 22.3 Example of a MDT single assessment tool

Multidisciplinary holistic single assessment
Reason for referral (who from, why now, any known previous history)
Client's perception (Why do they think they have been referred/are being assessed? What do they hope to gain from the meeting?)
Emotional health (mental health state, coping styles, etc.)
Social health (accommodation, finances, relationships, genogram, employment status, ethnic background, support networks, etc.)
Physical health (general health, illnesses, previous history, appetite, weight, sleep pattern, diurinal variations, alcohol, tobacco, street drugs; list any prescribed medication with comments on effectiveness)
Spiritual health (Is religion important? If so, in what way? What/who provides a sense of purpose?)
Intellectual health (cognitive functioning, hallucinations, delusions, concentration, interests, hobbies, etc.)
Risk assessment (self-harm, suicidal ideation, history/treats of violence, environment/relationship abuse)
Summary/formulation of difficulties (to include nursing diagnosis where possible)
Action plan (outcome of assessment, who else involved or to be contacted, follow-up appointment, etc.)

It is therefore postulated that a high carbohydrate load leads to increased tryptophan levels (precursor of serotonin) in the brain and may therefore elevate mood.[19,20] However, currently there is no evidence that this occurs in humans.[21] Folic acid deficiency has been shown to lower brain serotonin in rats and may have some effect in humans, whilst Benton and Donohue in 1999 also associated poor thiamine status with low mood.[18,21]

Caffeine intakes in excess of 600 mg/day can produce anxiety, psychomotor agitation, excitement and rambling speech. It is proposed that caffeine may elevate mood through increasing noradrenalin release and excessive consumption may even precipitate mania. Depressed patients may be more sensitive to the anxiogenic effects of caffeine, creating tolerance. Withdrawal symptoms develop when doses are reduced.[22]

This emerging data suggest that correction of deficiencies, ensuring a balanced diet and in some cases using nutritional supplementation, may be a helpful strategy in the management of psychiatric disease states. Future studies are needed to evaluate the reliability of initial findings and to investigate the long-term safety of supplementation within various subpopulations of psychiatric patients. Where the balance of possible benefit outweighs risk, supplementing multivitamin/minerals, and omega-3 oils (500 mg/day) may be seen as good practice in the vast majority of cases and routine supplementation in mood disorders is now more common in trust nutrition policy and prescribing guidelines.[22]

Managing behaviour change in mental illness

Behaviour change work within mental health must be underpinned by enhanced dietetic skills in motivational, behavioural and cognitive approaches. Working with complex needs or serious mental illness such as personality disorders and eating disorders requires skills in both cognitive behavioural and dialectical behavioural approaches and a high level of clinical supervision.[23] Therefore specialist dietetic postgraduate training in the area of MH and supervision by experienced practitioners or peers is essential. In addition to clinical supervision, psychological supervision is also recommended. Psychodynamic phenomena such as transference, counter-transferance and splitting are common in teams and individuals that work with mental illness. One of the primary tasks of psychological supervision is to help understand and manage the complexities of the setting and multiprofessional working, in order that the clinical work can be thought about and understood. This type of supervision may be offered from within the team and/or externally by regional networks.

Specialist and masters level training in the areas of assessment, treatment and psychological approaches that underpin working in MH can be accessed locally or nationally. The Mental Health Specialist Group (MHG) of the British Dietetic Association have developed courses in MH, learning disabilities and eating disorders at masters level, which dovetail with the accredited behaviour change training developed by Dympna Pearson, to form a complete postgraduate training package within this area. For further guidance, refer to the Chapter 3 on changing behaviour, by Dympna Pearson.

Working with personality disorders and borderline personality disorder

Personality disorders are a set of disorders characterised by deeply rooted patterns of thoughts, feelings and relating. Life experiences such as early and severe trauma, carers abusing drugs or alcohol, carers having MH problems, poor parenting skills, sexual abuse or neglect can lead to a child with a damaged personality and multiple problematic core beliefs develop. These may then interact with certain biological and genetic factors to form adult personality disorders.

Personality disorders are difficult to treat because they involve deeply rooted patterns of thoughts, feelings and relating. Research shows that people with personality disorders may change, although this may take a number of years and the focus may be more on managing current behaviours and feelings than on exploring the past. Psychological treatments include dialectical behavioural therapy (DBT), cognitive behavioural therapy (CBT), psychodynamic therapy, social skills training and problem solving.[23] Treatment should begin with minimising the biggest risks to self as outlined in Table 22.4.

People with a personality disorders are not easy to work with. They can challenge morally and emotionally

Table 22.4 Strategies for the treatment of eating disorders

Example from binge eating

Decrease suicide risk—focus on making life worth living	
Decrease therapy interfering behaviours	
Decrease behaviours that interfere with the quality of life	Stop binge eating Regular eating Chain analysis
Improve self-esteem	Eliminate mindless eating Decrease cravings, urges and preoccupation with food Emotional regulation
Set individual goals and targets	Decrease capitulating (giving up and acting as if there is no alternative to binge eating) Decrease 'apparent irrelevant behaviours' (buying favourite binge foods for friends/family)

Adapted from Wiser and Telch (1999).[23]

and can create feelings in those working with them of self-doubt, anxiety, helplessness, avoidance, guilt, shame and dependence.

The dietitian should be aware that people with serious mental illness, eating disorders, PD or BPD could exhibit the following:

- Behaviour experienced by others as manipulative, selfish or dishonest;
- Behaviours that cause the splitting of teams; showing very different aspects of personality to different team members;
- Passivity or inappropriate activity (e.g. cutting); taking little responsibility or ownership of the problem, but instead tries to make others responsible;
- Engagement in self-defeating behaviours that perpetuate the problem;
- Voicing of threats or incitement of guilt when problems are not resolved;
- If they do take ownership, they can become obsessive and extreme, e.g. with exercise and diet; individuals exhibiting this behaviour may also have obsessive compulsive PD;
- Request for something that will make them look and feel special and different to others, e.g. a nutritional supplement, a Halal meal, more time even when not clinically or ethnically indicated;
- Behaviours such as food refusal as a means of control or self-harm to demonstrate distress;
- Eating disorders behaviours, which are relatively common, particularly amongst females with BPD and those who self-harm;
- Easily dissociate and may not have heard what you have said;
- Impulsive behaviours that alleviate difficult feelings in the short term, e.g. drinking, drugs, self-harm, binging, vomiting or starvation;
- Dysfunctional and damaging relationships; and
- Making of multiple formal complaints and can be very litigious.

Dietitians working with these client groups require close supervision, peer support and skills in CBT and DBT approaches. The following points should be considered:

- Recovery is always possible; there is always hope.
- Treatments may involve team risk-taking and creative thinking.
- Service users with mental illness may need more clinic time and take longer to build rapport with. Diet changes need to be clearly linked to what is important in the day-to-day life of the service user. Change may be slow and all goals must be realistic.
- During an acute phase of mental illness such as depression, mania or psychosis, the service user will be mainly inaccessible to establishing rapport, dietary assessment and management. They may become non-attendees and so appointments need to be rearranged when the service user is better able to engage. Delusional or paranoid beliefs about food cannot be changed by logical argument or scientific evidence. The dietitian must work with the belief until the patient is more cognitively accessible. Service users experiencing withdrawal and lack of motivation will be very difficult to communicate with and elicit change.
- The involvement of support workers, family, friends, carers and other HCPs is vital in the assessment and planning of change. Always work as a team, do not work in isolation and agree approaches and boundaries. If possible, interview the service user with another member of the team, preferably their primary nurse or key worker.
- Always speak to a member of the team for an update prior to a dietetic consultation and feed back to the rest of the team after an interview.
- Set boundaries clearly and keep to them. Make sure service users are aware of the scope of your involvement and that you are part of the team and as such will share information.
- Do not treat individuals favourably over others or give in to demands when not clinically indicated.
- Build rapport and trust, be warm but firm. Show resolve, perseverance and consistency.
- Be prepared and well planned.
- Give plenty of warning for a change of appointment or dietitian and avoid frequent changes of any staff.
- Try to effect a small change early on to demonstrate that change is possible and use this to refer back to.
- Keep accurate and full written records.

Eating disorders

Eating disorders (ED) are highly complex disorders that involve psychological, physical, behavioural and psychosocial problems. Professionals working in this field need to be experienced within it, trained and supervised well. Multidisciplinary working is key as all professionals need to work as a team.

The role of the dietitian with ED is multifaceted and employs a wide range of advanced skills and knowledge. This cannot be discussed fully within the scope of this chapter; therefore the focus is on ways of working and the complexity of work.

The Quality Improvement Scotland (QIS) report of 2006 entitled 'Eating Disorders in Scotland: Recommendations for Management and Treatment' outlines the broad areas of work that dietitians are involved in:[24]

- Dietetic treatment should be offered to both in-patients and outpatients;
- The dietitian has an essential role in assessment, treatment and monitoring;
- Poor eating patterns and unhealthy views are primary symptoms that need addressing; and
- The dietitian has a key role in diet and weight management.

Most patients with anorexia nervosa can be managed on an outpatient basis with psychological component, medical monitoring and dietetic advice.

Dietitians working in child and adolescent MH and eating disorder services work with the patient (and families) on all food-related issues, thus enabling other therapists to work on the underlying issues of the disorder without being distracted by food-related issues.

Dietitians also have a critical role to play in helping service users meet their nutritional needs to ensure normal physical development and growth, establish normal eating behaviours, develop normal attitude to food, stop compensatory behaviours, develop appropriate responses to hunger and satiety cues and ultimately help patients to trust food again.

Ways of working in eating disorders

Anorexia nervosa is egosyntonic in nature, closely bound to a sufferer's identity and core values, and experienced as a solution to their problems. Therefore, behaviour change in this client group is difficult and treatment is often fraught by ambivalence about change.

Ways of working within eating disorders are underpinned by enhanced communication skills, which necessitate the use of motivational interviewing and cognitive behavioural approaches. Embedding these principles and practices into dietetics is essential for advanced level working. The following are some examples of how these can be achieved:

- Focusing on biological/global aspects of nutrition and separating out the emotional entanglement;
- Establishing expectations of self-monitoring and client responsibility as part of treatment;
- Presenting both sides of the picture and discussing choices in an open and honest way;
- Validating current experiences and ways of coping, whilst pushing towards the future and change;
- Discussing behaviours in the context of associated thoughts and feelings;
- Explaining and interpreting symptoms, giving alternative explanations for events or beliefs;
- Reframing and challenging beliefs about food and the body;
- Exploring the function of food rules and safety behaviours;
- Exploring the current situation in detail, eliciting associated thoughts, feelings and motivation;
- Planning, goal setting and problem solving;
- Increasing self-efficacy by giving practical advice to support self-efficacy—portioning, shopping, cooking;
- Setting up behavioural experiments around specific beliefs about food and weight;
- Using step-wise and graded approach to behaviour change;
- Being curious and noticing rather than judging;
- Establishing boundaries such as 'safe' diet, fluid and weight;
- Psycho-education, for example exploring specific behaviours such as binges and their meaning (dieting/deprivation punishing/ opportunity/pleasure, etc);
- Identify trigger foods/situations;
- Teaching distress tolerance techniques/active alternatives alongside MDT members; and
- Identifying and dealing with cravings.

Multidisciplinary working is essential and close liaison in designing a co-ordinated rehabilitation service is the cornerstone to effective patient centred working. Professional roles vary from team to team and will inevitably overlap. Patient centred working, good communication, liaison and team working allow for fluid boundaries between disciplines without effecting professional integrity or moving towards generic working.

Eating disorders assessment

Decision making is a whole team approach, driven by psychological formulation and based upon careful ongoing assessment of needs and the service user's wishes. In 2007 the Scottish Dietitians Eating Disorders Clinical Forum (SDEDCF) produced documentation for the initial dietetic assessment of patients with eating disorders, which aims to standardise assessment practice and provide dietitians with a means to collect the relevant information required to make a thorough assessment (see Appendices 22.3 and 22.4). Additional advanced assessment techniques for eating disorders include a detailed timeline of weight from childhood onwards matched across to significant life events and detailed description of family mealtimes and their meaning. The dietetic assessment should be summarised and fed back to the patient, forming part of early motivational enhancement work.

Refeeding at low weights

The challenge of refeeding in anorexia nervosa at very low weight, combined with the psychological needs of the service user who is extremely distressed or even under section, is enormous. MDT assessment and involvement is essential. The decision to nasogastrically feed is a difficult one and needs careful planning. A range of treatment options should be considered after a risk assessment of each option. Indicators for nasogastric feeding are:

- Life threatening low weight (BMI of < 13.5) and weight falling;
- High physical risk;[25]
- Minimal nutritional intake with no recent increase;
- Disengagement with psychological work;
- Poor cognitive functioning; and
- All other options exhausted.

NICE guidelines of 2004 states:

> Feeding against the will of the patient should be an intervention of last resort ... is a highly specialised procedure requiring expertise in the care and management of those with severe disorders and the physical complications associated with it.[26]

Assessment for feeding should include consideration of refeeding risk as outlined in Table 22.5.

Table 22.5 Considerations in the treatment of refeeding syndrome

Physiology—the following are high risk situations:

- Excess exercise and low weight;
- Frequent vomiting or blood in vomit;
- Electrolyte derangement;
- Laxative abuse or liver function tests increasing;
- Poor fluid intake;
- Chronic low weight;
- Type of food restriction (high protein/low carbohydrate); and
- Rapid weight loss (> 0.5 kg/week).

Risk assessment-based protocol/care pathways

The safest way to minimise risk in this situation is to use a refeeding protocol that details a step-wise guide to assessment, treatment and monitoring, with risks and steps taken to minimise risk highlighted. The development of such a tool will include input from pharmacy, doctors, nurses and psychologists. (An example of this can be found in Appendix 22.5.) It must take into account the practicalities of feeding at low weights, electrolyte regulation, use of magnesium, potassium and phosphate supplementation, and glucose/insulin dysregulation at low weights.[27]

All assessments and events involved in the refeeding process should be explained to the service user, and where possible options and risks discussed in an honest and supportive way. At very low weights (BMI< 13.5) a service user's options may be extremely limited due to the urgent need to act. Dietitians may need to switch role, for example from a supportive facilitator of behaviour change in outpatients to the key instigator of nasogastric feeding in an in-patient setting. The change from high to low service user choice, autonomy and control can potentially be damaging to the therapeutic relationship if not done with extreme care and due attention.

It is important to remain psychological in approach at all times and use language and approaches that emphasise you are working with the service user to overcome the disease and behaviours displayed by the service user, not the service user per se.

Ensure that time is taken for each feeding option and its consequences to be discussed. Where any choice exists that does not compromise safety, it is essential to try and give the service user some autonomy and return control and choice where possible.[28] For example they may wish to decide what time the feed commences, or what nostril the tube is inserted into.

Evidence suggests that tube feeding in the correct way does not impact on the therapeutic relationship, and indeed some have managed to use supplementary tube feeding as a self-managed, safe and acceptable treatment options for weight gain throughout in-patient treatment.[29,30] However, most current literature focuses on tube feeding as a life-saving intervention, or as a last resort, which is used to safely correct medical risks.[24] Working with the service user to support the reintroduction of food and return control and choice at the earliest possible point is crucial in enabling the service user to move towards accepting further treatment.

New developments for dietitians in mental health services

There are now many AHPs working within specialist MH roles. Their particular skills and expertise can be an important factor in helping people develop and maintain their independence through both physical and mental rehabilitation. A unique contribution of AHPs to MH is their ability to meet the combined mental and physical needs of service users.[2]

NWW makes specific recommendations for AHPs working in MH.[2] Dietitians working at an advanced practice level should consider these carefully when designing services, outcome measures, audit and research:

- Dietitians should use the Skills for Health competence-based approach to service delivery (http://www.skillsforhealth.org.uk) and the Creating Capable Teams Approach to MDT working.[31]
- Dietitians need to demonstrate to commissioners the cost-effective contribution that their specialist skills can make to improve the health and well being of service users and their carers.
- Dietitians should extend links with local authority and other services to ensure clinical protocols and care pathways for service delivery across organisational boundaries are in place.

- Dietitians should take advantage of their transferable skills in order to lead service development across MH services. Dietitians should make explicit the contribution they can make to improve a person's quality of life through reducing their reliance on services and by promoting health and well being.

Service users and carers should be actively involved in the development and delivery of training and education, and as partners in their care (at both individual and service levels). The ten essential shared capabilities underpinning values for all MH staff (http://www.nimhe.csip.org.uk) should be integral to the training, induction and continuous professional development of all AHP professionals and support staff.

Key points

- The way in which MH services are delivered is changing. New ways of working and an increased emphasis on physical health are key drivers of change.
- Dietitians need to demonstrate to commissioners the cost-effective contribution their specialist skills can make to improving the health and well being of service users and their carers.
- Dietitians may have to work at a strategic level to influence service user health through policy and strategy.
- Dietitians should use their transferrable skills to take on extended practice roles.
- There is increasing evidence directly linking improved nutrition to better MH.
- Eating disorders are highly complex. Dietitians working in this field should have a good understanding of the physical, psychological, behavioural and psychosocial facets of the disorder.
- Refeeding low weight patients with anorexia nervosa is a highly skilled process and should be undertaken by an experienced team in an appropriate setting.
- Dietitians should develop enhanced communication skills and skills in psychological approaches to support behaviour change in MH.
- Dietitians working in MH must undertake further specialist training, and have regular supervision and MDT support.

Case studies (multidisciplinary)

Carol is a 55-year-old mother of three children. Each has a different father, all of whom are now estranged. She had a difficult and unhappy childhood as her mother suffered MH problems, and her father was controlling and highly critical and cruel at times. Her eating problems began as a teenager when she oscillated between periods of starvation and binging. Despite her difficulties she achieved well at school and went on to further study, pushing herself to achieve academically. Her weight fluctuated greatly from quite underweight to at time being overweight. She was always surprised at pregnancy as her menstrual cycle was erratic. In the past she has also used drugs and alcohol in varying amounts and made superficial cuts to her arms. She adores her children and tries her best to be a good mother. She has been on antidepressants for years and juggles two very difficult jobs and the care of her three children. They are the only reason she gives for not committing suicide. She has lost contact with most friends and relatives and spends her time alone drinking. She never eats with the children and will spend weeks restricting to 500 calories a day, followed by three- or four-day binges in which she spends the month's food budget and consequently she has large debt problems. After vomiting until she nearly passes out, she will drink until she falls asleep. She is careful to hide these behaviours, and only does this when the children are at school or asleep. Her mood is low and she is again contemplating suicide. She has recently started seeing a community MH team and has agreed to consider a short period of in-patient treatment if her sister can have the children for a few weeks.

QUESTIONS

1. (a) In what order should treatment be offered?
   (b) What broad psychological approaches could be used to support this lady?
2. What MDT members should be involved?
3. At what point could dietetic involvement begin?
4. What would the dietetic aspect of treatment focus on?
5. What skills would be needed by the members of the team?

ANSWERS

1. (a) In what order should treatment be offered?
   The priority is to reduce the risk of suicide and interventions should focus on crisis resolution before moving towards long-term management. Generally alcohol misuse should be tackled before the eating difficulties. Binge eating is a distressing symptom and service users usually wish to gain control of this, so it may be that this is addressed next through self-monitoring, regulating eating patterns and acquiring skills in distress tolerance. However, it is important that binge eating is not simply replaced by regular but restrictive eating, so close monitoring of weight and mood is required. Skills training in emotional regulation and distress tolerance skills, followed by longer term work to explore core beliefs and maladapted thinking patterns, should be undertaken alongside dietetic input.
   (b) What broad psychological approaches could be used to support this lady?
   Approaches such as cognitive behavioural therapy, interpersonal therapy and didactical behavioural therapy are all valid evidenced-based techniques and using tools from any one or a combination of all may be useful in treatment.

2. Which MDT members could be involved?
   - Psychiatrist;
   - GP;
   - Psychologist;
   - Nurse therapist;
   - MH dietitian;
   - Occupational therapist;
   - CBT or DBT therapist;
   - Psychotherapist; and
   - Social worker.

3. At what point could dietetic involvement begin
   Assessment can begin at any point, but until the current crisis is resolved dietetic input may be limited to meal planning should inpatient treatment go ahead. Once risk of suicide decreases, dietetic interventions to support the service user in stopping specific behaviours can begin.

4. What would the dietetic aspect of treatment focus on?
   Assessment and motivational enhancement work. Behavioural analysis, managing cravings, identifying triggers, graded exposure to trigger foods and problem solving, supported by service user self-monitoring. Self-efficacy can be enhanced by supporting skills in meal planning, meal preparation and shopping, problem solving and goal setting. Psycho-education around food, weight, physiology and behavioural analysis can support relapse prevention work.

5. What skills would be needed by the members of the team?
   An understanding of MH services; a sound knowledge of MH developmental and treatment theories; experience in working with eating disorders; a good understanding of CBT/DBT approaches, psychological formulation and behavioural analysis.

References

1. Department of Health. *Choosing Health: Supporting the Physical Health Needs of People with Severe Mental Illness.* London: Department of Health; 2006.

2. Department of Health. *New Ways of Working for Psychiatrists: Enhancing Effective, Person-Centered Services through New Ways of Working in Multidisciplinary and Multi-agency Contexts.* DH Publication Ref 270394A/B/C. London: 2005.

3. Parliamentary Report. *The Link between Diet and Behaviour: The Influence of Nutrition on Mental Health.* Report of an inquiry held by associate parliamentary food and health forum. London: 2008.

4. Quality Improvement Scotland. *National Overview—Standards for Food, Fluid and Nutritional Care in Hospitals.* NHS QIS; 2006.

5. National Institute for Health and Clinical Excellence. *Nutrition Support for Adults Oral Nutrition Support, Enteral Tube Feeding and Parenteral Nutrition.* London: NICE; 2006.

6. Weissman MM, Bland RC, Canino GJ, et al. Cross-national epidemiology of major depression and bipolar disorder. *JAMA.* 1996;276:293–299.

7. Westover AN, Marangell LB. A cross-national relationship between sugar consumption and depression? *Depress Anxiety.* 2002;16:118–120.

8. Peet M. International variations in the outcome of schizophrenia and the prevalence of depression in relation to national dietary practices: an ecological analysis. *Br J Psychiatry.* 2004;184:404–408.

9. Hibbeln JR. Cross-national comparison of seafood consumption and rates of bipolar disorder. *Am J Psychiatry.* 2003;160:2222–2226.

10. Zanarini M, Frankenburg F. Omega-3 fatty acid treatment of women with borderline personality disorder: a double blind placebo controlled pilot study. *Am J Psychiatry.* 2003;160:167–169.

11. Parker G, Gibson NA, Brotchie H. Omega-3 fatty acids and mood disorders. *Am J Psychiatry.* 2006; 163:969–978.

12. Freeman MP, Hibbeln JR, Wisner KL. Omega-3 fatty acids: evidence basis for treatment and future research in psychiatry. *J Clin Psychiatry.* 2006;67:1954–1967.

13. Lin PY, Su KP. A meta-analytic review of double-blind, placebo-controlled trials of antidepressant efficacy of omega-3 fatty acids. *J Clin Psychiatry.* 2007;68: 1056–1061.

14. Hibbeln JR. Fish consumption and major depression. *Lancet.* 1998;351: 1213.

15. Noaghiul S, Hibbeln JR. Cross-national comparison of seafood consumption and rates of bipolar disorder. *Am J Psychiatry.* 2003; 160:2222–2226.

16. Edwards R, Peet M, Shay J, Horrobin D. Omega 3 polyunsaturated fatty acid levels in the diet and in red blood cell membranes of depressed patients. *J Affect Disord.* 1998;48:149–155.

17. Lin PY, Su KP. A meta-analytical review of double blind placebo-controlled trials of antidepressant efficacy of omega 3 fatty acids. *J Clin Psychiatry.* 2007;68(7):1056–1061.

18. Young SN. The use of diet and dietary components in the study of factors controlling affect in humans: a review. *J Psychiatry Neurosci.* 1993;18:235–244.

19. Wurtman J. Depression and weight gain: the serotonin connection. *J Affect Disord.* 1993;29:183–192.

20. Markus CR, Panhuysen G, Tuiten A, Koppeschaar H, Fekkes D, Peters ML. Does carbohydrate-rich, protein-poor food prevent a deterioration of mood and cognitive performance of stress-prone subjects when subjected to a stressful task? *Appetite.* 1998;31:49–65.

21. Benton D and Donohoe RT. The effects of nutrients on mood. *Public Health Nutritio.* 1999;2 (3):403–410.

22. Taylor D, Paton C, Kerwin R. *The Maudsley Prescribing Guidelines: The South London and Maudsley NHS Trust & Oxleas NHS Trust.* London: Taylor and Francis; 2006.

23. Wiser S, Telch C. Dialectical behaviour therapy for binge eating disorder. *J Clin Psychol.* 1999;55(6): 755–768.

24. Quality Improvement Scotland. *Eating Disorders in Scotland: Recommendations for Management and Treatment.* London: NHS QIS; 2006.

25. Treasure J. *A Guide to Medical Risk Assessment for Eating Disorders.* London: Maudsley; 2004.

26. National Collaborating Centre for Mental Health. *Eating Disorders: Core Interventions in the Treatment and Management of Anorexia Nervosa, Bulimia Nervosa and Related Eating Disorders.* Leicester: British Psychological Society; 2004.

27. Casper RC. Carbohydrate metabolism and its regulatory hormones in anorexia nervosa. *Psychiatry Res.* 1996;62:85–96.

28. Tan J, Hope T, Stewart A, Fitzpatrick R. Control and compulsory treatment in anorexia nervosa: the views of patients and parents. *Int J Law Psychiatry.* 2003;26:627–645.

29. Sarfaty M, McCluskey S. Compulsory treatment of anorexia nervosa and the moribund patient. *Eur Eating Disord Rev.* 1998;6: 27–37.

30. Zuercher JN, Cumella EJ, Woods BK, Eberly M, Carr JK. Efficacy of voluntary nasogastric tube feeding in female inpatients with anorexia nervosa. *JPEN J Parenter Enteral Nutr.* 2003;27(4): 268–276.

31. Department of Health. *Creating Capable Teams Approach: Best Practice guidance to support the implementation of New Ways of Working (NWW) and New Roles.* London: Department of Health; 2007.

Further reading/bookshelf

Mental Health Act 1983. HMSO. Information at http://www.dh.gov.uk.

Mental Capacity Act 2005 (came into force in two stages, April and October 2007). The Act and Code of Practice can be found at http://www.dca.gov.uk/menincap/legis.htm

National Service Framework in Mental Health. Department of Health; September 1999.

ICD-10 Classification of Mental and Behavioural Disorders. World Health Organization.

DSM-1V: Classification of Mental Disorders. American Psychiatric Association.

NICE Clinical Guidelines. *Topic: Mental Health and Behavioural Conditions. Clinical Guidelines on Anxiety, Bipolar Disorder, Dementia, Depression, Obsessive Compulsive Disorder, Self Harm Schizophrenia.* Available at: http://www.nice.org.uk/guidance

Useful links and organisations

Alzheimer's Society. http://www.alzheimers.org.uk

Dietitians in Mental Health. http://www.dietitiansmentalhealthgroup.org.uk

Sainsbury Centre for Mental Health. http://www.scmh.org.uk

Royal College of Psychiatrists. http://www.rcpsych.ac.uk

National Electronic Library for Mental Health. http://www.nelh.nhs.uk

National Institute for Mental Health in England. http://www.nimhe.csip.org.uk

Web4health. Sponsored by the European Commission. http://www.web4health.info

Mind. http://www.mind.org.uk

Rethink (formerly National Schizophrenia Fellowship). http://www.rethink.org

SAGB—Schizophrenia Association of Great Britain. http://www.sagb.co.uk

Sustain. Alliance for Better Food and Farming. http://www.sustainweb.org/

Food and Behaviour Research. http://www.fabresearch.org

Skills for Health: Better Skills, Better Jobs, Better Health. Sector Skills Council. UK Commission for Employment and Skills. http://www.skillsforhealth.org.uk

Appendix 22.1 Mode of action and influence of medication on nutritional status

Class of Drugs	Action	Possible nutritional consequence
Antidepressants		
Tricyclic antidepressants (TCA) • Amitriptyline • Amoxapine • Imipramine • Nortriptyline	Blocks the re-uptake of serotonin and norepinephrine to increase the level of neurotransmitter at the receptors	Nausea and vomiting Increased appetite and weight gain Dry mouth Constipation Blood glucose changes May also cause drowsiness, blurred vision and difficulty with micturition
Selective serotonin re-uptake inhibitors (SSRIs) • Citalopram • Fluoxetine • Fluvoxamine • Paroxetine • Sertraline	Their action is to block the re-uptake of the neurotransmitter serotonin to increase its level at central synapses to facilitate neurotransmission These have fewer side-effects than TCA	Nausea and vomiting Anorexia and weight loss Dry mouth and altered taste Other GI symptoms such as abdominal pain Headaches and anxiety may also occur
Serotonin and noradrenaline re-uptake inhibitors (SNRIs) • Venlafaxine • Duloxetine	Their action is to block the re-uptake of the neurotransmitters serotonin and norepinephrine into brain cells	Nausea and vomiting Anorexia and weight loss Dry mouth Other GI symptoms such as diarrhoea or constipation Headaches, fatigue and dizziness may also occur
Selective inhibitors of noradrenaline re-uptake • Reboxetine • Atomoxetine	Their action is to block the re-uptake of the neurotransmitters norepinephrine (noradrenaline) into brain cells. Effective in schizophrenia and ADHD	Nausea Anorexia Dry mouth Other GI symptoms such as constipation
Monoamine oxidase inhibitors (MAOIs) • Moclobemide (a reversible MAOI) • Isocarboxazid • Phenelzine	Act by inhibiting the breakdown of neurotransmitter, mainly serotonin and norepinephrine (noradrenaline)	A sudden rise in blood pressure may occur if taken with foods rich in tyramine, such as cheese, meat pies, yeast extract, stock cubes, red wine and soya Nausea and vomiting Increased appetite and weight gain Dry mouth and constipation

Mood stabilisers

Lithium salts	Thought to act by inhibiting protein kinase-C activity within the brain	Nausea, vomiting diarrhoea
• Lithium carbonate		Has a sedative effect that is increased with alcohol intake
• Lithium citrate		Excreted in breast milk, affecting baby
		Weight gain may occur
		Levels affected by salt intake so avoidance of sudden changes in diet advised
		A good fluid intake is also advised

Anticonvulsant, anxiolytic and hypnotic drugs

Phenytoin	Inhibits electrical stimulation in the brain	Nausea and vomiting until toleration develops Megaloblastic anaemia with prolonged use, due to its influence on folate absorption and metabolism
Benzodiazepines • Diazepam • Lorazepam • Temazepam	Enhances the inhibitory effect of the neurotransmitter gamma-aminobutyric acid (GABA) at GABA receptors, having a depressant effect on the central nervous system (CNS)	May occasionally cause diarrhoea, nausea, vomiting, consitipation or dry mouth Not suitable for use during breast feeding Also causes fatigue
Sodium valproate	Increases GABA activity to depress CNS activity	Loss of appetite, nausea and vomiting are reported as is weight gain and an adverse effect on the liver with long-term use

Appendix 22.2 Nutrition screening tool (Reproduced with permission from The State Hospital)

The State Hospital – Nutrition Screening Tool

Screening Date		Screening undertaken by	

SECTION 1 - Patient's Details	
Patient Name	
Patient Date of Birth	
CHI	
Ward	

SECTION 2 - Calculating BMI

Weight (kg) = _ _ _

Height (m) = _ _ _

BMI = _ _ _ (from BMI chart on separate sheet)

BMI SCORES	
<15	2
15–18.4	1
18.5–24.9	0
25–29.9	1
30–34.9	2
35–39.9	3
≥40	4

SECTION 2 score from above table (maximum score 4) = _ _ _

(BMI ranges taken from SIGN 8 guideline)

SECTION 3 - Weight Change

Has the patient's weight changed in the last 3–6 months?

☐ YES

☐ NO *(score 0 for this section and skip to section 4)*

☐ UNKNOWN *(score 0 for this section and skip to section 4)*

If yes, by how much?

☐ LOSS _ _ _ kg

☐ GAIN _ _ _ kg

Using the "Weight Change Chart", please enter the weight change score below.

SECTION 3 score (maximum score 2) = _ _ _

The State Hospital – Nutrition Screening Tool

SECTION 4 - Nutritional Assessment		Comments/ Details
1. Has the patient been prescribed an antipsychotic, antidepressant or mood stabiliser?	☐YES = 1 ☐NO = 0 ☐UNKNOWN =0	
2. Does the patient have any ongoing therapeutic reason for a special diet or require assistance. (Examples are allergies, diabetes, constipation, high cholesterol, ethnic or religious needs, physical or learning disability)?	☐YES = 1 ☐NO = 0 ☐UNKNOWN =0	
3. Is the patient currently experiencing any short-term acute illness, disease or treatment which may limit their ability to meet their current nutritional requirements?(examples are vomiting and diarrhoea, flu, infection, chemotherapy)	☐YES = 1 ☐NO = 0 ☐UNKNOWN =0	
4. Does the patient have difficulty chewing, swallowing, or digesting food? *(If swallowing difficulties reported, refer directly to Speech and Language Therapist)*	☐YES = 1 ☐NO = 0 ☐UNKNOWN =0	
5. Does a global assessment of the patient suggest inappropriate nourishment? (loose/tight fitting clothes, fragile skin, poor wound healing, apathy, wasted muscles, poor appetite, altered taste sensation, altered/heavy smoking habits)	☐YES = 1 ☐NO = 0 ☐UNKNOWN =0	
6. Does the patient indicate a disordered eating pattern (e.g. bingeing, restricting food) or pre-empt thoughts for food, and/or refuse 2 or more meals a day?	☐YES = 1 ☐NO = 0 ☐UNKNOWN =0	

SECTION 4 score (maximum score 6) = _ _ _

Please copy the patient's score from each section in the appropriate space below and enter total. Match the overall score to Management Grid scores and note action required.

SECTION 5 - Overall Score and patient management	
Section 2 score	_ _ _
Section 3 score	_ _ _
Section 4 score	_ _ _
TOTAL	_ _ _

	SCORE	0	1–2	3–5	6–8
MANAGEMENT GRID	RISK	Minimal Risk	Low Risk	Medium Risk	High Risk
	ACTION	No action required, routine care	Observe, Healthy Eating Diet	Referral to Dietician Set up weight trigger points	Urgent Referral to Dietitian
	SCREENING	Annually	Quarterly	Monthly	Monitor and review weekly

Appendix 22.3 SDEDCF Dietetic Assessment (Reproduced with permission from SDEDCF)

The Scottish Dietitians Eating Disorders Clinical Forum (SDEDCF) has produced documentation for the initial dietetic assessment of patients with eating disorders.

The documentation aims to:

- Standardise assessment practice; and
- Provide dietitians with a means to collect the relevant information required to make a thorough assessment.

Scottish Dietitian's Eating Disorders Dietetic Assessment Form

1. PATIENT DETAILS	
Date of referral: Source of referral Date of assessment:	Dietitian's name: Dietitian's Signature Co-workers:
Patient name:	D O B:
Address:	Telephone number:
GP:	General/Psychiatric Unit No:　　　(delete as appropriate) CHI No:

2. DIAGNOSIS
ICD10

3. CURRENT MEDICATION

4. RELEVANT MEDICAL AND PSYCHIATRIC HISTORY

5. HAVE YOU BEEN REFERRED TO A DIETITIAN BEFORE?

Yes - if yes, who, where and when

No

6. PATIENT'S VIEW OF REFERRAL

7. CLINICAL / PHYSICAL SYMPTOMS

GI tract – constipation, diarrhoea, bloating, irritable bowel, other - specify	☐
Skin changes – Colour, dryness, broken skin, pressure sores, poor healing	☐
Feel cold – susceptibility to cold hands or feet	☐
Hair changes – Hair loss, dryness, lanugo hair	☐
Pins and needles – mouth, hands, feet	☐
Menstruation – yes/no, pre-pubertal, amenorrhoea, check if patient on OCP	☐
Dental problems	☐
Swollen parotid glands	☐
Blood pressure – high or low, reading checked	☐
Bone scan – yes, no, results, date of last scan	☐
ECG – abnormal	☐
Low mood, disturbed sleep, anxiety	☐
Concentration – poor	☐
Relevant biochemistry/haematology	☐

8. FAMILY SITUATION

Parents/Guardians/Partner	Dependents	Siblings

9. SOCIAL SITUATION

Contact with peer group
Social life
Social support
Issues regarding socialising

10. DIET HISTORY current			
Diet History	**Weekdays**	**Weekends**	**Perfect Day**
Typical day – all food & fluid	Breakfast		
	Mid Morning		
	Lunch		
	Mid Afternoon		
	Dinner		
	Evening		

Eating Pattern		
	Avoids Meals	☐
	Snacks rather than meals	☐
	Eats alone	☐
	Chaotic	☐
	Rigid regime	☐
	Check labels	☐
	Weigh food	☐

Estimated kcals/day (intake) Estimated fluid/day (intake) Estimated alcohol (intake)		
Caffeine		
Fizzy drinks		
Nutritional supplements		
Estimated kcals from supplements		
Vitamin supplements	Yes/No If yes, name & dose:	
Estimated kcal/day (requirements) Estimated fluid /day (requirements		

11. MEALS

Who shops and prepares the food?		
What are mealtimes like?		
Where do you eat?		
Do you?	Eat alone	Yes/No
	With family	Yes/No
	Take lunch to school/work	Yes/No
	Buy food /eat out at lunch	Yes/No
	Eat with friends/colleagues	Yes/No

12. EATING BEHAVIOUR AND ATTITUDES TO FOOD

Food Choice	Safe foods
	Difficult foods/foods generally avoided
	Binge foods
	Identify trigger foods

Food Groups	Over concern with
	• Food groups – fats, carbohydrates, protein, dairy, fruit and veg
	• Label checking
	• Weighing food

Allergies – own beliefs	
Allergies and food intolerances – medically diagnosed	
Vegetarian / vegan When did this begin	
Multi cultural	
Food cravings Comments	Yes/No
Recognition of hunger Comments	Yes/No

13. PREVIOUS EATING HABITS AND DIETS (from childhood onwards)

14. FAMILY HISTORY OF WEIGHT, DIETING AND EATING DISORDERS

15. EXERCISE HISTORY

a) everyday activity e.g. housework

b) planned exercise

c) twitching, shaking, standing, restless

16. WEIGHT HISTORY

Height:	Per centile:	BMI: % weight for height (child / adolescent):
Weight : (date) Weighed in clothes Weighed in underwear	Per centile:	Healthy weight range:
Percentage weight loss: Over what period of time		
Last menstrual period:		
Highest weight	Lowest weight:	Patient's 'ideal weight
Do you weigh yourself? How often?		

Relevant weight history (incl. pregnancies)

17. OTHER EATING DISORDERED BEHAVIOUR		Comments
Food restriction	Yes/No	
Bingeing	Yes/No	
Purging-vomiting	Yes/No	
Laxatives	Yes/No	
Diuretics	Yes/No	
Appetite suppressants	Yes/No	
Alcohol	Yes/No	
Drugs	Yes/No	
Other eating disordered behaviour (refer to guidelines sheet)	Yes/No	
Dietary rules (refer to guidelines sheet)		

18. PATIENT'S AIMS OF CONTACT

19. MOTIVATION TO CHANGE   Comments

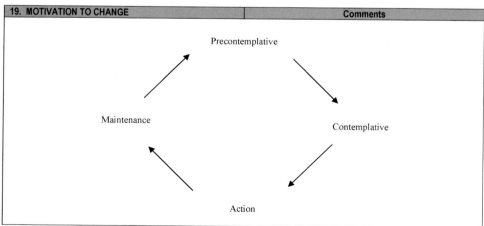

20. AGREED TREATMENT PLAN

Main Concerns

Agreed Treatment Plan
        Aims of Dietetic Contact

        Focus of Treatment

        Number of Sessions Before Planned Review

Date of Next Appointment

Handouts / Information Given

Initial Goals Set

Appendix 22.4 SDEDCF Dietetic Assessment Completion Guidelines (Reproduced with permission from SDEDCF)

The following guidance notes have been developed to help you complete the assessment form in Appendix 22.3.

Please note that:

- Completion of the assessment may take more than one interview session; and
- Questions may not be applicable to your patient and may be omitted.

Section 1: Patient details

- Co-workers

This section ought to include a note of any other health/social care professionals involved in assisting the patient with the eating disorder problem. Some examples might be psychologist, psychiatrist, community psychiatric nurse (CPN), counsellor, cognitive behaviour therapy (CBT) therapist, etc. It may be useful to have their phone numbers and/or location too.

- Community health index (CHI) number

The community health index (CHI) number is the national unique number for any health communication related to a given patient. The CHI number will be used on correspondence including sample bottles and request forms for labs, prescriptions from pharmacy, radiology requests and outpatient and inpatient correspondence.

The CHI is a ten-digit number created from a patient's date of birth and four other numbers, e.g. 0101256420. All patients who register with a GP will be allocated a CHI number.

The CHI number must be used on all health correspondence for all patients from visiting their GP surgery to visiting hospitals.

Section 2: Diagnosis

The following table shows the main classifications of eating disorders by the International Classification of Diseases (ICD). If the patient has been diagnosed as having an eating disorder, record the ICD-10 diagnosis on the assessment form.

ICD-10	Description
F50.0 Anorexia nervosa	A disorder characterised by deliberate weight loss, induced and sustained by the patient. It occurs most commonly in adolescent girls and young women, but adolescent boys and young men may also be affected, as may children approaching puberty and older women. The disorder is associated with a specific psychopathology whereby a dread of fatness and flabbiness of body contour persists as an intrusive overvalued idea, and the patients impose a low weight threshold on themselves. There is undernutrition of varying severity with secondary endocrine and metabolic changes and disturbances of bodily function. The symptoms include restricted dietary choice, excessive exercise, induced vomiting and purgation and use of appetite suppressants and diuretics
F50.1 Atypical anorexia nervosa	Disorders that fulfil some of the features of anorexia nervosa but in which the overall clinical picture does not justify that diagnosis. For instance, one of the key symptoms, such as amenorrhoea or marked dread of being fat, may be absent in the presence of marked weight loss and weight-reducing behaviour. This diagnosis should not be made in the presence of known physical disorders associated with weight loss
F50.2 Bulimia nervosa	A syndrome characterised by repeated bouts of overeating and an excessive preoccupation with the control of body weight, leading to a pattern of overeating followed by vomiting or use of purgatives. This disorder shares many psychological features with anorexia nervosa, including an overconcern with body shape and weight. Repeated vomiting is likely to give rise to disturbances of body electrolytes and physical complications. There is often, but not always, a history of an earlier episode of anorexia nervosa, the interval ranging from a few months to several years

ICD-10	Description
F50.3 Atypical bulimia nervosa	Disorders that fulfil some of the features of bulimia nervosa, but in which the overall clinical picture does not justify that diagnosis. For instance, there may be recurrent bouts of overeating and overuse of purgatives without significant weight change, or the typical over concern about body shape and weight may be absent
F 50.4	Overeating associated with other psychological disturbances
F50.5	Vomiting associated with other psychological disturbances
F50.8	Other eating disorders
F50.9	Eating disorder, unspecified

DSM-IV has a proposed category of binge eating disorder which is similar to bulimia nervosa, but without compensatory behaviours. In ICD-10 this would normally be subsumed into F50.3, F50.4, F50.8 or F50.9.

Section 3: Current Medication

- You may have this information already from the referral. If no information with referral ask patient.
- List medicines and dose if known, in box.

Section 4: Relevant Medical and Psychiatric History

- You may have this information already from the referral. Check with the patient.
- List conditions and dates if applicable: e.g. diabetes, thyroid problems, allergies, Crohn's disease, IBS, eating disorder, depression, substance abuse, self-harm.
- Note any hospital admissions, NHS or private for treatment of eating disorder.

Section 5: Have You Been Referred to a Dietitian Before? Yes/No (comment box)

Section 6: Patient's view of referral (comment box)

Section 7: Clinical/Physical Symptoms

Start by asking a general open question, e.g. 'Have you noticed any changes in your physical condition?' Use examples from the following lists to expand as necessary. Record any symptoms which are relevant either by circling the checklist or making brief notes on the assessment sheet. Examples of symptoms are:

- GI tract: e.g. constipation, diarrhoea, bloating, irritable bowel, heartburn/indigestion, stomach cramps;
- Skin changes: e.g. colour, dryness, broken skin, pressure sores, poor healing, cracked, parched skin, and transparency of skin;
- Feel cold; always cold, cold extremities;
- Hair changes: e.g. hair loss, dryness, lanugo;
- Pins and needles: where? (Mouth, hands, feet) worse at certain times?
- Menstruation: does the patient menstruate? Primary of secondary amenorrhoea? Regular or irregular periods? If amenorrhoea, for how long? Check if on oral contraceptive pill;
- Dental: significant dental problems? Regular contact with dentist?
- Swollen parotid glands;
- Blood pressure: normal, high or low? Postural hypotension? Any report of dizziness?
- Bone density: has this ever been done? If so where, when and results? Refer to QIS guidelines for Eating Disorders November 2006 or SNDRI pack for recommendations on DXA scanning;
- Mood lower: lethargic, unmotivated, isolated, irritable, tearful, etc.
- Sleeping: is sleep pattern disrupted? are they uncomfortable in bed? Sleeping more/sleeping less?
- Anxiety: is this present? Has it worsened? Heart palpitations, fainting, shortness of breath, sweating palms, increased senses, nausea;
- Low mood: e.g. reported poor sleep, anxiety;
- Concentration: e.g. poor, reduced;
- Relevant biochemistry of haematology results.

Section 8: Family Situation (boxes for parents/guardian; dependents; siblings)

Section 9: Social Situation (boxes for peer group; social life; social support; socialising issues)

Section 10: Diet History—Current

A Perfect Day?

This question forms part of the diet history. After asking the patient about a typical day, weekdays and weekends etc., a very useful question is to ask about a 'perfect day'. This establishes what the patient sees as being a good day for them and can help assess their motivation to change. A good way of wording this question is as follows:

'Imagine you could plan tomorrow and it turned out to be a "perfect day" eating-wise, a day where you went to bed at night feeling very content, what would you eat tomorrow?'

Section 11: Meals (i.e. food preparation; location of meals; eating company)

Section 12: Eating Behaviour and Attitudes to Food (food choice; concern with food groups; allergies; cultural food habits; hunger)

Section 13: Previous Eating Habits (from childhood onwards)

This section is designed to collect information about the patient's eating habits prior to being ill and to clarify how the eating problem developed.

- How would patient describe their eating pattern as a child/before onset of problems? Was patient a 'fussy' eater? Briefly describe variety/range/regularity of foods taken at this time.
- How did eating habits change as problems started to develop?
- Were any specific diets followed? When did this occur?

Section 14: Family History of Weight, Dieting and Eating Disorders (bland comments box)

Section 15: Exercise History (usual patterns of activity)

Section 16: Weight History (table for completion)

% weight for height

It is important to note that only growth charts and BMI charts specifically for children and young people under the age of 18 years should be used in any assessment of growth and development. These can be obtained from the Child Growth Foundation.

The aim is to re-establish a healthy body weight range somewhere between the 25th and 75th BMI centile.

A helpful tool for calculating weight-for-height ratios in children and young people is the Cole Calculator obtained from the Child Growth Foundation. At 95–100% weight-for-height, most girls reach ovarian maturity, but this can vary.

Section 17: Other Eating Disordered Behaviour

In this section, details of other unhelpful eating disorder behaviours and dietary rules can be recorded.

It is useful to have patients identify these behaviours for themselves using different self-assessment handouts. See the two attached handouts.

This section can be completed in different ways, depending on the patient:

- Go through lists in session as part of assessment; or
- By giving lists as a homework exercise.

Section 18: Patient's Aims of Contact (blank box)

Section 19: Motivation to Change (diagram for guidance)

Section 20: Agreed Treatment Plan

Under this heading the dietitian should document:

- Main concerns—areas of greatest concern to the dietitian regarding the patient;
- What has been agreed with the patient with regards to future dietetic contact;
- What the aims of dietetic contact and focus of treatment will be;
- Number of sessions to be offered before planned review;
- Date of next appointment;
- If not being offered another appointment, reasons for this and details of any follow up arrangements with other professionals;

- Details of any handouts or other information given; and
- Details of any initial goals set.

Ending the Assessment

Begin by giving the patient a lot of positive feedback for having taken steps to come along and seek help. Emphasise that you understand how difficult it must have been for them to come along to the consultation and to speak openly about having a problem with eating.

Parrot back the gist of what has been said along the lines of 'I understand that the problem began back when ... that this was more of a problem during times when you were under pressure from exams ... that your weight history was approximately ... etc., etc.' to demonstrate careful listening, attention and that you are keen to rectify anything that has been misunderstood in the recording.

Thank them for sharing the information with you. If arranging another appointment, give them some indication as to what will be looked at or discussed at that time. Tell them whether there is anything that you want them to do before the next appointment, e. g., fill out a food diary. However, due to the complexity of eating disorders and the amount of information to be gathered it is more usual to spend one or two consultations collecting information prior to offering advice to the patient. If you have concerns about the patient's physical health, e.g. frequency of vomiting, high use of laxatives, rapid weight loss, you may advise them to see their GP for physical examination and/or blood tests.

May 2007

Appendix 22.5   Refeeding Protocol (Feeding protocol reproduced with permission)

This protocol has been developed to offer guidelines in the care of a recently admitted patient with severe anorexia nervosa (defined as Body Mass Index < 15), for the physicians, psychiatrists, nursing staff and dietitians involved in their care.

Most patients with anorexia nervosa should be managed on an outpatient basis but, if there is a significant deterioration in their physical condition or mental state, then in-patient care should be considered.

It is important, prior to admission, to agree with both the patient and the care team the aims of the admission, for example, admission for weight restoration or management of significant risk of suicide or self-harm.

Nasogastric feeding is associated with significant physical risks, including refeeding syndrome. The setting for tube feeding should be an MDT decision, e.g. if physical risk is high, one may consider refeeding patients on a medical ward. However, staff experienced in managing patients with an eating disorder should be present, which may require mental health nursing staff to assist patients on the medical ward.

By the nature of their illness, these patients require care from various professionals and regular multidisciplinary reviews are vital to coordinate this care.

These are guidelines rather than rigid rules, and have been based on the care offered to patients within the specialist eating disorder service.

We are aware that this is based on a specialised service, and therefore some of the recommendations may not be possible in other settings.

These guidelines are not intended to replace the liaison role with the specialist eating disorder service.

1. Assess patient for nasogastric feeding or oral diet.
2. Initiate nasogastric feeding if:
   a. Planned admission for NG feeding;
   b. BMI < 12 and/or poor compliance with oral diet;
   c. Deteriorating LFTs;
   d. Deteriorating electrolytes;
   e. Deteriorating ECG; and
   f. As deemed medically necessary.

Prior to Commencing Feed

1. Weigh patient and calculate BMI;
2. Book ECG if no recent result available;

3. Take bloods e.g. FBC, U&Es, LFTs, albumin, CRP, phosphate, magnesium and calcium;
4. Call dietitian, liaison psychiatry and book mental health nurses if needed; and
5. Pass NG tube in accordance with hospital policy. Use Mental Health Act if necessary.

Commencing Nasogastric Feed

6. Commence feed according to plan below.
7. Do not allow to eat. Do not attempt to negotiate meal plans or arrange supplemented drinks.
8. Try not to rehydrate using IV fluids—insulin stimulation with dextrose administration precipitates refeeding syndrome. Double-ended port on the end of nasogastric feed can be used to rehydrate whilst feeding if needed.
9. Prescribe necessary electrolyte supplementation as medically necessary and commence administration as nasogastric feed commences, and run concurrently to feed.
10. Prescribe and administer immediately before feed commences and then daily vitamin supplements as per Table 1.
11. Start fluid chart.
12. Start stool chart (consider use of a commode).

Table 1 Commence with feeding

Thiamine	200–300 mg/day pre-feed
Vitamin B Co-strong	1–2 tablets t.d.s
Multivitamin tablet (e.g. Forceval)	Once a day
Magnesium glycerophosphate	Once a day after feeding begins for first 5–7 days
Sandophosphate	Once a day after feeding begins for first 5–7 days

Monitoring

U&Es, FBC, albumin, CRP, LFTs, phosphate, magnesium and calcium	Daily or as medically directed
Fluid balance chart	Daily
Temp, pulse, BP	Daily or as medically directed
Weight	Daily in night clothes in morning for first 10 days then twice weekly
ECG	On admission then as medically directed
Stool	Daily
Blood glucose	Only if breaks in feeding. Consider monitoring 4 hourly

Electrolyte Supplementation

Electrolyte	Oral	Intravenous
Hypokalaemia		
Mild 3.1–3.6 mmol/L Moderate 2.5–3.0 mmol/L Severe < 2.5 mmol/L	Sando K 4–8 tablets per day (each tablet 12 mmol of K$^+$)	As medically necessary
Hypophosphataemia		
Mild 0.7–0.8 mmol/L Moderate 0.7–0.32 mmol/L Severe < 0.32 mmol/L	Phosphate Sandoz 4–6 tablets daily (each tablet 16 mmol of PO$_4$)	Phosphate polyfusor = 50 mmol phosphate 81 mmol sodium 10 mmol potassium
Hypomagnesaemia		
Mild 0.55–0.74 mmol/L Moderate 0.40–0.55 mmol/L Severe < 0.4 mmol/L	Maalox suspension 10–20 mL daily	As medically necessary

Feeding Regimen

Addressograph: -   Authorised by _____
                     Date Commenced _____

DAY 1
300 mL 1 kcal/mL high fibre feed at 13 ml/hour for 24 hours.
DAY 2
400 mL 1 kcal/mL high fibre feed at 17 ml/hour for 24 hours.
DAY 3
600 mL 1 kcal/mL high fibre feed at 25 ml/hour for 24 hours.
DAY 4
800 mL 1 kcal/mL high fibre feed at 35 ml/hour for 24 hours.
DAYS 5–7
1000 mL 1 kcal/mL high fibre feed at 50 ml/hour for 20 hours.
DAY 8
1300 mL 1 kcal/mL high fibre feed at 65 ml/hour for 20 hours.
DAY 9
1600 mL 1 kcal/mL high fibre feed at 80 ml/hour for 20 hours.
DAY 10
2000 mL 1 kcal/mL high fibre feed at 100 ml/hour for 20 hours.

Maintain at this rate until Dietitian review. Once biochemically stable the following increases in feeding rate are possible.

2000 mL 1 kcal/mL high fibre feed at 100 ml/hour for 20 hours.
Rest for 4 hours.
2000 mL 1 kcal/mL high fibre feed at 125 ml/hour for 16 hours.
Rest for 8 hours.
2000 mL 1 kcal/mL high fibre feed at 150 ml/hour for 13½ hours.
Rest for 11½ hours.
Further increases in rate and feed may be necessary.

In the Interest of Patient Safety:

- Check stomach PH prior to commencing feed
- Feeding tube must be flushed before and after each feed/bolus and before and after the administration of medication

- For NG tubes, aspirate using a 50-mL syringe to check position (see Trust guidelines)
- To decrease the risk of aspiration keep the head of the bed elevated 30°–45°
- Hang feed for no longer than 12 hours (see infection control policies)
- A new giving set should be used every 24 hours

Nursing Assessment and Care Plan Formulation

The rationales behind the points covered in the Care Plan are:

- Bed rest: Required in view of compromised physical state of patient;
- Fluids: Often patients drink large amounts of fluid causing dangerous fluid overloading and electrolyte disturbance or drink very little;
- Supervise showers and washes: Due to patient's compromised physical state monitor for abnormal behaviours, and consider monitoring temperature;
- Toilet supervision: Due to patient's compromised physical state and consider monitoring for abnormal behaviours;
- Meals: Supervisor to give support to patients and to model normal eating patterns;
- Leave: Dependent upon physical well being;
- Physical observations: Patients vulnerable to hypothermia and hypoglycaemia. As well as physical observations ensure room is kept warm.

Problem Solving

Problem	Consider
Rapid weight gain (< 1.5 kg/week after re-hydration)	Review fluid chart and daily overall calorie and fluid intake, especially carbohydrate Reduce feed if necessary Reduce oral fluid intake if necessary or any additional fluids Spot weight to ensure patients not manipulating weight
Slow weight gain	Check feed is up to 70–100 kcal/kg. If weight gain still slow, feed is being tampered with, or vomiting/over activity. Book mental health nurse if needed for 24-hour supervision/support for patient
Suspected fluid loading/manipulation of weight	Spot weight checks. 24-hour 1-1 nursing
Patients wishing to negotiate regarding feed regimen, eating or drinking	Liaise with specialist unit. Not usually appropriate during initial refeeding phase
Patient wanting laxatives	Check history of previous abuse and stool chart
Suspicion of vomiting Raised potassium and bicarbonate	Use commode Book mental health nurse
Patient is over active (e.g. pacing) or standing up all day	Book mental health nurse Agreed short (5-min), supervised and purposeful walks once medically stable

Points to Consider in Nursing Care Plan Formulation

	Severe anorexia		Low-risk anorexia
	BMI < 13—high risk	BMI 13–15—moderate risk	BMI 15–16.9
Bed rest	24 hours Risk assessment for tissue viability Liaise with tissue viability nurse re: special mattress	6 hours (divided 3 × 2 hour periods) Social rest (patients to take responsibility for their own well being)	Social rest (patients to take responsibility for their own well-being)
Fluids	Input and output to be measured (supervised) Liaise with dietitian Water supply in room to be turned off to reduce fluid overloading if this is problematic	Liaise with dietitian re: fluid balance May need to consider turning off water to reduce fluid overloading	Liaise with dietitian re: fluid balance
Showers/washes	Supervised washes *only* within bedroom area recommended	Supervised showers recommended to monitor physical well-being and activity	Unsupervised showers (depending on physical well-being)
Toilet	Supervised to ensure physical safety and accurate fluid balance	Unsupervised (but fluid balance may be required) Liaise with dietitian	Unsupervised (depending on physical well-being)
Nutrition	Liaise with dietitian regarding NG feeding Supervised (and up to 1 hour post-meal supervision) All meals to be advised by dietitian Monitor for effects of refeeding syndrome	Supervised (and up to 45 minutes post-meal supervision) All meals to be advised by dietitian	Unsupervised (depending on behaviours, physical well-being and need for support) Liaise with dietitian
Leave	No leave when on medical ward Short period wheelchair leave when on psychiatric ward	Short periods in wheelchair where appropriate (depending on physical well-being)	Unescorted/escorted (as appropriate)
Physical obs	BP, pulse and temp (×4 daily) BMs (×4 daily using BM machine and finger prick)	BP, pulse and temp (×2 daily) BMs (×1 daily—depending on physical well-being)	BP, pulse, temp and BMs (depending on physical well-being)

Further Reading

Birmingham C, Alothman A, Goldner E. Anorexia nervosa; refeeding and hypophosphataemia. *Int J Eat Disord.* 1996;20:211–213.

British Dietetic Association Parenteral and Enteral Nutrition Group. *Pocket Handbook: Guidelines for Preventing Refeeding Syndrome.* 2001.

Casper RC. Carbohydrate metabolism and its regulatory hormones in anorexia nervosa. *Psychiatry Res.* 1996;62:85–96.

Crook MA, Hally V, Panteli J. The importance of the refeeding syndrome. *Nutrition.* 2001;17(7–8):632–637.

Faintuch J, Garcia F, Ladeira J, et al. Refeeding procedures after 43 days of total fasting. *Nutrition.* 2001;17(2):100–104.

Fisher M, Simpser E, Schneider M. Hypophosphataemia secondary to oral refeeding in anorexia nervosa. *Int J Eat Disord.* 2000;28:181–187.

Flesher M, Archer K, Leslie B, McCollum R, Martinka G. Assessing the metabolic and clinical consequences of early enteral feeding in the malnourished patient. *JPEN J Parenter Enteral Nutr.* 2004;29:108–117.

Klein C, Stanek G, Wiles C. Overfeeding macronutrients to critically ill adults: metabolic complications. *J Am Diet Assoc.* 1998;98(7):795–806.

Kraft M, Btaiche I, Sacks G. Review of refeeding syndrome. *Nutr Clin Pract.* 2005;20:625–633.

Marinella MA. Refeeding syndrome and hypophosphatemia. *J Intensive Care Med.* 2005;20:155–159.

Melchior JC. From malnutrition to refeeding during anorexia nervosa. *Curr Opin Clin Nutr Metab Care.* 1998;1(6):481–485.

Mental Health Act Commission Guidance Note3. *Guidance on the Treatment of Anorexia Nervosa under the Mental Health Act 1983.* 1997.

National Institute for Health and Clinical Excellence. *Eating Disorders: Core Interventions in the Treatment and Management of Anoxia Nervosa, Bulimia Nervosa and Related Eating Disorders.* 2004.

National Institute for Health and Clinical Excellence. *Nutrition Support in Adults: Oral Nutrition Support, Enteral Tube Feeding and Parentral Nutrition.* 2006.

Index